Ultrasound for Surgeons

Second Edition

Ultrasound
for Surgeons
Second Edition

EDITORS

Junji Machi, M.D., Ph.D.

Professor
Department of Surgery
University of Hawaii
John A. Burns School of Medicine
Honolulu, Hawaii

Edgar D. Staren, M.D., Ph.D., M.B.A.

Professor
Department of Surgery
Medical Director, MCO Cancer Institute
Medical College of Ohio
Toledo, Ohio

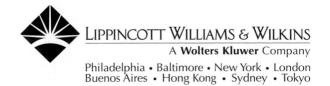

LIPPINCOTT WILLIAMS & WILKINS
A **Wolters Kluwer** Company

Philadelphia • Baltimore • New York • London
Buenos Aires • Hong Kong • Sydney • Tokyo

Acquisitions Editors: Brian Brown and R. Craig Percy
Developmental Editor: Michelle M. LaPlante
Production Manager: Robert Pancotti
Production Editor: Richard Rothschild, Print Matters, Inc.
Manufacturing Manager: Benjamin Rivera
Cover Designer: Andrew Gatto
Compositor: Compset, Inc.
Printer: Edwards Brothers

© 2005 by LIPPINCOTT WILLIAMS & WILKINS
530 Walnut Street
Philadelphia, PA 19106 USA
LWW.com

Machi: *Ultrasound for Surgeons,* first edition; copyright Igaku-Shoin, 1997.
Staren: *Ultrasound for the Surgeon,* first edition; copyright Lippincott–Raven Publishers, 1997.

Printed in the USA

Library of Congress Cataloging-in-Publication Data
Ultrasound for surgeons / editors, Junji Machi, Edgar D. Staren. — 2nd ed.
    p. ; cm.
    Rev ed. of: Ultrasound for surgeons / [edited by] Junji Machi, Bernard Sigel. 1997 and Ultrasound for the surgeon / editor, Edgar D. Staren. 1997.
    Includes bibliographical references and index.
    ISBN 0-7817-4291-9
    1. Ultrasonics in surgery. 2. Operative ultrasonography. I. Machi, Junji. II. Staren, Edgar D. III. Ultrasound for the surgeon.
    [DNLM: 1. Surgical Procedures, Operative—methods. 2. Ultrasonography—methods. WO 500 U47 2004]
RD33.7.U475 2004
617'.05—dc22

                            2004048430

10 9 8 7 6 5 4 3 2 1

To my wife, Takako, and my children, Stephanie, Raymond, and Alex.

JM

To my wife, Lisa, and my children, Ed, Dan, John, Tony, Mikey, and Helen.

EDS

CONTENTS

Reid B. Adams, M.D.
Associate Professor and Chief
Hepatobiliary and Pancreatic Service;
Director, Gastrointestinal Oncology Program
Department of Surgery
University of Virginia Health System
Charlottesville, Virginia

Maurice E. Arregui, M.D.
Director of Fellowship in Advanced Laparoscopy
Endoscopy and Ultrasound
St. Vincent Hospital
Indianapolis, Indiana

James P. Bonar, M.D.
Assistant Professor of Surgery;
Lt. Colonel, U.S.A.F., M.C.;
Department of Surgery
R. Adams Cowley Shock Trauma Center
University of Maryland
Baltimore, Maryland

David L. Coffman, D.O.
Clinical Fellow, Surgical Trauma
Section of Trauma, Surgical Critical Care
Yale University School of Medicine;
Surgical Critical Care Fellow
Yale–New Haven Hospital
New Haven, Connecticut

Daniel J. Deziel, M.D.
Professor of Surgery
Department of Surgery
Rush Medical College of Rush University;
Senior Attending Surgeon
Rush—Presbyterian—St. Lukes Medical Center
Chicago, Illinois

Heidi L. Frankel, M.D.
Associate Professor of Surgery
Section of Trauma
Surgical Critical Care
Yale University School of Medicine;
Director, Surgical Intensive Care Unit;
Attending Staff in Trauma Surgery
Yale–New Haven Hospital
New Haven, Connecticut

William R. Fry, M.D., R.V.T., R.D.M.S.
Trauma Director
Department of Surgery
Penrose Hospital
Colorado Springs, Colorado

Nancy L. Furumoto, M.D.
Assistant Professor
Department of Surgery
University of Hawaii
John A. Burns School of Medicine
Honolulu, Hawaii

Sara Goddu, R.D.M.S.
Department of Radiology
Medical College of Ohio
Toledo, Ohio

Jay K. Harness, M.D.
Medical Director
Comprehensive Breast Center;
Department of Surgery
St. Joseph Hospital
Orange, California

Tina J. Hieken, M.D.
Assistant Professor of Surgery
Department of Surgery
Rush Medical College of Rush University
Attending Surgeon
Rush—Presbyterian—St. Lukes Medical Center
Chicago, Illinois

M. Margaret Knudson, M.D.
Professor of Surgery
Department of Surgery
University of California, San Francisco
Attending Trauma Surgeon
Department of Surgery
San Francisco General Hospital
San Francisco, California

Mark J. Lybik, M.D.
Staff Physician
Division of Gastroenterology
St. Vincent Hospital and Health Care Center
Indianapolis, Indiana

Junji Machi, M.D., Ph.D.
Professor
Department of Surgery
University of Hawaii
John A. Burns School of Medicine
Honolulu, Hawaii

Michael R. Marohn, Col., U.S.A.F., M.C., F.S.
Uniformed Services University
Bethesda, Maryland;
Malcolm Grow U.S.A.F. Medical Center
Andrews Air Force Base, Maryland

Lawrence P. McChesney, M.D.
Associate Professor of Surgery and Chief
Division of Transplantation
Medical College of Ohio;
Associate Attending Surgeon
Medical College of Ohio Hospital
Toledo, Ohio

Andrew J. Oishi, M.D.
Assistant Professor
Department of Surgery
University of Hawaii
John A. Burns School of Medicine
Honolulu, Hawaii

Robert H. Oishi, M.D.
Associate Professor
Department of Surgery
University of Hawaii
John A. Burns School of Medicine
Honolulu, Hawaii

David B. Pilcher, M.D.
Professor of Surgery
Department of Vascular Surgery
University of Vermont College of Medicine
Burlington, Vermont

Stanley J. Rogers, M.D.
Assistant Professor
Department of Surgery
University of California, San Francisco
Co-Director, Minimally Invasive Surgery
Department of Surgery
San Francisco General Hospital
San Francisco, California

Theodore J. Saclarides, M.D.
Professor of Surgery
Department of Surgery
Rush Medical College;
Head, Section of Colon and Rectal Surgery
Rush–Presbyterian–St. Luke's Medical Center
Chicago, Illinois

David C. Ouliai, M.D.
Department of Surgery
University of California at San Francisco
East Bay Program
Oakland, California

Bruce D. Schirmer, M.D.
Professor and Chairman
Department of Surgery
University of Virginia Health System
Charlottesville, Virginia

Alex Senchenkov, M.D.
Chief Resident in Surgery
Department of Surgery
Medical College of Ohio
Toledo, Ohio

Steven R. Shackford, M.D.
Stanley S. Fieber Professor and Chairman
Department of Surgery
University of Vermont;
Surgeon-in-Chief
Fletcher Allen Health Care
Burlington, Vermont

Amy C. Sisley, M.D., M.P.H.
Assistant Professor of Surgery and
Director, Physician Education
Department of Surgery
R. Adams Cowley Shock Trauma Center
Baltimore, Maryland

R. Stephen Smith, M.D., R.D.M.S.
Professor
Department of Surgery
University of Kansas School of Medicine–Wichita
Wichita, Kansas

Nathaniel J. Soper, M.D.
Professor and Vice-Chair for Clinical Affairs
Director of Minimally Invasive Surgery
Northwestern University Feinberg School of Medicine
Northwestern Memorial Hospital
Chicago, Illinois

Edgar D. Staren, M.D., Ph.D., M.B.A.
Professor
Department of Surgery
Medical Director, MCO Cancer Institute
Medical College of Ohio
Toledo, Ohio

José M. Velasco, M.D.
Professor of Surgery
Rush Medical College;
Chairman, Department of Surgery
Rush North Shore Medical Center;
Senior Attending Physician
Rush–Presbyterian–St. Luke's Medical Center
Skokie, Illinois

Nitzet Velez, M.D.
Chief Resident in Surgery
Department of Surgery
Medical College of Ohio
Toledo, Ohio

Thomas Walsh, M.D.
Associate Professor of Cardiology
Division of Cardiology
Medical College of Ohio
Toledo, Ohio

Emily R. Winslow, M.D.
Department of Surgery
Washington University School of Medicine
St. Louis, Missouri

Nicholas Zyromski, M.D.
Department of Surgery
Medical College of Ohio
Toledo, Ohio

FOREWORD

When I was a surgical resident, surgeons did surgery and radiologists read radiographs. This categorical arrangement or "specialization," initially recommended by E. A. Codman in the early 20th century (1), was how modern medicine was practiced. It was reasoned that repeated exposure to a particular disease made a physician more adept at managing it. Radiologists were considered to be particularly adept at interpreting images and, when given the patient's history and clinical findings, they could greatly assist clinicians in the diagnosis and treatment of many illnesses. Interpreting images was the radiologist's practice domain, while cutting patients open and removing or repairing diseased or damaged viscera was the surgeon's practice domain.

Surgeons, while carefully observing the boundaries of the practice domain, have always considered themselves to be responsible for and in charge of the total management of the patient. My mentors considered themselves "internists who operated" and they taught me to manage the complex medical comorbidities of my patients. They also encouraged my participation in diagnostic imaging. For example, I dutifully completed the radiograph requisition slip, placed my patient on the gurney, wheeled the patient off to the radiology suite, and patiently waited until the study was completed. I frequently reviewed the study with the radiologist (while providing him or her with additional clinical information) so that I would be prepared to present the patient to my attending physician, who would invariably ask, "Did you review the films yourself?" That query (I later found) is a universal one characteristic of all surgical residencies and it has instilled in all surgeons a compulsion to carefully review all of the images and diagnostic studies on their patients in preparation for an operation. Since surgeons are ultimately responsible for the patient, they cannot rely solely on the reading of a radiologist without seeing the studies that are critical to the diagnosis or treatment of their patients.

Just when we thought that we were practicing modern medicine, technology arrived and practice domains began to blur. Computed tomography revolutionized the practice of medicine and surgery. It affected a host of specialties within surgery, from neurosurgery to otolaryngology. For general surgeons, computed tomography brought a unique visualization of abdominal disease processes (such as appendicitis and splenic rupture) and soon surgeons were comfortable reading the images. Computed tomography also allowed the accurate localization of intraabdominal abscesses. So accurate was the localization that abscesses could be drained percutaneously, by radiologists (2). Radiologists were now directly intervening in the course of a disease that had been traditionally managed by surgeons. Surgeons welcomed this blurring of practice domains because it improved the management of their patients. Radiologists recognized this unique role as it was evolving and those who specialized in "intervening" saw themselves as neither fish (radiologist) nor fowl (surgeon)—they became "interventionalists."

Technology continued to advance and continued to blur practice domains. Ultrasound imaging, like computed tomography, is a product of this advanced technology. The rapid evolution of microcircuitry facilitated the development of compact ultrasound instrumentation. This compactness made ultrasound machines cheaper and more transportable such that they could easily be used at the bedside, in the emergency room, or in the office. Ultrasound now comes to the patient, not the other way around. Sonographic images have become crisper and instrumentation has become increasingly user-friendly, so userfriendly that ultrasound, once solely in the practice domain of obstetrics and radiology, is now being used by virtually all the specialties of medicine. Surgeons, traditionally conservative, have been one of the last specialties to embrace ultrasound, but when they did so, the response was swift and direct (3). The response was facilitated, in large part, by the leadership of the American College of Surgeons, who provided not only a forum for the development of educational programs in ultrasound for surgeons, but also the organizational support and imprimatur for the hospital credentialing of surgeons to perform ultrasound studies (4). The College also encouraged the creation of the American College of Surgeons National Ultrasound Faculty, a group of surgeons with recognized expertise in ultrasound and recognized expertise in education, to oversee the quality of the educational programs and to assure that the programs would keep pace with this evolving technology.

Ultrasound and surgeons have a natural affinity. Ultrasound imaging requires skillful use of the hands and allows real-time acquisition of images, which assuages the compulsion to view one's own patient studies. Surgeons have unique skills at assessing spatial relationships and possess a comprehensive knowledge of anatomy. These skills and this knowledge are required to acquire and interpret sonograms. Thus, surgeons are well suited to use ultrasound and that is probably why they can learn it so quickly (5).

Ultrasound has become an extension of the physical exam for surgeons. Furthermore, when surgeons use ultrasound they often have a specific clinical question in mind: for instance, is there blood in this abdomen or are there stones in this gall bladder? They know what they want to learn about their patients and they can focus their exam on that specific question. Such focused exams expedite management and benefit patients.

Ultrasound for Surgeons, second edition, is a compendium of current information on ultrasound, edited by two pioneers in ultrasound education. The authors of the chapters are equally credentialed; most are members of the National Ultrasound Faculty of the American College of Surgeons. The book covers all of the essentials, from the physical principles underpinning ultrasound imaging to clinical applications that bear on all fields of surgery to practical matters, such as education, credentialing, and billing. Because of its comprehensive approach to the field, *Ultrasound for Surgeons*, second edition, should become an essential component of the personal library of all surgical residents and practicing surgeons. Equally important, *Ultrasound for Surgeons*, second edition, should be read cover to cover by surgical leaders—academic and nonacademic chairs of surgical departments—so that they can appreciate that modern surgery includes ultrasound imaging and that their support is necessary in order for surgeons to be credentialed to perform it.

Steven R. Shackford, M.D., F.A.C.S.
Stanley S. Fieber Professor and Chairman
Department of Surgery
University of Vermont
Surgeon-in-Chief
Fletcher Allen Health Care
Burlington, Vermont

REFERENCES

1. Codman BA. A resume of the results of Dr. F. B. Harrington's service, Massachusetts General Hospital, from June 1 to Oct. 1, as seen in the following June or later. *Boston Med Surg J* 1904;150:618–620.
2. Halasz N, Van Sonenberg E. Drainage of intraabdominal abscesses. Tactics and choices. *Am J Surg* 1983;146:112–115.
3. Shackford SR. Focused ultrasound examinations by surgeons: the time is now. *J Trauma* 1993;35:181–182.
4. Statement on ultrasound examination by surgeons. *Bull Am Coll Surg* 1998;83:37–40.
5. Shackford SR, Rogers FB, Osler TM, et al. Focused abdominal sonogram for trauma: the learning curve of nonradiologist clinicians in detecting hemoperitoneum. *J Trauma* 1999;46:553–564.

PREFACE

Only a decade ago, few surgeons in the United States were performing ultrasound examinations by themselves: this despite ultrasound being well recognized as one of the principal imaging methods in clinical medicine. Since then, innovations in ultrasound technology and instrumentation, together with increased awareness of its benefit to various surgical fields, have led to greater ultrasound use by surgeons. Such advances include computer-enhanced, high-quality ultrasound images, user-friendly, portable, and versatile machines, variably shaped and sized transducers designed for specific surgical applications, ultrasound needle guidance equipment, and ongoing developments such as 3-D, harmonic, and contrast-enhanced imaging.

To bring ultrasound progress to the attention of the larger surgical community, in 1997, we independently published two books, *Ultrasound for Surgeons* and *Ultrasound for the Surgeon*. Together with numerous surgical colleagues, many of whom are members of the National Ultrasound Faculty of the American College of Surgeons, we have attempted to facilitate ultrasound education and training for surgeons and surgical residents. Ultrasound is being applied in an ever-broadening variety of surgical practices and is now commonly used in the office, at the bedside, in the emergency room, in the endoscopic suite, and in the operating theater. This explosive growth convinced us of the need to combine our efforts and publish a second edition of *Ultrasound for Surgeons* to update surgeons on the most current applications and information of this evolving modality.

This book is directed at both practicing surgeons and surgeons in-training, whether they are ultrasound neophytes or relatively experienced ultrasonographers. Surgeons who will find this book of interest include: general surgeons, breast surgeons, head/neck surgeons, vascular surgeons, trauma surgeons, surgical intensivists, emergency room physicians, hepatobiliary/pancreatic surgeons, laparoscopic/endoscopic surgeons, transplant surgeons, and colorectal surgeons.

The first chapter addresses the past, present, and future education of ultrasound for surgeons. Chapters 2 and 3 describe the basic principles, instrumentation, and techniques for ultrasound use. An overview of interventional ultrasound is summarized in Chapter 4, which helps to clarify such topics presented in more detail in subsequent specialty chapters. Chapters 5 through 8 deal with so-called "small parts" ultrasound, including breast, thyroid and parathyroid, head and neck, and vascular ultrasound. Chapters 9 and 10 address the broad topic of critical care ultrasound including ultrasound for trauma and ultrasound in the acute setting. Ultrasound for abdominal diseases starts with Chapter 11. Transabdominal ultrasound is discussed in detail in Chapters 11 and 12, intraoperative and laparoscopic ultrasound in Chapters 13 through 17, transplant ultrasound in Chapter 18, and endoluminal ultrasound in Chapters 19 and 20. Chapter 21 introduces the reader to new ultrasound technologies. A general discussion on how to get started is presented in Chapter 22. The final chapter summarizes the coding and billing of ultrasound commonly used by surgeons. Technical and methodological aspects, indications, and clinical results are emphasized in each of the clinical chapters. Substantial numbers of carefully selected sonograms are shown so that surgeons can use this book as an atlas as well as a text. Tables of important points are included in each chapter as a summary of useful information.

The introduction, engagement, and expansion of ultrasound practice in various surgical fields will definitively improve surgical decision-making, patient care, and cost-effectiveness in management of surgical diseases. Surgeons need to understand the basics and evolving areas of ultrasound so that they might apply surgeon-performed ultrasound appropriately and effectively in their practice. We hope that this book will be viewed as a valuable tool for surgeons in this exciting endeavor.

Junji Machi, M.D., Ph.D.
Edgar D. Staren, M.D., Ph.D., M.B.A.

ACKNOWLEDGMENTS

This second edition would not have been possible without the cooperation and support of a number of individuals. The editors are especially grateful to each of the authors, whose expertise and diligence have contributed to the excellent quality of this book. Most contributors in this edition are members of the National Ultrasound Faculty of the American College of Surgeons; their dedication to the continuing medical education of surgeons is notable and greatly appreciated. We particularly appreciate Sandy Chu, Dory Ichinotsubo, Dale Ichinotsubo, Barbara Padgett, Meghan West, and Dana Earnest for their efficient, professional work in the preparation of this book. Our acknowledgment is extended to Dr. Bernard Sigel, co-editor of the first edition, for his pioneering work on intraoperative ultrasound and surgical ultrasound training. The preparation of this book was supported by Surgical Education, Inc., Honolulu, Hawaii.

Junji Machi, M.D., Ph.D.
Edgar D. Staren, M.D., Ph.D., M.B.A.

Ultrasound for Surgeons

Second Edition

Education and Training in Ultrasound for Surgeons

M. Margaret Knudson

Ever since Douglass Howry suspended a patient in a water tub and obtained the first medical ultrasound images a half century ago, diagnostic ultrasound has resided primarily in the domain of radiologists. With the exception of German surgeons, who are required to demonstrate proficiency in ultrasound to obtain their surgical boards, few surgeons appreciated the value of performing a focused, ultrasound examination to answer a clinical question. In fact, with the widespread use of computed tomography (CT) and magnetic resonance imaging (MRI) techniques, it was once largely believed that medical ultrasound would soon be of interest only for historical purposes. However, several factors converging together have instead pushed ultrasound to its current position of popularity, especially among nonradiologists.

The relatively recent addition of digital, computer-enhanced technology to ultrasound machines has resulted in the production of images that are clearer and easier to interpret. Surgeons comfortable with reading the cross-sectional images generated by the CT scanner can easily translate that knowledge to ultrasound imaging. Machines equipped with multiple probes of varying frequencies and configurations, including color flow and Doppler capabilities, are now less expensive, portable, and more versatile. The ability to obtain a focused ultrasound examination at the point of contact with the patient has great appeal for practicing surgeons. In the emergency setting, the detection of hemorrhage in the peritoneal, pericardial, or pleural cavity by bedside ultrasound scanning allows for rapid triage as well as prompt, efficacious, and cost-effective surgical intervention (1–3). Office-based breast imaging, including ultrasound-guided biopsy capabilities, offers the surgeon an efficient method of evaluating a lesion, often alleviating substantial delay and anxiety on the part of the patient. In vascular surgery, ultrasound has emerged as the preferred method of diagnosing, measuring, and following patients with aneurysmal disease. The laparoscopic surgeon can visu-alize biliary stones, stage cancer, and guide ablative therapy using specially designed surgical ultrasound probes. Portable machines bring ultrasound to the bedside in the critical care unit, where it can be used to assist in draining fluid, placing lines, diagnosing deep venous thrombosis, and detecting other disease processes. Ultrasound has even recently become available on the space station!

Given this enthusiasm for an ever-expanding role for ultrasound in surgical practice, surgical educators have of necessity taken on the responsibility of assuring that surgeons are trained in the proper use of this modality. Surgeons must be able to both obtain and interpret high quality ultrasound images, while appreciating the applications, advantages, and limitations of the exam. Most importantly, surgeons must be responsible for ensuring patient safety during ultrasound imaging. The American Board of Surgery has recommended that candidates have a working knowledge of ultrasound of the head and neck, breast, and abdomen (including transabdominal, intraoperative, and laparoscopic), as well as endorectal ultrasound (4). Sonographic images are now appearing on the qualifying examinations. To date, however, only a limited number of surgical residency programs formally incorporate ultrasound training into their curriculum. This chapter is intended to outline educational and training methods for the practicing surgeon and trainee in the use of ultrasound.

BACKGROUND

In order to address the need for ultrasound education for physicians other than radiologists, a number of professional societies have issued position statements and guidelines. The American Institute of Ultrasound in Medicine (AIUM) is a large society that represents primarily radiologists but includes many members from other disciplines who utilize medical ultrasound (i.e., cardiology, obstetrics and gynecology, emergency medicine, surgery). The

AIUM position statement on training guidelines for physicians who evaluate and interpret diagnostic ultrasound examinations is summarized below (5). The AIUM recommends that physicians performing diagnostic ultrasound examinations meet at least one of the following criteria:

1. Complete an approved residency program, fellowship, or postgraduate training that includes 3 months of supervised scanning (minimal 300 examinations).
2. In the absence of formal fellowship or postgraduate or residency training, documentation of clinical experience to include (a) 100 hours of American Medical Association (AMA) category 1 continuing medical education (CME) activity dedicated to diagnostic ultrasound in the area of practice; and (b) evidence of being involved in at least 300 examinations per 3-year period, under the supervision of a qualified physician.

As can be appreciated, meeting the AIUM criteria would be a formidable task for most surgeons.

Another society that has come forward with guidelines specific for surgeons in the use of ultrasound is the Society of American Gastrointestinal Endoscopic Surgeons (SAGES) (6,7). SAGES recognized that during surgical training all surgeons obtain extensive exposure to spatial relationships of organs as well as intensive experience in pathophysiology, natural history, and management of disease processes. This background should facilitate the incorporation of ultrasound skills into a surgeon's practice. In addition, the surgeon can verify the sonographic findings with those found at surgical exploration, thus rapidly improving interpretation skills by hands-on, immediate feedback. SAGES recommends that residents who wish to perform ultrasound after training document their hands-on experience with laparoscopic and/or endoscopic ultrasound before privileges are granted in this area. For those seeking training outside of residency, courses incorporating both didactic and hands-on training are recommended, followed by a minimum of 25 supervised ultrasound examinations and continued monitoring of each surgeon's performance. (See Chapter 22 for a more detailed discussion of credentialing and verification for surgeons using ultrasound).

Guidelines for training in ultrasound have also been compiled by the American Association of Emergency Physicians (AAEP) (8). In their statement, the authors outlined the scope of ultrasound practice for emergency medicine to include trauma ultrasound, emergency ultrasound in pregnancy, emergency echocardiography for assessment of the presence of cardiac activity and pericardial effusion, assessment for abdominal aortic aneurysm, biliary ultrasound for stones, renal ultrasound for obstruction, and procedural ultrasound (e.g., line placement) in their scope of practice. The recommended pathways for training included didactic courses (level I proficiency), training with supervision (level II proficiency), proficiency as judged by an expert (level III proficiency), credentialing within a local hospital, and CME. In general, a minimum of 25 examinations in each of the applications listed above is required. The AAEP indicated that only those physicians who had obtained level III proficiency should be using ultrasound for clinical decisions.

The American Society of Breast Surgeons has developed guidelines for the specific application of breast ultrasound. Moreover, this organization has developed a certification process through the society itself. Similar guidelines can be found for ultrasound training in other nonradiology fields, including obstetrics and gynecology and cardiology.

The Statement on Ultrasound Examinations by Surgeons published by the American College of Surgeons (ACS) helped to facilitate the incorporation of ultrasound into surgical practice by members of the College (9). The recognition of the importance of ultrasound in surgery set the stage for the development of the educational program in ultrasound sponsored by the ACS (see below). The statement on ultrasound by the ACS is summarized in Figure 1.

ESSENTIALS OF ULTRASOUND EDUCATION

The surgeon sonographer must be able to obtain a high-quality ultrasound image as well as be proficient in interpreting that image. These capabilities require an understanding of the physics of ultrasound as it affects the quality of the image. *Acquisition* of the image requires an understanding of how to enhance the image by selecting the proper frequency and probe, positioning the patient appropriately, making adjustments on the machine (gain, focus, and so forth), and locating the "windows" used to view certain organs. Labeling and annotation of images is also important. *Interpretation* of the image requires an understanding of probe orientation as well as the characteristic echo pattern of the area of interest. Surgeon sonographers should recognize ultrasound artifacts that may contribute to misinterpretation of ultrasound findings. To ensure patient safety, the bioeffects of ultrasound must also be appreciated. Finally, the surgeon must understand the indications for and limitations of focused ultrasound examinations.

Most of these basic ultrasound principles can be provided in a didactic lecture-style course, and such a course is essential for all surgical trainees and novice surgeon sonographers. Following the lectures, most courses include some experience with supervised hands-on scanning. Volunteer models are frequently employed for the hands-on session, but occasionally patients with known

American College of Surgeons Ultrasound Examinations by Surgeons

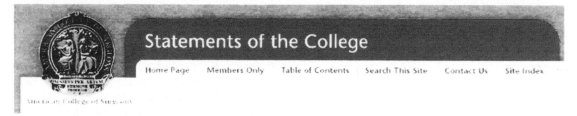

[ST-31] Ultrasound Examinations by Surgeons

[by the American College of Surgeons]

    Application for Ultrasound Verification

The following statement was developed by the College's Committee on Emerging Surgical Technology and Education (CESTE) and was approved by the Board of Regents at its February 1998 meeting.

Introduction

Ultrasonography is a technology applicable in a wide variety of surgical practices and surgical specialties, and has become a routine tool for noninvasive evaluation of many organ systems and targeting areas for intervention. Examples include ultrasonic evaluation of the eye, the neck, reproductive organs, and the vascular, nervous, and musculoskeletal systems. Clinical applications of ultrasound require unique knowledge and skill.

To ensure that surgeons who use ultrasound are qualified and that the ultrasound facilities and equipment they use are appropriate for the medical application and meet and maintain quality standards, a voluntary verification process has been made available to Fellows. There are several components to this process: first, the surgeon must meet the requirements for education and/or experience; second, the facilities and equipment should meet recommended standards; third, the surgeon should maintain qualifications through continued experience and formal continuing medical education in the technique and its applications; and fourth, surgeons' outcomes using ultrasound should be assessed through a program of continuous quality improvement.

American College of Surgeons' Voluntary Verification Program for Surgeons in the Use of Ultrasound

FIGURE 1. Statement on Ultrasound Education from the American College of Surgeons.

pathology (i.e., peritoneal fluid, pericardial effusion, gallstones, breast masses) can be found for the course (Table 1). Courses that include intraoperative, endoscopic, and laparoscopic ultrasound applications require animal facilities. After successful completion of both the didactic and hands-on session, the surgeon is ready for continued hands-on training and supervised practice.

TRAINING AND PRACTICUM

Developing competence in any surgical skill requires a period of practice under supervision. The same is true for the use of ultrasound by surgeons. There is a variable learning curve for focused ultrasound examinations, which is defined to some extent by the skills of the surgeon sonographer. Perhaps even more important to gaining competence in ultrasound examination is the inherent degree of difficulty of different types of ultrasound studies. Smith, Fry, and others developed a grading scale for ultrasound examinations that should be considered when planning the time frame for supervised practice (10). As can be seen in Table 2, performance of a transcutaneous focused trauma examination is considered elementary when compared with scanning the pancreas or performing and interpreting a vascular examination. However, despite this important contribution to the surgical literature, Smith and his coinvestigators were un-

▶ **TABLE 1 Essential Elements of a Basic
Ultrasound Course**

Physics of Ultrasound
    Wave properties
    Piezoelectric principle
    Pulse-echo principle
    Impedance
    Attenuation
    Doppler effect
Instrumentation/Scanning Techniques
    Labeling and annotation of images
    Transducer selection, frequency selection
    Resolution
    Gain and time–gain compensation, focus
    Image artifacts
    Bioeffects/machine maintenance
Clinical Application of Surgical Ultrasound
    Breast
    Head/neck
    Vascular
    Trauma/acute care
    Abdominal/intraoperative/laparoscopic
Hands-on Practical Sessions
    Models/patients
    Deep scanning and small parts scanning

able to demonstrate a learning curve for surgical residents performing trauma examinations at their institution, and they questioned the need for extensive proctoring after the initial training period. It should be noted that their residents received 11.5 hours of hands-on and didactic instruction in their initial course and 8 additional hours each academic year. In addition, in their analysis of the sensitivity, specificity, accuracy, and predictive values for their surgical residents, they evaluated only the trauma ultrasound exam.

In contrast, Rozycki and her colleagues found that the accuracy of trauma ultrasound examinations was definitely influenced by the surgeons' experience and that the false-negative rate dropped to nearly 0% once 200 examinations had been performed (11). Similarly, Forster et al.

▶ **TABLE 2 Relative Difficulty for
Ultrasound Examinations**

Examination	*Degree of Difficulty*
Trauma (FAST)	1
Breast	2
Thyroid	2
Hepatobiliary/laparoscopic	3
Pancreas	5
Vascular	5

Modified from Smith RS, Fry WR, Helmer SD. Institutional learning curve for surgeon-performed trauma ultrasound. *Arch Surg* 1998;133:530–536.

reported that surgeons with a learning period of less than 1 year had a positive predictive value of only 60% when performing ultrasound for trauma (12). After one year, however, the positive predictive value rose to 76% and reached 92% after 3 years of experience. In another report it was noted that the sensitivity for surgeon-performed trauma examinations was nearly 100% after the first 100 patients (13). More recently, McCarter and others reported that five attending trauma surgeons newly trained in focused assessment for the sonographic examination of the trauma patient (FAST) initially achieved a 90% accuracy (14). However, it was acknowledged that there was some variability even among these five surgeons.

Shackford and coinvestigators observed performance of the FAST examination by surgeons and emergency physicians (15). These physicians first received a formal ultrasound course with 4 hours of didactic and 4 hours of "hands on" instruction. Following the course, the initial error rate was 17%, but decreased to only 5% after just 10 examinations. Importantly, the authors recognized that the number of examinations required to obtain proficiency would depend on the prevalence of the target disease among the patients studied (i.e., the number of positive examinations). They suggested that for a disease prevalence of less than 20%, 50 additional examinations (after the first 10) should be proctored. However, if the disease prevalence is greater than 20%, only 30 observed examinations might be needed to achieve an error rate of less than 5%.

In another study, Gracias et al., using peritoneal dialysis patients as models, tested the ability of surgeons to recognize increasing amounts of fluid during the FAST exam (16). They began by rating the surgeons on their previous experience with FAST; minimal exposure was defined as fewer than 30 patients studied, moderate as 30 to 100 studies, and extensive as more than 100 studies. The sensitivity of those with minimal, moderate, and extensive experience to detect less than 1 L of fluid was 45%, 87%, and 100%, respectively. The ability to estimate the quantity of fluid also increased with experience. From this limited study it appeared that the learning curve for FAST flattens out between 30 and 100 examinations.

While most investigations regarding ultrasound learning curves have focused on the trauma examination, similar numbers are recommended for other areas of study as well. For endoscopic examinations, SAGES recommends at least 25 supervised cases (6,7). The learning curve of transrectal ultrasound has also been described (17). The accuracy of transrectal ultrasound was 58% for the initial 12 studies performed by surgeons versus 87.5% at the completion of 36 examinations.

The criteria developed by the American Society of Breast Surgeons for certification in breast ultrasound are

▶ **TABLE 3 Criteria for Certification in Breast Ultrasound**

- Appropriate training in breast ultrasound
- A minimum of 1 year experience in performance/interpretation
- Documented 100 examinations per year with a review of 100 mammograms
- A minimum of 80 diagnostic and 20 interventional examinations
- Completion of 15 AMA category 1 credits in breast ultrasound

outlined in Table 3 (18). It is likely that other societies will make similar recommendations for training, practicum, and certification for the use of ultrasound in their specialty. In the interim, after completion of a didactic and hands-on ultrasound course, the novice surgeon sonographer should seek out a proctor who is willing to directly supervise his or her examinations. Ideally, this mentor would be an experienced surgeon sonographer within the department. If no such surgeon exists, mentors should be recruited from other departments (i.e., radiology, cardiology, gynecology, emergency medicine). A registered diagnostic medical sonographer (RDMS) might also be helpful. After a period of direct observation by the proctor, additional examinations can be recorded on video (ideally) or photographed for future review. During the practicum, a log should be kept of all examinations performed including the indications for and interpretation of the examination, and a comparison to other studies obtained on that patient (e.g., CT scans, mammograms, and operative findings). All errors (false positive, false negative) require review by the mentor until he or she has signed off on the student's competence. After that, identified errors should be part of the department's performance improvement monitoring process. During the learning process, the student sonographer should seek out opportunities to scan patients with known pathology, such as a breast cyst previously identified by a qualified sonographer, or peritoneal fluid seen on an abdominal CT scan. After this period of education and practice, the surgeon may seek privileges to perform ultrasound in his or her hospital. The criteria for privileges are listed in Table 4.

▶ **TABLE 4 Criteria for Hospital Privileges in the Use of Ultrasound**

- Documented education in ultrasound
- A period of monitoring by an experienced sonographer
- A period of practice with documented good results
- An identifiable performance improvement process
- Continued CME credits in ultrasound

INNOVATIVE METHODS OF TRAINING IN ULTRASOUND

Although gaining ultrasound experience on patients is the best way to train, learning can be accelerated by other methods that can rapidly introduce a wide variety of pathologic images. One such method involves training in ultrasound using a simulator. The UltraSim ultrasound simulator (MedSim, Fort Lauderdale, FL) is composed of a modified ultrasound machine that displays patient data in three dimensions and a medical mannequin (Fig. 2). By scanning on the mannequin, the student can reconstruct the patient images in real time. In a study that compared surgical residents who trained on a simulator to those who trained on patients/volunteers, simulator training compared favorably to the more traditional method (19). Residents can practice in simulation without supervision; this practice period may enhance their ability to recognize a pathologic process. As simulation becomes an integral part of surgical training, the use of simulators for education in ultrasound will undoubtedly be included.

As a result of the scarcity of time available for training residents and practicing surgeons, as well as the expenses incurred with traveling to and sponsoring educational courses, web-based education is becoming increasingly popular. An extensive CD-ROM–based interactive program in ultrasound has been developed by HealthStream (Nashville, TN) (20). This program incorporates sound,

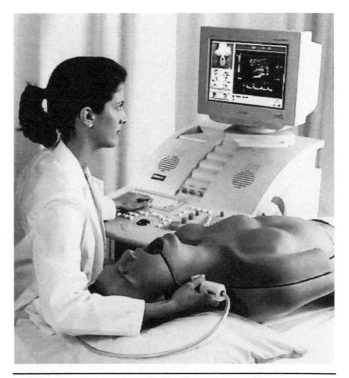

FIGURE 2. UltraSim medical ultrasound simulator.

color, streaming video, and a large number of normal and abnormal ultrasound images. Interactive components include measurements, gain adjustments, probe position, and labeling images. Self-tests and extensive references are also available. This program and others likely to follow are well suited for introducing basic ultrasound principles and images to surgeons prior to their participating in more advanced, hands-on courses.

A method for training surgeons in laparoscopic ultrasound that includes inanimate and ex vivo training models followed by live animal models has also been described (21). In this model, hepatic metastases were simulated to provide practice in performing laparoscopic biopsies. For quite some time German and more recently U.S. medical schools have incorporated cross-sectional anatomy into a medical school curriculum to introduce clinical anatomy and ultrasound imaging (22). Both cadavers and animal models have been used to introduce the FAST examination to surgical residents (23,24). Some investigators have found dynamic ultrasound videos to be more realistic than animal models during hands-on sessions (25). Others have recommended extensive use of phantoms or excised specimens suspended in a water bath (26).

EVALUATION OF EDUCATIONAL PROGRAMS IN ULTRASOUND

Whatever method is chosen for training, ongoing evaluation of the program is essential. Mandavia and others developed an excellent course for emergency physicians, which included didactic and hands-on training over a period of 16 hours (27). After the course, 18 resident physicians were followed for 10 months during which they performed 1,138 ultrasound examinations. After 10 months, their accuracy was 94.6%, sensitivity was 92.4%, and specificity was 96.1%. There did not appear to be any diminution of skills over the observation time. In another study of emergency physicians, 456 taped studies were independently reviewed by blinded cardiologists (for echocardiography) or radiologists (for abdominal scanning) (28). The overall accuracy of these studies was 90%. In a study from England, ultrasound examinations performed by urologists in training were evaluated; 50 patients (100 kidney units) had renal ultrasound performed by urology trainees on acute admission (29). The results were compared with subsequent definitive radiologic investigations. Of 100 kidney scans, only 7 results were discordant (2 false negatives and 5 false positives) achieving 97% specificity and 84% sensitivity.

Sisley and others used the objective structured clinical examination (OSCE) to assess physician performance in ultrasound for trauma (30). In this study, participating surgery and emergency medicine physicians were first given a precourse OSCE test that required interpretation of videotaped ultrasound examinations presented along with a clinical scenario. The students then attended a formal ultrasound course that included both didactic and hands-on sessions. At the completion of the course, the OSCE videotape was presented again. Significant improvements in postcourse OSCE scores were observed for both factual knowledge and ultrasound interpretation. The authors suggested that the OSCE should be considered not only in evaluating courses but also in assessing physician competency in ultrasound.

AMERICAN COLLEGE OF SURGEONS ULTRASOUND EDUCATION PROGRAM

To address the needs of surgeons who wish to perform focused ultrasound examinations, the ACS has developed an extensive educational program (see also Chapter 22). The program is modular in design, beginning with a basic course that concentrates on physics, principles, instrumentation, scanning techniques, and clinical applications. After completion of the basic course, the student achieves level I verification and is then qualified to take an advanced course in their area of interest (Fig. 3). Available advanced courses include head/neck, vascular, breast, acute (emergency/critical care), and abdominal (transabdominal, intraoperative, and laparoscopic) ultrasound. Written and hands-on tests are included in the advanced modules. After successful completion of the

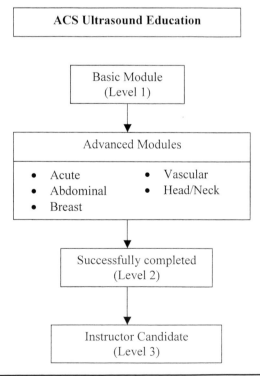

FIGURE 3. American College of Surgeons Modular Ultrasound Education Program.

course, the student receives a level II verification. Surgeons with extensive ultrasound experience can apply for instructor–level III verification. An evaluation of the ACS program is currently being conducted. The College remains committed to conducting both educational and verification programs in surgeon-performed ultrasound.

CONCLUSIONS

Focused ultrasound examinations performed by surgeons have emerged as an important procedure in many areas of surgical practice. Surgeons are encouraged to embrace this technology, but only after proper education, training, and a period of supervised practice. The ACS has taken a leadership role in ensuring that surgeons have access to ultrasound education and is collaborating with surgical specialty societies to develop criteria for verification and certification. As such, the role of ultrasound in the evaluation of the surgical patient will continue to expand, and surgeons will continue to bring the latest technology to the bedside of the patients we serve.

REFERENCES

1. Branney SW, Moore EE, Cantrill SV, et al. Ultrasound based key clinical pathway reduces the use of hospital resources for the evaluation of blunt abdominal trauma. *J Trauma* 1997;42:1086–1090.
2. Patrick DA, Bensard DD, Moore EE, et al. Ultrasound is an effective triage tool to evaluate blunt abdominal trauma in the pediatric population. *J Trauma* 1998;45:57–83.
3. Boulanger BR, McLellan BA, Brenneman FD, et al. Prospective evidence of the superiority of a sonography-based algorithm in the assessment of blunt abdominal injury. *J Trauma* 1999;47:632–637.
4. *Bull Am Coll Surgeons* 1998; 83:37–40.
5. American Institute of Ultrasound in Medicine. Training guidelines for physicians who evaluate and interpret diagnostic ultrasound examinations. 2000. http://www.aium.org/consumer/statement.
6. Society of American Gastrointestinal Endoscopic Surgeons. Granting of endoscopic ultrasonography privileges for surgeons. Los Angeles, CA, 1992. http://www.sages.org.
7. Society of American Gastrointestinal Endoscopic Surgeons. Framework for post-residency education and training: a SAGES guideline. *Surg Endosc* 1994;8:1137–1142.
8. American College of Emergency Physicians. Use of ultrasound imaging by emergency physicians. *Ann Emerg Med* 2001;38:469–470.
9. Statement on ultrasound examinations by surgeons. *Bull Am Coll Surg* 1998;37–40.
10. Smith RS, Kern SJ, Fry WR, et al. Institutional learning curve for surgeon-performed trauma ultrasound. *Arch Surg* 1998;133:530–536.
11. Rozycki GS, Ochsner MG, Jaffin JH, et al. Prospective evaluation of surgeons' use of ultrasound in the evaluation of trauma patients. *J Trauma* 1993;34:516–527.
12. Forster R, Pillasch J, Zielke A, et al. Ultrasonography in blunt abdominal trauma: influence of the investigators' experience. *J Trauma* 1992;34:264–269.
13. Thomas B, Falcome RE, Vasquez D, et al. Ultrasound evaluation of blunt abdominal trauma: program implementation, initial experience, and learning curve. *J Trauma* 1997;42:384–390.
14. McCarter FD, Luchette FA, Molloy M, et al. Institutional and individual learning curves for focused abdominal ultrasound for trauma: cumulative sum analysis. *Ann Surg* 2000;231:689–700.
15. Shackford SR, Rogers FB, Osler TM, et al. Focused abdominal sonogram for trauma: the learning curve of nonradiologist clinicians in detecting hemoperitoneum. *J Trauma* 1999;46:553–564.
16. Gracias VH, Frankel HL, Gupta R, et al. Defining the learning curve for the focused abdominal sonogram for trauma (FAST) examination: implications for credentialing. *Am Surg* 2001;67:364–368.
17. Carmody BJ, Otchy DP. Learning curve of transrectal ultrasound. *Dis Colon Rectum* 2000;43:193–197.
18. American Society of Breast Surgeons. Breast ultrasound certification. 2002. http://www.breastsurgeons.org/members only/ultrasoundcert.
19. Knudson MM, Sisley AC. Training resident using simulation technology: experience with ultrasound for trauma. *J Trauma* 2000;48:659–665.
20. Kendall JL, Deutchman M. *Ultrasound in emergency medicine and trauma.* Nashville, TN: HealthStream, 2001.
21. Velez PM, Robertson DW. A method for training surgeons in laparoscopic ultrasound. *Endosc Surg Allied Technol* 1994;2:155–160.
22. Teicheraber UK, Meyer JM, Poulssen NC, et al. Ultrasound anatomy: a practical teaching system in human gross anatomy. *Med Educ* 1996;30:296–298.
23. Frezza EE, Solis RL, Silich RJ, et al. Competency-based instruction to improve the surgical resident technique and accuracy of the trauma ultrasound. *Am Surg* 1999;65:884–888.
24. Han DC, Rozycki GS, Schmidt JA, et al. Ultrasound training during ATLS: an early start for surgical interns. *J Trauma* 1996;41:208–213.
25. Salen PH, Melenson SW, Heller MB. The focused abdominal sonography for trauma (FAST) examination: considerations and recommendations for training physicians in the use of a new clinical tool. *Acad Emerg Med* 2000;7:162–168.
26. Shackford SR, Ricci MA, Hebert JC. Education and credentialing. *Probl Gen Surg* 1997;14:126–132.
27. Mandavia DP, Aragona J, Chan L, et al. Ultrasound training for emergency physicians: a prospective study. *Acad Emerg Med* 2000;7:1008–1014.
28. Lanoix R, Leak LV, Gaeta T, et al. A preliminary evaluation of emergency ultrasound in the setting of an emergency medicine training program. *Am J Emerg Med* 2000;18:41–45.
29. Nargund VH, Cumming JA, Jerwood D, et al. Ultrasound in urological emergency: results of self audit and implications for training. *Int Urol Nephrol* 1996;28:267–271.
30. Sisley AC, Johnson SB, Erickson W, et al. Use of an objective structure clinical examination (OSCE) for the assessment of physician performance in the ultrasound evaluation of trauma. *J Trauma* 1999;47:627–631.

Ultrasound Physics and Principles

William R. Fry and R. Stephen Smith

What is sound, and how does it interact with biologic tissue? Ask a simple question and, in this case, get a book chapter (1–3).

Sound is defined as the propagation of pressure through matter (Table 1). Since sound requires a substance through which to propagate, it cannot move through a vacuum. It moves in a straight line until it interacts with a different medium. In order for sound to propagate through a medium, such as air or biologic tissues, an energy transfer must occur. Sound energy causes the molecules of the medium to move. This mechanical transfer of energy allows the sound wave to propagate. The motion of the sound wave and the particles affected both move in the same direction. These properties lead sound waves to be classified as longitudinal mechanical waves. By comparison, waves moving on the surface of water are referred to as perpendicular waves because the motion of the water and the motion of the waves are at 90-degree angles to each other (Fig. 1).

Sound can be described in several ways. Frequency, measured in hertz (Hz), is the number of cycles per second that pass a given point. When sound is below 20 Hz, it is inaudible to humans and is therefore called *infrasound*. Sound above human hearing (i.e., above 20,000 Hz) is classified as *ultrasound*. Medical ultrasound is typically in the range of 1 million to 15 million cycles/sec or 1 to 15 megahertz (MHz). It is noteworthy that as the frequency increases, the wavelength decreases; that is, frequency and wavelength are inversely related. This relationship can be expressed such that:

$$\text{Wavelength } (\lambda) = \frac{\text{Speed of Sound } (v)}{\text{Frequency } (f)}$$

The speed with which sound moves through biologic tissue is dependent on the tissue density (Table 2). Sound moves slowly (e.g., 330 m/sec) through less dense materials such as air. Of human tissues, the highest propagation speed is through high-density bone (e.g., 4,050 m/sec). Most soft tissues have a relatively similar density and thus a similar propagation speed of sound. The ultrasound machine assumes that the speed of sound in soft tissue is 1,540 m/sec.

ATTENUATION

As a sound wave moves through a medium, it loses energy, or becomes attenuated (Table 3). The loss of sound energy is a function of the medium through which the sound wave travels. Numerous examples in our daily life remind us of the basic physical principle. The farther away we get from a sound source the weaker it becomes due to attenuation. We are less able to hear the sound energy the farther we are from the source. In diagnostic ultrasound, this effect is doubled because the sound, which is "listened to," travels the distance twice. Unlike listening to sound from a radio, where the sound is generated in one place and travels to our ear, diagnostic ultrasound is based on evaluating sound emitted from a source (e.g., transducer) that is sent to tissues and is reflected back.

The energy of sound can be expressed in two ways: power and intensity. *Power*, expressed in watts, is the rate at which work is done. *Intensity* is the power per unit area and is expressed in watts per square centimeter. These are both dependent on the amplitude of the sound wave.

Attenuation of sound is expressed in decibels (dB). It is related to the ratio between the powers of sound at two different points.

$$\text{Attenuation Decibels (dB)} = 10 \log \frac{\text{Power at point A}}{\text{Power at point B}}$$

For a 50% decrease in power or a 50% attenuation:

$$\text{Attenuation} = 10 \log \tfrac{1}{2} = 10 \log 0.5 = 10\,(0.3) = 3 \text{ dB}$$

The sound frequency is also related to the amount of attenuation such that:

$$\text{Attenuation (dB)} = \tfrac{1}{2}\,[\text{frequency (MHz)}]\,[\text{distance traveled (cm)}]$$

The following example dramatically illustrates the clinical importance of ultrasound transducers of differ-

▶ **TABLE 1** **What Is Ultrasound?**

- Sound is a longitudinal mechanical wave measured in frequency of cycles per second.
- Humans can hear sound between 20 and 20,000 cycles/sec or Hz.
- Ultrasound has a frequency greater than 20,000 Hz.
- Diagnostic ultrasound measurements are expressed in millions of cycles per second or megahertz (MHz).
- Diagnostic frequency range is 1 to 15 MHz:
- As the frequency increases, the wavelength decreases.
- Ultrasound machines assume the speed of sound at 1,540 m/sec.

▶ **TABLE 2** **Speed of Sound in Human Tissues**

Substance	Speed of Sound (m/sec)
Air	330
Lung	650
Soft tissue:	
Fat	1,459
Average	**1,540**
Liver	1,550
Kidney	1,560
Muscle	1,580
Blood	1,575
Bone	4,050

ent frequencies. Differences in attenuation between a 5-MHz and a 10-MHz transducer (also called a "probe") used to evaluate a mass 10 cm deep in the liver yield the following:

$$\text{For 5 MHz: } \tfrac{1}{2} \text{ (5 MHz) (10 cm) = 25 dB}$$
$$\text{For 10 MHz: } \tfrac{1}{2} \text{ (10 MHz) (10 cm) = 50 dB}$$
$$50 \text{ dB} - 25 \text{ dB} = 25 \text{ dB}$$
$$10^{2.5} = 316$$

This 25-dB difference translates to more than a 300-fold difference in power! Lower frequency ultrasound is less attenuated than its higher frequency counterpart as a result of traveling a given distance. This higher attenuation rate for higher frequency ultrasound transducers is what causes them to be ineffective at greater depths. The sound wave is attenuated at greater depths such that there is no significant sound energy returning to the machine for analysis. Therefore, different-frequency ultrasound transducers are required for optimal examination of different areas of the body.

Sound energy interacts with biologic tissue in many ways other than propagation of the sound wave. Absorp-

tion and scattering are the primary causes of attenuation. Absorption occurs as the molecules of tissue are set in motion. There is not 100% transmission of the sound energy through tissue. Some of the sound energy is converted to heat, through vibration, and is lost from the sound transmission wave. The properties of a tissue primarily determine, for any given frequency of ultrasound, the degree of attenuation of the sound wave going through it (Table 4).

Higher attenuation coefficients correspond to a higher rate of attenuation for a given distance of sound traveled. Blood is the most efficient transmitter of sound energy and lung the least. These differences have clinical importance in the creation of artifacts.

IMPEDANCE

Diagnostic ultrasound relies on analysis of sound waves that are reflected back to the ultrasound transducer. What causes the sound waves to be reflected back rather than dying a quiet death of attenuation within the tissues through which they travel? The answer is differences in impedance (Table 5). Impedance is dependent on the speed of sound in the tissue and the density of the tissue:

$$\text{Acoustic impedance } (Z) = \text{Density } (\rho) \times \text{velocity } (v)$$

If one visualizes a series of compartments that are sequentially set in motion by vibration, it becomes evident

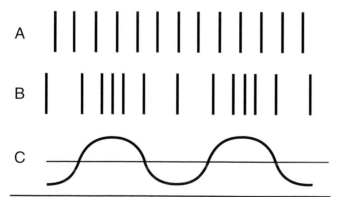

FIGURE 1. Propagation of sound. **A, B.** One representation of a sound wave is shown. **(A)** shows an undisturbed medium while **(B)** shows the compression and rarefaction of the medium with a sound wave propagating through it. **C:** This is a more typical representation of a waveform. Within the context of sound, **(C)** is a graphic representation of pressure changes that occur as a sound wave propagates through a medium.

▶ **TABLE 3** **Attenuation and Frequency**

- Attenuation: loss of sound energy as sound wave propagates through a medium
- Measured in decibels (dB): a logarithmic scale 50% attenuation = 3 dB
- Attenuation (dB) = ½ [(transducer frequency (MHz)] [distance traveled (cm)]
- Lower frequency ultrasound attenuates less than higher frequency ultrasound for given distance

▶ **TABLE 4** **Ultrasound Attenuation Coefficients of Human Tissues**

Tissue	Attenuation Coefficient at 1 MHz
Blood	0.021
Fat	0.069
Kidney	0.115
Muscle (across fibers)	0.380
Brain	0.098
Liver	0.103
Lung	4.600
Skull bone	2.300

From Hedrick WR, Hykes DL, Starchman D. *Ultrasound physics and instrumentation.* St. Louis: Mosby–Year Book, 1992:18.

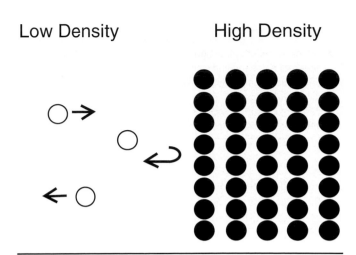

FIGURE 2. Low-density to high-density impedance.

that unless two adjacent compartments are very similar to each other in density, the vibration does not propagate from one compartment to the next. When a less dense substance is propagating a sound wave to a denser one, the inertia of the less dense substance cannot overcome the inertia of the more dense substance. The sound wave from the less dense substance bounces off the more dense substance (Fig. 2). This contrasts with sound propagating from a denser substance to a less dense substance. If one considers inertia, one might expect the more dense substance, having more inertia, to plow through the less dense substance. This is not a contest between a bowling ball and a bowling pin, where the bowling ball is moving at a velocity that creates momentum that overwhelms the pin. When an ultrasound wave causes a more dense substance to move, molecular bonds keep it from "rolling down the alley." This causes the dense substance to vibrate within a confined space. When the vibrations of the sound wave reach the boundary with the less dense substance, the denser substance has fewer molecules to interact with than within its own substance (Fig. 3). The kinetic energy of the sound wave cannot be transferred to the less dense substance because it cannot interact with it. The kinetic energy in the more dense substance stretches the molecular bonds at the edge. With an inadequate number of new molecules with which to interact, the molecular bonds stretch out maximally and then snap back. This causes the sound energy to be propagated back through the denser substance. The amount of energy that is transmitted to the next tissue is contingent

on how similar it is to the density and compliance of the tissue trying to transfer the sound energy. The term *reflector* is used to denote an area of *acoustic impedance mismatch* where sound is reflected back to an ultrasound transducer.

PIEZOELECTRIC EFFECT

When a pressure wave, in this case an ultrasound wave, deforms a certain type of crystal, a voltage is generated; the reverse also happens. This phenomenon, referred to as the piezoelectric effect (Table 6), is the principle that underlies clinical ultrasound. When a certain crystal has a voltage applied to it, the crystal vibrates, generating a pressure wave. Crystals that have this capability include amber, quartz, and lead zirconate titanate (PZT). PZT is the most common material used for crystals in ultra-

▶ **TABLE 5** **Impedance and Reflector**

- Acoustic impedance difference between two materials is what makes sound reflect back to the transducer.
- Impedance is related to the material's density.
- Reflector denotes an area where an acoustic impedance mismatch exists.

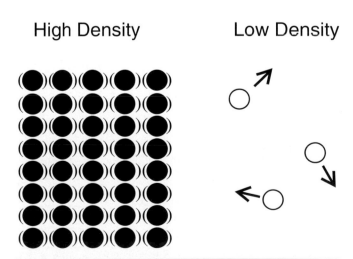

FIGURE 3. Sound does not propagate from a high-impedance to low-impedance substance.

▶ **TABLE 6** **Piezoelectric Effect**

- Piezoelectric effect: the properties of a crystal, when deformed, generate a voltage and vice versa.
- Ultrasound transducers' piezoelectric crystals are made of lead zirconate titanate.
- Different crystal thicknesses and voltages applied to them create different ultrasound frequencies.

▶ **TABLE 7** **Factors in Ultrasound Transmission and Reception**

- In a transducer, the same crystals send out a sound impulse and then wait for reflected sound waves.
- Assume that average speed of sound in human tissues is 1,540 m/sec.
- Range equation:

    Reflector distance from transducer =
    ½ round-trip time × 1,540 m/sec
- Duty factor is the amount of fraction of time the transducer sends out sound waves versus "listening" for their return (0.01 to 0.001).

sound transducers. By altering the voltage applied as well as the thickness of the PZT crystal, different ultrasound frequencies can be generated.

The ultrasound crystals can both generate sound and receive (e.g., "listen to") sound (Fig. 4). In essence, the ultrasound crystals first act as a megaphone by sending out a sound wave. In diagnostic scanning, it is the sound that is reflected back to the transducer that provides clinically relevant information.

FACTORS IN THE UTILIZATION OF ULTRASOUND IN DIAGNOSTIC IMAGING (TABLE 7)

In order to use sound to generate images, we must know where to place the amplitude of a returning echo on the image screen. To do this, an assumption must be made about the speed of sound in tissue. The ultrasound machine assumes that the speed of sound is 1,540 m/sec, which is the approximate velocity of sound in most human soft tissues. By measuring the time it takes from the origination of the sound wave to be sent from the ultrasound transducer until its return, the distance of the reflector from the transducer can be calculated. This is accomplished by the following equation, called the range equation:

Reflector distance from transducer = ½ round-trip time × 1,540 m/sec

SENDING AND RECEIVING SOUND

The ultrasound crystals used in diagnostic ultrasound do not constantly send out sound waves. If sound were constantly being transmitted, there would be ambiguity in interpretation of the returning sound with regard to depth. The ability to time the round trip would be lost. This is because sound waves would continually be returning to the transducer. There would be no ability to discriminate sounds that were sent earlier from those that were transmitted later. The range equation would therefore become useless. Ambiguity of returning sound would make it impossible to place a returning echo in its proper location on the display.

In order to solve this problem, the ultrasound probe spends most of its time "listening for" (i.e., receiving) returning sound waves and only a small amount of time sending them. The amount of time that the transducer spends sending out sound is called the *duty factor*. It is the amount of time that sound is "sent out" as a fraction of the total time of a cycle of "sending" and "listening." Average duty factors are 0.01 to 0.001, which means that sound is being sent out only 1/100th to 1/1000th of the time. Conversely, the transducer is listening 99% to 99.9% of the time (Table 7).

MAKING AN ULTRASOUND TRANSDUCER

The majority of ultrasound transducers contain several hundred crystals, although some are made up of only a single crystal (Table 8). A single-crystal transducer is generally attached to an oscillating or rotating arm. The transducer sends out a sound wave, listens for returning waves, and then moves to another spot where the process is repeated. This kind of transducer can generate an image that is close to real time because the speed of

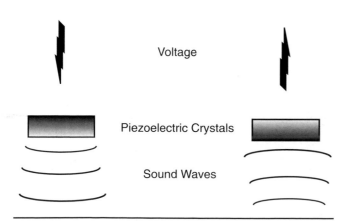

Voltage

Piezoelectric Crystals

Sound Waves

FIGURE 4. Piezoelectric effect. Graphic representation of voltage applied to a piezoelectric crystal creating wave and vice versa.

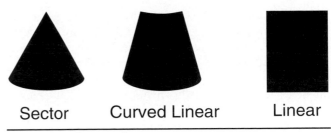

FIGURE 5. Ultrasound image types.

▶ TABLE 8 Type of Transducer

Mechanical sector (single crystal)
Electronic phased (multiple crystals)
  Linear
  Curved linear
  Sector

sound is very fast relative to the distance it has to travel. For example, if imaging to a depth of 8 cm, the total round trip distance is 16 cm; 0.016 m × 1 sec/1,540 m = 1.04×10^{-5} sec. Since such a short time is needed for the sound wave to make one round trip, constructing an image is possible using just one piezoelectric crystal. Obviously this doesn't take into consideration the time necessary to move from place to place, but the concept of how fast things are moving should be appreciated. Each time the piezoelectric crystal transmits and receives a reflected set of sound waves, the data are used to create a scan line. Multiple scan lines are assembled to create an image. With a crystal that is attached to a swinging arm, the image generated is called a sector image; the transducer is called a mechanical sector type. However, this type of transducer has some disadvantage. Due to the fast speed that the transducer's motor must rotate the crystals around, the motor becomes susceptible to breakage.

To overcome this problem, many ultrasound crystals are cut from a single block of PZT with each individual crystal given electrical connections. This allows each crystal to function independently. By coupling crystals together electronically, they can be used to send out sound waves and listen for returning sound waves in a coordinated fashion (a process called *phasing*). Phased transducers cover an area determined by their width. Rather than having a motor to move the crystals around, the phasing of the crystals accomplishes the same thing. By electronically stimulating a small number of crystals synchronously to transmit and receive sound, a portion of the image is acquired with each phased set of crystals. Again, because of the speed of sound relative to the distances traveled, the image can be assembled so as to appear as a "real time" image. This type of transducer has several advantages over mechanical types. First of all, it has no moving part to burn out. Furthermore, the sound waves can be electronically focused to different depths by changing the phasing routines. This focusing helps improves lateral resolution. Phased transducers are faster than mechanical ones because there are no moving parts, thereby giving a more flowing and real-time image. Finally, phased electronic transducers can readily provide differently shaped images depending on the scanning needs.

Phasing is typically done in three different patterns (Fig. 5). A linear transducer has a flat surface in contact with the patient. It constructs scan lines that are parallel to each other and perpendicular to the contact surface (face) of the transducer. A curved linear or curvilinear (convex) transducer has a curved face in contact with the patient. It constructs scan lines that diverge from each other in relation to the face of the transducer. While a sector transducer has a flat face in contact with the patient, it constructs scan lines that diverge from each other. The sector transducer's scan lines diverge from a single point on the transducer's face rather than the entire face as occurs with a curved linear transducer. Current ultrasound scanners mostly use electronic transducers rather than mechanical transducers.

There are numerous other factors that must be considered in transducer design. The transducer is more than just a housing for piezoelectric crystals and wiring. Since impedance differences cause sound to be reflected and piezoelectric crystals have significantly different impedance than biologic tissue, a material must be put between the two to allow the majority of the generated sound to go into the body and back out of the body. Otherwise the majority of the sound would be reflected at the interface (point of substantial impedance mismatch) between the crystals and the skin. The gray material that is present on the face of the transducer that comes in contact with the patient is called the matching layer. This layer "matches" the impedance differences between the two materials so as to maximize sound transmission to the body and back out to the crystal(s) (Fig. 6).

While an ultrasound transducer is often labeled at a specific frequency (e.g., 4 MHz), this does not necessarily

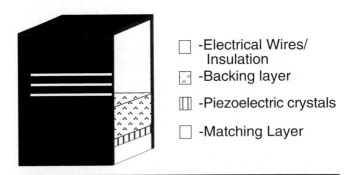

☐ -Electrical Wires/
      Insulation
☒ -Backing layer
▥ -Piezoelectric crystals
☐ -Matching Layer

FIGURE 6. Anatomy of an ultrasound probe.

mean that the transducer only produces the same frequency. A piezoelectric crystal has inertia to overcome just like any object at rest. When a voltage is applied to a piezoelectric crystal it vibrates in an accelerated fashion up to the desired frequency. This can cause a series of frequencies to be generated. This series of frequencies is called the bandwidth. The broader the bandwidth, the greater is the number of frequencies present.

There are two approaches to this dilemma. One approach is to utilize the broad bandwidth to get the highest frequency available for a given depth of penetration, with the goal of obtaining the best resolution possible. These types of transducers are usually labeled with a range, such as 2 to 5 MHz. The other approach is to tighten the bandwidth as much as possible toward the desired frequency. While not yet perfected, this method screens the frequencies received by the machine and listens to the desired frequency.

RESOLUTION

Optimal resolution, or clarity of the image, is an important goal of diagnostic ultrasound (Table 9). Three types of resolution are important in day-to-day scanning (Table 9). Axial resolution refers to the ability to distinguish an object from another, deeper one. Axial resolution is dependent on the frequency of the sound wave. Lateral resolution refers to the ability to distinguish an object from another object at the same depth; it is dependent on ultrasound beam width and independent of ultrasound frequency. The third type of resolution is temporal resolution, referring to the ability to distinguish closely spaced events. Temporal resolution is independent of frequency and beam width, but is dependent on frame rate.

Axial Resolution

Axial resolution is directly related to the frequency of the sound wave. That is, as the transducer frequency increases, so does the axial resolution. The ultrasound transducer only transmits a sound impulse for a brief period. This

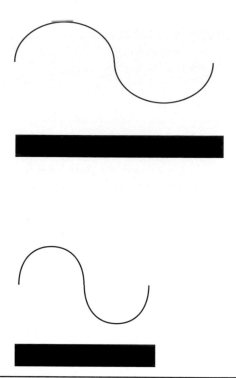

FIGURE 7. Axial resolution. The ultrasound pulse takes up physical space. This pulse length has a measurable length, called the spatial pulse length. The spatial pulse length acts like a ruler to measure distances in the axial plane. The lower the frequency, the longer is the spatial pulse length. Because of the sound wave traveling to and reflecting back from an impedance difference, the ability to distinguish two objects in the axial plane is dependent on one half of the spatial pulse length.

impulse takes up a certain distance, which is called the spatial pulse length. If the number of cycles in an ultrasound pulse is held constant, then the distance of the spatial pulse length is dependent on the wavelength, which in turn is dependent on the frequency. The spatial pulse becomes a ruler to measure distances. Since the sound wave is sent out and reflected back, the axial resolution is equal to one half of the spatial pulse length (Fig. 7). The spatial pulse length's effect on discrimination of two reflectors in the axial plane is shown in Figure 8.

The voltage applied to piezoelectric crystals causes them to vibrate. Like a bell, however, the crystals vibrate for a while after being struck. This has a negative effect on the spatial pulse length. In order to shorten the spatial pulse length, a layer of material is placed on the nonpatient side of the crystals to stop the vibrations from continuing in an unwanted fashion; this is called the backing layer (Fig. 6).

Lateral Resolution

Lateral resolution, or the discrimination of two objects located side by side, is dependent on the width of the ultrasound beam. The best method of controlling the width

TABLE 9 Resolution

Axial: differentiating one object from another that is deeper
    Depends on ultrasound frequency
    Higher frequency = higher resolution
Lateral: differentiating one object from another that is beside it
    Depends on beam width
    Independent of frequency
Temporal: perception of real-time motion
    Depends on frame rate

Influenced by depth, other modalities such as Doppler that are used.

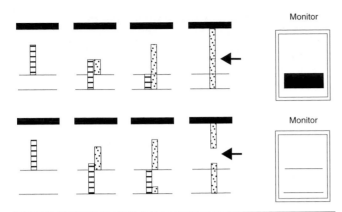

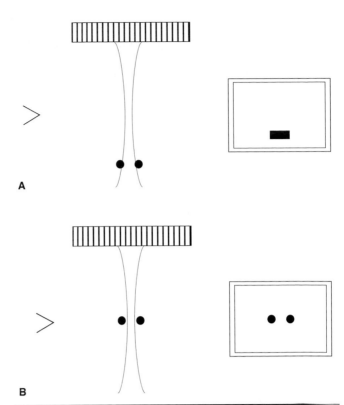

FIGURE 8. Axial resolution. The top and bottom show an ultrasound probe (*black*), the spatial pulse length (*striped*), the returning pulse (*stippled*), and the reflectors (*horizontal lines*). At the top, the two reflectors are too close to each other in the axial plane and the returning echoes overlap (*see arrow*). Without a gap between the two returning echoes, the ultrasound machine cannot interpret any difference between the two pulses since they overlap and displays them as a single reflector. At the bottom when the reflectors are more than one half the spatial pulse length, the reflectors can be displayed separately.

FIGURE 9. Lateral resolution is determined by the beam width, which is narrowest at the focal point. As demonstrated in **A**, if the ultrasound beam is wider than the lateral distance between two objects, the returning signal cannot differentiate the two objects and displays them as one. In **B**, the beam width is narrower than the lateral distance between the two objects. This correctly interprets that there are two objects.

of the ultrasound beam is by focusing. In the case of older, nonphased ultrasound probes, the beam is focused at a particular point by an acoustic lens. In this case, the focal point is fixed and can only be changed by changing the focusing lens. While more complex, the current method of focusing an ultrasound beam relies on phasing of multiple piezoelectric crystals (Fig. 9).

If the face of an ultrasound transducer were a single piezoelectric crystal, the width of the beam at its narrowest point would be equal to the width of the crystal. With a lens to focus the beam, this distance could be reduced somewhat, but it then becomes fixed at that depth. However, if the transducer face is made up of several hundred ultrasound crystals, multiple focal zones can be generated. Furthermore, by activating only a small number of piezoelectric crystals at a time, the ultrasound beam can be focused electronically to a very narrow width, thereby improving lateral resolution.

Temporal Resolution

When we look at a series of images shown in sequence, we perceive real time when we cannot distinguish one image from the next one. In video, a frame rate of 30 images per second causes our brain to see what we perceive as real-time full-motion video. As the frame rate decreases the motion becomes less smooth, and we perceive a hesitation or a jerky transition from one ultrasound image to the next. How is it that the acquisition of ultrasound images is synthesized to give the appearance of real-time video?

One must recall that the speed of sound is very fast relative to the distances traveled. Sequential generation of 100 separate beams to a depth of 10 cm would take only 0.013 second. The time needed to generate 30 images would be 0.39 second, much faster than the rate of full-motion video of 30 images per second.

Unfortunately, image acquisition isn't quite as fast as the above example because the sound wave portion of ultrasound is only one part of acquiring an image. An impulse generator must initiate the voltage impulses sent to the piezoelectric crystals. The returning voltages also have to be analyzed for amplitude. In order to make the data easier to analyze, the amplitude data are converted to a scale based on relative brightness, or B mode. Considering the B-mode data along with the travel time data, the area of reflected sound can then be placed on the video image in the proper location. This is repeated for each set of piezoelectric crystals that are phased together. Since the speed of sound is constant, it is the availability of faster computer processing for analysis and construction of the ultrasound video image that has increased the speed and quality of current ultrasound machines.

Factors that affect temporal resolution include the depth of the structure evaluated and which ultrasound modalities are used. If a greater depth of tissue is studied, more time must be spent waiting for the reflected sound to return before the next sound pulse can be sent out. This has the additive effects of slowing down image acquisition and frame rate.

Other modalities that are used include color Doppler, power Doppler, and spectral Doppler (see Chapter 8 for a discussion about how these modalities work). All of these modalities slow the frame rate. In the past, one set of sound waves was sent out to generate the B-mode image. This image would then be frozen to allow placement of the spectral Doppler in the correct location. The subsequent sound waves sent out would be ignored for B-mode analysis and only be used for Doppler frequency shifts in the selected area. With faster processing power, a real-time B-mode image and a spectral Doppler or color Doppler overlay could be displayed. This requires one set of ultrasound waves being sent out to acquire a B-mode image with a second set of waves sent out to acquire a Doppler shift from the selected area that is superimposed on the gray scale image. This process has been accelerated even more with faster processing. In routine B-mode imaging, returning sound information contains frequency shifts caused by interaction with moving objects. However, until the advent of faster and more powerful computing power, these data were ignored. With faster computing, the returning beam can be split into two data sets. One set of information can be analyzed for amplitude data (B mode), the other analyzed for frequency shift data (Doppler). By not having to send out separate sets of data for each type of information requested, image acquisition is further accelerated.

▶ **TABLE 10** **Various Ultrasound Artifacts**

Reverberation
Ring down (comet tail)
Mirror image
Posterior enhancement
Acoustic shadowing
Edge shadowing
Side lobe artifact

PHYSICS OF ARTIFACTS

While ultrasound generally works well, problems do arise. Some of the structures within the ultrasound image are not real. These "artifacts" arise because the ultrasound machine makes assumptions that are not always true. These assumptions include the following: (a) The speed of sound is 1,540 m/sec and (b) ultrasound pulses travel in a straight line from the transducer, reflect off of an interface, and then return straight back to the probe. As a general rule of thumb, if there is uncertainty regarding whether part of an image is real or an artifact, one should scan the center of the area under question from different directions. If the area disappears, it is probably an artifact.

ARTIFACT DUE TO TIMING ERRORS (TABLE 10)

Reverberation Artifact

Reverberation artifact is one of the more common ultrasound artifacts. One should remember that sound is re-

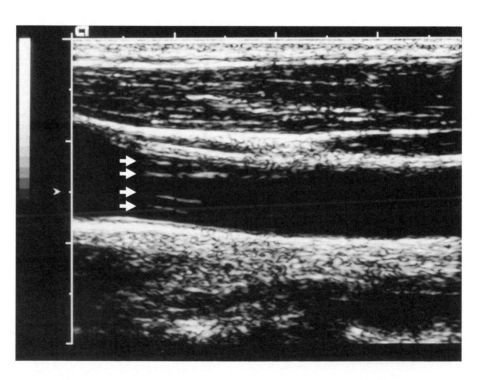

FIGURE 10. Reverberation artifact (*arrows*) in a longitudinal image of the common carotid artery.

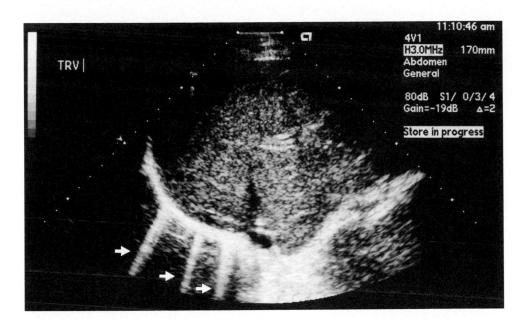

FIGURE 11. Ring-down artifact (*arrows*) in a transverse image of the liver and diaphragm.

flected at the interface of two tissues of different impedances. This not only occurs when the sound is traveling out into tissue but also on the way back to the transducer. Sound can get "trapped" between two interfaces and bounce back and forth. Some of this temporarily trapped sound energy may eventually return to the transducer. It takes time for sound waves to bounce back and forth. When this sound energy returns to the transducer, the delay in returning is interpreted as an impedance interface that is deeper than the first one; however, such an

interface does not exist. As the sound continues to bounce back away from the transducer and then back toward the transducer, more returning sound amplitude is displayed at regular intervals deeper and deeper on the screen. The appearance of a reverberation artifact is that of a ladder with brighter or hyperechoic lines representing the rungs of a ladder. Reverberation can make cystic structures appear to have a solid inner component, such as a breast cyst, or an artery have an intimal flap (Fig. 10).

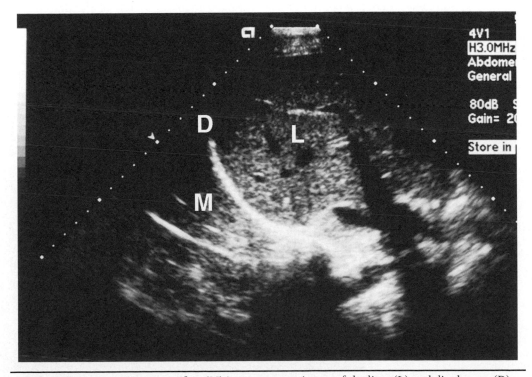

FIGURE 12. Mirror image artifact (M) in a transverse image of the liver (L) and diaphragm (D).

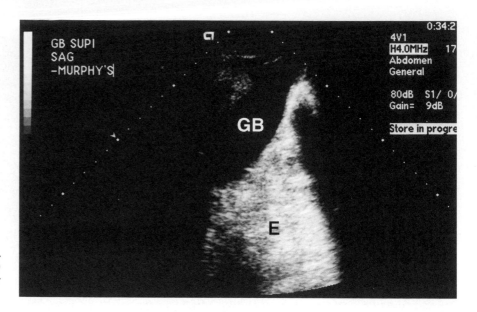

FIGURE 13. Posterior enhancement (E) in a longitudinal image of the gallbladder (GB).

Ring-Down Artifact

The ring-down artifact, which is also a common artifact, is sometimes referred to as the comet tail artifact. Ring down occurs when the ultrasound transducer strikes an object, such as a piece of metal or gas bubbles. These objects act as a bell and the ultrasound wave is the clapper. The object then "rings" much longer than the time of contact between the sound wave and the object. Again the sound energy generated by this interaction goes back to the probe. As with reverberation, the ultrasound machine interprets delays in returns as having traveled to a greater depth. Due to the "ringing" nature of this artifact, there is a constant return of sound energy, so the ladder rungs are much closer together and look more like a flashlight beam emanating from the gas bubble or metallic object (Fig. 11).

Mirror Image Artifact

If the sound wave reflects off of a curved surface rather than off of a flat surface oriented perpendicular to the direction of the sound wave, the sound can be reflected multiple times in different directions before returning to the transducer. Like reverberation artifacts, the sound impulse takes longer to return to the transducer. The reflected echoes then are placed at a deeper, and often more lateral, location than the real source of the reflection, since the re-reflected sound has to travel a longer distance. Most of the time this occurs when imaging involves a view of the diaphragm or a full urinary bladder. These curved structures act like an acoustic mirror to redirect sound back to the transducer (Fig. 12).

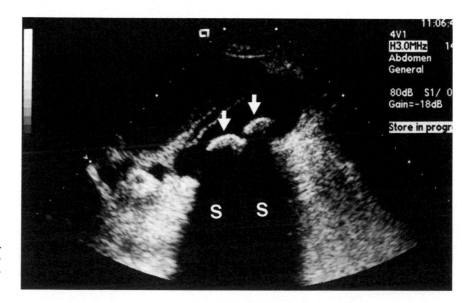

FIGURE 14. Posterior shadowing (S) behind a longitudinal image of the gallbladder with gallstones (*arrows*).

ARTIFACTS DUE TO ATTENUATION ASSUMPTIONS

Posterior Enhancement

Some autocorrection of attenuation is built into most ultrasound machines. This assumes that the tissue is uniform in its ability to attenuate sound. But this is not always the case. The most common example of this problem occurs during imaging of a fluid-filled structure. Water and other bodily fluids are not compressible. This makes them efficient transmitters of sound energy with relatively little energy loss. An efficient sound transmitter minimizes attenuation. The ultrasound machine assumes a constant rate of attenuation and compensates for it. If the rate of attenuation is decreased, structures deep to the fluid-filled structure have a higher than expected amplitude. This greater returning amplitude translates to a brighter B-mode display of that area. Since the brighter display is behind or deep to the fluid-filled structure, this artifact is called posterior enhancement (Fig. 13).

Posterior enhancement deep to a very small cyst cannot be explained well by a decreased rate of attenuation. With a small distance traveled, it is unlikely that the small decrease in attenuation can create significant posterior enhancement. One explanation is that the cystic structure acts like an acoustic lens to focus the sound toward the center. With more acoustic intensity directed at one location, a higher returning amplitude results, which is displayed as posterior enhancement.

ARTIFACTS DUE TO A DECREASE OR NO RETURNING SOUND WAVES

Acoustic Shadowing

When sound strikes an interface with a large acoustic impedance difference, virtually all of the sound energy is reflected back in the direction of the transducer. If this very high acoustic impedance mismatch covers the entire surface of the transducer, no image is obtained below this level. One common example of this is no image at all. This is a result due to air between the matching layer of the probe and the body, with no sound transmission into the body. Another example occurs with imaging an extremity with bone being below the soft tissue.

When this high acoustic impedance difference does not involve the entire image, there may be an area deep to the high acoustic impedance difference where no information is obtained. Because there is no information obtained in this area, the machine defaults to showing this area as black. Sound waves diverge beyond the focal zone, giving the data void an appearance of a shadow. This is most commonly seen with ultrasound of gallstones (Fig. 14).

Edge Shadowing

The best surface to examine with ultrasound is one that is perpendicular to the ultrasound beam. As the surface under study becomes parallel to the ultrasound beam, less acoustic energy is reflected back to the transducer. When the surface and the ultrasound beam are completely parallel, no sound is reflected back to the transducer. The most common example of this is a structure that is round, such as a transverse image of a blood vessel or the gallbladder. The tangent of that section of the curve affects ultrasound waves coming in contact with a curved surface. The sound waves traveling through the center of a circle encounter a tangent perpendicular to the direction of the sound wave. This causes the amplitude of the reflected waves to be reflected directly back to the transducer. As the sound waves sent from the transducer go farther away from the center, the tangent becomes more oblique. This causes less reflected amplitude of the waves back to the transducer and more wave amplitude to be reflected perpendicular to the tangent, which is away from the transducer. Just before the edge where the tangent is parallel to the direction of the sound wave, the tangent reflects all of the returning sound amplitude away from the transducer. At this point, the ultrasound machine gets no information regarding amplitude and distance. So like shadowing from gallstones, a shadow is displayed at this area of the curve (Fig. 15).

IMAGE AVERAGING ARTIFACT

Image averaging artifact is also called slice thickness or beam width artifact. The ultrasound beam has a thickness, which is least at the focal zone. As with computed tomographic scanning, where the image has a specified thickness, the ultrasound image incorporates volume averaging for a given image. When evaluating a cystic structure on a tangent, the volume averaging of fluid and solid structures can cause the material within the cystic structure to appear echogenic rather than echolucent, or anechoic. This causes the supposed fluid within a cystic structure to look like more solid material. Depending on the anatomic area imaged, this can be misinterpreted as thrombus within an artery or complexity within a cyst.

A variant of this artifact is called a side lobe artifact. The ultrasound beam is more powerful in its center and weaker at its edges. Early in its propagation into the body, the lateral portion of the wave is refracted away from the main beam; it can be reflected off a structure entirely different from the main portion of the beam. When the lateral portion of the beam returns to the transducer, this set of information is assumed to have traveled in a straight line from the transducer. This results in an artifact being displayed on the image, usually an echo-

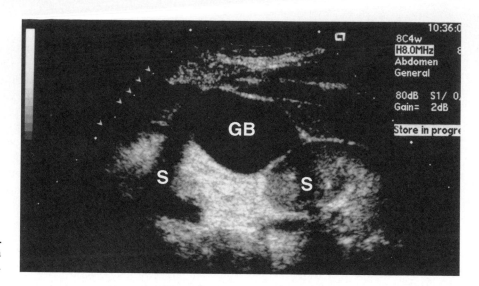

FIGURE 15. Edge shadowing (S) of a transverse image of the gallbladder (GB).

genic line. If it is superimposed on an image of an artery, it could be interpreted as an intimal flap (Fig. 16). It can also mimic septations in a cystic structure.

HARMONICS

As sound waves impact tissue in the body, they do more than just vibrate at the frequency imparted by the transmitted sound wave, or fundamental frequency. Resonance or harmonic frequencies develop. These harmonic frequencies are multiples of the fundamental frequency. The first harmonic is two times the fundamental frequency, the second harmonic is three times the fundamental frequency, and so on. These harmonic frequencies are weaker than the amplitude of the fundamental sound wave.

Harmonic frequencies had been difficult to evaluate until recently when increased computer power became available to electronically isolate the harmonic frequency; this has enabled a newer ultrasound imaging technology known as *tissue harmonic imaging*. The harmonic frequency can be isolated by electronically subtracting the fundamental frequency of the returning sound impulse. More recently, digital encoding of the fundamental frequency has allowed for improvement in harmonic imaging. Digital encoding takes advantage of

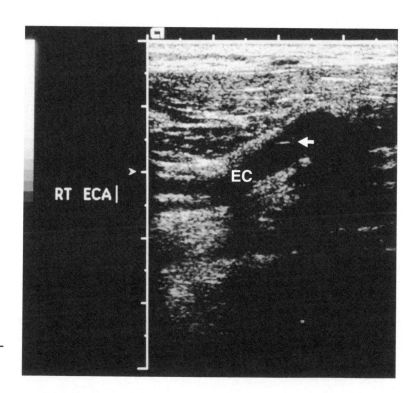

FIGURE 16. Side lobe artiface (*arrow*) of a longitudinal image of the external carotid artery (EC).

the fact that harmonic waves are out of phase with the fundamental sound wave. This allows the fundamental frequency to be canceled out while the harmonic frequency propagates undisturbed back to the transducer.

In using ultrasound harmonics, the first harmonic is utilized. If harmonic is used with a 2-MHz transducer, the frequency listened for on the returning sound impulse is 4 MHz. This is the advantage of harmonics. Remember that the higher the frequency, the faster the rate of attenuation. By sending out a lower frequency sound impulse that in essence is converted to a higher frequency wave, axial resolution is improved. This occurs because the pulse length becomes shorter due to a shorter wavelength.

Harmonics also clean up reverberation artifacts by deleting the fundamental frequency. When the fundamental frequency causes reverberation, this information is not processed. The harmonic frequency is only generated in the tissues. The fact that the harmonic wave makes a one-way trip and is of low amplitude reduces any significant reverberation artifacts. Remember that higher frequency sound is attenuated more quickly than lower frequency sound waves. Harmonics are maximized at an area called the sweet spot. This tends to be in the middle of the image. It is like an inverse of the focus with fewer harmonics above and below the sweet spot.

CONCLUSIONS

The physics of ultrasound is a complex and confusing subject. In fact, volumes are written regarding the physics of ultrasound images. This chapter serves as an introduction to the basic principles of ultrasound physics. By knowing these basic tenets, one can generally determine why objects appear the way they do on an ultrasound image, as well as what is real and what is not.

REFERENCES

1. Harness JK, Wisher DB, eds. *Ultrasound in surgical practice: basic principles and clinical applications.* New York: John Wiley and Sons, 2001.
2. Hikes DL, Hedrick WR, Starchman DE. *Ultrasound physics and instrumentation.* St. Louis: Mosby-Year Book, 1992.
3. Kremkau FW. *Diagnostic ultrasound: principles and instruments,* 4th ed. Philadelphia: WB Saunders, 1989.

Instrumentation and Scanning Techniques

Stanley J. Rogers and M. Margaret Knudson

Ultrasound can be an extremely useful tool for the surgeon, but image acquisition requires both an understanding of the principles of physics and a working familiarity with the components of the machine itself. The quality of the image obtained is dependent on a number of factors, including the choice of the appropriate transducer, the quality of the returned signal, the selection of an acoustic "window," and the position of the patient. In addition, all images must be labeled and stored in a secured area for future reference, and the equipment must be properly maintained. Finally, the surgeon must understand the potential biohazards associated with the use of ultrasound in the clinical setting.

TERMINOLOGY

The term *echogenicity* refers to the appearance of tissues and adjacent structures relative to each other as determined by ultrasound. The American Institute of Ultrasound in Medicine standardized the definitions of the patterns of images as seen in gray scale scanning (Table 1). For example, *anechoic* refers to the property of appearing echo free or without echoes on a sonographic image. In Figure 1, the gallbladder lumen is noted to be anechoic or *hypoechoic* (i.e., with fewer echoes) when compared with the liver. The term *hyperechoic* describes a region in a sonographic image where echoes are brighter than surrounding structures (Fig. 2). Differences in echogenicity allow us to identify interfaces between two structures. For example, the hyperechoic appearance of Gerota's fascia helps to define the edge of the right lobe of the liver from the cortex of the right kidney, both of which have similar echogenic properties (Fig. 3).

SELECTION OF EQUIPMENT

Obtaining an ultrasound image begins with providing a path for transmission of the sound wave between the transducer and the object being imaged. This process is termed *coupling* and is usually accomplished by replacing the air between the transducer and the object with a fluid (as with saline in intraoperative ultrasound) or, more commonly, with a gel for surface imaging (contact coupling). Standard ultrasound gels can be heated to enhance coupling and improve patient comfort. More important than heating, however, is the amount of gel applied. Figure 4 demonstrates a poor-quality image secondary to lack of coupling gel. The gel can be applied directly to the transducer or to the skin over the area to be imaged. Occasionally, when imaging superficial structures such as peripheral blood vessels, thyroid gland, or breast, a standoff device is placed between the transducer and the skin so that ultrasound imaging can be performed without some of the artifacts that would arise in contact scanning (Fig. 5). Standoff devices can be either liquid or solid but should be very low in attenuation in order to avoid any loss of amplitude as the sound wave travels through it to the object of interest.

Next, the surgeon must choose the transducer that will obtain the best image. Transducers are described thoroughly in Chapters 2 and 13. For the purposes of this discussion, the sonographer should appreciate that linear transducers give the best view of structures superficial surfaces such as peripheral blood vessels, breast, and thyroid gland. Convex or sector designs facilitate obtaining images between ribs or within limited spaces and are generally preferred for transabdominal and cardiac scanning (Fig. 6). The frequency of the transducer determines the depth of sound penetration and the resolution of the image. In general, transducers of higher ultrasound frequencies provide high resolution but lose their signal strength quickly and therefore provide poor penetration in deeper tissue (1). Conversely, lower frequency transducers demonstrate good penetration but the image resolution diminishes considerably. The transducer selected should be of the highest frequency possible for imaging the target organ. Table 2 describes the uses for various frequency transducers.

▶ **TABLE 1 Glossary of Ultrasound Terminology**

Acoustic power: acoustic energy transported per unit time, expressed in watts

Amplifier: a device that magnifies the amplitude or power of its input signal

Anechoic: the property of appearing echo free or without echoes on a sonographic image

Attenuation: the decrease in amplitude or intensity as sound travels through a material caused by absorption, scattering, and beam divergence

Contact coupling: acoustic coupling of a transducer by direct contact with the skin, using liquid or gel to exclude air from the space between the transducer and the skin

Echogenic: describes a structure or medium that is capable of producing echoes

Frame rate: the rate at which pictures are refreshed on the display of a real-time system

Freeze frame: control setting of sonographic equipment that causes the most recent image to be stored in a scan converter memory and continuously displayed on a monitor

Gain: ratio of the output to the input of a system, generally an amplifying system, expressed in decibels

Gray scale: a display technique in which echo amplitude or intensity information is recorded as variations in brightness (shades of gray)

Hard copy: a permanent visual record stored on materials such as paper, radiographic film, or photographic film

Hyperechoic: describes a region in a sonographic image in which the echoes are brighter than normal or brighter than surrounding structures

Hypoechoic: describes a region in a sonographic image in which the echoes are not as bright as normal or less bright than surrounding structures

Phantom: a device that simulates some parameters of the human body, allowing measurements of ultrasound system parameters or visualization of simulated anatomic features

Standoff: a device placed between a transducer and the skin so that ultrasound imaging can be performed without some of the artifacts that would arise in contact scanning

Time–gain compensation (TGC): increase in receiver gain with time introduced to compensate for loss in echo amplitude, usually due to attenuation with depth

Adapted from *Recommended Ultrasound Technology*, 2nd Ed. American Institute of Ultrasound in Medicine, 1997.

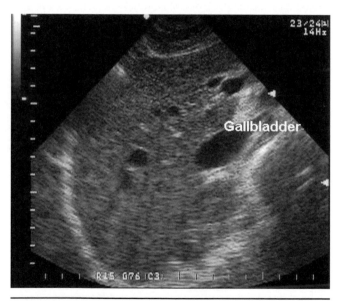

FIGURE 1. The gallbladder lumen appears *hypoechoic* in comparison with the surrounding liver tissue.

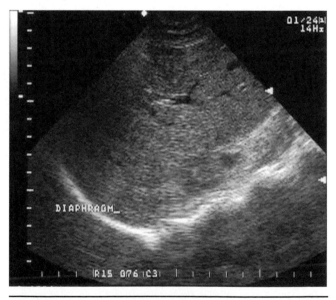

FIGURE 2. The diaphragm is a *hyperechoic* structure in comparison with the lung (*left posterior side of the screen*) and the liver.

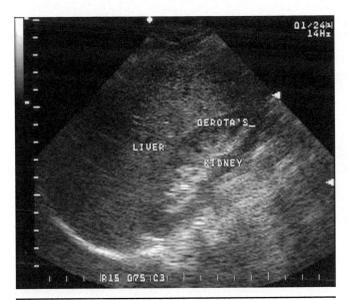

FIGURE 3. The hyperechoic stripe of Gerota's fascia separates the liver from the kidney.

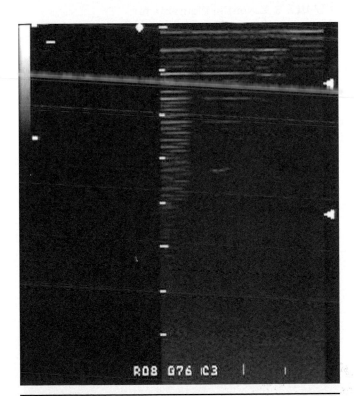

FIGURE 4. Image obtained without gel coupling. Note the linear stripes produced by the presence of air between the transducer and the skin causing reverberation artifact.

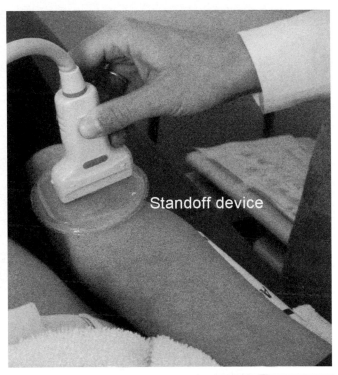

FIGURE 5. A standoff device can be used to improve the visualization of superficial structures such as peripheral vessels.

All ultrasound machines have annotation keys for labeling images. Annotation is performed when the image is "frozen" on the screen. It is essential to type in the date of the scan, the patient's name and record number, and the plane of the image being obtained (i.e., transverse versus sagittal; see below) (Table 3). Image orientation has been standardized such that when one is scanning in the sagittal plane, the patient's head is located on the left side of the screen (Fig. 7). When scanning in transverse, the left side of the screen corresponds to the right side of the patient (Fig. 8). Images can be printed on photographic paper, on film, or stored digitally, but protection of the patient's privacy must be guaranteed.

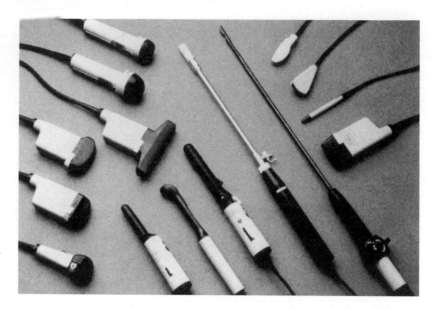

FIGURE 6. Various types of transducers that are chosen according to the type of ultrasound examination being performed.

▶ **TABLE 2** Uses for Transducers of Various Frequencies

Transducer (MHz)	Application
2.25	Deep abdominal; obese patients
3.5	General abdominal, renal, obstetrics
5.0	Neonates/pediatric patients; peripheral vascular
7.5	Cerebrovascular; breast, testicle thyroid, intraoperative, laparoscopic
10	Ocular, vein mapping superficial soft tissue

▶ **TABLE 3** Essential Elements for Documentation/Image Labeling

Patient's name/ID Number
Date of examination
Type of preset selected (e.g., cardiac, abdomen)
Orientation of the transducer (e.g., transverse, oblique)
Additional comments: patient characteristics, symptoms, comparison studies

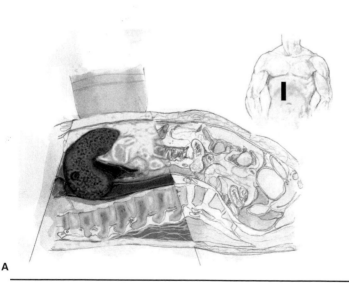

A

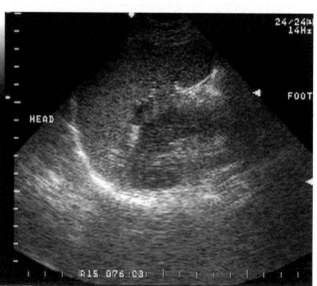

B

FIGURE 7. A. Transducer held with a sagittal orientation in the right upper quadrant and underlying area of the body visualized in this plane and position. **B.** Ultrasound image obtained with a sagittal orientation of the transducer in this position. Note that the patient's head is on the left side of the screen, with the feet on the right. Illustration by Nicolas Villarreal.

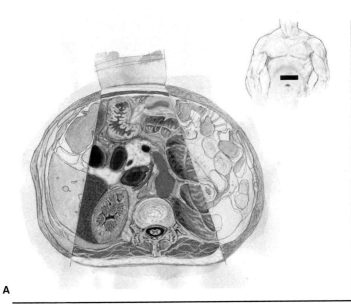 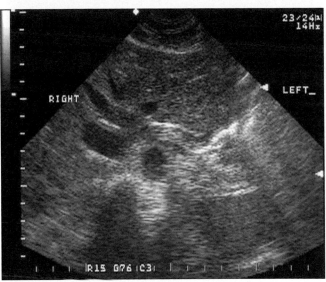

A

B

FIGURE 8. **A.** Transducer held in a transverse orientation in the epigastric area and underlying area of the body visualized. **B.** Ultrasound image obtained with a transverse orientation in the epigastric area. Note that the patient's right side is on the left side of the screen. Illustration by Nicolas Villarreal.

IMAGE REFINEMENT

Echo or signal amplification is necessary because the returning echoes are too weak to be displayed. Echoes can be strengthened by increasing the intensity of the transmitted signal (i.e., the power) or by increasing the amplification of the transmitted signal by increasing the gain. The enhancement of the returning echoes can be "preset" into the machine for each type of scan (e.g., breast/abdominal), and the sonographer can simply select a particular preset. In general, presets include the lowest power that results in a high-resolution image. Although increasing the power allows a brighter display from all reflectors and visualization of very weak reflectors that are not normally seen, it also increases the acoustic exposure of the patient. Presets also determine the frame rate at which pictures are displayed on the screen. For certain types of scanning, such as vascular imaging, faster frame rates are required (2).

The overall brightness of the image displayed on the screen can be adjusted by controlling the degree of amplification of the returning echo or the "gain" (Fig. 9). When initiating the scan, the sonographer should adjust the gain so that a structure known to be anechoic (such as a ventricle or blood vessel) appears black on the screen. Gain is the ratio of output power to input power, expressed in decibels. The gain increases the amplitude of the returning ultrasound signal strength, which is analogous to turning up the volume on a stereo. However, if the gain is too high, additional image artifacts will be created (Fig. 10). Similarly, if the gain is set too low, some structures may not be visualized at all (Fig. 11).

Because the ultrasound wave becomes attenuated as it passes deep into tissue, the returning signal from the deepest regions are the weakest, creating an imbalance of the signal from the far field compared to the near field that is closest to the transducer. In order to adjust for this, the time–gain compensation (TGC) controls can be utilized to enhance the brightness of the structure of interest. These controls are often "slide pots" on the console (Fig. 9). Adjustments in the TGC pots and the corresponding changes in the image are demonstrated in Figure 12. The skilled sonographer will also learn to adjust the "depth of focus"

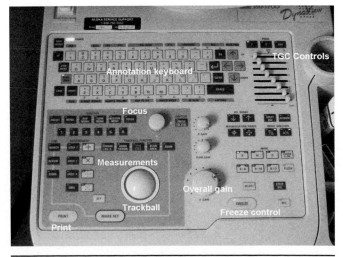

FIGURE 9. Console of a typical ultrasound unit, describing the function of the various controls.

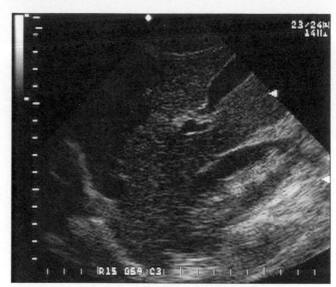

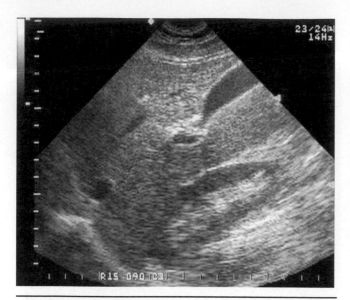

FIGURE 10. An image of the right upper quadrant obtained with the gain set too high.

FIGURE 11. An image of the right upper quadrant obtained with the gain set too low.

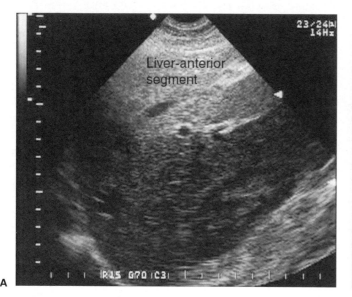

A

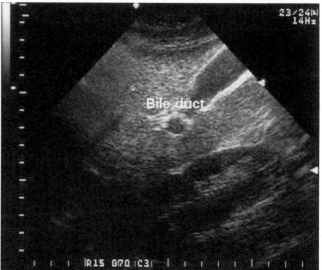

B

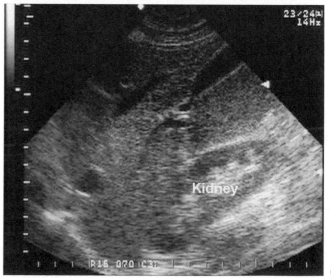

C

FIGURE 12. **A.** The upper time–gain compensation (TGC) slide pots have been moved to the right in order to enhance the image of the anterior segment of the right lobe of the liver. **B.** The middle TGC slide pots have been moved to the right in order to brighten up the region of the bile duct. **C.** The lower TGC slide pots have been moved to the right in order to enhance the returning echoes from the kidney.

control, which allows the most sensitive area of the sound wave to query the structure of interest. The region close to the probe (near field) is characterized by great variation in ultrasound intensity from one wave to the next (3). By contrast, the far field has more uniform intensity between wave fronts but the wave fronts start to diverge. Thus, the best images are obtained in the areas where there is a transition from the near field to the far field (focal region).

Most commonly, acquired ultrasound images are displayed in gray scale (B mode or "brightness modulation") (4). Gray scale displays echo intensity as brightness-modulated dots along a scale from black to gray to white. In contrast, spectral analysis displays the "spectrum" of Doppler-derived velocities or frequencies plotted against time as shades of gray. The more "scatterers" detected at a given velocity (frequency), the more white and the less gray the image will appear. Spectral broadening indicates turbulence, and increased velocities suggest vessel narrowing. Color flow is produced by computer transformation of Doppler-derived direction and velocity. Conventionally, flow away from the transducer is blue and flow toward the transducer is red. Velocity is displayed as hues or shades of color, with darker hues indicating reduced velocities and brighter hues corresponding to higher velocities.

Viewing of ultrasound images is made possible by the scan converter. The scan converter stores the images from individual beams and converts the scanned images to a format that can be viewed on the video monitor or other output device (VCR, digital cameras, and so forth). Once the desired image is obtained, the freeze button is activated and image labeling can occur using the annotation keys. Some ultrasound machines are equipped with a "cine loop," which allows the sonographer to view sequential images obtained just before freezing by rolling the track ball. This is particularly useful in vascular imaging. Printing or capturing the image requires that the image be frozen. Measurements, using digital calipers, can also be obtained on the frozen image, including linear and elliptical and volumetric measures (Fig. 13).

PATIENT POSITION AND IMAGE ACQUISITION

Knowledge of anatomy is essential for attainment of high-quality ultrasound images, and having such knowledge is characteristic of surgeons. The surgeon sonographer has an innately well-developed understanding of three-dimensional anatomy allowing natural creation, reconstruction, and interpretation of ultrasound images. However, finding acoustic windows in order to optimize the image requires practice and considerable patience. The organ or area of interest should be visualized in at least two planes (sagittal and transverse); occasionally, oblique views are also helpful (see below). Learning to apply the right amount of pressure between the transducer and the surface of the body or organ (in the case of intraoperative scanning) in order to obtain the optimal image also requires considerable practice. Many novice sonographers will pick up the transducer in order to move it around, or quickly change position rather than change the angle of inquiry. Transducers should be "slid" across the surface of the skin or organ rather than lifted off (Fig. 14). Once over the area of interest, a rocking motion (change of direction parallel to the scanning plane), or tilting motion (change of direction perpendicular to the scanning plane), or rotating motion will help to optimize the image (Fig. 14) (5).

As important as obtaining optimal images are patient factors. Whenever possible, patients should be made comfortable and imaged in a quiet and private environment. Administration of analgesics is recommended in some circumstances, such as when scanning for the evaluation of acute appendicitis. A calm and cooperative patient helps to minimize motion artifacts and can assist when position changes are required. Change of position is often required when ultrasound examinations are performed in the emergency setting when the patient has not been fasted and intestinal gas obscures the view. A graded compression may also be used to reduce bowel gas artifacts (6). Visualization of the spleen may require that the patient hold his or her breath to eliminate interference from the ribs. Other helpful "pearls," as outlined by Rozycki and others, are summarized in Table 4 (7).

Most commonly, scans are performed with the patient in a supine position and the sonographer on the right side of the patient. However, decubitus positions as well as prone and sometimes even upright imaging are occasionally required (8). Figure 15 demonstrates the anatomic landmarks on the body that are used as references for scanning. Using these references, the abdominal surface areas of the body can be divided into nine regions (9).

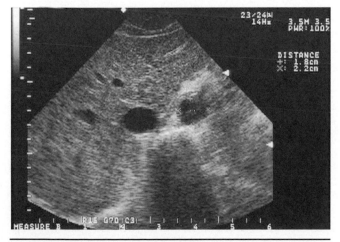

FIGURE 13. The aorta is outlined with measurement calipers. Note the distances between calipers are seen on the right side of the screen (1.8 × 2.2 cm).

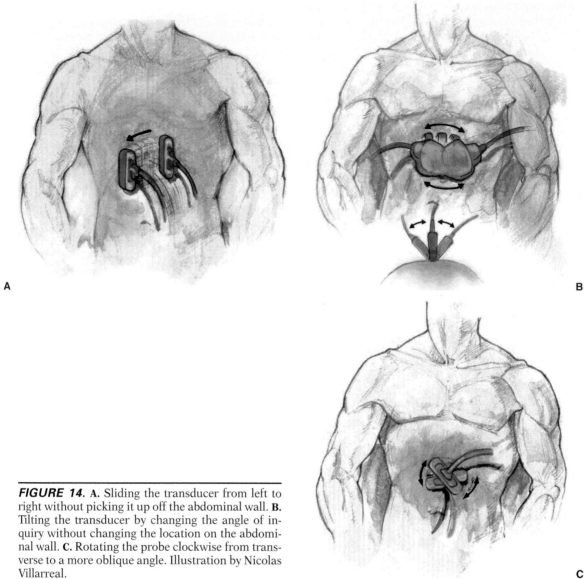

A

B

C

FIGURE 14. **A.** Sliding the transducer from left to right without picking it up off the abdominal wall. **B.** Tilting the transducer by changing the angle of inquiry without changing the location on the abdominal wall. **C.** Rotating the probe clockwise from transverse to a more oblique angle. Illustration by Nicolas Villarreal.

▶ **TABLE 4 Tips for Enhancing Ultrasound Images**

Darken the room as much as possible.
Interact with the patient to gain cooperation.
Enhance the gain, TGC, and depth of focus for optimal imaging.
Be liberal with the use of the coupling gel.
Use gentle but firm compression.
Scan a "normal area" first; then the area of interest.
Scan in at least two different planes.
Learn to slide, rock, tilt, and rotate the transducer.
Reposition the patient as needed.
Decrease gas interference by graded compression.
Consider placement of a nasogastric tube for scanning in
    emergency situations.
Changes in respiration may be helpful.

When images are obtained with the transducer positioned parallel to the long axis of the body, the image is "sagittal." Using a line drawn through the midline of the body, images obtained while moving toward the midline are termed medial, whereas those moving away from the midline are lateral (Fig. 16). Images obtained with the orientation of the probe at right angles to the body are "transverse" images. Transverse images toward the head are proximal, whereas those toward the feet are distal (Fig. 17). Images obtained at other angles are "oblique" images. "Coronal" planes divide the body into anterior and posterior sections. Coronal planes can be anterior or posterior, inferior or superior (Fig. 18) Thus, it can be appreciated that image labeling for future reference must include the plane of orientation.

Regions of the body

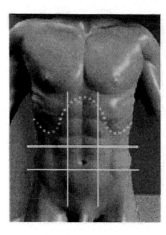

Landmarks

- Xiphoid process
- Costal margins
- Umbillicus
- Rectus muscles
- Iliac crests

Regions

- Right hypochondrium
- Left hypochondrium
- Epigastric
- Right lumbar
- Left lumbar
- Umbilical
- Right iliac fossa
- Left iliac fossa
- Hypogastric

FIGURE 15. Anatomic landmarks on the body and the resulting nine regions describe the abdominal area being scanned. (Reproduced from Kendall JL, Deutchman M. *Ultrasound in emergency medicine and trauma.* Nashville, TN: HealthStream, 2001, with permission.)

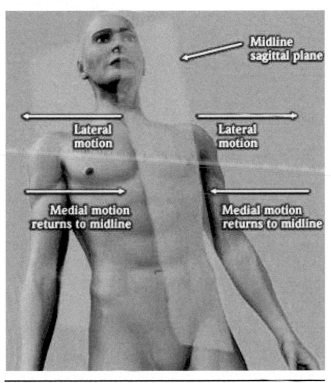

FIGURE 16. Visualization of the sagittal plane and the resulting medial and lateral directions. (Reproduced from Kendall JL, Deutchman M. *Ultrasound in emergency medicine and trauma.* Nashville, TN: HealthStream, 2001, with permission.)

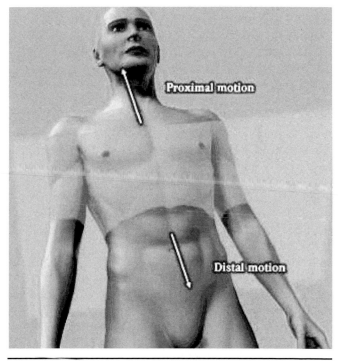

FIGURE 17. Visualization of the transverse plane with proximal and distal directions. (Reproduced from Kendall JL, Deutchman M. *Ultrasound in emergency medicine and trauma.* Nashville, TN: HealthStream, 2001, with permission.)

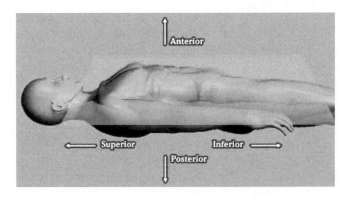

FIGURE 18. Orientation of the coronal plane with anterior, superior, inferior, and posterior directions. (Reproduced from Kendall JL, Deutchman M. *Ultrasound in emergency medicine and trauma.* Nashville, TN: HealthStream, 2001, with permission.)

SAFETY AND BIOHAZARDS OF ULTRASOUND

In general, medical ultrasound is associated with few side effects (Table 5). However, ultrasound can result in generation of sufficient heat to be harmful. Heat is proportional to the power applied to the beam or "pulse" and to the duration of exposure. Recent-generation scanners provide "real time" assessment of the potential risk of bioeffects due to heating by calculating the thermal index for a given transducer in a particular mode doing a preset scan. The thermal index and exposure time should be minimized. Cavitation results when the pressure oscillations produced by sound create gas bubbles from the air dissolved in tissue fluids. Oscillations that are rapid and intense can cause the bubbles to expand and contract, causing local shear stresses or cavitation. Modern scanners provide assessment of the potential risk of bioeffects due to cavitation by calculating the mechanical index for a given transducer in a particular mode doing a preset scan. The mechanical index is inversely proportional to the square root of the frequency of the transducer. Although there have been no documented biohazards to patients using medical ultrasound, the ALARA principle is generally endorsed ("as low as reasonably achievable") in reference to power and exposure time while acquiring the necessary clinical information (10). On the other hand, it is possible to shock both patients and sonographers if the transducer housing is cracked or there are breaks in the insulation. Dropping probes is an excellent method of damaging the housing. Machines should be well maintained and checked frequently for safety hazards and well as for accuracy. Adjustments in the machines for distance accuracy and resolution require scanning of phantoms at periodic intervals but at least annually (Table 6). Sterilization procedures must be followed carefully for intraoperative applications. Probes should always be cleaned after patient use by washing and/or application of cleansers and disinfectants. (Note: One should check with the manufacturer to get a list of safe cleaners that can be used with transusers and particular machines.) These principles are particularly important when machines are used in the emergency or intensive care setting to avoid transmission of disease from patient to patient. Finally, the surgeon sonographer should be an active participant in quality monitoring of

▌**TABLE 5 Biohazards of Ultrasound**

Heat
Cavitation
Electric shock
Disease transmission
Misinterpretation due to poor-quality images

▌**TABLE 6 Quality Control for Ultrasound Equipment**

Ensure maximal depth of visualization and hard copy recording with a tissue-mimicking phantom.
Ensure distance accuracy: vertical and horizontal.
Ensure uniformity.
Ensure anechoic void perception.
Ensure ring-down and dead space determination.
Optimize lateral resolution.
Optimize axial resolution.
Obtain data logs on system performance and examples of results.
Assure adherence to universal infection control precautions.

ultrasound images for accuracy in comparison with the "gold standard." By adhering to these principles, surgeon sonographers can continue to advance the field of surgical ultrasound by obtaining high-quality images while ensuring that their patients are not being harmed.

CONCLUSIONS

The most successful surgeon sonographers have learned to incorporate science, art, and safety into their ultrasound practice. Important scientific principles include the appreciation of the echogenicity of various organs, the ability to select the most appropriate transducer for the examination to be performed, and a thorough knowledge of anatomy and spacial planes. Obtaining the highest quality images also requires thoughtful adjustments of overall gain, TCG, and focus. Mastery of the art of steering the transducer with sliding, rotating, rocking, and tilting, while developing the proper touch when applying pressure on the skin or organ and optimizing the patient's position to obtain a high-quality image, will only come with practice. Finally, patient safety and confidentiality must be maintained, and are best accomplished by proper maintenance of equipment and leadership by surgeons in performance improvement programs in ultrasound.

REFERENCES

1. Case RD. Ultrasound physics and instrumentation. *Surg Clin North Am* 1998;78:197–217.
2. American College of Surgeons. *Ultrasound for surgeons.* Basic ultrasound course syllabus, Chicago, 2001.
3. Heller M, Jehle D. *Ultrasound in emergency medicine.* Philadelphia: WB Saunders, 1995.
4. Zagzebski JA. *Essentials of ultrasound physics.* St. Louis: Mosby–Year Book, 1996.
5. American College of Surgeons. *Abdominal ultrasound: transabdominal/intraoperative/laparoscopic.* Course syllabus, Chicago, 2002.
6. Puylaert JBCM. Acute appendicitis: US evaluation using graded compression. *Radiology* 1986;156:355–360.

7. Rozycki GS. Ultrasonography: surgical applications. In: Wilmore DW, Cheung Lyk, Harkin AH, et al., eds. *American College of Surgeons ACS Principles and Practice*. New York, 1999:1–14.

8. Tempkin BB. *Ultrasound scanning: principles and protocols,* 2nd ed. Philadelphia: WB Saunders, 1999:18.

9. Kendall JL, Deutchman M. *Ultrasound in emergency medicine and trauma*. Nashville, TN: HealthStream, 2001.

10. Statement on Ultrasound Examinations by Surgeons. *Bull Am Coll Surg,* 1998(June):37–40.

Interventional Ultrasound

Junji Machi, Maurice E. Arregui, and Edgar D. Staren

Ultrasound can be used not only as a diagnostic imaging modality but also as a guide for various procedures. Ultrasound that is used to assist or guide procedures or surgeries is called "interventional ultrasound" or "invasive ultrasound."

The potential value of interventional ultrasound was recognized quite early, dating back to the early 1960s. In 1961, Berlyne used ultrasound as an imaging guide for renal biopsy (1); he performed 20 such biopsies with excellent accuracy. In 1972, both Holm, a Danish urologist, and Goldberg, an American radiologist, independently developed ultrasound transducers equipped with built-in central canals dedicated for interventional procedures (2,3). That same year, Rasmussen used one of these biopsy-dedicated transducers to perform ultrasound-guided biopsies of hepatic metastases (4). Yokoi and colleagues, in 1974, reported on ultrasound-guided biopsy of masses of the breast and of the thyroid (5). In 1975, Hancke and associates used ultrasound not only to guide biopsies of masses of the pancreas as a diagnostic aid but also to guide drainage of a pancreatic cyst as a therapeutic intervention (6).

With advances in ultrasound instrumentation and refinement of biopsy and drainage techniques, the field of percutaneous interventional ultrasound expanded dramatically in the 1980s and 1990s. Furthermore, the introduction of ultrasound to the operating room in the 1980s initiated an additional avenue of ultrasound use; with intraoperative interventional ultrasound, various surgical procedures were wholly or partially guided by ultrasound (7,8). For example, certain hepatic resections may now be more often successfully completed because of the assistance of intraoperative ultrasound guidance (8).

Initially, the principal use of interventional ultrasound was as a diagnostic adjunct (i.e., guidance of biopsies). Currently, interventional ultrasound is used to guide therapeutic interventions as well; examples include drainage, injection, ablation, or tissue dissection. The use of ultrasound in such settings directly affects the therapeutic outcome. In this chapter, general principles of interventional ultrasound, mainly for needle, catheter, and cannula placement, are discussed. The specific applications of interventional ultrasound in different organs are described in relevant chapters. Intraoperative and laparoscopic ultrasound guidance is described in detail in Chapter 13 and subsequent chapters.

INDICATIONS

Indications for interventional ultrasound are many, variable, and expanding. Various indications of ultrasound-guided procedures can be categorized as shown in Table 1.

Interventional procedures guided by ultrasound for needle placement include biopsy, aspiration, and injection. Both fine needle aspiration (FNA) cytology and core needle biopsy can be guided by ultrasound. Ultrasound-guided FNA cytology is usually indicated for neck masses, including thyroid nodules, parathyroid nodules, cervical or other lymph nodes, and pancreatic lesions. On the other hand, ultrasound-guided core needle biopsy is indicated more commonly for breast lesions, abdominal diseases such as liver tumors, retroperitoneal or pelvic masses, prostate lesions, and transplanted organs. Ultrasound is indicated for FNA of serendipitously discovered thyroid nodules or the dominant nodule in a patient with an otherwise multinodular goiter (Fig. 1) (9). Ultrasound may be used to guide FNA for diagnosis and confirmation of a hyperplastic or adenomatous parathyroid gland (10); such a procedure is usually reserved for a patient with recurrent or persistent hyperparathyroidism. Determining the presence of abnormal cervical adenopathy is an important diagnostic discriminant for a variety of neoplasms of the head and neck (11). Ultrasound is used to accurately guide FNA of suspicious neck masses in such cases, thereby influencing the subsequent therapeutic plan (12). On occasion, suspicious axillary lymph nodes may be imaged in the course of evaluating a patient with breast tumors. Ultrasound-guided FNA of such lymph nodes can be performed concomitant to ultrasound-guided biopsy of the primary breast lesion (13).

TABLE 1 Indications for Interventional Ultrasound

1. Needle guidance
   Biopsy: fine needle aspiration cytology, core needle biopsy
   Aspiration: fluid (e.g., paracentesis), cyst, etc.
   Injection: contrast, ethanol, etc.
2. Catheter guidance
   Drainage: fluid, abscess, cyst, biliary, etc.
   Vascular access
3. Cannula or probe guidance
   Thermal ablation, cryoablation
4. Tissue dissection guidance
   Intraoperative or laparoscopic procedures

FNA cytology has been used for the diagnosis of breast lesions (14). However, recently the preferred approach has been to perform core needle biopsy to obtain histologic specimens (Fig. 2) (13–15). For both FNA and core needle biopsy, interventional ultrasound facilitates the diagnosis and management of nonpalpable breast lesions, particularly breast cancer. A vacuum-assisted core needle biopsy system for breast lesions is currently available for use under ultrasound guidance (16). Ultrasound-guided biopsy of the liver can be performed percutaneously in most circumstances and is frequently indicated for definitive diagnosis of liver tumors (Fig. 3) (17). Percutaneous biopsy of intraabdominal, retroperitoneal, or pelvic masses

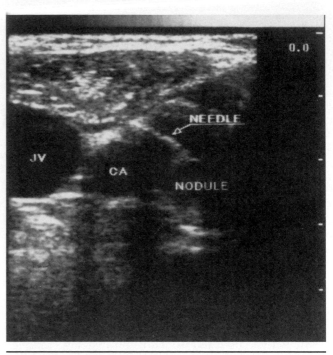

FIGURE 1. Ultrasound-guided fine needle aspiration biopsy of a right thyroid nodule. CA, carotid artery; JV, jugular vein.

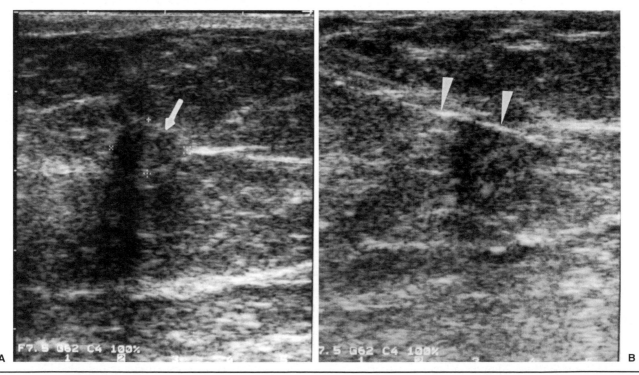

FIGURE 2. Ultrasound-guided core needle biopsy of a breast lump. **A:** A 9 × 6 mm lesion (*arrow*). **B:** A 16-gauge needle (*arrowheads*) through the lesion.

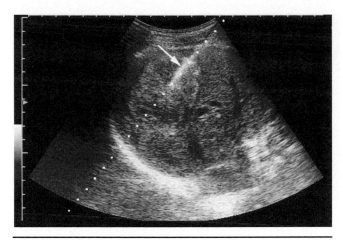

FIGURE 3. Percutaneous ultrasound-guided core needle biopsy of a liver tumor. An arrow indicates a hyperechoic needle in the tumor on a needle guide line (*white dotted line*).

can be guided by ultrasound as well as computed tomography (CT). Percutaneous ultrasound-guided biopsy of tumors of the liver or extrahepatic abdomen may confirm metastatic or unresectable disease, thereby avoiding unnecessary laparotomy in a patient with incurable malignancy (17,18). Ultrasound can be used to biopsy retroperitoneal masses including lymph nodes (19); even preventing unnecessary laparotomy in a patient with

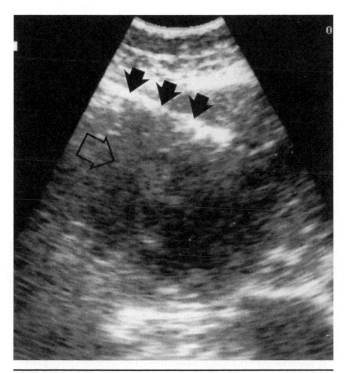

FIGURE 4. Percutaneous ultrasound-guided core needle biopsy (*three solid arrows*) of a large retroperitoneal lymphoma (*single open arrow*).

retroperitoneal lymphoma (Fig. 4). Ultrasound-guided core needle biopsy of transplanted organs such as the liver, kidney, and pancreas is indicated for histologic diagnosis of possible transplant rejection or other transplantation-related complications (20).

Ultrasound-guided needle placement is also indicated for aspiration of various fluids and cystic lesions involving the thoracic and abdominal cavities as well as other areas of the body. Ultrasound-guided aspiration is performed for both diagnostic and therapeutic purposes. For differential diagnosis of pleural effusion and ascites, needle aspiration is indicated. These thoracenteses and paracenteses are more safely and accurately performed by ultrasound guidance than by the "blind" method. Ultrasound-guided pericardiocentesis can be life saving in cases such as traumatic cardiac tamponade. Cystic lesions that can be aspirated by ultrasound-guided needle placement are numerous and include, but are not limited to, thyroid cyst, breast cyst, and abdominal and retroperitoneal cystic lesions such as liver cyst, renal cyst, and pancreatic cystic lesions (Fig. 5) (21). Although not commonly used currently, gallbladder aspiration can be performed using ultrasound guidance for diagnostic purposes.

Following needle placement, various agents can be injected under ultrasound guidance. Such agents include blue dye, radiographic contrast, or therapeutic agents such as alcohol. Blue dye injection may be used for marking the tissue. Contrast can be injected into cystic lesions or biliary ducts for radiographic contrast studies (e.g., percutaneous transhepatic cholangiography). Ultrasound-guided alcohol injection has been used for management of hepatomas, parathyroid adenomas, thyroid nodules, and other diseases (22).

Ultrasound-guided needle aspiration may be followed by ultrasound-guided catheter placement for drainage of various diseases. Pleural effusion or ascites can be drained continuously (Fig. 6). Intraabdominal or pelvic abscesses and cystic lesions such as pancreatic pseudocyst are drained by ultrasound-guided catheterization (23). Other percutaneous interventions of catheter placement for drainage guided by ultrasound include percutaneous cholecystostomy, as well as percutaneous transhepatic cholangiography and drainage (PTCD), percutaneous nephrostomy, percutaneous gastrostomy, and others (24). Ultrasound-guided catheterization is also useful for vascular access. Ultrasound-guided subclavian or internal jugular venous catheterization is an accurate and safe method, particularly in the difficult-to-access patient (see Chapter 8, Figs. 25 and 26) (25,26).

Tumor ablation has become increasingly popular for management of various types of cancers. Cryoablation and thermal ablation have been extensively described for the management of liver tumors (27). A cryoprobe for

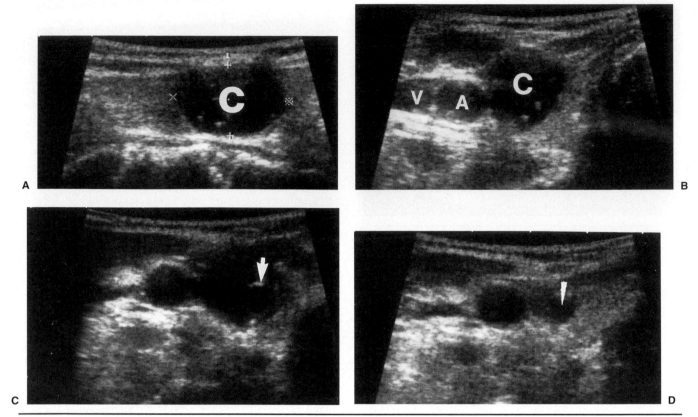

FIGURE 5. Ultrasound-guided aspiration of a thyroid cyst. **A:** Sagittal view of a cyst (C) of the right thyroid lobe. **B:** The same cyst (C) in a transverse view. V, jugular vein; A, carotid artery. **C:** A fine needle (*arrow*) was inserted into the cyst under ultrasound guidance. **D:** After aspiration, the cyst almost disappeared (*arrowhead*).

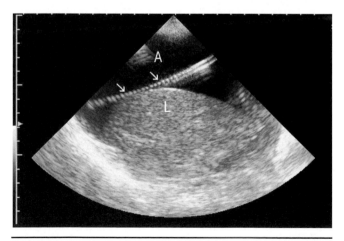

FIGURE 6. Percutaneous ultrasound-guided drainage of ascites. Arrows indicate a drainage catheter introduced in ascites (A) over the right lobe of the liver (arrow).

cryoablation and an electrode cannula for radiofrequency thermal ablation are most accurately, expeditiously, and conveniently guided by ultrasound (Fig. 7). Following ultrasound-guided cannula or probe placement, the ablation process is also monitored by ultrasound. Radiofrequency-ablated or cryoablated lesions become hyperechoic associated with shadowing. Ultrasound-guided ablation has been used or is under investigation for management of benign and malignant tumors of various organs such as prostate, kidney, bone, brain, lung, and breast (28).

Surgical procedures or tissue dissection can be guided by ultrasound (7). This is a unique intraoperative indication of ultrasound, and is described in detail in Chapter 13 and subsequent chapters. It is likely that the list of indications for interventional ultrasound will continue to expand concomitant with its increased utilization and also in association with new surgical technologies or with laparoscopy, endoscopy, and other minimal-access procedures.

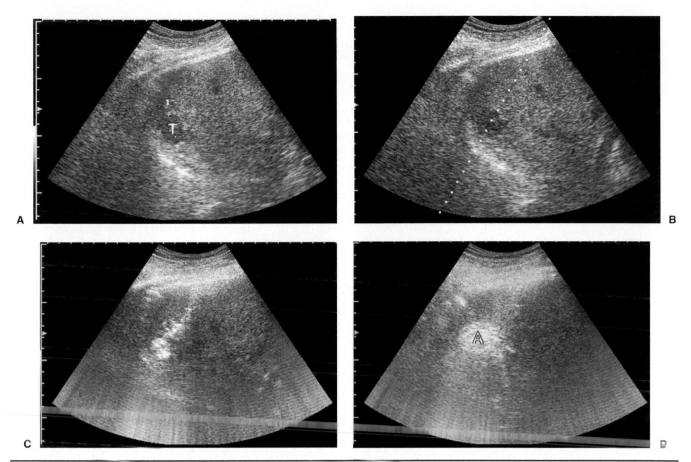

FIGURE 7. Percutaneous ultrasound-guided radiofrequency thermal ablation of a metastatic liver tumor. **A:** A 2-cm tumor (T) was located in segment 7 of the liver just under the diaphragm. **B:** A needle guide line was seen to guide an electrode cannula into the tumor. **C:** After the electrode was placed in the tumor, radiofrequency ablation was started. Note hyperechoic changes. **D:** After complete ablation, the ablated lesion (A) became hyperechoic.

CONTRAINDICATIONS

Contraindications to interventional ultrasound are limited but rather definite (29). Ultrasound should not be used as an imaging guide when no safe pathway is demonstrable on diagnostic evaluation. For example, therapeutic drainage of an intra-abdominal abscess located in the mid-abdomen has an excessively high risk of passage of a large-bore dilator through several loops of bowel with potentially catastrophic consequences. A previous history of significant bleeding in association with minor surgical procedures or a known coagulopathy should be viewed as a relative contraindication to many, particularly advanced, interventional ultrasound procedures. Although percutaneous interventional ultrasound is risky in the face of bleeding diathesis, ultrasound-guided procedures can be performed once open intraoperative ultrasound is used (e.g., open liver biopsy) because bleeding is then controlled by routine surgical methods. The disoriented or uncooperative patient should not undergo interventional ultrasound unless the patient can be otherwise controlled, such as with general anesthesia.

ADVANTAGES AND DISADVANTAGES

There are several advantages of ultrasound in guiding procedures over other imaging modalities as summarized in Table 2 (30,31). The most significant advantage it is its visualization of an interventional procedure in real time, which allows for precise needle or cannula placement (31). With the exception of fluoroscopy, other image guidance modalities (e.g., CT and magnetic resonance imaging) require assessment of static images and, when necessary, subsequent adjustment of needle placement prior to rescanning; of course, this is time consuming. Needle, catheter, cannula, and probe placement

▶ **TABLE 2 Advantages of Ultrasound-
          Guided Procedures**

1. Real-time visualization, which facilitates precision
2. Quick
3. Safe (no ionizing radiation)
4. Repeatable (confirmation of procedures or detection of complications)
5. Color Doppler imaging
6. Portable
7. Widely available (generally inexpensive)
8. Intraoperative capability

under ultrasound guidance can be performed as a dynamic study, making controlled placement possible in real time. Ultrasound is a highly expeditious method of guiding interventional procedures, which generally does not add greatly to the time necessary for performance of the diagnostic examination. The real-time feature often simplifies placement of a needle or cannula within the desired location.

Ultrasound involves no ionizing radiation. Therefore, its use is permissible in circumstances in which image guidance would otherwise not be possible; examples include pregnant patients or radiation-sensitive areas (e.g., ultrasound-guided aspiration of amniotic fluid). Compared to blind needle placement, ultrasound-guided needle placement is considered much safer. Because ultrasound demonstrates surrounding structures such as blood vessels or ducts (e.g., pancreatic duct or bile duct), inadvertent puncture of these structures can be avoided, thereby reducing associated complications such as bleeding, pancreatic or bile leakage. Because of its ease, safety, and quickness, an ultrasound examination is amenable to repetition during procedures. At the end of the procedures, ultrasound can be repeated so as to confirm the satisfactory and safe completion of the procedure. Successful aspiration of the fluid or drainage can be confirmed. Tumor-ablative procedures can be monitored by continuous ultrasound examination during the operation. During or at the end of the procedure, ultrasound may be used to detect early complications such as bleeding at the needle insertion site or hematoma formation (Fig. 8). The availability of color Doppler imaging may be quite helpful during interventional ultrasound. Because flow within blood vessels can be easily identified, color Doppler imaging may assist the performance of safe in-

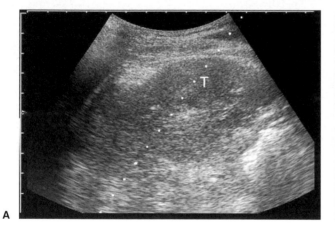

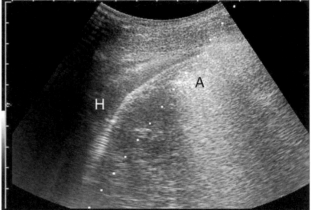

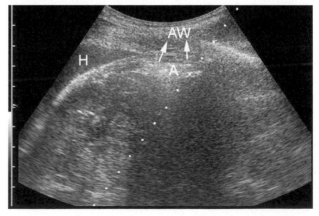

FIGURE 8. Detection of bleeding complication during percutaneous radiofrequency ablation of a liver tumor by repeat ultrasound examination. **A:** A tumor (T), primary hepatoma, was located in segment 6 of the liver. Note needle guide line. **B:** During radiofrequency ablation, the ablated area (A) became hyperechoic. A fluid accumulated in the subphrenic space from the area of ablation, suggesting hematoma formation or bleeding complication (H). **C:** The ablated lesion (A) was pulled toward the abdominal wall (AW) by pulling the electrode needles (*arrows*). After that, the amount of fluid or hematoma (H) did not increase. The patient remained stable, and laparotomy was not required for this bleeding complication. Ultrasound was helpful in detecting and monitoring this complication.

terventional procedures by demonstrating normal as well as aberrant or pathologic vasculature (32). Color Doppler imaging may allow for better visualization of a needle or catheter (33).

Most ultrasound machines are designed to be readily portable. As such, they can be transported for use at a patient's bedside. Such access is especially important in cases of critically ill patients not capable of leaving an intensive care unit or intermediate care facility (34). This decreases the risk and resources required for transporting such patients to the radiology department. Because of the portability, ultrasound has had increased utilization in the office or ambulatory setting, emergency room, and procedure room (35). Bedside use of interventional ultrasound as well as diagnostic ultrasound is likely to increase. Particularly relevant, given the current escalation of health care costs, is the fact that ultrasound is considerably less expensive than other imaging studies. Ultrasound-guided intervention is cost effective as compared with intervention guided by CT. Ultrasound machines are often widely available in the hospital; therefore, ultrasound-guided procedures can generally be performed on short notice when required. During open surgical procedures, ultrasound is the optimal imaging modality available to guide various procedures in the operating room (7,8).

Like any imaging method, ultrasound has disadvantages (36). Because ultrasound does not penetrate bone or air well, ribs or air within the lung limit its use in evaluating the chest. Similarly, gas within the bowel lumen limits the value of ultrasound in evaluating the mid-abdominal region. Therefore, in most circumstances CT guidance is required for intervention in these areas. Ultrasound and CT are considered complementary in their use for guidance of interventional procedures. Whenever either modality can be used, ultrasound should be the preferred choice because of the aforementioned advantages. The cumbersome mechanism for disinfection and sterilization of ultrasound transducers is a minor impediment to their use. Current transducers have limited tolerance to high temperature, preventing their sterilization by autoclaving. Alternative techniques necessitate time-consuming cold gas sterilization or soaking procedures with or without the use of sterile drape covers.

PATIENT PREPARATION

History and Consent

As with any interventional procedure, routine background information with attention to a history of bleeding disorders, liver disease, and medications is required (31,36). Patients need careful inquiry regarding medica-

tion use (e.g., platelet-inhibiting drugs). We generally do not obtain laboratory studies in patients without a positive history of the above. However, in those patients who do indicate a bleeding history, liver disease, or use of a medication that might inhibit normal blood coagulation, we obtain prothrombin time (PT) and partial thromboplastin time (PTT) as well as a platelet count and bleeding time.

Informed consent is somewhat straightforward for most interventional ultrasound procedures and involves discussion of alternatives to the procedures, rare potential morbidity, and extremely rare mortality. When interventional procedures of the abdomen are evaluated carefully, the most common morbidity is hemorrhage, but the possibility of pancreatitis, pneumothorax, bile or pancreatic leak, visceral injury, and other even less common complications exists (37,38). Concern about the potential for needle track seeding is frequently expressed. It would appear that such a complication is extremely rare and, if it does occur, is likely to be clinically irrelevant to the overall clinical course. Several studies have evaluated the potential for mortality with percutaneous interventional ultrasound procedures. Even with more advanced procedures involving the deeper viscera, the risk of major complications and death has been exceedingly low, varying from approximately 0.01% to 0.0006% (37–40).

Patient Position

In most cases, optimal patient position for interventional ultrasound procedures is the same as that used for diagnostic ultrasonography of the area. In general, one should attempt to take the shortest possible path to a lesion. For example, to optimally visualize lesions in the abdomen (such as the liver) it may be necessary to move the patient from the supine to the left lateral decubitus position (17,18). Exposure of the liver may be further enhanced by raising the patient's right arm over the head, thereby moving the rib cage in a more cephalad direction. Such maneuvers may be required to optimally visualize and access a liver mass. Similarly, most interventional procedures of the breast require positioning the patient as for the diagnostic study. Generally, the patient is placed in the supine position with the ipsilateral arm behind the head. In the case of laterally placed lesions, moving the patient to a lateral decubitus position may rotate the breast toward the midline. This decreases the distance between the skin and the lesion, resulting in a more direct access. Our recommendation for most interventional ultrasound procedures is to perform a brief diagnostic scan of the patient prior to setting up for the planned intervention. This preliminary maneuver confirms the safest and most direct route to the area in question. When such a position is ascertained, the patient can be prepared in the usual manner.

Skin Preparation

Skin preparation for ultrasound-guided procedures varies from routine painting with alcohol or povidone-iodine (Betadine) solutions to sterile gowning and gloving of the surgeon, followed by wash and paint with sterilizing solutions and full operative drape of the patient and ultrasound equipment. The method will vary according to the nature and severity of the planned interventional ultrasound procedure. Routine preparation of the patient with simple painting and the surgeon's using sterile gloves is satisfactory for most circumstances of ultrasound-guided needle placement procedures (Fig. 9). On the other hand, prolonged ultrasound-guided procedures such as catheter, cannula, or probe placement (e.g., biliary drainage, tumor ablation) or open surgical procedures require full operative settings (Fig. 10).

For acoustic coupling between the transducer and the skin, sterile ultrasound coupling gel can be used. For short procedures, povidone-iodine or alcohol solution can suffice as an acoustic coupler. During open surgical procedures, saline solution is used in the operative field for acoustic coupling.

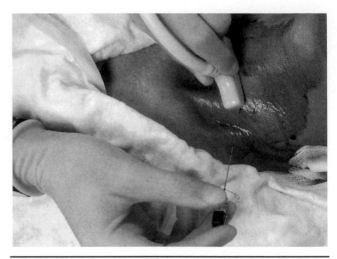

FIGURE 9. Ultrasound-guided fine needle aspiration of a nodule of the left thyroid lobe. The skin is simply prepped with povidone-iodine without a formal draping. Ten percent of providone-iodine is used for acoustic coupling. A fine needle is inserted under ultrasound guidance.

Anesthesia

The use and type of anesthesia varies depending on the nature and extent of the procedure and the anxiety and cooperation of the patient (31). Most percutaneous inter-

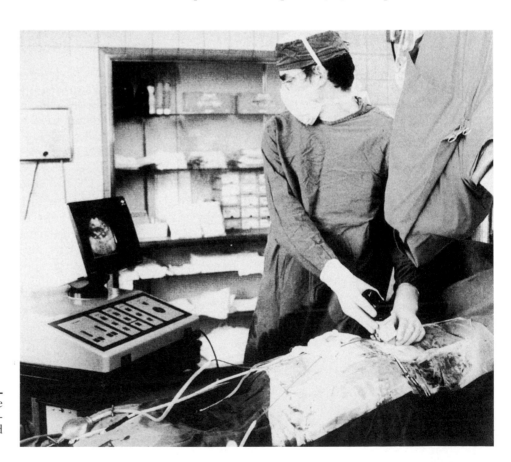

FIGURE 10. Complete sterile draping of patient and surgeon during an interventional ultrasound procedure.

ventional ultrasound procedures are accomplished readily with simple instillation of local anesthetic. In fact, for aspiration of superficial lesions such as thyroid or breast cysts, no local anesthetic may be needed. For more complex procedures, such as drainage of an intraabdominal abscess or percutaneous biliary drainage, or for patients with anxiety, intravenous sedation using narcotics and/or tranquilizers is generally required. Prolonged ultrasound-guided procedures, such as liver tumor ablation, are more frequently performed under general anesthesia.

For so-called conscious sedation, intravenous fentanyl, morphine, or meperidine is commonly used for analgesia, and diazepam or midazolam is frequently used as a tranquilizer. When using these agents, careful drug titration and constant monitoring of blood pressure, heart rate, respiration rate, and oxygen saturation are required to avoid complications such as respiratory compromise or hypotension. Moreover, it is absolutely necessary to have resuscitatory equipment and personnel trained in cardiopulmonary resuscitation readily available when using intravenous sedation. Therefore, it is recommended to restrict those procedures requiring sedation to the ambulatory department or operating room rather than the office setting, unless such equipment and personnel are available in the office.

ULTRASOUND GUIDANCE METHODS

Various ultrasound guidance methods are utilized to optimally guide a needle, cannula, or probe as summarized in Table 3 (31,36).

Indirect ultrasound guidance is basically a blind method because a needle or cannula is inserted without real-time visualization by ultrasound. However, ultrasound is used to select the site and the angle of needle insertion. First, the size and the exact location of the lesion are evaluated by ultrasound. The needle puncture site is selected and marked with a marking pen or other convenient tool. The direction and depth of the needle insertion are determined by ultrasound. The site is then prepared in the usual manner. The needle is inserted from the predetermined site without concomitant use of ultrasound visualization (Fig. 11). As such, the indirect ultrasound guidance method is less precise than the direct ultrasound guidance method. However, skin and equipment preparation is easier because disinfection or sterilization of the ultrasound transducer is not needed. An indirect ultrasound guidance method is generally used when the target lesion is relatively large, e.g., aspiration or drainage of large fluid collections such as ascites, pleural effusion, a large cystic lesion, or biopsy of a large tumor.

Direct ultrasound guidance methods allow real-time needle visualization and therefore more precise needle placement. There are two techniques of needle insertion in relation to the ultrasound scanning plane along the long axis of the transducer (Fig. 12). The better and preferred technique is to insert and advance a needle in the plane parallel to the long axis of the transducer (i.e., ultrasound scanning plane) (Fig. 13). This allows for constant visualization of the shaft and tip of the needle throughout its entire path to the target (Figs. 1 to 4). This is a safer and more accurate method because the needle tip is always demonstrated on the ultrasound monitor. The second and less preferable technique is to insert the needle perpendicular to the long axis of the transducer (Fig. 14). This technique increases the difficulty of needle tip visualization because the tip is not seen until it enters the ultrasound scanning plane (Fig. 15). This increases the risk of significant past pointing of the needle tip, which may lead to complications such as pneumothorax, hemorrhage, and so on. For this reason, the use of this second technique should be limited to the situation in which the placement of transducer or access of the needle to the target cannot be achieved by the first technique.

Direct ultrasound guidance methods are performed either by a "freehand" technique or by using the needle guidance system (so-called biopsy guide). In the freehand technique, the needle can be placed either adjacent to (Fig. 16) or remote from the transducer (Fig. 17), and parallel or perpendicular to the ultrasound scanning plane as described above (Figs. 13 and 14). Another advantage of the freehand technique is that it allows independent movement of the transducer and the needle. For example, after placement of the needle, scanning can be continued at a different location or different direction by moving the transducer independently. In addition, the needle can be placed perpendicular or almost perpendicular to the ultrasound beam, which improves needle visualization (see also Figs. 37 and 38). The main disadvantage of the freehand technique is that it is sometimes difficult to keep or advance the needle within the ultrasound scanning plane for needle visualization.

Various types of needle guidance systems are available as described below. The principle of needle placement using a needle guidance system is shown in Figure 18. Such a system greatly facilitates maintenance of the needle within the small ultrasound scanning plane (approximately

text continues on page 49

▶ **TABLE 3** **Ultrasound Guidance Methods**

1. Indirect method
2. Direct method: freehand technique
3. Direct method: needle guidance system

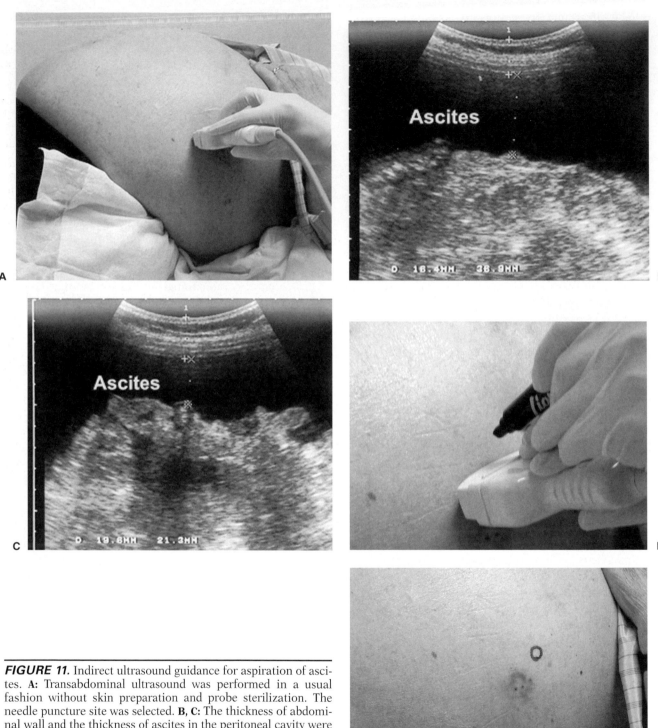

FIGURE 11. Indirect ultrasound guidance for aspiration of ascites. **A:** Transabdominal ultrasound was performed in a usual fashion without skin preparation and probe sterilization. The needle puncture site was selected. **B, C:** The thickness of abdominal wall and the thickness of ascites in the peritoneal cavity were measured. The safe accessible site for the needle puncture was selected. **D, E:** The selected needle puncture site was marked using a black marking pen. **F, G:** The site was prepared and draped. A needle with catheter was inserted at the predetermined angle in the peritoneal cavity. The ascites was drained.

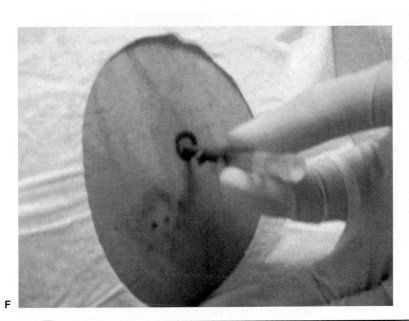
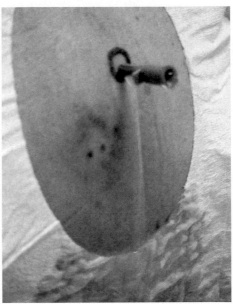

F   G

FIGURE 11. *Continued.*

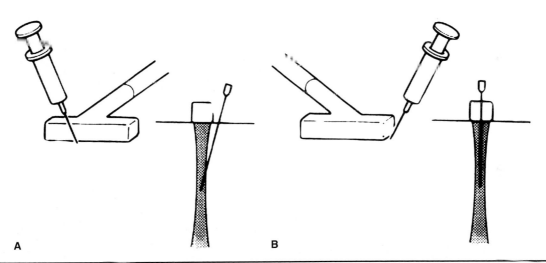

A   B

FIGURE 12. Two techniques of needle insertion under direct ultrasound guidance. **A:** A needle is inserted perpendicular to the long axis of the transducer. **B:** A needle is inserted parallel to the long axis of the transducer. This is the preferred needle guidance technique. (Courtesy of Dr. Masatoshi Makuuchi.)

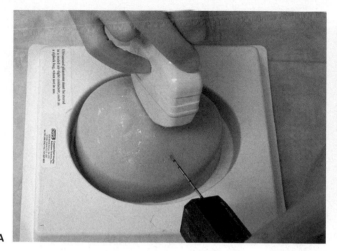

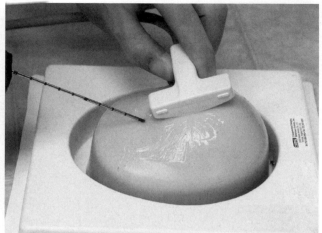

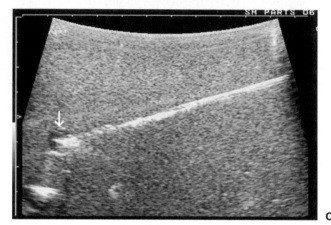

FIGURE 13. Ultrasound guidance of a needle that is inserted in the plane parallel to the long axis of the transducer (ultrasound scanning plane). **A:** A core needle insertion using a transabdominal convex probe and a phantom. **B:** A core needle insertion using a small-parts intraoperative ultrasound probe and a phantom. **C:** An image of the phantom showing the entire shaft and tip (*arrow*) visualized by ultrasound. The tip of the needle is in a small cystic structure of the phantom.

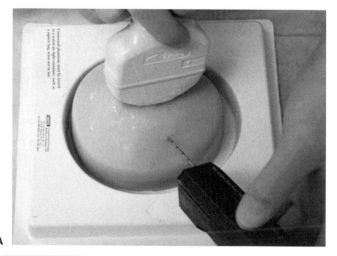

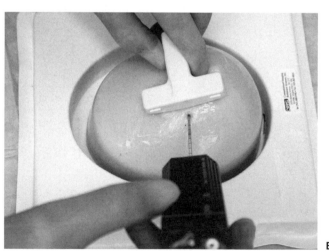

FIGURE 14. Ultrasound guidance of a needle that is inserted perpendicular to the long axis of the transducer. **A:** A core needle insertion using a transabdominal convex probe and a phantom. **B:** A core needle insertion using a small-parts intraoperative ultrasound probe and a phantom. **C:** An image of the phantom showing a part of the shaft or the tip of the needle (*arrow*), which is outside of a small cystic structure located posteriorly.

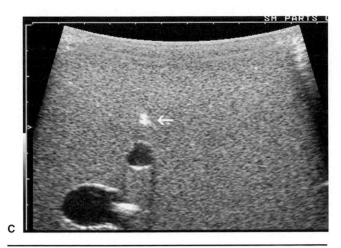

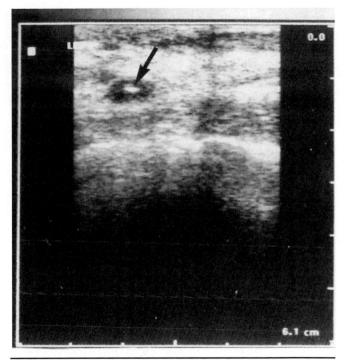

FIGURE 14. *Continued*

FIGURE 15. Hyperechoic needle tip (*solid arrow*) within a 7-mm hypoechoic breast mass.

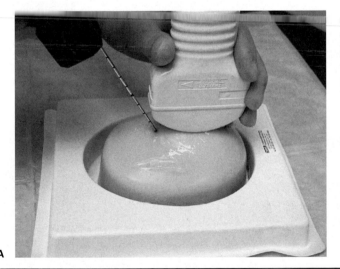

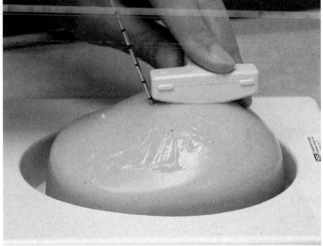

FIGURE 16. Direct ultrasound guidance method by a freehand technique. **A:** A core needle insertion using a transabdominal convex probe. The needle is inserted adjacent to the transducer. **B:** A core needle insertion using an intraoperative ultrasound probe. The needle is inserted adjacent to the transducer.

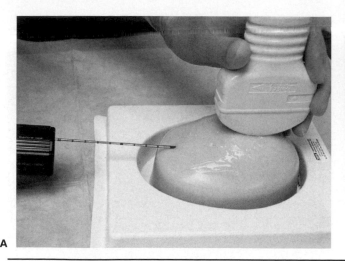
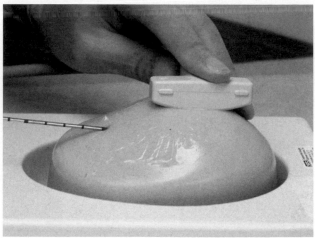

A

B

FIGURE 17. Direct ultrasound guidance method by a freehand technique. **A:** A core needle insertion using a transabdominal convex probe. The needle is inserted far remote from the transducer. **B:** A core needle insertion using an intraoperative ultrasound probe. The needle is inserted remote from the transducer. Note that the needle is placed almost perpendicular to the ultrasound beam (almost parallel to the transducer surface).

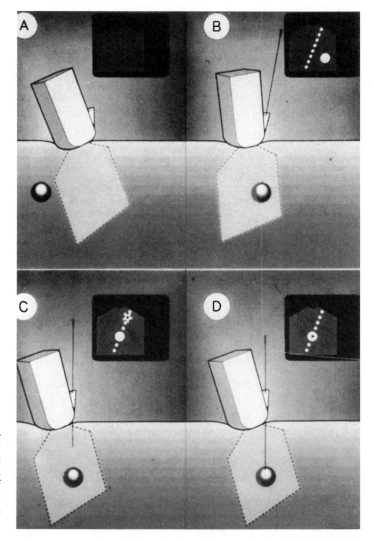

FIGURE 18. Principle of ultrasound-guided needle placement using a needle guidance system. **A:** Target outside image plane. Target not visualized. **B:** Transducer moved and target visualized in the image plane. **C:** Fine adjustment of transducer position. Target transected by a needle guide line. Needle inserted through needle guide attachment. Needle-tip echo indicates actual needle position. **D:** Target hit.

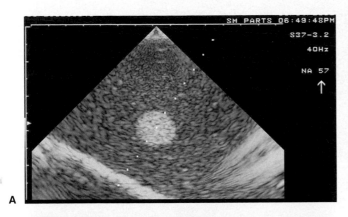

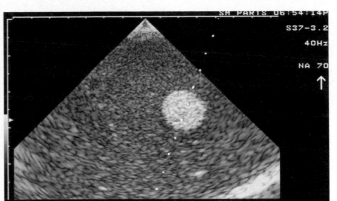

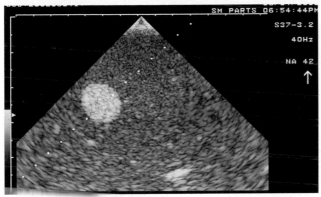

FIGURE 19. Ultrasound needle guidance using an angle-adjustable needle guidance system and a needle guide line on the ultrasound monitor. **A:** A hyperechoic target is in the center of the image, and a needle guide line is positioned through this target. Note that the angle of the line (*small arrow*) is 57 degrees. **B:** A target is located at the right side of this image. A needle guide line on the monitor is moved to the target. The angle is 70 degrees (*arrow*). **C:** A target is located at the left side of this image. A needle guide line is moved to the target. The angle is 42 degrees (*arrow*).

1.5 mm in width) of the ultrasound beam. By holding the needle in place, this guidance system allows for placement of the needle precisely along a predetermined course into the target site, which is often displayed as a needle guide line on the ultrasound monitor (Figs. 19 and 20; see also Figs. 3 and 7). However, the use of a needle guidance system attached to the transducer can be cumbersome. In addition, the needle must be placed adjacent to the transducer and cannot be placed from a remote site (Fig. 21).

The use of either a freehand technique or a needle guidance system depends on the size and location of the target lesion and on the experience of the surgeon. In general, more superficially located organs or lesions such as the thyroid or breast can be approached by the freehand technique (Fig. 9). On the other hand, deeply situated lesions in locations such as the intraabdominal organs often require a needle guidance system to access (Fig. 22). Advantages of the use of a needle guidance system are often not

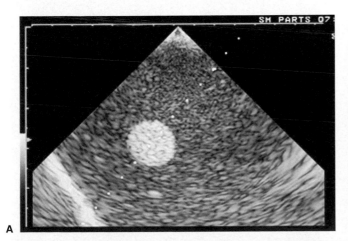

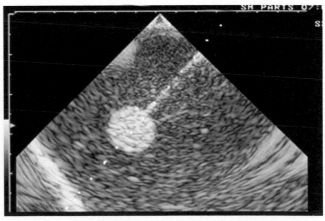

FIGURE 20. Ultrasound-guided needle placement using a needle guidance system with a needle guide line on the monitor. **A:** A hyperechoic target is visualized. A needle guide line is placed through the target. **B:** The angle of needle insertion is adjusted so that a needle is advanced along this line. A hyperechoic needle is inserted in the target along the line.

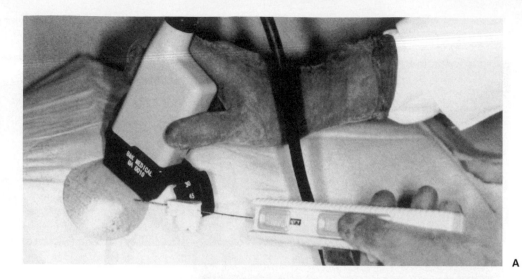

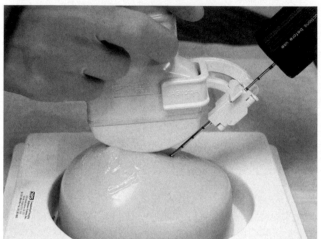

FIGURE 21. A: Ultrasound-guided core needle biopsy of a breast mass using a needle guidance system. **B:** Ultrasound-guided needle placement into a phantom using a needle guidance system. Note that the site of needle insertion is adjacent to the transducer.

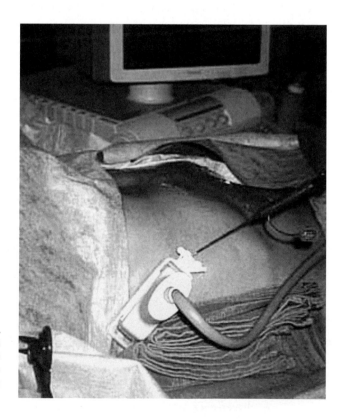

FIGURE 22. Ultrasound-guided needle placement using a needle guidance system to access intraabdominal organs. This shows placement of an electrode cannula into the liver tumor for radiofrequency ablation under ultrasound guidance using a needle guidance system.

as apparent for the more experienced surgeon sonographer as compared with the ultrasound neophyte. In certain situations, a needle guidance system may limit the angle of approach to a desired area, which will necessitate a freehand technique for optimal ease and safety. Because the individual performing interventional ultrasound procedures needs to be facile with both techniques, switching of each technique as necessary should not pose a problem.

EQUIPMENT PREPARATION

Interventional ultrasound procedures often do not require that the transducer come in direct contact with the area actually involved in needle insertion. This is particularly true when using a freehand technique. As such, transducers are usually cleaned with germicidal wipes and then soaked for 10 to 20 minutes in alcohol or dialdehyde (glutaraldehyde) solutions prior to the procedures (41). True sterilization, such as that required for intraoperative ultrasound, necessitates more prolonged (10 hours or longer) soaks in dialdehyde solutions, ethylene oxide gas sterilization, or covering with sterile sheets or drapes (Fig. 23). Although use of these drapes results in a definite, albeit minimal, decrease in resolution of the ultrasound image, we have found this method to be the best compromise for transducer preparation when sterility is required (29). Furthermore, we generally recommend a routine 10- to 20-minute soak in a dialdehyde solution, despite use of these covers, because occasionally the covers tear during an operative procedure. Recently, some manufacturers have developed transducers that are amenable to a low-temperature chemical sterilization method (e.g., Steris, Sterrad) by which instruments can be sterilized in 30 to 60 minutes (see Chapter 13, Fig. 4).

The transducers used for interventional ultrasound procedures have been either those that are biopsy dedicated or those that have the potential for needle guidance system (biopsy guide) attachment (2,3,42). Biopsy-dedicated transducers have fallen out of favor, primarily as a result of difficulty in needle visualization using such a transducer, but also because of the considerable difficulty in sterilizing the transducer's central canal.

Needle guidance systems are available in multiple shapes and sizes to accommodate various types of transducers (Fig. 24; see also Chapter 13, Figs. 38, 40, and 41). Most systems hold the needle firmly in place along a predetermined angle. Some have variable angles of insertion, which greatly facilitates appropriate and safe approach of the needle into targets (Fig. 25). Some systems

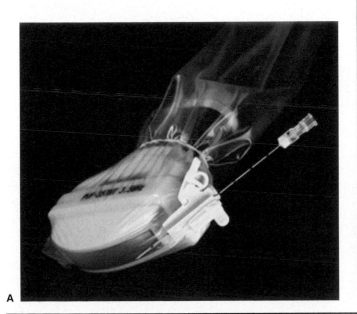

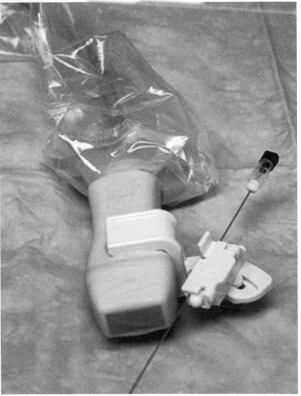

FIGURE 23. Preparation of ultrasound probes with sterile covers. **A:** A transabdominal convex probe. **B:** A transabdominal phased-array probe. Sterile needle guidance systems are attached outside of the cover. (Courtesy of Toshiba Medical.)

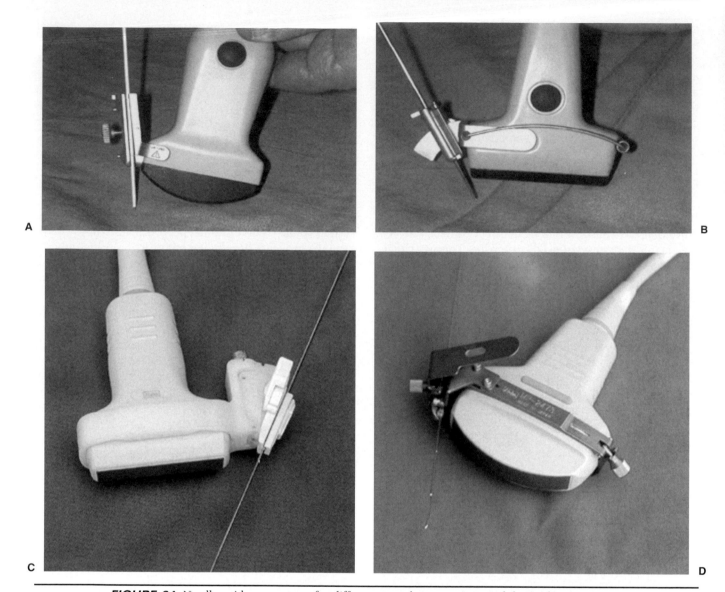

A   B

C   D

FIGURE 24. Needle guidance systems for different transducers. **A:** A transabdominal convex transducer. **B:** A small-parts linear array transducer. (Courtesy of B & K Medical.) **C:** A small-parts linear array transducer. **D:** A transabdominal convex transducer. (Courtesy of Aloka.)

keep the needle in the ultrasound scanning plane, but the insertion angle is not fixed (Fig. 26).

Reusable needle guidance systems necessitate sterilization by ethylene oxide gas, autoclaving, or prolonged soaking in dialdehyde solutions (36). Single-use, disposable needle guidance systems are now available; these have alleviated much of the criticism directed to the reusable type with their cumbersome sterilization requirements (Fig. 27).

For most interventional ultrasound procedures, the necessary associated equipment is contained in readily available kits (Fig. 28). These kits include essential items such as syringes and needles for instillation of local anesthetic and aspiration biopsy, skin preparation solutions (i.e., povidone-iodine), gauze sponges, a no. 11 blade, fenestrated drapes, and adhesive bandages. Sterile acoustic coupling gel also comes available as individually wrapped units.

text continues on page 56

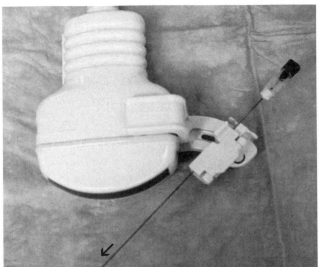

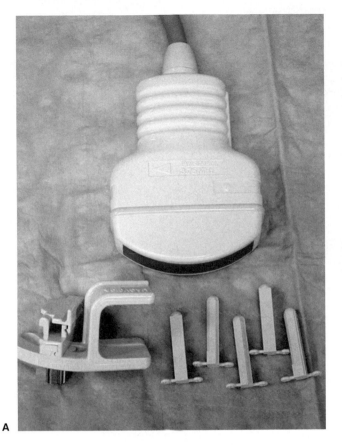

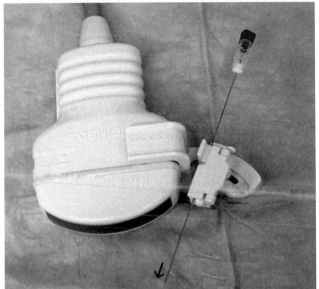

FIGURE 25. Angle-adjustable needle guidance system with variable calibers to accommodate various gauge needles. **A:** A transabdominal convex probe and its needle guidance system. **B, C:** The angle of insertion of a needle (*arrows*) is changed.

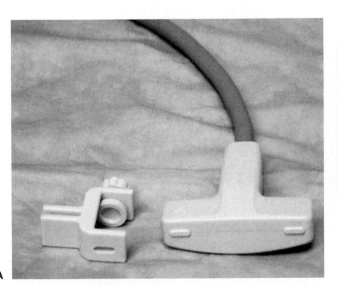

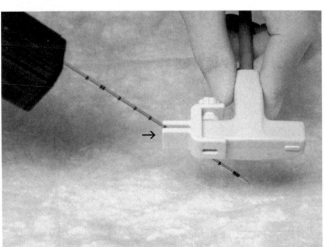

FIGURE 26. Needle guidance system without a fixed insertion angle. **A:** An intraoperative ultrasound probe with its needle guidance system. **B:** A core needle is inserted using this guidance system. This maintains the needle in the ultrasound scanning plane (*arrow*).

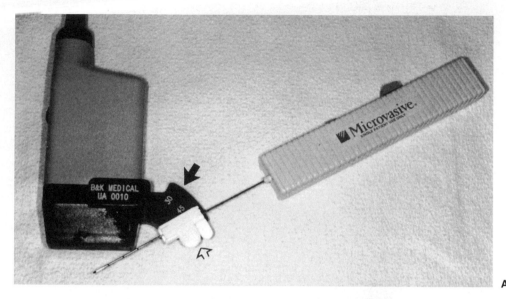

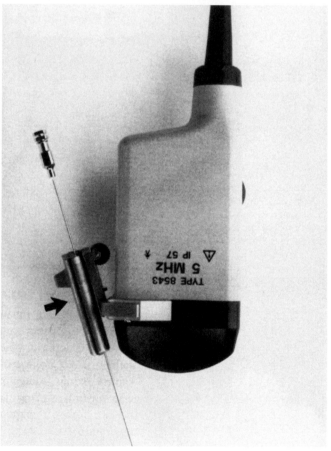

FIGURE 27. Needle guidance systems attached to transducer (*solid arrow*). **A:** Disposable attachment (*open arrow*). **B:** Nondisposable stainless steel needle guidance system (*solid arrow*).

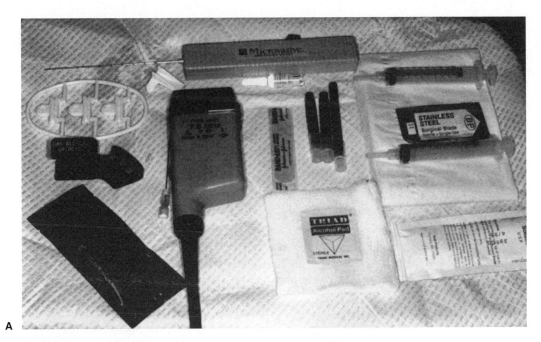

A

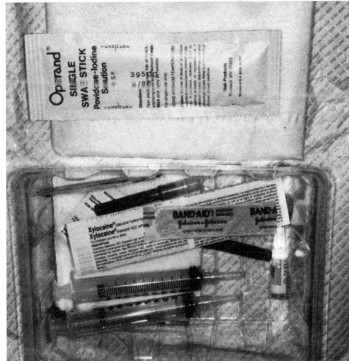

B

FIGURE 28. A,B: Disposable biopsy kits useful for interventional ultrasound–guided procedures.

NEEDLES

The needles used for interventional ultrasound vary from so-called thin to large bore (Fig. 29) (31,36,43). Biopsy techniques using these needles may involve needle aspiration from which cytologic, and occasionally histologic, specimens are obtained. Alternatively, a core biopsy technique may be used to obtain histologic information only. Although there are a variety of means for distinguishing needle types, the primary discriminant involves gauge or diameter. The thin needles are those with a gauge less than or equal to 20 to 22, while the large-bore needles are those with a gauge greater than or equal to 18. Needles smaller than 18-gauge may safely transverse the bowel without consequent damage, whereas 18-gauge and larger needles have the potential to injure the bowel wall with resultant laceration and leak.

Biopsy needles are available with several different tips (Fig. 30) (31, 36). The needle tips fall somewhere within a spectrum that includes the spinal needle, which has an acutely angled, beveled tip, and the Greene needle, which has a nonangled, circumferentially sharpened tip. Most needle tips are somewhere between these two and have a less acutely angled end. This group includes the Chiba needle, the Turner needle, the Westcott or Tru-Cut needle, the

Menghini needle, and Franseen needle. Beveled-tip needles usually yield more suitable specimens than nonbeveled ones. However, beveled-tip needles, particularly thin needles, tend to bend as they advance through tissues. The principle of biopsy using the Tru-Cut needle is shown in Figure 31.

Increasingly, the use of spring-loaded automated biopsy needles (so-called biopsy gun) is preferred to standard aspiration needles (Fig. 32; see also Fig. 29B) (31,44,45). The spring-loaded needles have been shown to reproducibly obtain histologic specimens. Such biopsy needles are available in a variety of gauges and specimen sizes and in both disposable and nondisposable forms; the latter may be used with single-use needles. These systems all work on the same basic two-phase, spring-loaded firing mechanism; that is, a sharpened outer cannula automatically fires over and subsequent to an inner notched sheath (Fig. 33). Specifically, once advanced to a desired lesion or tissue, the biopsy needle is in position to fire. When fired, the inner notched sheath advances forward followed rapidly by the outer cannula, about 15 to 25 mm from its nonfired position into the target. This results in a small piece of tissue being trapped within the notched area of the inner sheath (Fig. 34). This tissue is then available for pathologic evaluation.

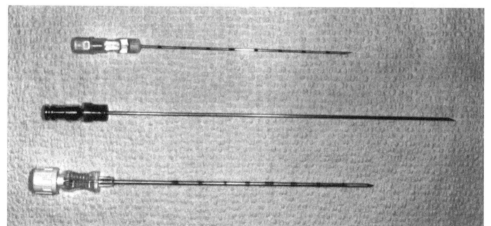

A

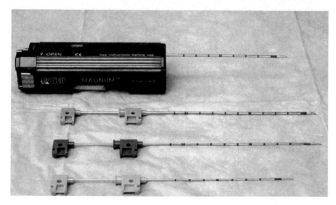

B

FIGURE 29. A: Variably gauged needles—from fine to large bore—used for ultrasound-guided needle aspiration and biopsy. B: A spring-loaded automated biopsy needle (biopsy gun) with various size and length of core needles.

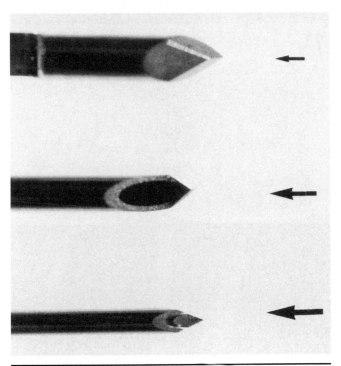

FIGURE 30. Variably shaped tips from a Tru-Cut (*small arrow*); spinal (*medium arrow*), and Franseen needle (*large arrow*), the latter with sheath in place.

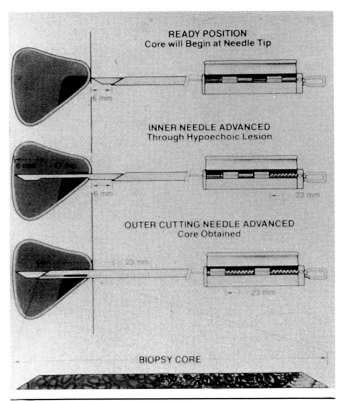

FIGURE 31. The Tru-Cut biopsy principle. The needle is advanced to the border of the target area. The inner trocar is advanced into the target. The outer cannula advancing over the trocar cuts the tissue sample, which is retrieved in a groove in the trocar.

The selection of needle depends on the type of procedure, the tissue type and location of targets, and operator preference. For aspiration of fluid, 20- or 22-gauge needles are usually appropriate. However, when fluid is viscous or purulent, 18-gauge or larger needles are sometimes needed. For FNA cytology, different types of thin needles of 20 to 27 gauge are used. For core needle biopsy

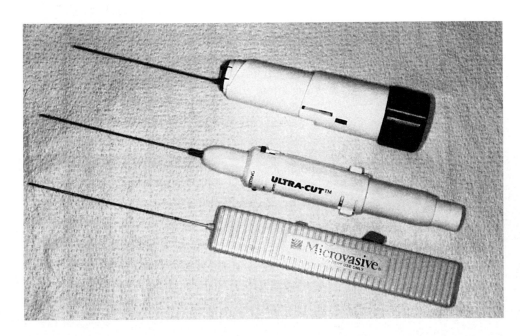

FIGURE 32. Examples of disposable core biopsy needles and automated spring-loaded firing guns.

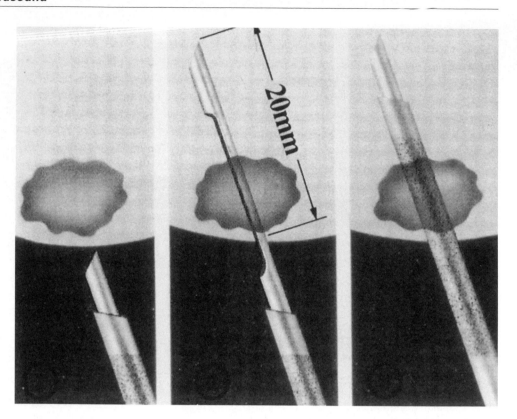

FIGURE 33. Demonstration of two-phase firing mechanism characteristic of automated biopsy guns and needles used for core biopsy.

for histologic examination, needles of 18 gauge or larger (up to 14 gauge) are usually required (31). A vacuum-assisted core needle biopsy system (i.e., Mammotome; Ethicon Endo-Surgery, Cincinnati, OH) employs needles as large as 11 or 8 gauge. In general, the larger the needle, the better the yield is with fewer false results. However, larger needles may be associated with a higher complication rate (e.g., bleeding).

CYTOLOGY VERSUS HISTOLOGY

Many studies have indicated that cytologic examination, while extremely accurate, is critically dependent on opera-

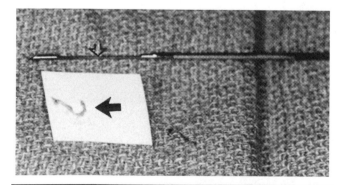

FIGURE 34. Histopathologic specimen (solid arrow) obtained from the notched area (*open arrow*) of a core biopsy needle.

tive technique and particularly on cytopathologic interpretation. As such, we and others have been more satisfied with histologic specimens for tissue evaluation whenever possible. Advantages of histology over cytology include the potential for obtaining a specific benign diagnosis rather than a more limited diagnosis such as "negative for malignancy." As an example, in interventional ultrasound of the breast, the availability of a histologic specimen allows the pathologist to make a definitive diagnosis of "fibroadenoma" rather than "benign breast epithelial cells," "myoepithelial cells," and so on. Such a diagnosis may prevent the unnecessary open surgical biopsy of such lesions. Histologic examination may allow for definitive designation of a specific cell type, which can have important implications regarding therapy. The most common example is cell typing for lymphoma. Ultrasound-guided core biopsy has prevented the need for laparotomy in many cases of lymphoma presenting as a retroperitoneal mass (Fig. 4). Histologic examination may allow for a more complete evaluation of specimens including flow cytometric and immunohistochemical studies; hormone receptor status may be determined easily in most cases.

Because of these and other advantages, even when performing FNA, we have endeavored to obtain histologic information rather than simple cytologic information whenever possible. We perform cell block as well as cytologic evaluation of FNA specimens; using both, we have found indeterminate diagnoses to be much less common than with cytology alone. With such techniques,

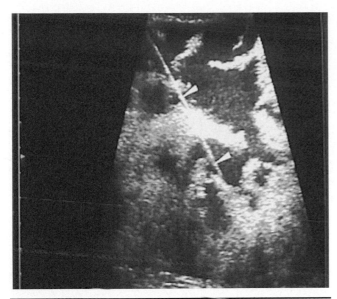

FIGURE 35. Better visualization of a needle in fluid. A needle was introduced into a complex cystic lesion of the liver for biopsy. The needle is better visualized in the fluid component (*arrowheads*) than in the soft-tissue component.

one might expect up to 95% accuracy of definitive histologic diagnoses (12). We have generally limited biopsy of suspicious lymph nodes, most thyroid nodules, and the lesions of the pancreas to FNA. For essentially all nonpalpable masses of the breast, liver tumors, retroperitoneal masses and others, we prefer to use automated biopsy needles to obtain core needle specimens.

NEEDLE VISUALIZATION

Optimal visualization of the needle, cannula, or probe is the key for successful interventional ultrasound. Needle visualization is determined by many factors, one of which is the type of tissue or fluid. In general, needle visualization is much better in fluid than in soft tissues (Fig. 35). Usually the tip of needle is better visualized than the shaft. A variety of methods can be used to facilitate the visualization of needles as shown in Table 4 (31).

First, it is important to optimize ultrasound images, particularly at the site where a needle is placed. Ultra-

▶ **TABLE 4 Methods to Facilitate
 the Needle Visualization**

1. Optimize ultrasound images
2. Use larger or echogenic needles
3. Insert perpendicular to the ultrasound beam
4. Move the needle or stylet
5. Use color Doppler imaging

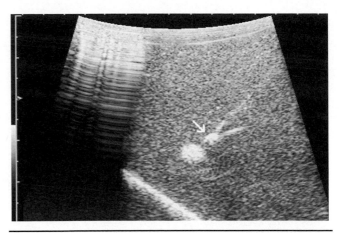

FIGURE 36. Echogenic tip needle. This is a 22-gauge needle with an echogenic-tip (*arrow*). Using a phantom, this needle is inserted under ultrasound guidance toward a hyperechoic lesion.

sound parameters such as transducer frequency and focal zone should be optimized to improve ultrasound image quality. When a needle is inserted in superficial soft tissues, such as the thyroid or breast, high-frequency ultrasound with a good near-field focal zone should be used.

Needles vary according to their echogenicity. The larger the needle diameter, the more easily it can be visualized by ultrasound. Therefore, if the needle size is not an issue, the larger gauge needle is preferable. This is particularly relevant for biopsy procedures because larger bore needles also produce better specimens. Needle echogenicity can be enhanced by maneuvers that roughen, scratch, or alter its outer surface, or by coating with materials such as Teflon (31,46). Such echogenic needles

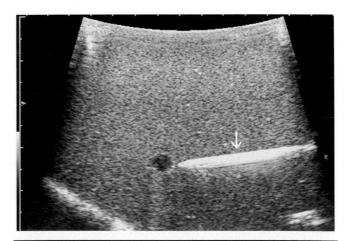

FIGURE 37. Better visualization of a needle placed perpendicular to the ultrasound beam. This is a 22-gauge needle inserted toward a cystic lesion of a phantom. The needle (*arrow*) is well visualized.

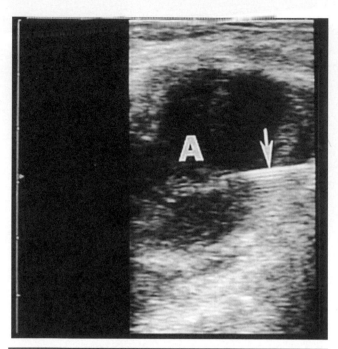

FIGURE 38. Well-visualized needle (*arrow*) placed close to perpendicular to the ultrasound beam. This shows intraoperative ultrasound-guided needle placement into an abdominal abscess (A) for aspiration and drainage.

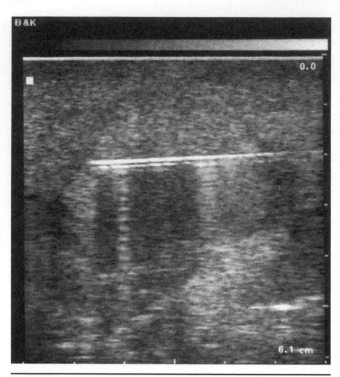

FIGURE 40. Relatively increased anechoic nature of the interior of a needle within a hepatic tumor resulting from instillation of saline into the lumen.

specifically made for ultrasound-guided procedures are commercially available (Fig. 36).

Visualization of needles is dependent on the angle of needle insertion in reference to the ultrasound beam because it is determined by reflection of the sound. When the needle is placed perpendicular (or close to perpendicular) to the ultrasound beam (i.e., parallel to the transducer surface), much of the sound is reflected back to the transducer, thus providing better needle visualization (Figs. 37 and 38; see also Fig. 17). On the other hand, the needle is less well visualized when its angle is more parallel to the ultrasound beam (Fig. 39; see also Fig. 16). Usually the needle can be more perpendicular to the ultrasound beam when it is placed by the freehand technique than by use of a needle guidance system because with the former the needle can be inserted from a remote location (Figs. 17 and 21B).

Moving of the needle or stylet is often helpful for needle visualization. Most needles come equipped with internal stylets or with dilators. The stylet is simply moved up and down gently in the needle, often improving needle visualization. The lumen of the needle may be made more anechoic relative to the needle wall by removal of the stylet and instillation of a fluid such as saline, thereby facilitating its visualization (Fig. 40). Alternatively, introducing a guidewire or filling the needle lumen with air or air-gel mixture can make the lumen more echogenic. Moving the needle itself back and forth in the tissue leading to visible movement of the lesion or adjacent tissue may help to locate the tip of the needle. When a needle is advanced toward a lesion but is not well seen, slight movement (sliding or tilting) of the transducer often allows visualization of the needle (Fig. 41).

The use of color or power Doppler imaging to detect minute movements of the needle may help needle visualization. After appropriate color Doppler settings, the stylet is moved within the needle or the needle is moved back and forth in the tissue. These movements produce

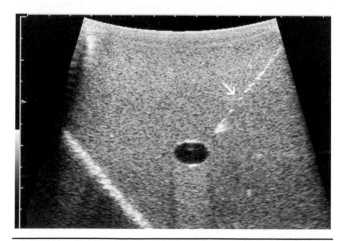

FIGURE 39. Not-so-good visualization of a needle inserted more parallel to the ultrasound beam. This is a 22-gauge needle, the same as that in Fig. 37. The shaft of the needle (*arrow*) is not optimally visualized.

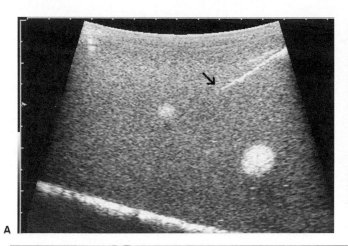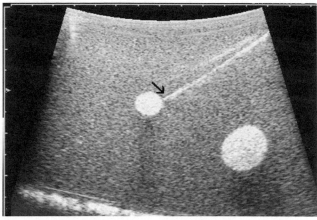

A

B

FIGURE 41. Adjustment of the ultrasound scanning plane for better visualization of a needle. **A:** A part of the shaft of a needle is seen in this scanning plane. After the point indicated by an arrow, the needle is not visualized. **B:** With slight movement, either sliding or tilting of the transducer, the scanning plane can be changed so that the entire shaft and the tip (*arrow*) of the needle are well visualized.

color motion marking (Fig. 42) (33). A special ultrasound unit (e.g., a vibrating needle system) that can detect minute movements of needles on color Doppler imaging has been developed (32,47). Such technical advances may be increasingly used in the future to facilitate needle placement into smaller and more deep-seated lesions.

TECHNICAL CONSIDERATIONS

Aspiration, Fine Needle Aspiration Cytology, and Biopsy

The basic ultrasound-guided technique for aspiration, biopsy, or drainage is the same, relying highly on precision

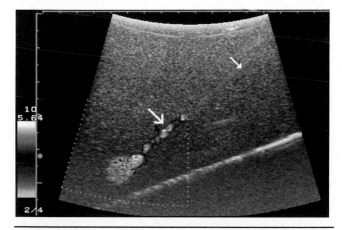

FIGURE 42. Color motion marking for better visualization of the location of the needle using color Doppler imaging. Under color or power Doppler imaging, a needle or a stylet is moved back and forth. This movement produces color motion marking (*large arrow*). This needle is not well visualized in the area of B-mode ultrasound imaging (*small arrow*). (See Color Plate 1.)

of needle placement under ultrasound guidance. For aspiration or biopsy (particularly when using a needle of 20 gauge or larger), the use of a stylet within the needle is recommended to prevent contamination or obstruction of the lumen by tissue or blood clot before it reaches the target.

When a relatively small amount of fluid is aspirated (e.g., aspiration of small cysts, diagnostic paracentesis), thin needles with or without stylets suffice using 5- to 20-mL syringes. Even with thin needles, when inserting through the skin is difficult, the skin may be punctured first using a no. 11 blade. When a large amount of fluid is aspirated (e.g., therapeutic paracentesis), the use of a flexible catheter (e.g., long angiocatheter) that is left in a fluid during aspiration is preferred because of a decreased risk of associated tissue injury. In addition, a three-way stopcock with tubing attached to a larger syringe (30 to 60 mL) is useful and convenient because the syringe need not be detached after each aspiration.

FNA cytology is performed by either an aspiration or a nonaspiration method (31,48). Under ultrasound guidance, a needle is placed in appropriate position, the stylet removed, and a syringe (usually 10 mL) attached. Several millimeters to 1 cm of negative suction is applied to the syringe. The needle is then moved in the target lesion; at least three to four passes are made by withdrawing and advancing back and forth 1 to 2 cm. The suction is then released and the needle withdrawn from the skin. The specimen is better if it is not aspirated into the syringe because this may cause fragmentation of cells. Gentle compression is applied at the biopsy site for hemostasis. The specimen is then placed on a slide and smeared. When the syringe is manipulated with one hand while the transducer is held with the other hand, some types of unorthodox grips can be used for aspiration, or an aspira-

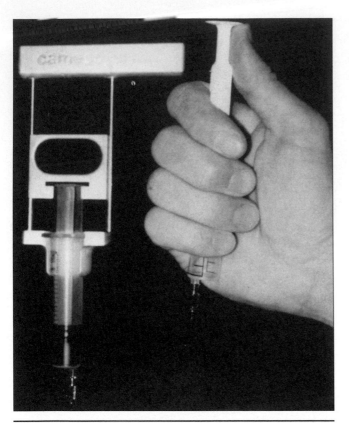

FIGURE 43. Aspiration techniques. Aspiration handle for a 10-mL syringe (*left*). Manual aspiration by an unorthodox grip on a 10-mL syringe (*right*).

tion handle may be used (Fig. 43). A nonaspiration cytology method is performed in a similar technique. After removal of the stylet, a syringe is not attached. Several back-and-forth movements are performed until a small amount of fluids returns to the hub of the needle. It is preferable for a cytopathologist to be available to examine the specimen immediately so that the adequacy of the specimen can be evaluated and determined.

Because of advantages of histology over cytology, even when performing FNA, it is more appropriate to obtain tissues or larger fragments rather than cells. This may be accomplished by moving the needle in the lesion in a rotatory motion. After withdrawal of the needle, the needle contents are expelled into saline or a fixative solution. The syringe and needle are also washed with the solution. A pathologist makes a cell block and processes it like a biopsy specimen.

When performing ultrasound-guided core needle biopsy with one hand holding the transducer and the other hand holding a needle, a nonautomated Tru-Cut needle or one of its variations is difficult to manipulate because an inner sheath and an outer cannula are separately advanced step by step with one hand. An automated spring-loaded biopsy needle is much easier to use by one hand. In addition, an automated biopsy nee-

dle may have advantages over regular Tru-Cut needles. One study showed that an 18-gauge automated needle used under ultrasound guidance demonstrated an excellent specimen retrieval rate and was associated with fewer complications than a 14-gauge Tru-Cut needle (49). For core needle biopsy, availability of a pathologist for immediate frozen-section examination is also helpful. If such an examination is not possible, at least three or four core needle specimens should be obtained from the lesion.

A variety of phantoms are available that may help the practitioner to rapidly develop an ultrasound-guided needle placement technique and accuracy (Figs. 13, 14, 16, 17, and 21B). Needles are, in general, easier to visualize in a phantom than in soft tissues of a human. These phantoms contain both solid and cystic lesions. The lesions are available in colors that are different from that of the surrounding material. This color difference allows for immediate feedback to the operator regarding the success rate for biopsy of a lesion within the phantom.

Drainage

Percutaneous drainage of various lesions or organs may be performed by ultrasound-guided catheterization technique. Needle and catheter placement can be performed under real-time ultrasound guidance, and at times final catheter placement can be confirmed by contrast radiography or fluoroscopy. Various types of catheters and needle–catheter systems are commercially available for drainage. Two fundamental ultrasound-guided catheter placement methods are a guidewire exchange technique and a trocar technique (Fig. 44) (31). A guidewire exchange technique (or Seldinger technique) is more commonly used. A needle (usually 18 gauge) is introduced into the target lesion or organ under ultrasound guidance. A guidewire is introduced through the needle, and the needle is removed. The tract is then progressively dilated over the wire. Once the tract is appropriately dilated, a catheter is introduced and advanced into the lesion or organ. Ultrasound can be used to confirm the location of the catheter in the lesion. This same technique can be performed for vein catheterization.

A trocar technique employs a special needle–catheter unit (e.g., McGahan drainage catheter), which includes a pigtail catheter, a cannula, an inner blunted obturator, and a sharp inner stylet (31,36). Under ultrasound guidance, the unit is inserted through the skin and advanced. Once the tip of the cannula is confirmed to be in the lesion or organ, the catheter is pushed from the cannula. Reformation of a loop of the pigtail catheter can be visualized by ultrasound. In general, catheters are more difficult to visualize than needles. The rapid injection of saline solution under color Doppler imaging can be helpful to confirm the presence of the catheter in the lesion.

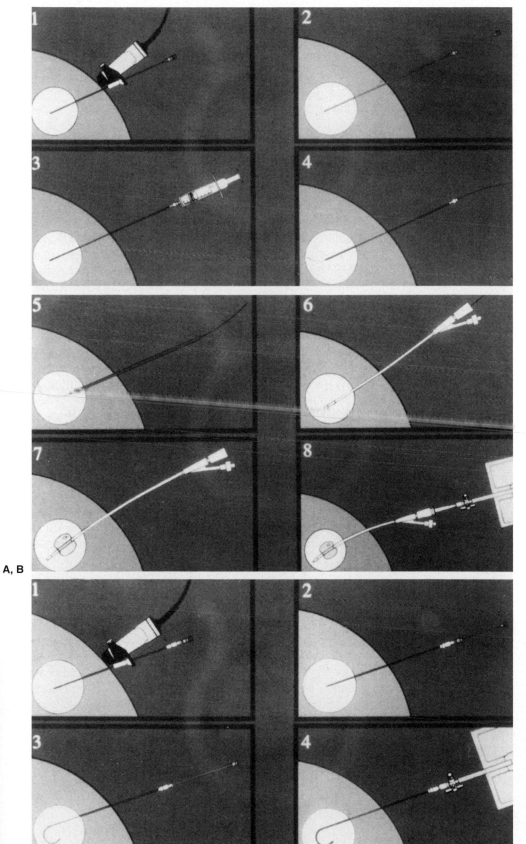

A, B

C

FIGURE 44. Principles of ultrasound-guided drainage. **A, B:** The guidewire exchange or Seldinger technique. A puncture needle is inserted into the target under ultrasound guidance. The stylet is removed and aspiration of fluid or pus verifies the indication for drainage. A guidewire is inserted and the balloon or pigtail catheter is placed over the guidewire. A dilator may be used (as illustrated) prior to the insertion of the catheter. The catheter is secured to the skin. **C:** The Trocar technique. A trocar catheter is inserted under ultrasound guidance. The stylet is removed and fluid or pus is aspirated. The catheter is advanced over the cannula or through the trocar and the pigtail curls up in the cavity.

▶ **TABLE 5 Advantages and Disadvantages of Various Approaches for Radiofrequency Thermal Ablation**

1. Percutaneous	Advantages:	Least invasive, possible outpatient procedure, needle guidance system (+)
	Disadvantages:	Less accurate cancer staging, some areas not accessible, possible adjacent organ thermal injury
2. Laparoscopic	Advantages:	Less invasive, better cancer staging with laparoscopic ultrasound, short recovery
	Disadvantages:	Technically demanding, lack of needle guidance system
3. Open surgical	Advantages:	Better cancer staging with intraoperative ultrasound, needle guidance system (+), inflow occlusion possible
	Disadvantages:	Most invasive, longer recovery

Ablation

Since the 1980s, percutaneous ethanol ablation and open surgical cryoablation have been used for management of various tumors, particularly liver tumors. Recently, use of these ablation methods seems to be decreasing with increased use of the radiofrequency thermal ablation method. Most of the ablation methods are performed under ultrasound guidance. The basic ultrasound guidance technique for needle, cannula, or probe placement for various types of ablations is the same.

Radiofrequency thermal ablation management of abdominal organs such as tumors of the liver can be performed percutaneously, laparoscopically, or open surgically (50). Advantages and disadvantages of each approach are summarized in Table 5. Surgeons should use different approaches appropriately depending on the condition of patients and tumors to be ablated. In the United States, three companies manufacture radiofrequency thermal ablation devices. RITA Medical (Mountain View, CA) and Radio Therapeutics (Mountain View, CA) use electrode cannulas with multiple retractable curved electrode needles (arrays), whereas Radionics (Burlington, MA) uses a cool-tip single-needle or a triple-needle cluster. The size of cannulas or needles ranges from 18 gauge to 14 gauge (Fig. 45). Under ultrasound guidance, cannulas or needles are inserted into the tumor. It is important to visualize the tips of needles and to understand their locations before ablation starts in order to obtain an adequate margin of ablation (Fig. 46). Depending on the size of the tumor and the achievable size of ablation, a single ablation or multiple overlapping ablation sessions are performed (Fig. 47; see also Fig. 7). The ablation process can be monitored by ultrasound imaging; the ablated lesion becomes hyperechoic because of outgassing from heated tissues (Figs. 7, 8, and 47). However, the hyperechoic area does not always correspond exactly to the ablated lesion. In addition, the hyperechoic area obscures the ultrasound images around the tumor. Therefore, it is critical to make a good plan for multiple ablation sessions before the first ablation starts. When the cannula is withdrawn at the completion of ablation, the cannula track is also ablated under ultrasound visualization to prevent bleeding and possible tumor seeding. If color or power Doppler imaging demonstrates intratumoral blood flow prior to ablation, Doppler imaging can be repeated after ablation to confirm loss of blood flow within the tumor. Percutaneous ultrasound-guided radiofrequency ablation is usually performed using a needle guidance system because the distance to the tumor is usually longer. Laparoscopic ultrasound-guided radiofrequency ablation should be performed by a freehand technique because of the lack of a needle guidance system with laparoscopic ultrasound transducer. Open surgical radiofrequency ablation can be performed either by a freehand technique or using a needle guidance system depending on the size, depth, and location of tumors.

CONCLUSIONS

Surgeons are becoming more and more involved in the use of ultrasound not only for diagnosis but also for in-

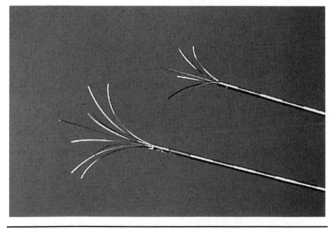

FIGURE 45. Electrode cannulas with needles for 3-cm and 5-cm radiofrequency ablation. (Courtesy of RITA Medical.)

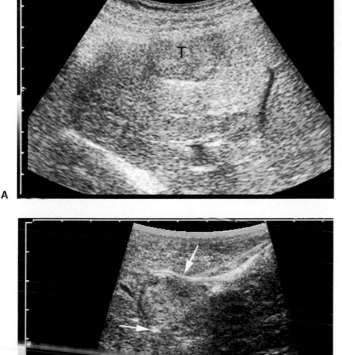

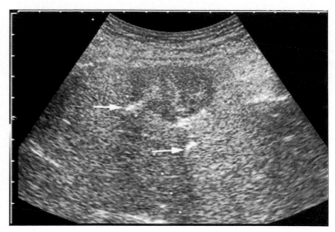

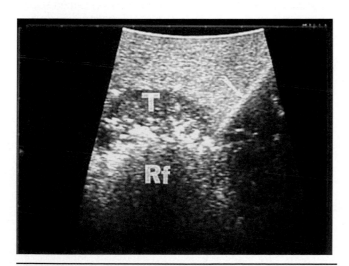

FIGURE 46. A: Percutaneous ultrasound-guided radiofrequency thermal ablation of a metastatic liver tumor. A: A metastatic liver tumor (T) was located near the surface of segment 8 of the liver. B: Under ultrasound guidance, an electrode cannula was inserted and needles were deployed. Note that the tips of the needles (*arrows*) were seen outside of the tumor. C: Open intra-operative ultrasound-guided radiofrequency ablation of a liver tumor. This shows the locations of needles (*arrows*) in relation to a metastatic tumor before ablation.

FIGURE 47. Multiple overlapping ablations for treatment of a large tumor. The posterior portion of the tumor on ultrasound imaging should be treated first because radiofrequency ablated lesion (Rf) becomes hyperechoic. For this particular tumor, the anterior (superficial) portion of the tumor (T) was not ablated yet. An arrow indicates the shaft of an electrode cannula.

terventional procedures. Both diagnostic and therapeutic interventional ultrasound are now widely accepted techniques that can be used as an adjunct in nearly all areas of the body. Indications for interventional ultrasound are numerous and expanding: needle aspiration, biopsy, drainage, catheterization, tumor ablation, and tissue dissection. There are many advantages of using ultrasound as the imaging modality to guide interventional procedures. In particular, the real-time feature, safety, relatively low cost, portability, and expediency make ultrasound an ideal modality to perform interventional procedures at various locations. Interventional ultrasound in the surgeon's office setting is acceptable and, moreover, convenient for the patient. More advanced interventional ultrasound, such as radiofrequency tumor ablation, should be performed by surgeons because it often involves laparoscopic or open surgical approaches. Introduction and availability of newer devices such as automated core biopsy needles have allowed for increased reliability in the performance of interventional ultrasound. The recent changes in the health care environment will further foster an expanded role for interventional ultrasound in clinical medicine. In such a clinical environment, surgeon-performed interventional ultrasound will be cost effective and beneficial for surgical patients.

REFERENCES

1. Berlyne GM. Ultrasonics in renal biopsy: an aid to determination of position. *Lancet* 1961;1:750.
2. Holm HH, Kristensen JK, Rasmussen SN, et al. Ultrasound as a guide in percutaneous puncture technique. *Ultrasonics* 1972;10:83–86.
3. Goldberg BB, Pollack HM. Ultrasonic aspiration transducer. *Radiology* 1972;102:187–189.
4. Rasmussen SN, Holm HH, Kristensen JK, et al. Ultrasonically guided liver biopsy. *Br J Med* 1972;2:500–502.
5. Yokoi H, Tatsumi T, Ito K. Clinical application of ultrasonic aspiration biopsy transducer for simultaneous tomogram method. *Proc Jpn Soc Ultrasonics* 1974;25:207–208.
6. Hancke S, Holm HH, Koch F. Ultrasonically guided percutaneous fine needle biopsy of the pancreas. *Surg Gynecol Obstet* 1975;140:361–364.
7. Machi J, Sigel B, Kurohiji T, et al. Operative ultrasound guidance for various surgical procedures. *Ultrasound Med Biol* 1990;16:37–42.
8. Makuuchi M, Torzilli G, Machi J. History of intraoperative ultrasound. *Ultrasound Med Biol* 1998;24:1229–1242.
9. Sanchez RB, vanSonnenberg E, D'Agostino HB, et al. Ultrasound-guided biopsy of non-palpable and difficult to palpate thyroid masses. *J Am Coll Surg* 1994;178:33–37.
10. Gooding GA, Clark OH, Stark DD, et al. Parathyroid aspiration biopsy under ultrasound guidance in the postoperative hyperparathyroid patient. *Radiology* 1985;155:193–196.
11. Simeone JF, Daniels GH, Hall DA, et al. Sonography in the follow-up of 100 patients with thyroid carcinoma. *AJR Am J Roentgenol* 1987;148:45–49.
12. Sutton R, Reading CC, Charboneau JW, et al. US-guided biopsy of neck masses in postoperative management of patients with thyroid cancer. *Radiology* 1988;168:769–772.
13. Staren ED. Surgical office-based ultrasound of the breast. *Am Surg* 1995;61:619–626.
14. Palombini L, Fulciniti F, Vetrani A, et al. Fine-needle aspiration biopsies of breast masses: a critical analysis of 1956 cases in 8 years (1976–1984). *Cancer* 1988;61:2273–2277.
15. Ballo MS, Sneiga N. Can core needle biopsy replace fine needle aspiration cytology in the diagnosis of palpable breast carcinoma: a comparative study of 124 women. *Cancer* 1996;78:773–777.
16. Parker SH, Klaus AJ. Performing a breast biopsy with a directional vacuum-assisted biopsy instrument. *Radiographics* 1987;17:1233–1252.
17. Welch TJ, Reading CC. Imaging-guided biopsy. *Mayo Clin Proc* 1989;64:1295–1302.
18. Schwerk WB, Durr HK, Schmitz-Moormann P. Ultrasound guided fine-needle biopsies in pancreatic and hepatic neoplasms. *Gastrointest Radiol* 1983;8:219–225.
19. Bernardino ME. Percutaneous biopsy. *AJR Am J Roentgenol* 1984;142:41–45.
20. Don S, Kopecky KK, Pescovitz MD, et al. Ultrasound-guided pediatric liver transplant biopsy using a spring-propelled cutting needle (biopsy gun). *Pediatr Radiol* 1994;24:21–24.
21. Gandini G, Grosso M, Bonardi L, et al. Results of percutaneous treatment of sixty-three pancreatic pseudocysts. *Ann Radiol* 1988;31:117–122.
22. Verges BL, Cercuell JP, Jacob D, et al. Results of ultrasonically guided percutaneous ethanol injection into parathyroid adenomas in primary hyperparathyroidism. *Acta Endocrinol* 1993;129:381–387.
23. vanSonnenberg E, D'Agostino HB, Casola G, et al. Percutaneous abscess drainage: current concepts. *Radiology* 1991;181:617–626.
24. McGahan JP, Lindfors KK. Percutaneous cholecystostomy: an alternative to surgical cholecystostomy for acute cholecystitis? *Radiology* 1989;173:481–485.
25. Machi J, Takeda J, Kakegawa T. Safe jugular and subclavian venipuncture under ultrasonographic guidance. *Am J Surg* 1987;153:321–323.
26. Nolsoe C, Nielsen L, Karstrup S, et al. Ultrasonically-guided subclavian vein catheterization. *Acta Radiol* 1989;30:108–109.
27. Seidenfeld J, Korn A, Aronson N. Radiofrequency ablation of unresectable primary liver cancer. *J Am Coll Surg* 2002;194:813–828.
28. Izzo F, Thomas R, Delrio P, et al. Radiofrequency ablation in patients with primary breast carcinoma. *Cancer* 2001;92:2036–2044.
29. Reading CC, Charboneau JW. US-guided biopsy. In: Rumack CM, Wilson SSR, Charboneau JW, eds. *Diagnostic ultrasound*. St. Louis: Mosby–Year Book, 1991:429–442.
30. McGahan JP. Advantages of sonographic guidance. In: McGahan JP, ed. *Controversies in ultrasound*. New York: Churchill Livingstone, 1987:249–267.
31. McGahan JP. Invasive ultrasound principles (biopsy, aspiration, and drainage). In: McGahan JP, Goldberg BB, eds. *Diagnostic ultrasound. A logical approach*. Philadelphia: Lippincott–Raven Publishers, 1998:39–75.
32. Taylor KJW, Burns PN, Wells PNT. *Clinical applications of Doppler ultrasound*. New York: Raven Press, 1987.
33. Kurohiji T, Sigel B, Justin JR, et al. Motion marking in color Doppler ultrasound needle and catheter visualization. *J Ultrasound Med* 1990;9:243–245.
34. McGahan JP. Aspiration and drainage procedures in the intensive care unit: percutaneous sonographic guidance. *Radiology* 1985;154:531–532.
35. McGahan JP, Anderson MW, Walter JP. Portable real-time sonographic and needle-guidance systems for aspiration and drainage. *AJR Am J Roentgenol* 1986;147:1241–1246.
36. McGahan JP, Brant WE. Principles, instrumentation, and guidance systems. In: McGahan JP, ed. *Interventional ultrasound*. Baltimore: Williams & Wilkins, 1990:1–20.
37. Fornari F, Civardi G, Cavanna L, et al. Complications of ultrasonically guided fine-needle abdominal biopsy: results of a multicenter Italian study and review of the literature. *Scand J Gastroenterol* 1989;24:949–955.
38. Nolsoe C, Nielsen L, Torp-Pedersen S, et al. Major complications and deaths due to interventional ultrasonography: a review of 8000 cases. *J Clin Ultrasound* 1990;18:179–184.
39. Smith EH. The hazards of fine needle aspiration biopsy. *Ultrasound Med Biol* 1984;10:629–634.
40. Livraghi T, Damascelli B, Lombardi C, et al. Risk in fine needle abdominal biopsy. *J Clin Ultrasound* 1983;11:77–81.
41. Reading CC, Charboneau JW, James EM, et al. Sonographically guided percutaneous biopsy of small (3 cm or less) masses. *AJR Am J Roentgenol* 1988;151:189–192.
42. Holm HH, Torp-Pedersen S, Juul N, et al. Instrumentation for sonographic interventional procedures. In: vanSonnenberg E, ed. *Interventional ultrasound*. New York: Churchill Livingstone, 1987:9–40.
43. Parker SH. Needle selection. In: Parker SH, Jobe WE, eds. *Percutaneous breast biopsy*. New York: Raven Press, 1993:7–14.
44. Parker SH, Hopper KD, Yakes WF, et al. Image-directed percutaneous biopsies with a biopsy gun. *Radiology* 1989;171:663–669.
45. Bernardino ME. Automated biopsy devices: significance and safety. *Radiology* 1990;176:615–616.

46. McGahan JP. Laboratory assessment of ultrasonic needle and catheter visualization. *J Ultrasound Med* 1986;5:373–377.

47. Jones CD, McGahan JP, Clark KJ. Color Doppler ultrasonographic detection of a vibrating needle system. *J Ultrasound Med* 1997;16:269–274.

48. Fagelman D, Chess Q. Nonaspiration fine-needle cytology of the liver: a new technique for obtaining diagnostic samples. *AJR Am J Roentgenol* 1990;155:1217–1219.

49. Mahoney MC, Racadio JM, Merhar GL, et al. Safety and efficacy of kidney transplant biopsy: Tru-Cut needle vs sonographically guided Biopsy gun. *AJR Am J Roentgenol* 1993;160:325–326.

50. Machi J, Uchida S, Sumida K, et al. Ultrasound-guided radiofrequency thermal ablation of liver tumors: percutaneous, laparoscopic and open surgical approaches. *J Gastrointest Surg* 2001;5:477–489.

Diagnostic and Interventional Breast Ultrasound

Nitzet Velez and Edgar D. Staren

Stimulated by various social and political factors, the number of mammographic screening examinations being performed increased substantially in the early 1970s. On the other hand, for quite some time, ultrasound evaluations of the breast were generally limited and, when used, dealt almost exclusively with the simple differentiation of a lesion's cystic, as opposed to solid, nature (1,2). Expanded use of ultrasound was hindered particularly by the relatively poor quality of the ultrasound image in the 1970s and the early 1980s. In the last two decades, significant technological improvements have been made in ultrasound imaging, resulting from computer enhancement, availability of high-frequency transducers, and other advancements (3,4). Such improvements were essential to allow for better evaluation of near-field images, so critical to accurate diagnostic breast ultrasound. In addition to allowing for ready differentiation of cystic and solid lesions, improved ultrasound images permitted identification of various characteristics useful in separating breast lesions into categories of relative risk (5–7). In recent years, ultrasound has played an increasing role in the assessment and management of breast disease and has gradually become an integral part of the workup of breast patients. In addition, the use of ultrasound has expanded beyond initial assessment and is now being employed more frequently as an interventional modality. Ultrasound-guided breast biopsy of nonpalpable abnormalities with spring-loaded core biopsy needles has become relatively routine. Increased tissue removal for biopsy, and in some circumstances excision, performed with hand-held vacuum-assisted devices, is another tool available in the arsenal against breast diseases. Moreover, the use of ultrasound to guide delivery of ablative therapy lies in the near horizon of breast care. This chapter provides a comprehensive review, from the basics of diagnostic breast ultrasound to the routine use of interventional breast ultrasound and even potential therapy.

DIAGNOSTIC BREAST ULTRASOUND

Indications

The many advances in ultrasound technology have led to continuously increasing indications for ultrasound of the breast (Table 1). Ultrasound is the primary means of evaluating mammographically detected, benign-appearing lesions, the solid (as opposed to cystic) nature of which is otherwise indistinguishable (Fig. 1) (3,8,9). Ultrasound of the breast may be helpful in evaluating patients with difficult physical findings but with negative or nonspecific mammographic examinations (4,10,11). A sonographically homogeneous dense pattern is strongly indicative of the benign nature of the area in question. Furthermore, when nonspecific asymmetries are demonstrated on two mammographic views, ultrasound evaluation is generally recommended (5,6). Demonstration of underlying cysts by ultrasound may obviate the need for further mammographic workup (12). Occasionally, solid nodules may be identified by ultrasound within these focal asymmetries (Fig. 2). Under such circumstances, these nodules should be treated based on their benign or suspicious characteristics. Ultrasound may be used to evaluate the breasts of patients with pathologic nipple discharge (13). Although ductography is considered by many to be the procedure of choice for evaluating nipple discharge, its use requires the ability to express secretions from the nipple and to identify and cannulate the appropriate duct. By scanning radially, parallel to its axis, ultrasound can often identify a dilated, fluid-filled duct (Fig. 3). In experienced hands, this may allow for detection of intraductal papillomas as well. Ultrasound is useful in the assessment of fluid collections such as postoperative seromas or hematomas (Fig. 4). Ultrasound is the diagnostic modality of choice to evaluate breast masses in pregnant women. It is also preferred in the evaluation of the breasts of younger women prior to the age at which mammographic exami-

▶ **TABLE 1** Indications for Breast Ultrasound

1. Evaluation of mammographically detected lesions
2. Evaluation of patients with difficult physical findings and negative or nonspecific mammography results
3. Evaluation of palpable lesions and guidance for needle aspiration
4. Evaluation of nipple discharge
5. Evaluation of postoperative changes
6. Evaluation of younger patients
7. Evaluation of pregnant patients
8. Evaluation of acute mastitis
9. Evaluation of implant leaks
10. Screening test for women with mammographically dense breasts
11. Guide for interventional procedures, including needle aspiration, core biopsy, and localization

nation is suggested (9). Ultrasound is particularly effective in the evaluation of acute mastitis in terms of identifying abscesses (Fig. 5). (14) Magnetic resonance imaging (MRI) is often viewed as the modality of choice for evaluating rupture of silicone breast implants. Nevertheless, ultrasound is useful in determining the presence of an implant leak or rupture. Furthermore, it is considerably more comfortable and cheaper for the patient (15). Whole-breast ultrasound is increasingly recommended for screening of women with very dense breasts in whom mammographic examination may miss lesions, particularly when such women have difficult physical examinations or strong family histories of breast cancer (10,11).

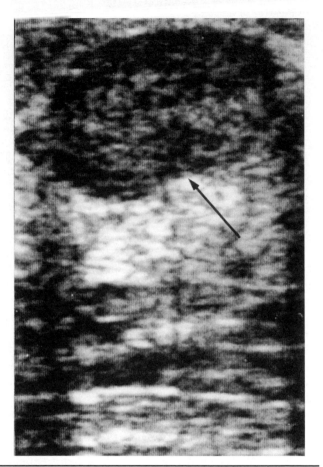

FIGURE 2. Homogeneous gray (hypoechoic) internal pattern of a solid lesion consistent with a fibroadenoma (*arrow*).

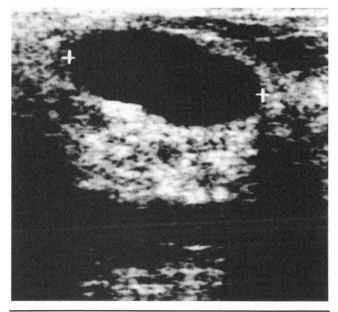

FIGURE 1. Homogeneous black (anechoic) interior of a breast lesion (cursors) consistent with a fluid-filled cyst.

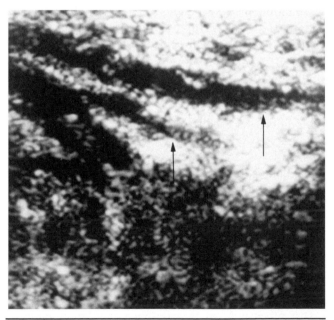

FIGURE 3. Ultrasound image of dilated ducts (*arrows*) in a lactating breast.

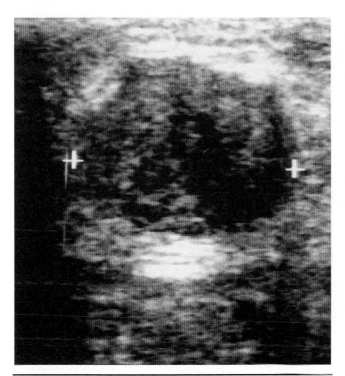

FIGURE 4. Postoperative sero-hematoma (*cursors*) after breast conservation therapy.

Finally, breast ultrasound is routinely used to guide percutaneous needle aspiration, core biopsy, and localization procedures (16–23).

Scanning Technique

An ultrasound scanning technique must be highly reliable and reproducible (Table 2). For screening breast ultrasound, the whole breast must be examined so that abnormalities are not inadvertently missed. The examiner must be sure to identify all normal structures as well. Un-

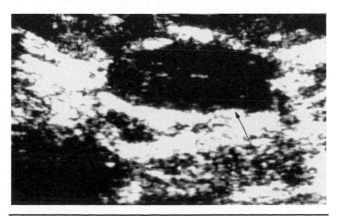

FIGURE 5. Resolving abscess (*arrow*) of the breast in a patient with mastitis.

▶ **TABLE 2 Important Points of Scanning Technique**

1. The whole breast must be examined with screening breast ultrasound.
2. Normal structures must be identified.
3. Image of nipple must be kept in left corner of screen.
4. It is necessary to use transducer with linear footprint.
5. Patient must be supine with ipsilateral arm above head.
6. The sonographer should begin at 12:00 position and move peripherally until no more breast tissue is found. This should be repeated radially around entire breast (radial scanning technique).
7. To image nipple-areolar complex, the sonographer should place probe at margin of areola and angulate toward the retroareolar area (tangential scanning technique).
8. A series of transverse or sagittal sweeps may be undertaken as a double check.

less this is accomplished, a complete report is not possible. To this end, we perform the radial scanning technique or "ductal echography" as described by Teboul in 1988 (Fig. 6A) (24). We prefer this technique because it respects the normal architecture of the breast and enables the examiner to view the breast lobes and the ducts in their full extent (Fig. 6B). The examination technique must be standardized to make it reproducible. For this reason, we advise keeping the image of the nipple in the upper left corner of the screen. This allows for precise localization of any finding, such as a solid lesion seen at 5 o'clock, 3 cm from the nipple, and at 1.5 cm depth. Other techniques (e.g., sagittal or transverse sweeps of the breast for routine scans) are also described in the literature. We often perform such a scan rather quickly upon completion of the radial scan as a double check.

Good breast ultrasound scanning with accurate interpretation is highly dependent on excellent equipment and technical skill. Significant advances in ultrasound equipment, including high-resolution transducers and computer-enhanced imagery, along with precise examination techniques, allow for depiction of the fine anatomy of the breast and, hence, recognition of changes or lesions in the breast even in relatively early stages. Dedicated equipment for ultrasound of the breast includes a high-frequency, real-time, linear array transducer of at least 7 to 8 MHz (Fig. 7). Transducers up to 15 MHz are available commercially, and increasingly transducers in the range of 10 MHz are used routinely. Nevertheless, a high-quality 7-MHz transducer is generally sufficient for a complete examination of the breast. The linear shape of the transducer footprint optimizes maintenance of contact with the breast skin. This footprint (or sole) must be of sufficient size (e.g., 4 to 6 cm) to cover the breast without an excessive number of sweeps but small enough to be comfortably held by the examiner.

EXAMINATION TECHNIQUE

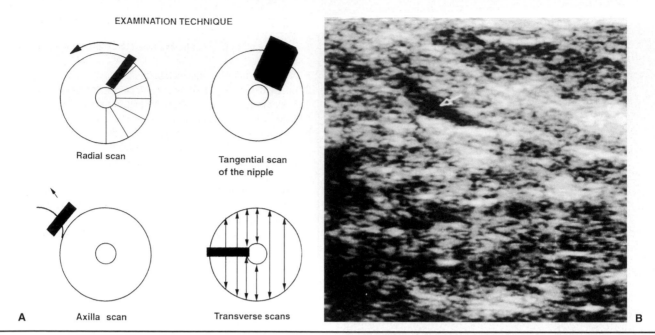

Radial scan

Tangential scan of the nipple

Axilla scan

Transverse scans

A

B

FIGURE 6. **A:** Breast ultrasound examination techniques. **B:** Longitudinal orientation of a duct (*arrow*) or "ductal echography" as seen using a radial scanning technique.

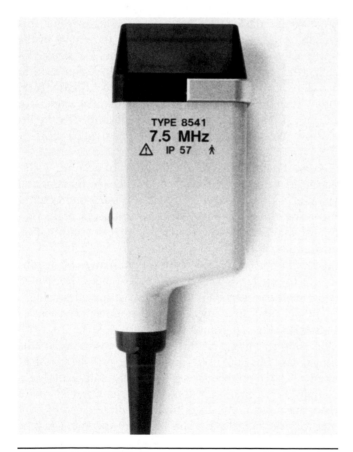

TYPE 8541
7.5 MHz
⚠ IP 57 🏃

FIGURE 7. A 7.5-MHz linear array transducer, ideal for ultrasound of the breast.

For diagnostic breast ultrasound, the patient should be lying in the supine position with the ipsilateral arm placed under her head (Fig. 8). This position helps to stabilize the breast. Moreover, because this is the position assumed for routine physical examinations, it may help the surgeon to relocalize questionably palpable lesions. For whole-breast ultrasound, we start the ultrasound examination by placing the transducer at the 12-o'clock position on the breast. We stay within the axis of this position while tilting the transducer slightly from left to right and moving it toward the periphery of the gland until no more breast tissue is visualized. We then move the transducer to the 1-o'clock position and repeat the procedure, moving clockwise around the breast until the entire breast is thoroughly examined. If a lesion is identified, it is examined in detail and images are recorded in at least two perpendicular dimensions (Fig. 9).

Imaging the nipple–areolar complex requires special maneuvering because of the dense connective tissue in the area (Fig. 10). This tissue may cause strong posterior acoustic shadowing, which limits imaging of underlying tissues. To avoid this image restriction, the transducer is placed adjacent to the nipple and the ultrasound beam is acutely angled into the retroareolar area (tangential scanning, Fig. 6A). The examiner may use his or her free hand to compress opposite to the transducer so as to optimize visualization.

To conclude the examination, a series of transverse or sagittal sweeps may be undertaken. This allows the examiner to assess the architectural harmony of the struc-

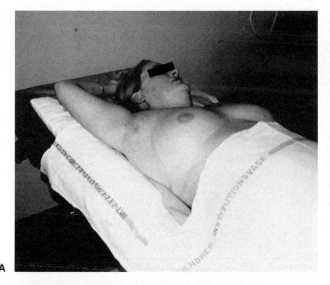

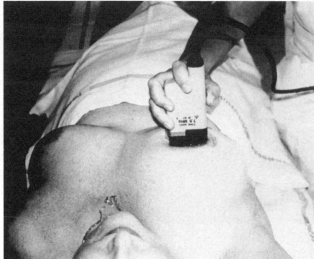

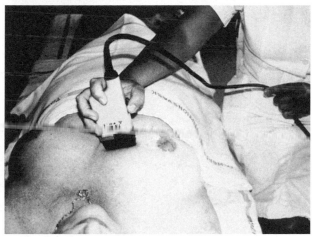

FIGURE 8. **A:** Standard position of the patient for ultrasound of the breast with patient lying supine and ipsilateral arm (in this case, right) behind the head. **B:** Initial orientation of transducer at the 3-o'clock position. Note how the transducer is placed so that the ultrasound image will have the nipple–areolar complex in the upper left portion; **C:** Transducer at the 3-o'clock position but moved out toward the periphery until no more breast tissue is visualized.

tures of the breast and appreciate the regularity of the criss-crossing of Cooper's ligaments. Occasionally, small tumors may be revealed in this sweep because they may appear as a disruption in the normal course of the ligaments (Fig. 11).

Sonographic Anatomy

"Anatomy of course does not change, but our understanding of anatomy and its clinical significance does change as do anatomical terminology and nomenclature."

—Frank H. Netter, M.D.

The breast is the quintessential feature of the mammalian class. It develops from ectodermal tissue that grows into the supporting tissues to form alveoli and ducts. In a female adult, the breast tissue extends from the second rib superiorly to the seventh to eighth rib infe-

riorly and from the lateral edge of the sternum medially to a variable extent laterally but usually to at least the midaxillary line. The axillary tail of Spence is an extension of breast tissue that extends into the anterior axilla. Breast anatomy can be described in layers from superficial to deep or as a "functional anatomy" that describes the alveolar-ductal unit and its supporting elements. The actual anatomy is a combination of these, but for the purposes of ultrasound it is the description of the layers of the breast that is most relevant.

Epidermis/Dermis

The major structures of the breast have characteristic sonographic features (Figs. 12 and 13), some of which will vary with age. The skin appears as a homogeneous, hypoechoic zone between two hyperechoic layers repre-

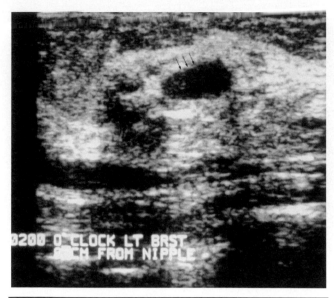

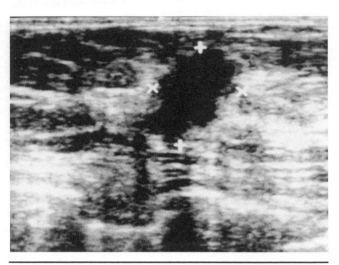

FIGURE 11. Small infiltrating carcinoma of the breast (*cursors*) identified secondary to disruption in the normal course of Cooper's ligaments.

FIGURE 9. Ultrasound of the breast with the nipple–areolar complex oriented toward the left upper portion of the image. Note how radial scan facilitates accurate specification of a lesion's (*arrows*) precise location.

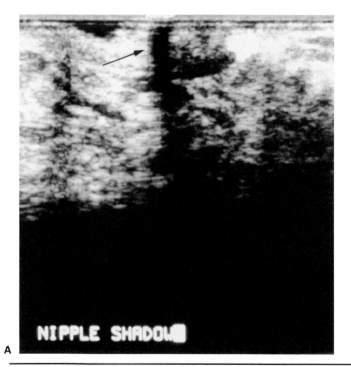

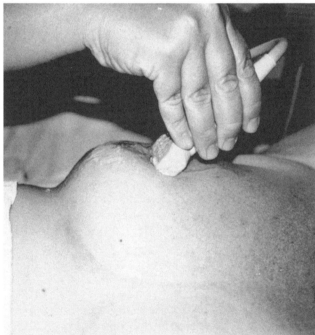

A

B

FIGURE 10. **A:** Nipple shadow (*arrow*), which results from the ultrasound transducer's being placed directly over nipple–areolar complex. **B:** Angled position of the transducer used to scan the nipple–areolar complex, thereby avoiding excessive shadow artifact.

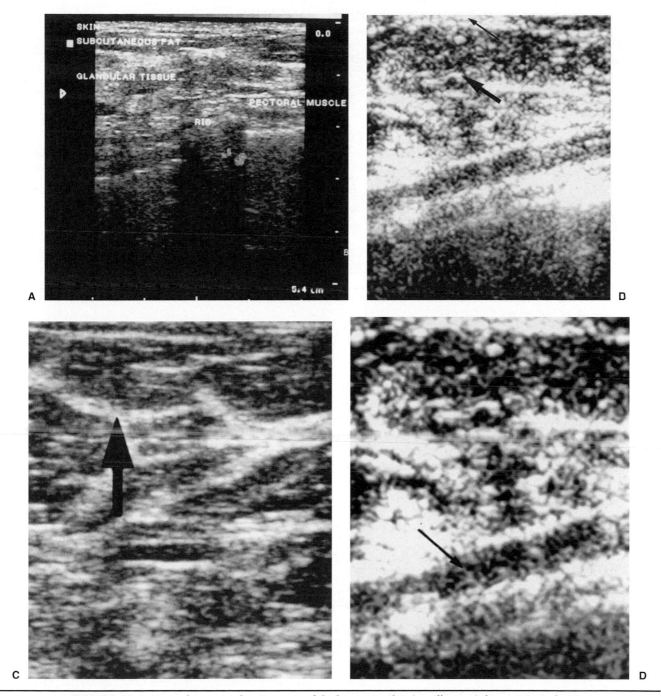

FIGURE 12. A: Normal sonographic anatomy of the breast. B: Skin (*small arrow*), breast parenchyma (*large arrow*). C: Cooper's ligament (*arrow*). D: Pectoral muscles (*arrow*).

senting the interfaces between the transducer and the skin and between the skin and subcutaneous tissues. Normally the entire complex measures up to 2 mm. The skin can be involved in various breast pathologies including invasive carcinoma, Paget's disease of the nipple, and others. Depending on the extent of growth and the location, the tumor can extend to and involve the skin. Clinically, this manifests itself as thickened, edematous-appearing skin, otherwise known as "peau d'orange." Microscopically this represents the plugging of dermal lymphatics with tumor (25). Sonographically this manifests as a thickening of the skin, often with an increased hypoechoic middle layer. A suspicious lesion deeper in the breast parenchyma may not be visualized. Paget's disease of the nipple generally is composed of intraductal carcinoma but may have an invasive component and typically involves both the nipple and the areola. Microscopically it is characterized by the identification of Paget cells in the epithelium (25).

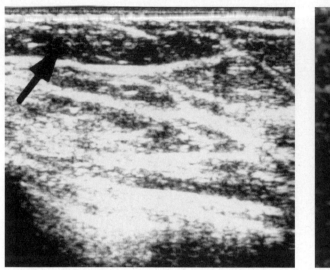
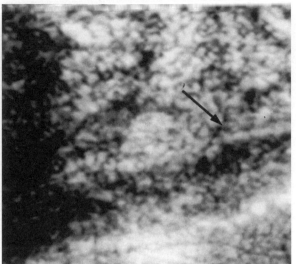

FIGURE 13. A: Hypoechoic subcutaneous tissue (*arrow*) just beneath skin. B: Thin, hypoechoic layer of retromammary fat (*arrow*).

Nipple/Areolar Complex

Areolar epithelium is variably pigmented. It contains radially arranged smooth muscle fibers that are embedded in connective tissue. Accessory glands of Montgomery empty onto the areola and produce small elevations otherwise known as Montgomery tubercles. The thickened connective tissue in this area makes the retroareolar region difficult to visualize on ultrasound unless the transducer is angulated toward the nipple from the edge of the areola.

Subcutaneous

Subcutaneous fatty tissue appears as a hypoechoic layer just beneath the skin complex (Fig. 13). Retromammary fat has the same appearance and, when seen, is found just above the pectoral muscle.

Parenchyma

The glandular region occupies the space between the two fat layers. The glandular and fibrous tissue structures are usually highly reflective (i.e., hyperechoic), whereas the intramammary fatty tissue is poorly reflective (i.e., hypoechoic). Small, linear, hypoechoic tubular lactiferous ducts can be identified in the parenchyma. Normally the ducts can range from 1 mm to 4 mm in diameter. Use of the radial scanning technique enables a thorough evaluation of the ducts; however, accurate detection of intraductal papillomas requires much experience. *Cooper's ligaments* appear as hyperechoic curvilinear structures representing planes of fibrous tissue (Fig. 12C). The ar-

chitecture of the breast varies considerably during a lifetime as changes occur in the hormonal milieu in which it exists. Distinct sonographic characteristics can be described for the juvenile, premenopausal, postmenopausal, and lactating breast.

Juvenile Breast

The juvenile breast is composed mainly of glandular tissue, thin fat layers, and very little intramammary fat (Fig. 14). On ultrasound the gland appears hyperechoic and homogeneous. (26)

Premenopausal Breast

The premenopausal, partly involuted breast appears with fat lobules distributed throughout the glandular tissue as well as increased amounts of subcutaneous and retromammary fat (Fig. 15). Fat lobules are usually well defined by their thin connective tissue envelopes and should not be mistaken for fibroadenomas or other hypoechoic solid masses.

Postmenopausal Breast

The postmenopausal, involuted breast has very little parenchyma (Fig. 16A). Cooper's ligaments are particularly prominent sonographically in these breasts. Shadowing can occur at the intersection of the Cooper's ligaments and must not be mistaken for retrotumoral acoustic shadowing (Fig. 16B).

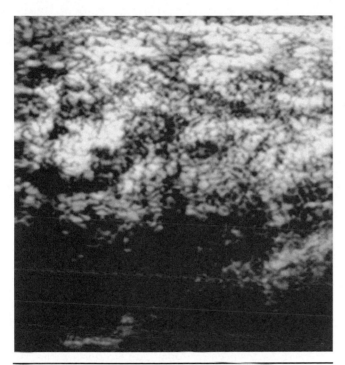

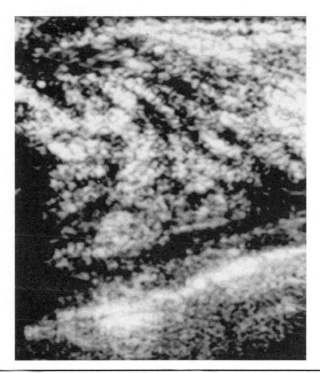

FIGURE 14. Juvenile breast demonstrating hyperechoic parenchyma with practically no fat.

FIGURE 15. Premenopausal, partly involuted breast demonstrating increased amounts of subcutaneous and intramammary fat.

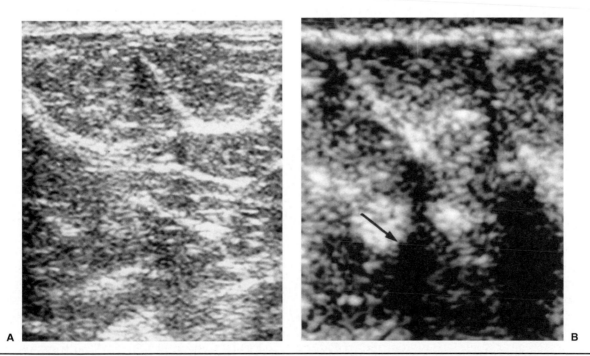

FIGURE 16. **A:** Postmenopausal, fully involuted breast demonstrating very little parenchyma with particularly prominent Cooper's ligament. **B:** Shadowing at intersections of Cooper's ligaments (*arrow*).

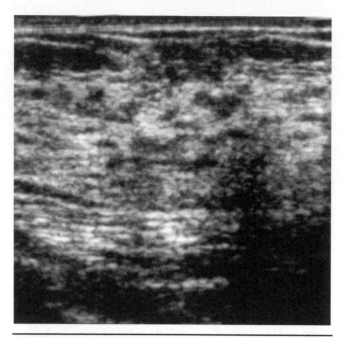

FIGURE 17. Hyperechoic glandular parenchyma in pregnancy with prominent ducts.

Pregnancy

The pattern during pregnancy and lactation is characterized by hypertrophy of the glandular tissue with compression of the fatty layers. Sonographically, this appears very similar to the juvenile breast. Lactiferous ducts can frequently be identified as prominent tubular structures (Fig. 17) (26).

Retromammary Fat

Occasionally, a thin layer of hypoechoic retromammary fat can be found posterior to the breast tissue and just anterior to the pectoralis fascia. It is not likely to be prominent in the adolescent breast (Fig. 13B).

Pectoral Muscles

The pectoralis major muscle arises from the middle third of the clavicle superiorly. Medially it arises from the lateral border of the sternum and from the cartilage of the first six ribs (27). The muscle inserts on the anterior surface of the humerus. It is covered entirely by pectoralis fascia. The pectoralis minor muscle lies posterior to the pectoralis major muscle and arises from the second to fifth or sixth rib and inserts superiorly and laterally at the coracoid process (27). The pectoralis major appears as a hypoechoic structure anterior to the ribs and separated from the breast tissue by a thin reflective hyperechoic zone (the anterior pectoralis fascia). The pectoralis

minor lies posterior to the pectoralis major and appears as a hypoechoic structure separated from the pectoralis major by a thin reflective hyperechoic zone representing the posterior pectoralis fascia and the anterior pectoralis minor fascia or clavicopectoral fascia (Fig. 12D).

Ribs/Intercostal Muscles

The ribs are identifiable as semilunar hyperechoic structures with strong acoustic shadowing (Fig. 12A), best seen at the most medial and lateral aspects of the breast. Between the ribs, hypoechoic intercostal muscles may be identified. The pleura is identified on ultrasound as a thin hyperechoic layer immediately beneath the ribs and intercostal muscles. With respiration, the motion of hyperechoic lung may be visualized in real time just under the pleura.

Lymph Nodes/Axilla

The axilla is bordered medially by the serratus anterior, anteriorly by the pectoralis major and minor muscles, superiorly by the axillary vessels, and inferiorly by skin and reflected fascia from the abdominal wall. When the breast examination is completed, the axillary region may be scanned for abnormal nodes (Fig. 18). Lymph nodes are generally visible in the axilla only if they have pathologic changes within them. Pathologic lymph nodes are increased in size (e.g., more than 1 cm), round, hypoechoic, with a well-defined border, and may lose the fatty hilar areas that appear normally as a hyperechoic line (28). In the axilla, the sonographer can easily visualize the axillary vessels by positioning the transducer in a transverse line to the long axis of the vessel and looking for the characteristic anechoic pulsation for an artery and a tubular compressible structure for a vein. He or she can easily differentiate the vessels from lymph nodes by rotating the transducer to demonstrate them as elongated pulsatile or compressible structures on real-time images. This can be confirmed using color flow imaging to identify blood flow but is generally not necessary. The entire examination should be repeated on the opposite breast and axilla.

Nitz et al. (29) described a method for ultrasound evaluation of the axilla. They described three levels of nodes. Level I was defined as those lymph nodes that were visualized when the thoracodorsal bundle and the axillary vein were visualized. Level II was defined as those lymph nodes that could be identified when the pectoralis muscle and the axillary vein were simultaneously visualized. Level III nodes were defined as those that could be visualized while inclining the transducer caudally from the position to view level II. They found that by using these sonographic views and combining that with the finding

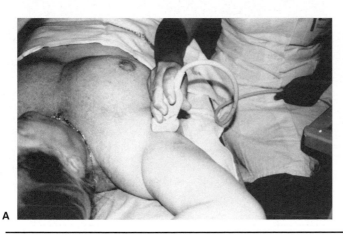

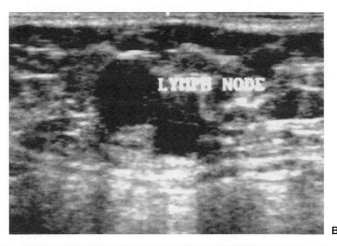

A   B

FIGURE 18. A: Sagittal sweep technique generally used for examining the axilla by ultrasound. B: Enlarged hypoechoic axillary lymph nodes shown to be positive for metastatic carcinoma of the breast.

of suspicious lymph nodes—defined by ultrasound criteria as an enlarged hypoechoic, ovoid structure—they were able to achieve a sensitivity and specificity of 83% and 89%, respectively, when correlated with histopathologic findings.

Breast Diseases

Fibrocystic Changes

Fibrocystic changes are nonproliferative changes that occur most commonly in the premenopausal breast. They can take several forms, varying from gross cystic changes to fibrosis, and can be viewed as different points on a time line (25). Investigation of these changes usually begins with a palpable mass. The classic breast cyst appears blue–brown due to its turbid fluid content. When such cysts rupture, they release their contents into the parenchyma, leading to scarring or fibrosis. Under such conditions the abnormality may be ill defined on palpation. On ultrasound examination, fibrocystic change may demonstrate simple cysts with smooth-walled, anechoic interiors and good through transmission, with posterior enhancement and edge shadowing (Fig. 19). Conversely, cysts may less often contain thick fluid with or without debris that will have a hypoechoic interior and variable internal regularity. In like manner, a fibrotic breast may have a variable character depending on the amount of fibrotic changes and associated fat in the parenchyma.

Abscess

Clinically, breast abscess can occur in the subareolar, subcutaneous, parenchymal, or retromammary locations. Infections that occur in the lactational period are most likely to be caused by *Staphylococcus aureus*, whereas those in the nonlactating breast are caused by a wider spectrum of infecting organisms (30). Milk provides a favorable environment for bacterial reproduction, and infections of the breast can quickly spread throughout the breast. Traditionally, the treatment has been open drainage of the abscess cavity, but recently ultrasound-guided percutaneous drainage has been highly successful (see "Interventional Breast Ultrasound" in this chapter). On

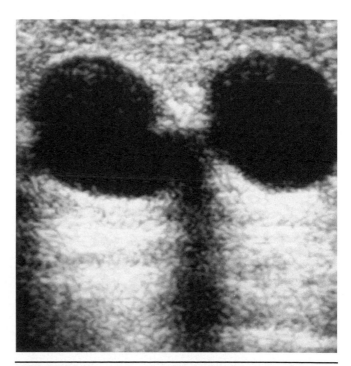

FIGURE 19. Two adjacent simple cysts; both with anechoic interiors, smooth borders, posterior enhancement, and edge shadowing.

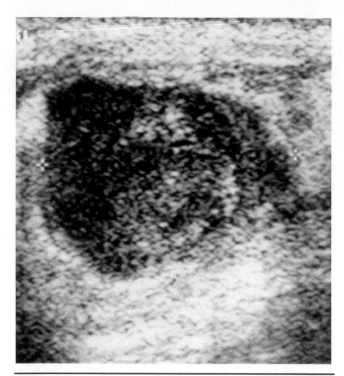

FIGURE 20. Ultrasound image of a hypoechoic, smooth-margined hematoma (*cursors*).

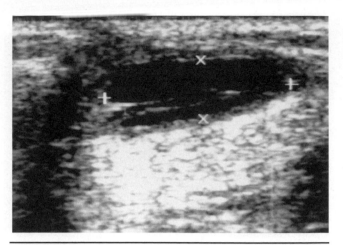

FIGURE 21. Ultrasound image of a seroma (*cursors*) subsequent to lumpectomy.

ultrasound examination, abscesses appear as multi-echoic lesions, which may demonstrate fluid/debris motion and posterior enhancement (Fig. 5). At times, the border or the extent of abscesses is not so well defined as cysts.

Trauma/Hematoma

Trauma to the breast can result in contusions or hematoma formation. Contusions are soft-tissue damage without a clear collection of fluid. They appear on ultrasound as alterations in echogenicity of several layers without a distinct fluid-filled cavity. In contradistinction, hematomas appear as a hypoechoic, homogeneous, smooth-bordered lesions on ultrasound (Fig. 20).

Seroma

Seromas are most often encountered in the postsurgical period and represent exudative fluid that occupies the space within the breast that has been previously occupied by the biopsied or excised mass. They usually present as a fluid-filled, smooth mass in the region of the biopsy. Seromas can be identified on ultrasound as cystic collections with a well-defined, hyperechoic outer layer and with posterior enhancement (Fig. 21).

Fibroadenoma

Fibroadenoma is a benign tumor that ranges in clinical presentation from a discrete, easily palpable abnormality to a simple asymmetry of the breast. It occasionally mimics malignancies with rapid growth and large size (30). Grossly, a fibroadenoma appears as a sharply circum-

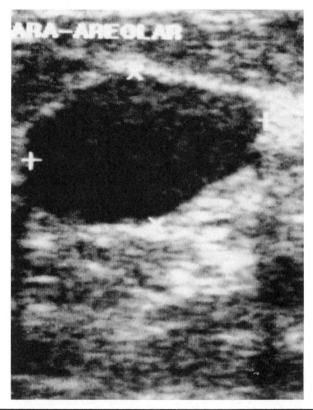

FIGURE 22. Smooth, well-defined margins of a benign fibroadenoma (*cursors*) of the breast.

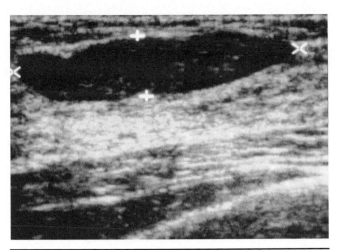

FIGURE 23. Very well-defined, hypoechoic lipoma (*cursors*) in subcutaneous tissue of the breast.

scribed mass; its cut surface is grainy and white. Microscopically, the tumor is composed of a fibroelastic stroma with glandular areas forming cystic spaces (25). On ultrasound examination, a fibroadenoma appears as an ovoid mass that is sharply circumscribed, has a homogeneous and hypoechoic internal pattern, and may display posterior enhancement (Fig. 22). Bilateral edge shadowing may occur and is related to bending of the sound wave on the edge of the fibroadenoma's smooth surface. On occasion, fibroadenomas, particularly those that are degenerating, can appear heterogeneous due to internal calcification.

Lipoma

Lipoma is a fatty tumor that occurs in the stroma of the breast. On ultrasound examination it appears as very well-circumscribed lesion that is isoechoic to fat (Fig. 23).

Intraductal Papilloma

Intraductal papilloma is a benign tumor that is usually located beneath the areola; it can grow to a large size and present as a palpable mass. Most often, it presents with bloody nipple drainage. Microscopically it is composed of a fibrovascular core of tissue that extends into the ducts. On ultrasound, it can be identified as an irregular hyperechoic solid mass within the ducts (Fig. 24).

Cancer

The defining sonographic characteristic of breast malignancy is that of irregularity. Carcinoma often has irregular margins, and is hypoechoic and heterogeneous in its interior resulting from areas of proliferation and necrosis that cause irregular posterior shadowing (Fig. 25). In ad-

dition, malignancies tend to violate tissue planes, making them "taller than they are wide," and frequently span several tissue layers. Inflammatory carcinoma demonstrates surrounding tissue edema that manifests as a thickened hypoechoic skin layer on ultrasound.

Phylloides Tumor

This stromal tumor is related to but distinct from fibroadenoma. Grossly, it is softer than fibroadenoma and appears more lobulated. It appears well defined on sections but can display invasion into the surrounding normal breast tissue. The cut surface is brown and necrotic (30). The diagnosis is made on both histologic examination and tumor size. Generally, microscopic examination reveals a tumor that is largely cellular and displays significant pleomorphism (25). On sonographic examination, it may be confused with fibroadenoma. Suspicion for phylloides tumor may be related to its increased size, heterogeneous interior, and invasive character.

Diagnostic Discriminants

Various sonographic characteristics occur predominantly in association with certain benign or malignant breast lesions and may suggest a differential diagnosis of an abnormal finding. Although none of these characteristics is

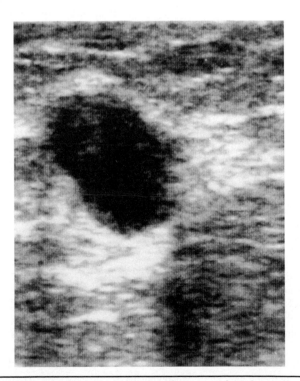

FIGURE 24. Ultrasound image of an intraductal papilloma demonstrating primarily cystic (anechoic) component but with substantial solid component as well.

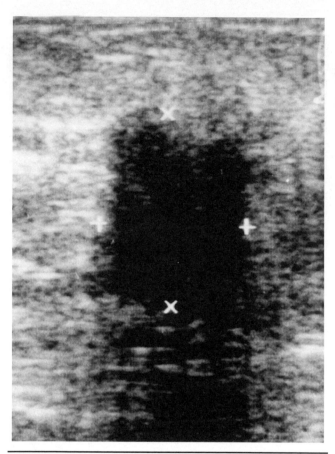

FIGURE 25. Ultrasound image of an infiltrating carcinoma (*cursors*) demonstrating irregular margins, hypoechoic heterogeneous interior, and posterior shadowing.

100% specific, these so-called diagnostic discriminants, combined with physical examination and mammography, may be useful in identifying lesions that are sufficiently suspicious to warrant histopathologic evaluation (5,31) (Table 3). For example, smooth, well-defined margins support the diagnosis of a benign lesion, whereas ir-

▶ **TABLE 3** **Diagnostic Discriminants of Ultrasonographically Visualized Breast Masses**

	Benign	Malignant
Margins	Smooth, sharp	Irregular, indistinct
Echogenicity	Anechoic or hypoechoic	Variable
Internal pattern	None or homogeneous	Heterogeneous
Retrotumoral phenomenon	None or posterior enhancement	Irregular shadowing
Lateral/ anteroposterior dimension	>1	<1

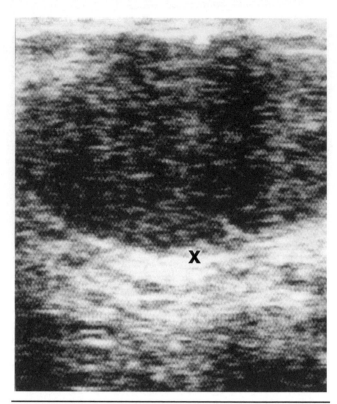

FIGURE 26. Homogeneous, hyporechoic internal pattern in lobular hyperplasia (*cursors*) of the breast in a pregnant patient.

regular or jagged margins, which may be quite indistinct, indicate a malignant lesion (Figs. 26 and 27). Although breast cancer may rarely have a cystic component, most malignant lesions of the breast are, of course, solid. An anechoic (or black-appearing) interior indicates a lesion's homogeneity and is most likely indicative of its being fluid filled (Fig. 21) (5,8). While there are exceptions in other organs, an entirely anechoic lesion of the breast is rarely anything other than a benign simple cyst. Solid breast nodules may be hyperechoic (or white) on ultrasound, although most commonly such nodules are hypoechoic (or gray). Benign solid nodules generally have a homogeneous internal pattern, whereas a heterogeneous internal pattern is more indicative of malignancy (Fig. 28) (5). Microcalcifications occasionally may be recognized with ultrasound when they are within a mass (32). Their detection in an otherwise suspicious mass is strongly suggestive of malignancy. Nevertheless, internal pattern is one of the least specific of the diagnostic discriminants because resolving abscesses, degenerating fibroadenomas, complex cysts, and other benign conditions have a heterogeneous internal pattern. Most benign masses in the breast, particularly cystic lesions, have good through transmission of sound waves resulting in posterior enhancement (Fig. 29). Posterior enhancement is evident in the majority of simple cysts (Fig. 30); exceptions include cysts located near the chest wall and smaller

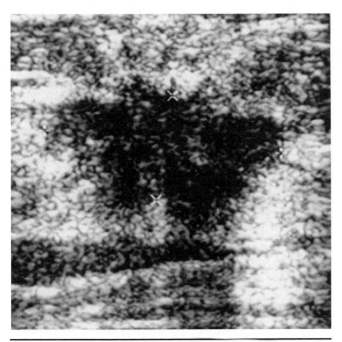

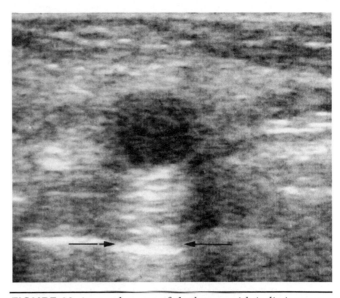

FIGURE 29. A complex cyst of the breast with indistinct margins, a heterogeneous internal pattern, and posterior enhancement (*arrows*).

FIGURE 27. Heterogeneous internal pattern of this invasive ductal carcinoma of the breast (*cursors*). Note the irregular, indistinct margins.

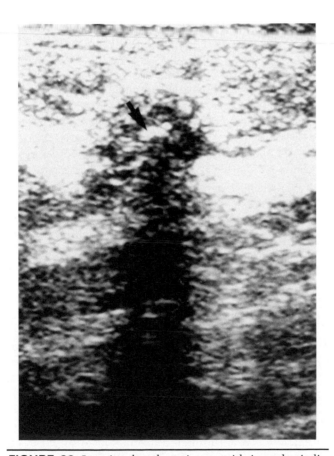

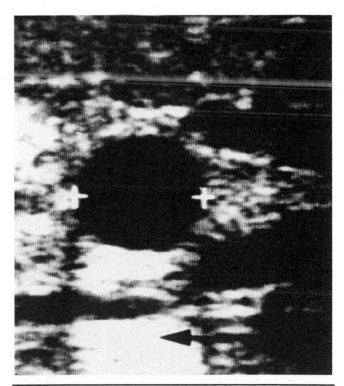

FIGURE 30. An incidentally identified cyst (*cursors*) demonstrating posterior enhancement (*arrow*).

FIGURE 28. Invasive ductal carcinoma with irregular indistinct margins, heterogeneous internal pattern, posterior shadowing, and microcalcifications (*arrow*).

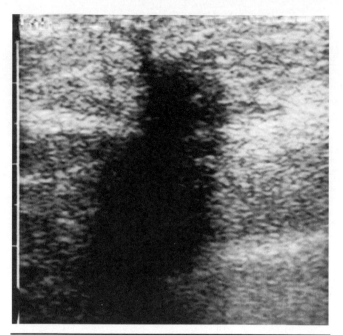

FIGURE 31. Postoperative scar after lumpectomy; note the irregular edges of the area as well as the posterior shadowing. This resembles a carcinoma.

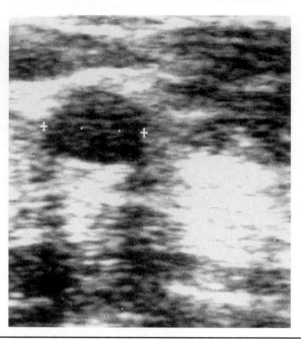

FIGURE 33. An increased lateral (*cursors*) versus anteroposterior dimension in this fibroadenoma of the breast.

cysts, such as those less than 5 mm in diameter. Approximately 25% of fibroadenomas have posterior enhancement. When there is no history of surgery or trauma, posterior shadowing strongly suggests malignancy (Fig. 31) (33). Malignant lesions tend to have irregular posterior

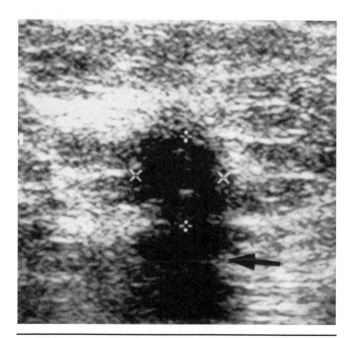

FIGURE 32. Invasive ductal carcinoma (*cursors*); note irregular, indistinct margins, heterogeneous hypoechoic and anechoic interior, and irregular posterior shadowing (*arrow*).

shadowing because of their heterogeneous internal echo pattern (Fig. 32). Sound attenuation or posterior shadowing is a feature of approximately 75% of breast cancers. However, there are exceptions. For example, medullary carcinomas of the breast show regular, smooth borders and may even demonstrate posterior enhancement. Benign lesions, particularly cysts, can generally be compressible, whereas solid lesions, particularly cancers, cannot. Finally, orientation of benign solid nodules of the breast is most often parallel to the skin; hence, the nodules do not appear to disrupt the normal anatomic structures of the breast. These lesions tend to have a lateral dimension that is greater than their anteroposterior (AP) dimension (Fig. 33). Consistent with their infiltrative nature, which disrupts normal architecture, malignant lesions often have a lateral AP dimension ratio that is less than 1 (i.e., taller than wide) (Figs. 25 and 32).

Ultrasound Classification

Using the diagnostic discriminants, breast masses can be classified with some reliability into various categories. Depending on the category in which a mass is placed, it may be selected for observation as opposed to aspiration or biopsy (Table 4). Most *simple cysts* are readily classified by their smooth, well-defined margins, anechoic interior, and good through transmission with posterior enhancement (Figs. 34 and 35) (5–9). On ultrasound, a classic *fibroadenoma* also has smooth, well-defined mar-

▶ TABLE 4 Categories of Ultrasonographically Visualized Breast Masses

	Simple Cyst	Fibroadenoma	Indeterminate	Suspicious
Margins	Sharp, smooth	Sharp, smooth	Usually sharp, usually smooth, may be indistinct	Irregular, indistinct, jagged
Echogenicity	Anechoic	Hypoechoic	Variable anechoic, hypoechoic	Almost anechoic, hypoechoic
Internal pattern	None	Homogeneous	Heterogeneous	Heterogeneous
Retrotumoral phenomenon	Posterior enhancement	Posterior enhancement, bilateral edge shadowing	Posterior enhancement	Irregular shadowing or none
Compressibility	Yes	None	Variable	None
Lateral/ anteroposterior dimension	Variable	>1	Variable	<1

gins and occasionally posterior enhancement (Fig. 36) (6,34). Most fibroadenomas have a homogeneous, hypoechoic internal pattern, although this can be variable. They may have bilateral, symmetric edge shadowing as well. The *indeterminate* category is characterized by complex cysts as well as by lesions for which ultrasound is ineffective in making a clear distinction between solid and cystic lesions (Fig. 37) (12). Difficulty in making this distinction may be encountered with thick, viscous, fluid-filled cysts particularly, which cause a hypoechoic inter-

nal feature but often demonstrate posterior enhancement. Even under real-time examination by an experienced sonographer using high-quality equipment, such a lesion may be relatively indistinguishable from a solid nodule. Atypical characteristics leading to a lesion being placed in the *complex* cyst category are identified in approximately 25% of cases of ultrasound-diagnosed breast cysts (20). Suspicious lesions are characterized by irregular, indistinct borders, and inhomogeneous internal patterns that are primarily hypoechoic or anechoic (Fig. 38) (5). These lesions are generally noncompressible, have ir-

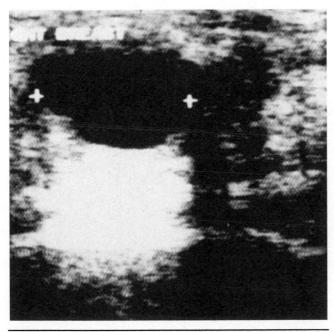

FIGURE 34. Simple cyst of the breast (*cursors*) characterized by smooth, well-defined borders, anechoic interior, and good through transmission with posterior enhancement.

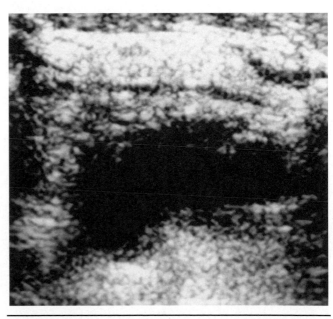

FIGURE 35. Cyst demonstrating posterior enhancement.

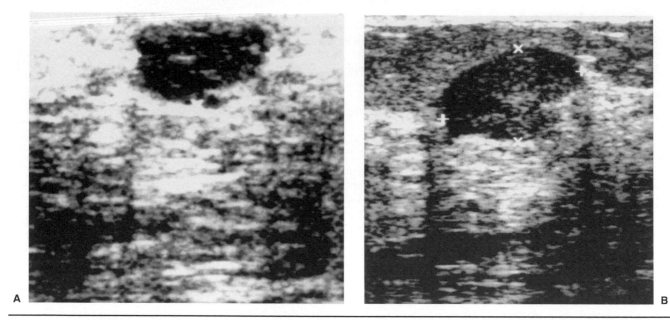

FIGURE 36. A: Fibroadenoma of the breast (*cursors*) demonstrating smooth, reasonably well-defined margins; a homogeneous, hypoechoic internal pattern; a lateral to anteroposterior ratio greater than 1; and bilateral symmetric edge shadowing. **B:** Atypical fibroadenoma (*cursors*) with irregular, notched borders.

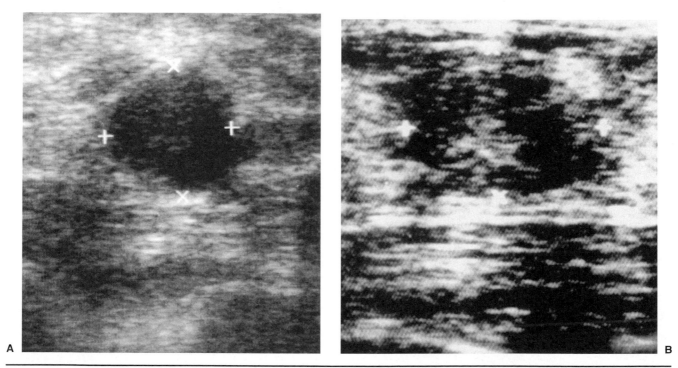

FIGURE 37. A: Indeterminate solid as opposed to cystic lesion (*cursors*) with hypoechoic, heterogeneous internal pattern and indistinct margins, but with posterior enhancement, which, on needle aspiration, was demonstrated to be a thick fluid-filled cyst. **B:** Complex cyst (*cursors*) shown to contain debris on dynamic ultrasound.

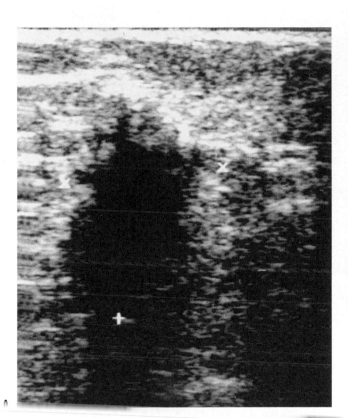
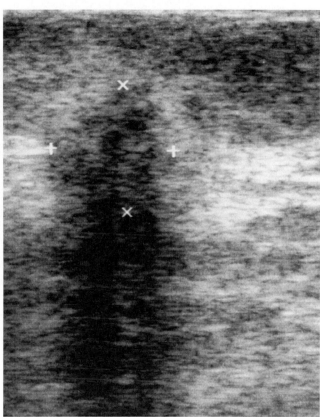

FIGURE 38. Invasive ductal carcinoma of the breast (*cursors*) characterized by irregular indistinct borders, a heterogeneous internal pattern. **A:** Primarily anechoic. **B:** Primarily hypoechoic; an increased anteroposterior versus lateral dimension, and irregular posterior shadowing.

regular posterior shadowing, and often have an increased AP dimension as compared with their lateral dimension.

Although there is some overlap in ultrasound characteristics and therefore in classification, these characteristics may also be used to separate probably solid breast lesions into groups of low, intermediate, or high risk for malignancy (6,12). Low-risk lesions are those with a homogeneous and hypoechoic interior, a well-circumscribed ovoid shape, sharp smooth borders, and a thin echogenic rim. They generally have strong posterior enhancement secondary to good through transmission. These are mostly fibroadenomas and fibrocystic breast, but also include a substantial number of thick fluid-filled cysts. Most of these lesions should undergo ultrasound-guided aspiration and/or core biopsy, if solid; if found to be benign, they may be safely observed. Intermediate-risk lesions are often lobulated with a heterogeneous, hypoechoic interior pattern. They are most frequently large fibroadenomas, and occasionally complex cysts; however, about 10% to 15% will be found to be cancerous (13,20). High-risk lesions correspond to the "suspicious" category. Essentially all high-risk and some intermediate-risk lesions require definitive excision. Ultrasound-guided bi-

opsy may be useful for better characterizing these lesions prior to open procedures, but only clearly benign lesions (i.e., cysts, fibroadenomas) may be safely observed.

NEW BREAST ULTRASOUND IMAGING MODALITIES

Color Doppler Ultrasound

Doppler ultrasound has been proposed for some time as an effective means to establish the vascularity of breast tumors (Fig. 39) (35). Since neoplastic growth requires neovascularization, the use of color Doppler to ascertain the presence of increased blood flow has been proposed as a tool both to differentiate malignant from benign lesions and to estimate the likelihood of axillary nodal metastases (36). In an early study by Srivastava et al. (35), Doppler flow was used to determine the presence or absence of vascularity in 108 discrete breast lumps. The histopathology was then correlated with the preoperatively determined vascular status. The authors found significantly higher Doppler flow signals in the malignant

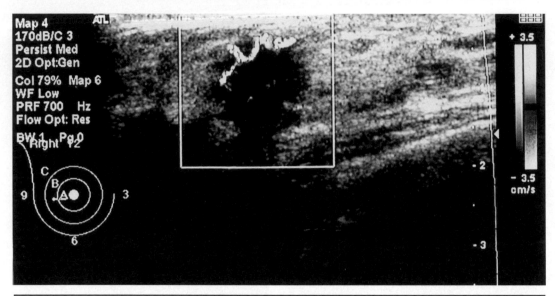

FIGURE 39. Color Doppler ultrasound of an infiltrating carcinoma of the breast demonstrating vascularity.

lumps as compared with benign lumps and normal breast.

The resistance index (RI) is based on a high velocity signal due to arteriovenous malformations within the tumor and low diastolic flow. The significance of the RI was previously investigated by Choi et al. (37) In this study, 106 breast masses were identified; 64 were benign and 42 were malignant. An RI greater than 0.7 was found in more than 80% of malignant tumors. Power Doppler ultrasound is a modality in which the energy of the signal and not its frequency is encoded (38); it is more sensitive to low-volume and low-velocity blood flow. Milz et al. classified tumors as being of low, intermediate, and high flow using this approach (39). Seventy-four percent of benign lesions were classified as either no or low flow, and 80% of invasive breast cancers were categorized as intermediate or high flow. Madjar et al. evaluated the flow characteristics of malignancies in 258 color Doppler examinations performed on clinical, mammographic, and ultrasound-detected breast abnormalities (40). The masses and the number of vessels emerging from the margin of the tumor were recorded, as were the RIs. Among 172 benign abnormalities, the majority were avascular; only 8% had more than three vessels. Among 82 cancers, none were avascular and only three cases involved fewer than two vessels. These studies have shown that color or power Doppler ultrasound may be helpful as an additional diagnostic discriminant to classify breast lumps.

THREE-DIMENSIONAL ULTRASOUND

Three-dimensional ultrasound is a relatively new modality that allows for three-dimensional reconstruction of two-dimensionally acquired images. This technique is somewhat similar to the means by which computed tomography allows for three-dimensional reconstructions. Recreation of the three-dimensional anatomy of the breast requires integration of multiple two-dimensional images. This information can then be used both for diagnosis and for ultrasound-guided interventions. Three-dimensional ultrasound obviates the need for the user to recreate the anatomy abstractly and may thereby circumvent interpretation ambiguity. Several types of three-dimensional ultrasound setups have been described, but they all require the ultrasound machine to obtain information regarding the precise location and orientation of each of the rapidly acquired two-dimensional images. To this end, mechanical scanners and freehand scanning, with and without position sensing, are required (41). Weismann et al. (42) evaluated the use of three-dimensional ultrasound in determining the correct position of the core biopsy needle within the target lesion. They suggested that in a significant number of cases three-dimensional ultrasound contributed important information regarding accurate needle positioning for core needle biopsy. Despite such reports, the specific indications for three-dimensional breast ultrasound are to date undefined and its use is primarily considered to be investigational.

INTERVENTIONAL BREAST ULTRASOUND

A direct corollary of the increase in mammographic screening examinations has been the identification of increased numbers of nonpalpable breast lesions that require further diagnostic evaluation, often including biopsy. The majority of patients with nonpalpable, mammographically detected lesions designated as sufficiently suspicious to warrant localization and biopsy are found to have benign diseases and therefore are subjected to an unnecessary operation (43–45). In fact, most series report a yield of only approximately 20% to 30% for malignant diagnosis. Stereotactic biopsy, pioneered by investigators in Sweden and then brought to the United States by Dowlatshahi, has been demonstrated to be an extremely accurate modality for the evaluation of nonpalpable breast lesions. The success of stereotactic needle biopsy appears to have been enhanced by the availability of spring-loaded, automated core biopsy needles and now by the availability of percutaneous vacuum-assisted biopsy devices. These have been shown to reliably obtain histologic specimens allowing for definitive diagnoses of both benign and malignant diseases of the breast (46,47). Nguyen et al. (48) reported a 99% sensitivity and 100% specificity with a false-negative rate of 1.7%. This false-negative rate is comparable to that recently reported by Jackman et al. (49).

Concurrent to this period of mammographic technical advancement, significant improvements have been made in ultrasound as well (50,51). The improved ultrasound image that resulted from developments such as computer enhancement and high- and multifrequency transducers allowed for better separation of breast lesions according to their relative risk of malignancy (6,7,52). By using this information in addition to that already gleaned from physical examination plus screening and diagnostic mammography, better decisions could be made as to the need for breast biopsy. Furthermore, when appropriate, ultrasound can also be used as a convenient guide for aspiration or biopsy (53–58). Ultrasound-guided core biopsy has been demonstrated to have a comparable accuracy to traditional needle localization and open breast biopsy. A logical transition of breast ultrasound from solely an imaging diagnostic tool to a safe, rapid, and reliable means of guiding tissue access for pathologic diagnosis and intervention has occurred.

Management (Table 5)

When a patient presents with a new or increasing-in-size breast mass detected by mammography, the next step should be a thorough physical examination to confirm that the lesion is nonpalpable (Table 5). Not infrequently, with orientation from the mammogram, an experienced examiner may be able to palpate a lesion previously thought to be nonpalpable. Should such a circumstance occur, then we would recommend management of the palpable nodule as is per routine (i.e., fine needle aspiration or core needle biopsy, followed by appropriate inter-

▶ TABLE 5 Indications for Interventional Breast Ultrasound

1. Needle guidance
   Biopsy: fine needle aspiration cytology, core needle biopsy
   Aspiration: cyst, fluid, etc.
2. Catheter guidance
   Drainage: abscess, fluid, etc.
3. Cannula or probe guidance
   Cryoablation
   Thermal (radiofrequency) ablation
4. Tissue dissection guidance
   Intraoperative guidance of biopsy or excision

vention if required). Ultrasound may be quite helpful when a vaguely palpable abnormality corresponds to a mammographically detected lesion. Certainly if no mass is palpable, we would usually perform an ultrasound of the breast at the time of the initial clinic visit.

If a nonpalpable breast lesion identified by mammogram is determined on diagnostic ultrasound to be a simple cyst, no further intervention is required (18,19). This is the case with the majority of lesions newly identified on screening mammography (57). It is our practice, however, to perform aspiration in patients with symptomatic

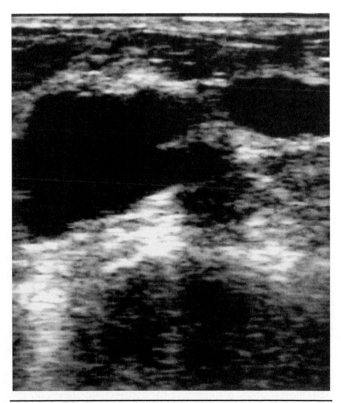

FIGURE 40. Multiple and superficial areas of gross cystic change demonstrated on ultrasound.

(i.e., painful) cysts and cysts sufficiently large as to interfere with optimal mammography and/or physical examination (Fig. 40). Ultrasound can be quite helpful in simplifying aspiration of painful cysts which, despite causing significant discomfort, may be difficult to locate precisely or to puncture due to an often thick wall.

As indicated previously, the need for an ultrasound-guided biopsy is determined on the basis of classification of the lesion according to various diagnostic discriminants and, therefore, levels of risk. While asymptomatic simple cysts may be safely observed, we recommend ultrasound-guided biopsy of most low-risk and all intermediate- and high-risk lesions. Therefore, we needle biopsy all indeterminate or suspicious lesions as well as lesions viewed as probable fibroadenomas on diagnostic ultrasound.

Technique of Ultrasound-Guided Aspiration

Like diagnostic ultrasound, interventional ultrasound of the breast is generally performed with the patient supine and with the ipsilateral hand placed behind the head. It may be helpful to have patients with large or pendulous breasts lie in a more lateral position, thereby rotating the breast toward the midline. This rotation is particularly helpful when evaluating more laterally placed lesions because it allows for thinning of the breast necessary for maximal sound transmission (1). We generally scan a

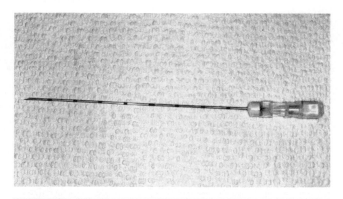

FIGURE 42. Ultra-Vu procedure needle with a roughened echogenic tip (Becton–Dickinson, Rutherford, NJ).

one-fourth to one-half wedge of the breast in a radial manner using the nipple as an axis around any mammographically detected lesion. It is important to scan a wide enough area of the breast to ensure adequate visualization; a nodule identified while a breast is compressed during mammographic examination may move quite a distance when that compression is removed.

For those lesions placed in the indeterminate category on diagnostic ultrasound, most often we first perform a fine needle aspiration to determine if the lesion is in fact cystic (Fig. 41). This is the case in nearly all of the presumed complex cysts and approximately half of the questionable solid as opposed to cystic lesions (58). It has been our practice to use a 20-gauge spinal-type needle with a roughened echogenic tip that is acutely angled for needle aspiration biopsy (Fig. 42). We have found a Franseen needle to be adequate for obtaining histologic as well as cytologic information for those lesions determined to be solid. However, in most circumstances where histologic examination is required, we prefer a spring-loaded automated needle to perform the biopsy.

Authors vary in their recommendations regarding the use of a freehand versus biopsy-guide technique for ultrasound-guided breast aspiration or biopsy (Fig. 43) (20, 57). The objective with both techniques is to maintain the needle in a longitudinal plane to the long axis of the transducer, thereby allowing for constant visualization of the needle along its path from the skin to the lesion (detailed in Chapter 4). Particularly when the operator is first beginning to perform ultrasound-guided procedures, the biopsy guide is useful because it greatly facilitates maintenance of the needle within this plane (21). However, even for an operator with relatively little experience, the attachment of the biopsy guide adds little to the procedure and may limit ease of altering the angle of approach. This is particularly true in those individuals with small, dense breasts and in whom a small lesion is located near the chest wall. Under such a circumstance, the

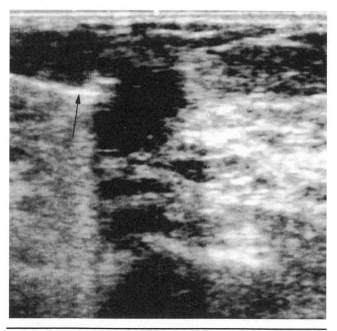

FIGURE 41. Ultrasound-guided fine needle aspiration of an indeterminate breast lesion. Note the hyperechoic line on the left (*arrow*) depicting the needle within the breast.

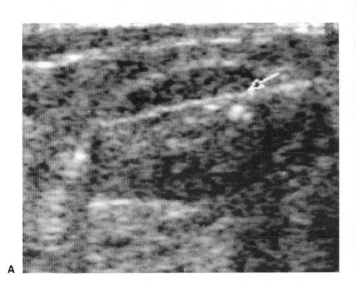
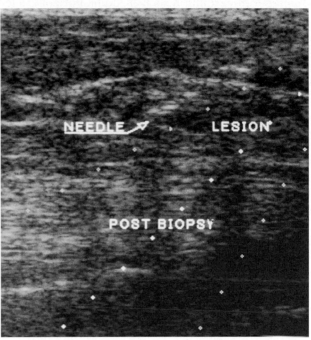

A

B

FIGURE 43. A: Hyperechoic white line representing a needle (*arrow*) entering a solid breast mass and utilizing a freehand technique. **B:** Demonstration of a biopsy needle maintained in a longitudinal axis along ultrasound cursors as a result of its placement through a biopsy guide.

freehand technique allows for an approach that avoids the possibility of "past pointing" the lesion into the chest wall with potential pneumothorax.

It has been our practice to routinely clean the ultrasound transducers between uses with germicidal wipes followed by a soak in a dialdehyde solution for approximately 10 minutes. While the transducer is soaking, the patient may be instructed as to the procedure and potential, albeit rare, associated complications.

When performing an ultrasound-guided aspiration/biopsy, we prefer to use one of the readily available minor-surgery or biopsy kits (Fig. 44). These kits include syringes for aspiration and local anesthetic instillation, needles of varying gauges, sterile gauzes, alcohol wipes, a

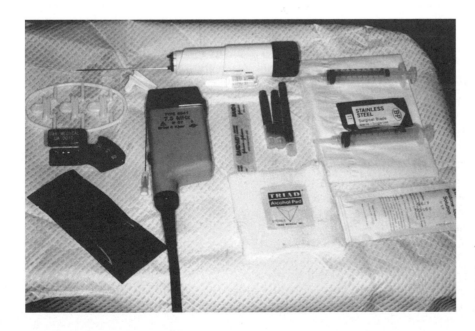

FIGURE 44. Ultrasound biopsy kit containing needles, fenestrated drape, iodine-povidone solution, syringes, no. 11 blade, alcohol wipes, gauze sponges, and adhesive bandage.

skin preparation solution such as iodine-povidone, a fenestrated drape, and an adhesive bandage. When the patient has been prepared and draped, we rescan the appropriate area briefly to determine the optimal orientation of the transducer for needle insertion. Even with fairly superficial lesions, we generally instill a small amount (2 to 3 mL) of local anesthetic under ultrasound guidance. This serves both to calm the patient as to the relative painlessness of the procedure and to numb much of the area involved should a larger needle (e.g., core) be required for biopsy. We then orient the lesion in the center of the monitor, anticipating the appropriate angle of approach. Under real-time imaging, we carefully monitor advancement of the long 20-gauge needle into the lesion. If the lesion is cystic, we aspirate until it is resolved. We generally discard fluid from simple cysts that does not have any appearance of blood. Fluid from complicated cysts with suspicious characteristics, such as those that do not completely resolve, and fluid that appears bloody is sent for cytologic examination.

Technique of Ultrasound-Guided Biopsy

Should the diagnostic ultrasound procedure result in identification of a solid nodule warranting biopsy or should the attempted fine needle aspiration of an indeterminate lesion determine that it is in fact wholly or partially solid, then we perform a core biopsy using a spring-loaded, automated biopsy device (Figs. 45 and 46A) (57). These biopsy devices work on a two-step firing mechanism that results in reliable procurement of a small piece of tissue. Rapid firing of a notched inner sheath is followed immediately by an outer cannula that traps a piece of tissue from within the lesion. In most circumstances, we use a large-gauge needle (i.e., 14-gauge) to perform these core biopsies and have found no increase in complications as compared with the smaller needles (i.e., 16 or 18 gauge). Furthermore, an advantage to using the larger gauge is a decrease in indeterminate pathology diagnoses caused by insufficient or inadequate tissue samples.

As is the case with fine needle aspiration, after briefly soaking the transducer in dialdehyde solution, we perform a quick ultrasound scanning of the relevant area of the breast to determine optimal transducer orientation for needle placement. If not done so already, this area is anesthetized from the skin down along the anticipated biopsy path, to and around the lesion to be biopsied. When using the larger gauge needle for core biopsy, it is necessary to make a very small nick approximately 2 to 3 mm long in the skin with a no. 11 stainless steel blade. This facilitates advancement of the needle through the otherwise resistant dermis and epidermis. A coaxial needle may be inserted and left in place as a tract for the biopsy

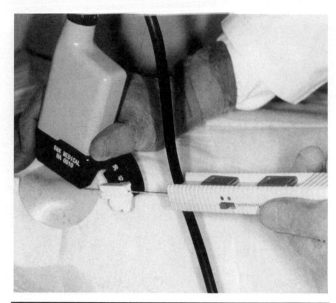

FIGURE 45. Technique of ultrasound-guided core needle biopsy of a breast lesion using a disposable biopsy guide attached to the transducer.

needle itself. The biopsy gun is advanced through the biopsy guide attachment (if utilized), skin, subcutaneous tissues, and breast parenchyma up to the lesion (Fig. 46B). It is then fired through the lesion a minimum of three times to ensure adequate sampling (Fig. 46C). We have found that it is seldom necessary to go through the lesion more than five passes at most, assuming adequate ultrasound image and evidence of an expected pathologic process. The specimen may then be sent for routine histopathologic evaluation or, rarely, a frozen section examination depending on the circumstances and desires of the patient and physician (Figs. 47 and 48). In general, frozen sections are not encouraged due to the small amount of tissue available and the expected distortion of specimens not evaluated by standard Hematoxylin and Eosin staining. When the procedure is complete, pressure is held over the biopsy area and skin nick for approximately 5 minutes. If no oozing is identified at that point, a simple adhesive bandage is placed over the wound.

Complications

A pathologically detected hematoma may occur after image-guided biopsy; however, this is seldom clinically relevant when appropriate caution regarding patient history and proper techniques are exercised. We have not had to drain a hematoma in any of the more than 1,000 patients on whom we have performed an ultrasound-guided needle aspiration or core biopsy. The possibility of pneumothorax exists with any needle biopsy of a breast mass. However, this complication is extremely rare, partic-

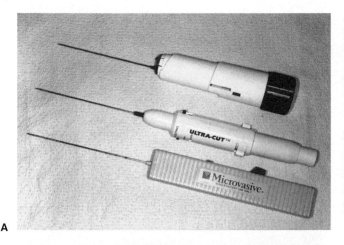

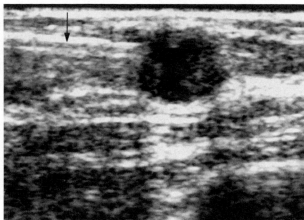

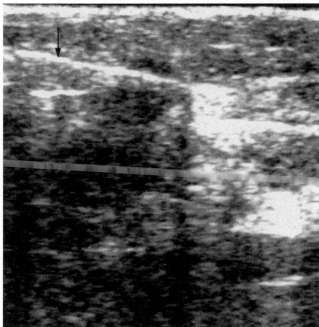

FIGURE 46. A: Examples of automated core needle biopsy guns. **B, C:** Ultrasound image using a freehand technique of a core needle biopsy (*arrow*) adjacent to (**B**) and through (**C**) of a small breast cancer.

ularly with appropriate angulation of the needle and constant ultrasound visualization of the needle throughout its path. Although infection is a potential complication of any interventional procedure, it has seldom been reported in association with ultrasound-guided needle biopsy of a breast mass. Patients may be told to expect very mild discomfort or ecchymosis of the breast in some cases.

Biopsy Accuracy

We and others have demonstrated the high degree of accuracy associated with ultrasound-guided biopsy of breast masses (Table 6). Fornage used ultrasound to guide fine needle aspiration of solid breast masses and reported 91% accuracy (20). In a more recent study, Parker and col-

leagues compared ultrasound-guided automated core biopsy with routine surgical biopsy of breast masses and reported 100% accuracy with this technique (22). In fact, because of its relative ease of use, rapid performance, lack of ionizing radiation, patient acceptance, and accuracy, those physicians familiar with both ultrasonographic and stereotactic biopsy techniques are increasingly expressing preference for the former with lesions identifiable by both modalities (20,21,59). Staren et al. evaluated ultrasound-guided core needle biopsy in the clinician's office (60). Of 210 patients who underwent the procedure, 53 of 55 cancer patients were found to have concordance of their needle and open biopsy pathology. No cancers were identified at a median follow-up of 18 months among those who had negative core needle biopsies.

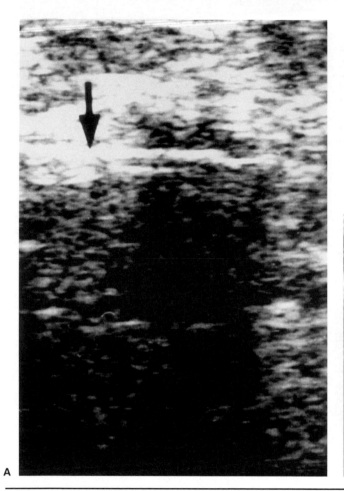

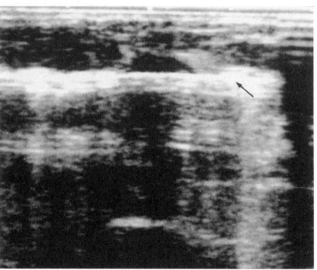

A   B

FIGURE 47. A: Ultrasound image of a core needle (*arrow*) incompletely penetrating a suspicious breast lesion, increasing the risk of an inadequate biopsy specimen. **B:** Satisfactory penetration of this lesion; note needle (*arrow*) completely firing through area in question.

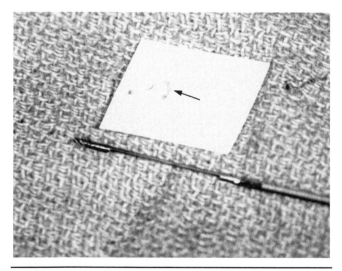

FIGURE 48. Tissue (*arrow*) obtained from a single pass of a core biopsy needle into a solid breast mass.

Visualization of a suspicious, nonpalpable breast lesion by both ultrasound and mammogram may be anticipated to occur in more than two thirds of cases. Diagnostic ultrasound may fail to identify mammographically

▶ **TABLE 6 Advantages of Ultrasound-Guided Breast Biopsy**

1. Ultrasound-guided biopsy uses real-time.
2. Ultrasound is accurate as stereotactic biopsy.
3. No ionizing radiation delivered.
4. Color Doppler is available to assess blood flow to lesion.
5. Ultrasound-guided biopsy is easier for elderly patients who have difficulty negotiating the position required for stereotactic biopsy.
6. Lesions that are difficult to biopsy stereotactically due to proximity to chest wall or skin, or which cannot be visualized stereotactically, may be more easily accessed with ultrasound.

identified lesions (masses) in approximately 10% of cases (57). Particularly problematic lesions are those that are small (≤0.5 cm). Stereotactic mammography is still the preferred method of localization and biopsy for lesions 5 mm or smaller, for indeterminate or suspicious microcalcifications of the breast not associated with a mass, and for any lesion not visualized by ultrasound (4,20,57).

INTERVENTIONAL BREAST ULTRASOUND: OTHER USES

Preoperative and Intraoperative Uses

As ultrasound-guided interventional procedures on the breast become more routine, the potential for expanded use increases dramatically (Table 7). For example, real-time ultrasound is increasingly being used as a localization procedure prior to definitive excision of nonpalpable pathologically "atypical" or "suspicious" lesions and breast cancers (Fig. 49). (18,23). The technique may be performed in the operating room immediately prior to the open excision with the patient placed on the same table and in the same position as for the operative procedure. This substantially decreases the overall time required for needle localization and open biopsy because the procedures can be performed in the same setting. It may also facilitate the surgical procedure itself because the wire can be placed in the most direct path to the lesion in question (61).

Moore et al. (62) discussed results of intraoperative ultrasound-guided breast biopsy in a study group of 51 patients with nonpalpable lesions determined to be malignant on needle biopsy. Those biopsies performed with the aid of intraoperative ultrasound yielded a significantly lower rate (3.5% versus 29%) of positive margins in this study.

Other Uses of Interventional Ultrasound

A newly described technique is that of ultrasound-guided biopsy using the traumatic hematoma created after needle biopsy as a localization guide. Smith et al. (63) described such a technique utilizing MRI in patients with nonpalpable breast lesions. The authors identified patients whose lesions were only visible on MRI and created a hematoma at the site of the lesion. The hematomas were then used as the target for biopsy under intraoperative ultrasound. Radiopaque and sonographically identifiable clips may also be deployed at the time of spring-loaded core needle or mammotome-type biopsy and used for identification of lesions intraoperatively.

Palpation is a relatively inaccurate method of identifying axillary lymph node involvement in patients with

TABLE 7 Other Uses for Interventional Breast Ultrasound

1. Pre- and intraoperative use
   Localization and excisional guidance
2. Lymph node fine needle aspiration
3. Abscess drainage
4. Tumor ablation
   Cryoablation
   Thermal (radiofrequency) ablation

breast cancer. However, when axillary lymph nodes are identified by ultrasound in such a patient, the majority will be found to contain metastatic disease. Yang et al. (64) reported a sensitivity and specificity of 84.1% and 97.1%, respectively, for identifying positive nodes in 114 patients with breast carcinoma. Parker et al. (65) described a technique for identification of involved axillary nodes in breast cancer that utilizes both technetium-labeled sulfur colloid and ultrasound. Ultrasound was utilized to identify sonographically abnormal nodes; if none were present, they then utilized the ultrasound to direct the placement of a hook wire into the radiolabeled lymph node so as to facilitate excision. Verbanck et al. (66) reported 92% sensitivity and 95% specificity in detection of malignant nodes in patients with breast cancer. For ultrasound-guided biopsy of suspicious adenopathy, fine needle aspiration should be used rather than automated core biopsy due to the close proximity of vessels and nerves. We generally use a 20-gauge cutting-type needle to obtain histologic as well as cytologic evidence.

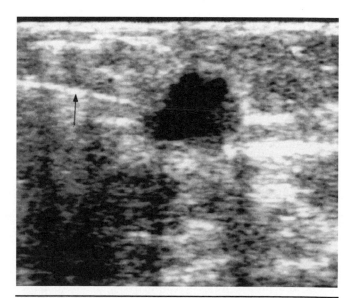

FIGURE 49. Ultrasound-guided placement of a localization wire (*arrow*) into a suspicious breast mass prior to open surgical excision.

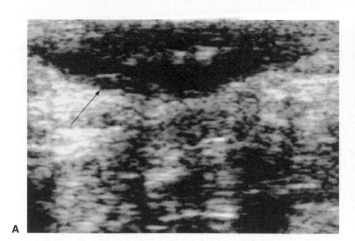
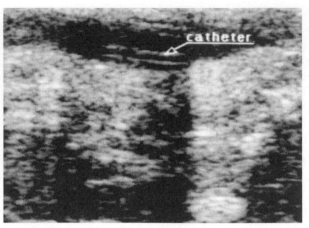

FIGURE 50. **A:** A 4-cm superficial abscess (*arrow*) in a nonlactating breast. **B:** Ultrasound-guided placement of a drainage catheter (*arrow*) into a breast abscess.

Standard treatment of breast abscesses is a surgical incision under general anesthesia, wound packing, stopping lactation if applicable, and antibiotics. In addition to being traumatic, this procedure is associated with anesthetic risk and generally poor aesthetic results. Karstrup and colleagues reported on 20 breast abscesses in 19 patients treated successfully by ultrasound-guided drainage (Fig. 50) (14). Transducers were equipped with a puncture attachment through which a 5.7- to 7-Fr one-step pigtail catheter could be introduced. The catheter was advanced under ultrasound guidance through a small skin nick made using local anesthesia. When pus was aspirated, the catheter was connected to a closed drainage system and the cavity was flushed with saline until the effluent was clear. The patient was released to home and instructed to flush the cavity six times daily. The instillation of antibiotics did not prove to be necessary. The cavity was evaluated by ultrasound two or three times per week until it collapsed and the clinical condition had normalized. It was not necessary to interrupt lactation. In this series, 95% of patients were cured. In one patient, the catheter fell out and open surgical drainage was required. With follow-up of 2 to 60 months, there were no recurrences and the cosmetic results were excellent.

Numerous reports have demonstrated that ultrasound-guided placement of sclerosing agents (e.g., alcohol) and particularly thermal ablative tools may be used to manage primary and secondary neoplasms in organs such as liver, prostate, parathyroid, and kidney (67,68). In our laboratory we have used cryotherapy to ablate inducible and transplantable mammary adenocarcinomas in rat and mouse models, respectively. In addition, we have demonstrated that ultrasound-guided cryosurgery of hyperplastic breast tissue in large animal models is well tolerated with a high correlation between the ultra-

sound-visualized ice ball and the subsequent area of histopathologic necrosis. This technique is currently being evaluated as a treatment for select patients with early-stage breast cancer (Fig. 51). Cryoablation techniques cause tumor cell death by causing crystallization within the tumor cell. Rui et al. examined the thermal variables that optimize crystallization and therefore cell death (69). They found that increased cooling rates were associated with a higher probability of causing intracellular crystallization. Moreover, they found that a double freezing cycle was more effective for achieving complete cell death. With this in mind, we have used the "double freeze–thaw cycle" under ultrasound monitoring of the freezing progress. A zone of frozen tumor is created that expands radially from the tip of the probe and can be visualized with real-time ultrasound as a heterogeneous hypoechoic region with posterior shadowing (70). Patient selection for these modalities is currently being defined, but it is accepted that the optimal tumors for which these modalities can be attempted should be smaller than 2 cm in diameter and must be amenable to visualization by ultrasound. Preliminary reports suggest 100% tumor necrosis in properly selected patients.

Radiofrequency ablation of breast cancer was initially described by Jeffrey et al. (71). The proposed mechanism of action of this technique is that heat is generated as a result of friction caused by tissue ions following high-frequency alternating current. Radiofrequency ablation of breast tumors has been carried out under ultrasound guidance followed by lumpectomy or mastectomy. M.D. Anderson Cancer Center reports a 100% tumor cell necrosis in 94% of patients enrolled in their study (72). This group has initiated a multiinstitutional trial evaluating radiofrequency ablation of breast cancers left in situ after treatment.

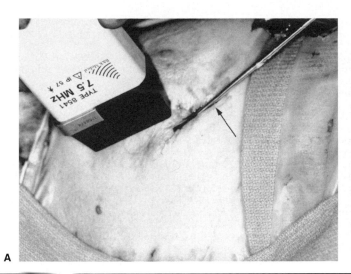
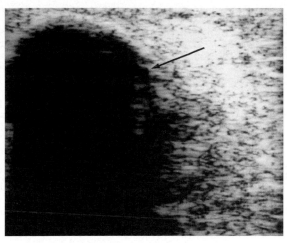

A   B

FIGURE 51. **A:** Ultrasound-guided placement of cryoprobe (*arrow*) in a breast lesion. **B:** Ultrasound image of cryolesion (i.e., "ice ball") (*arrow*) formed during cryotherapy of a breast cancer. This cryolesion is associated with posterior shadowing.

CONCLUSIONS

It is clear that ultrasound is settling into a well-established role in the diagnosis and management of breast abnormalities. In addition to the radiology department, it is now common to find ultrasound equipment in the surgeon's office or even in the operating room; it has been shown to be effective in their hands. The future holds much promise regarding new methods of delivering local therapy for breast cancer. In addition, further investigations and refinements in technique could help to identify sentinel lymph nodes and be used to direct decisions regarding axillary lymph node dissections. Its noninvasive real-time imaging character and lack of ionizing radiation make ultrasound an attractive alternative to other imaging methods, and in many cases it can be used for definitive management of breast diseases.

REFERENCES

1. Jackson VP. The role of US in breast imaging. *Radiology* 1990;177:305–311.
2. Bassett LW, Kimme-Smith C. Breast sonography. *AJR Am J Roentgenol* 1991;156:449–455.
3. Dempsey PJ. Breast sonography: historical perspective, clinical application, and image interpretation. *Ultrasound Q* 1988;6:69–90.
4. McSweeney MB, Murphy CH. Whole-breast sonography. *Radiol Clin North Am* 1985;23:157–167.
5. Leucht W. *Teaching atlas of breast ultrasound*. New York: Thieme, 1992.
6. Jackson VP, Rothschild PA, Kreipke DL, et al. The spectrum of sonographic findings of fibroadenoma of the breast. *Invest Radiol* 1986;21:34–40.
7. Jackson VP. Sonography of malignant breast disease. *Semin Ultrasound Comput Tomogr Magnet Reson* 1989;10:119–131.
8. Mendelson EB. Breast sonography. In: Rumack CM, Wilson S, Charboneau JW, eds. *Diagnostic ultrasound*. St. Louis: Mosby–Year Book, 1998:751–789.
9. Hackeloer B-J, Duda V, Lauth G. *Ultrasound mammography: methods, results, diagnostic strategies*. New York: Springer-Verlag, 1989.
10. Guyer PB, Dewbury KC. Ultrasound of the breast in the symptomatic and X-ray dense breast. *Clin Radiol* 1985;36:69–76.
11. Jackson VP, Hendrick RE, Feig SA, et al. Imaging of the radiographically dense breast. *Radiology* 1993;188:297–301
12. Staren ED. Surgical office-based ultrasound of the breast. *Am Surg* 1995;61:619–626.
13. Stavros AT, Dennis MA. An introduction to breast ultrasound. In: Parker SH, Jobe WE, eds. *Percutaneous breast biopsy*. New York: Raven Press, 1993:95–109.
14. Karstrup S, Nolsoe C, Brabrand K, et al. Ultrasonically guided percutaneous drainage of breast abscesses. *Acta Radiol* 1990;31:157–159.
15. Levine RA, Collins TL. Definitive diagnosis of breast implant rupture by ultrasonography. *Plast Reconstr Surg* 1991;87:1126–1128.
16. Fornage BD, Faroux MJ, Simatos A. Breast masses: US-guided fine-needle aspiration biopsy. *Radiology* 1987;162:409–414.
17. Staren ED. Ultrasound-guided biopsy of nonpalpable breast masses by surgeons. *Ann Surg Oncol* 1996;3:476–482.
18. Kopans DB, Meyer JE, Lindfors KK, et al. Breast sonography to guide cyst aspiration and wire localization of occult solid lesions. *AJR Am J Roentgenol* 1984;143:489–492.
19. Meyer JE, Christian RL, Frenna TH, et al. Image-guided aspiration of solitary occult breast "cysts." *Arch Surg* 1992;127:433–435.
20. Fornage BD. Interventional ultrasound of the breast. In: McGahan JP, ed. *Interventional ultrasound*. Baltimore: Williams & Wilkins, 1990:71–83.
21. Fornage BD, Coan JD, David CL. Ultrasound-guided needle biopsy of the breast and other interventional procedures. *Radiol Clin North Am* 1992;30:167–185.
22. Parker SH, Jobe WE, Dennis MA, et al. Ultrasound-guided automated large core breast biopsy. *Radiology* 1993;187:507–511.
23. Schwartz GF, Goldberg BB, Rifkin MD, et al. Ultrasonography: an alternative to x-ray-guided needle localization of nonpalpable breast masses. *Surgery* 1988;104:870–873.

24. Teboul M. A new concept in breast investigation. echo-histo-logical acino-ductal analysis or analytic echography. *Biomed Pharmacother* 1988;42:289–295.

25. Lester SC, Cotran RS. The breast. In: Cotran RS, ed. *Robbins pathologic basis of disease*, 6th ed. Philadelphia: WB Saunders, 1999:1093–1120.

26. Lanfranchi ME. *Breast ultrasound*. New York: Marban Books, 2000.

27. Hollinshead WH, Rosse C. *Textbook of anatomy*, 4th ed. Philadelphia: Harper and Row, 1985.

28. Bruneton JN, Caramella E, Hery M, et al. Axillary lymph node metastases in breast cancer: preoperative detection with US. *Radiology* 1986;158:325–326.

29. Nitz U, Kuner R, Rezai M, et al. Axillary sonography in preoperative staging of breast cancer. In: Madjar H, Teubner J, Hackeloer B-J, eds. *Breast ultrasound update: proceedings of the 8th International Congress on the Ultrasonic Examination of the Breast*. Basel: Karger, 1994:220–225.

30. Hughes LE, Mansel RE, Webster DJT. *Benign disorders and diseases of the breast. Concepts and clinical management*, 2nd ed. London: WB Saunders, 2000.

31. Heywang SH, Lipsit ER, Glassman LM, et al. Specificity of ultrasonography in the diagnosis of benign breast masses. *J Ultrasound Med* 1984;3:453–461.

32. Kasumi F. Can microcalcifications located within breast carcinomas be detected by ultrasound imaging? *Ultrasound Med Biol* 1988;14(Suppl 1):175–182.

33. Mendelson EB. Evaluation of the postoperative breast. *Radiol Clin North Am* 1992;30:107–138.

34. Fornage BD, Lorigan JG, Andry E. Fibroadenoma of the breast: sonographic appearance. *Radiology* 1989;172:671–675.

35. Srivastava A, Webster DJT, Woodcock JP, et al. Role of Doppler ultrasound flowmetry in the diagnosis of breast lumps. *Br J Surg* 1988;75:851–853.

36. Chao TC, Luo YF, Chen SC, et al. Color Doppler ultrasound in breast carcinomas: relationship with hormone receptors, DNA ploidy, S-phase fraction, and histopathology. *Ultrasound Med Biol* 2001;27:351–355.

37. Choi HY, Kim HY, Baek SY, et al. Significance of resistive index in color Doppler ultrasonogram: differentiation between benign and malignant breast masses. *Clin Imaging* 1999;23:284–288.

38. Bude RO, Rubin JM. Power Doppler sonography. *Radiology* 1996;200:21–23.

39. Milz P, Lienemann A, Kessler M, et al. Evaluation of breast lesions by power Doppler sonography. *Eur Radiol* 2001;11:547–554.

40. Madjar H, Sauerfrei W, Mundinger A, et al. Color Doppler flow assessment of breast disease. In: Madjar H, Teubner J, Hackeloer B-J, eds. *Breast ultrasound update: proceedings of the 8th International Congress on the Ultrasonic Examination of the Breast*. Basel: Karger, 1994:298–307.

41. Fenster A, Downey DB, Cardinal HN. Three-dimensional ultrasound imaging. *Phys Med Biol* 2001;46:R67–R99.

42. Weismann CF, Forstner R, Prokop E, et al. Three-dimensional targeting: a new three-dimensional ultrasound technique to evaluate needle position during breast biopsy. *Ultrasound Obstet Gynecol* 2000;16:359–364.

43. Sailors DM, Crabtree JD, Land RL, et al. Needle localization for nonpalpable breast lesions. *Am Surg* 1994; 60:186–189.

44. Wilhelm MC, de Paredes ES, Pope T, et al. The changing mammogram. A primary indication for needle localization biopsy. *Arch Surg* 1986;121:1311–1314.

45. Miller RS, Adelman RW, Espinosa MH, et al. The early detection of nonpalpable breast carcinoma with needle localization. Experience with 500 patients in a community hospital. *Am Surg* 1992;58:193–198.

46. Dowlatshahi K, Yaremko ML, Kluskens LF, et al. Nonpalpable breast lesions: findings of stereotaxic needle-core biopsy and fine-needle aspiration cytology. *Radiology* 1991;181:745–750.

47. Parker SH, Lovin JD, Jobe WE, et al. Nonpalpable breast lesions: stereotactic automated large-core biopsies. *Radiology* 1991;180:403–407.

48. Nguyen M, McCombs MM, Ghandehari S, et al. An update on core needle biopsy for radiologically detected breast lesions. *Cancer* 1996;78:2340–2345.

49. Jackman RJ, Nowels KW, Rodriguez-Soto J, et al. Stereotactic, automated, large-core needle biopsy of nonpalpable breast lesions: false negative and histologic underestimation rates after long-term follow-up. *Radiology* 1999;210:799–805.

50. Jokich PM, Monticciolo DL, Adler YT. Breast ultrasonography. *Radiol Clin North Am* 1992;30:993–1009.

51. Bassett LW, Kimme-Smith C. Breast sonography: technique, equipment, and normal anatomy. *Semin Ultrasound Comput Tomogr Magnet Reson* 1989;10:82–89.

52. Sickles EA, Filly RA, Callen PW. Benign breast lesions: ultrasound detection and diagnosis. *Radiology* 1984;151:467–470.

53. Hatada T, Aoki I, Okada K, et al. Usefulness of ultrasound-guided, fine-needle aspiration biopsy for palpable breast tumors. *Arch Surg* 1996;131:1095–1098.

54. Gordon PB, Goldenberg SL, Chan NHL. Solid breast lesions: diagnosis with US-guided fine-needle aspiration biopsy. *Radiology* 1993;189:573–580.

55. Hieken TJ, Velasco JM. A prospective analysis of office-based breast ultrasound. *Arch Surg* 1998;133:504–507.

56. Parker SH. Percutaneous large core breast biopsy. *Cancer* 1994;74:256–262.

57. Velez N, Earnest DE, Staren ED. Diagnostic and interventional ultrasound for breast disease. *Am J Surg* 2000;180:284–287.

58. Louie L, Velez N, Earnest D, Staren ED. Management of nonpalpable ultrasound-indeterminate breast lesions. *Surgery* 2003;134:667–674.

59. Parker SH, Stavros AP. Interventional breast ultrasound. In: Parker SH, Jobe WE, eds. *Percutaneous breast biopsy*. New York: Raven Press, 1993:129–146.

60. Staren ED, O'Neill TP. Ultrasound-guided needle biopsy of the breast. *Surgery* 1999;126(4):629–634.

61. Feig SA. Localization of clinically occult breast lesions. *Radiol Clin North Am* 1983;21:155–171.

62. Moore MM, Whitney LA, Cerilli L, et al. Intraoperative ultrasound is associated with clear lumpectomy margins for palpable infiltrating ductal breast cancer. *Ann Surg* 2001;233:761–768.

63. Smith LF, Henry-Tillman R, Harms S, et al. Hematoma-directed ultrasound-guided breast biopsy. *Ann Surg* 2001;233:669–675.

64. Yang WT, Ahuja A, Tang A, et al. High resolution sonographic detection of axillary lymph node metastases in breast cancer. *J Ultrasound Med* 1996;15:241–246.

65. Parker SH, Dennis MA, Kaske TI. Identification of the sentinel node in patients with breast cancer. *Radiol Clin North Am* 2000;38:809–823.

66. Verbanck J, Vandewiele I, De Winter H, et al. Value of axillary ultrasonography and sonographically guided puncture of axillary nodes: a prospective study in 144 consecutive patients. *J Clin Ultrasound* 1997;25:53–56.

67. Kane RA. Ultrasound-guided hepatic cryosurgery for tumor ablation. *Semin Intervent Radiol* 1993;10:132–142.

68. Ravikumar TS, Kane R, Cady B, et al. A 5-year study of cryosurgery in the treatment of liver tumors. *Arch Surg* 1991;126:1520–1523.

69. Rui J, Tatsutani KN, Dahiya R, et al. Effect of thermal variables on human breast cancer in cryosurgery. *Breast Cancer Res Treat* 1999;53:185–192.

70. Staren ED, Sabel MS, Gianakakis LM, et al. Cryosurgery of breast cancer. *Arch Surg* 1997;132:28–33.

71. Jeffrey SS, Birdwell RI, Ikeda DM, et al. Radiofrequency ablation of breast cancer: first report of an emerging technology. *Arch Surg* 1999;134:1064–1068.

72. Simmons RM, Dowlatshahi K, Singletary SE, et al. Percutaneous ablation of breast cancer. *Contemp Surg* 2002;58: 61–71.

Ultrasound of the Thyroid and Parathyroid Glands

Jay K. Harness and David E. Sahar

Surgeons clearly have a key role in the evaluation and treatment of patients with diseases of the thyroid and parathyroid glands. Despite this, most patients needing surgery for endocrine diseases have been extensively evaluated and often have an established diagnosis prior to referral to a surgeon. Given this to be the case, one might rightly ask why general or endocrine surgeons would need to know how to perform ultrasound examinations on their patients.

Ultrasound examinations by physicians often serve as an adjunct to the physical examination. Performing their own real-time ultrasound examination of the neck allows surgeons to mentally construct a picture of what will be encountered in the operating room. For surgeons exploring and resecting endocrine glands, real-time ultrasound examinations may assist in demonstrating the three-dimensional anatomy of the target organ(s). In the authors' practice, we use ultrasound to image the target gland (i.e., a thyroid nodule or parathyroid adenoma), evaluate the apparently uninvolved opposite thyroid lobe and/or isthmus (i.e., looking for occult disease), and perform ultrasound-guided fine needle aspiration (FNA) biopsies of thyroid pathologic lesions, enlarged cervical lymph nodes, and parathyroid glands. The superficial location of the thyroid and parathyroid glands allows the normal anatomy and pathologic conditions to be imaged with remarkable clarity using high-frequency, high-resolution ultrasound.

EQUIPMENT AND TECHNIQUE

Ultrasound examinations of the thyroid and parathyroid glands should be performed with high-frequency, linear array transducers of 7.5 to 13 MHz. Linear array transducers provide a wide near-field view of the superficial anatomy of the neck. Occasionally, convex (curvilinear) array transducers are used for small-parts examination, but most surgeons prefer linear array transducers.

Ultrasound examination of the neck is typically performed with the patient in a position similar to that used in operative exposure of the thyroid and parathyroid glands. The patient is placed in the supine position with a pillow under the shoulders and with the neck extended. The examiner may stand or sit lateral or cephalad to the patient. The region of the thyroid gland, the parathyroid glands, and the jugular chain of lymph nodes should always be examined in at least two planes (transverse and longitudinal) (Fig. 1).

Prior to detailed examination, a brief survey of the anterior structures of the neck is performed. The entire thyroid gland and isthmus is examined. The gland should be imaged from the superior poles (including the superior pole vessels) through the most inferior portions of the lower poles. Examination of the inferior lobes may on occasion be assisted by having the patient swallow. The examination should also be focused laterally to include the internal jugular veins, the internal jugular lymph nodes, and the carotid arteries. If thyroid carcinoma is suspected, then the ultrasound examination of the cervical lymph nodes should be thorough and complete (see Chapter 7).

PARATHYROID ANATOMY

Normal parathyroid glands vary only slightly in size and are generally spherical and somewhat flattened or oval. The average size of a parathyroid gland is $5 \times 3 \times 1$ mm and the average weight 20 to 50 mg. An ultrasound scan will not demonstrate normal parathyroid glands in most patients due to their small size and similar echogenicity to adjacent structures (1–3). When scanning for parathyroid glands, surgeons should remember the basic principles of surgical exploration for parathyroid glands, namely, that the position of abnormal parathyroids can vary because of "migration" of enlarged glands and embryologic variation in their location. The percentage of

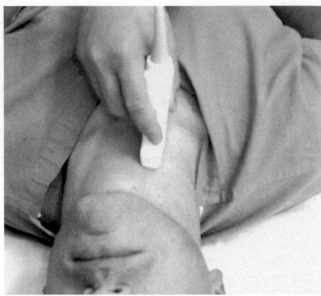

FIGURE 1. Photograph of examination of the thyroid and parathyroid glands with transducer in the transverse (**A**) and longitudinal (**B**) positions.

patients with supernumerary glands ranges from 2.5% to 22% (4).

Superior parathyroid glands are usually located in the posteromedial aspect of the thyroid gland near the tracheal–esophageal groove (Fig. 2). They are often within an area 2 cm in diameter, about 1 cm above the intersection of the inferior thyroid artery and the recurrent laryngeal nerve. Enlarged superior parathyroid glands (either adenomas or hyperplasia) may migrate posteriorly and inferiorly as far as the posterosuperior mediastinum.

The locations of inferior parathyroid glands are more widely distributed than superior glands (5). These glands

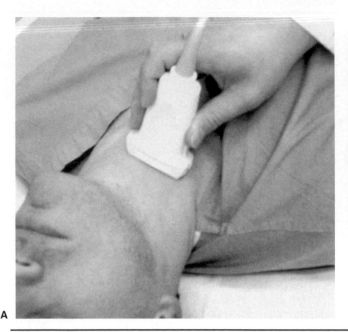

FIGURE 2. An 11-mm, intrathyroidal, parathyroid adenoma (*cursors*) located in the posteromedial aspect of the thyroid gland, shown in the longitudinal view.

can be found on the posterolateral aspect of the lower pole of the thyroid gland; inferior to the thyroid gland; at the carotid bifurcation; in the thyrothymic ligament; within the cervical portion of the thymus; in the anterior mediastinum; and within the substance of the thyroid gland (6,7). Intrathyroid parathyroid glands are considered to be inferior glands (6). If inferior parathyroid glands fail to descend during embryonic development, they may be found above the level of the superior thyroid pole in the carotid sheath.

THYROID SONOGRAPHY

The normal cross-sectional anatomy of the thyroid gland (including the isthmus), trachea, and carotid arteries is shown in Figure 3. The skin and subcutaneous fat are easily seen. The strap muscles are seen as relatively thin, hypoechoic bands anterior to each thyroid lobe. The sternocleidomastoid muscles are seen as larger hypoechoic bands lateral to the thyroid lobes and anterior to the jugular veins. Normal thyroid parenchyma has a homogeneous, medium- to high-level echogenicity (8); the homogeneous nature facilitates identification of hypoechoic or cystic (anechoic) lesions. The capsule of the thyroid gland may appear as a thin hyperechoic line. The normal gland is from 4 to 7 cm in length and less than 2 cm in thickness. The isthmus is generally less than 5 mm thick. The trachea is a useful reference point, appearing as a hyperechoic, crescent-shaped, midline ring with an anechoic interior and posterior shadowing. Just

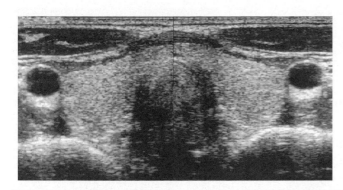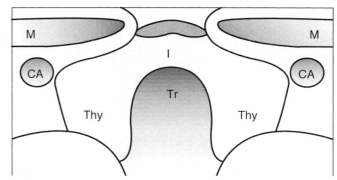

FIGURE 3. Transverse image of the thyroid gland and carotid arteries. Thy, thyroid glands; I, isthmus; Tr, trachea; Ca, carotid arteries; M, muscles. (From Harness JK, Wisher DB, eds. *Ultrasound in surgical practice: basic principles and clinical applications*. New York: Wiley–Liss, 2001, with permission.)

lateral to the thyroid are the anechoic carotid artery and jugular vein. Scanning in the longitudinal plane allows the surgeon to identify the bifurcating superior thyroid arteries and veins at the superior pole of each lobe. The identification of these vessels can usually be done in B-mode ultrasound, but the use of color Doppler (duplex) may facilitate their identification. The same is true for the inferior thyroid veins at the lower poles of each lobe. The esophagus is visualized just to the left and posterior to the trachea; it has a characteristic "bull's eye" appearance that may be identified by peristalsis with swallowing.

CLINICAL APPLICATIONS OF THYROID ULTRASOUND

The clinical applications of high-resolution ultrasound in patients with thyroid disease are several (Table 1). Ultrasound helps to determine the exact location of vaguely palpable neck masses. Furthermore, ultrasound allows the examiner to better characterize a palpable mass (i.e., cystic, solid, mixed; thyroid gland, lymph node, vascular mass, other masses; benign or malignant features) (Fig. 4). Ultrasound can be used to evaluate the apparently uninvolved portion of the thyroid gland (i.e., the isthmus

and the contralateral lobe). It may be useful in locating occult thyroid nodules in high-risk patients (i.e., with a history of head and neck irradiation or a history of familial thyroid carcinoma). Ultrasound is sensitive in detecting recurrent or metastatic carcinoma (see Chapter 7 on cervical lymph nodes). Finally, it is of great assistance in guiding FNA biopsies of thyroid nodules and suspicious cervical lymph nodes (Fig. 5).

> **TABLE 1 Applications of Thyroid Ultrasound**

1. Exact localization of vaguely palpable neck mass
2. Characterization of palpable neck mass:
   - Thyroid versus other mass
   - Cystic, solid, mixed
   - Benign versus malignant
3. Evaluation of the contralateral lobe, isthmus
4. Screening for occult thyroid nodules in high-risk patients
5. Detection of recurrent or metastatic thyroid cancer, e.g., lymph nodes
6. Guidance of fine needle aspiration

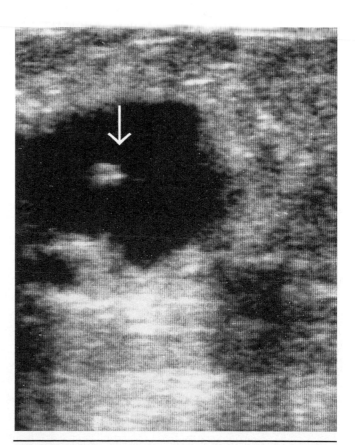

FIGURE 4. Ultrasound image demonstrating mixed solid-cystic nature (*arrow*) of a palpable thyroid nodule.

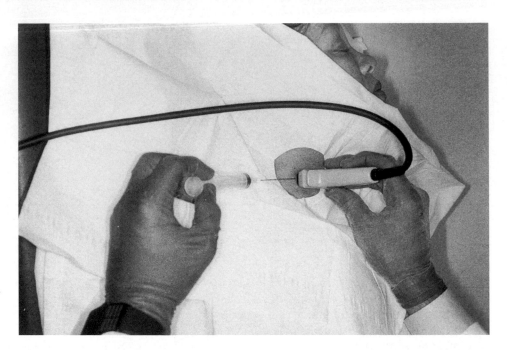

FIGURE 5. Ultrasound-guided fine needle aspiration biopsy of a thyroid nodule.

Thyroid Nodules

Because of their high incidence, the evaluation of thyroid nodules is a common problem for both endocrinologists and endocrine surgeons. These nodules are more common in women (9), and the vast majority are benign. The ultrasound appearance of benign thyroid lesions is summarized in Table 2. Their significance must be balanced against the fact that occult, nonpalpable thyroid carcinomas have been found in autopsy series in the United States in up to 12% of cases.

Most nodular thyroid disease arises from hyperplasia of the thyroid gland secondary to iodine deficiency, hereditary thyroid disease, and poor use of iodine as a result of medication (10). Thyroid hyperplasia can result in the formation of a thyroid goiter (Fig. 6A, B). As the hyperplasia continues, macronodules and micronodules develop. These nodules may then undergo liquefactive degeneration with the accumulation of colloid and serous fluid. Many cystic lesions of the thyroid are nodules that have undergone liquefactive degeneration. With cystic degeneration, fibrosis and calcification may result (11).

On ultrasound imaging, most hyperplastic nodules appear isoechoic as compared with normal thyroid tissue (8). A thin, hypoechoic halo may be seen to surround the nodule (Fig. 7). These nodules may become hyperechoic from multiple cycles of hyperplasia and involution, resulting in the development of numerous interfaces between cells and colloid substances (12).

True epithelial thyroid cysts rarely occur (1). Most cysts are really degenerating adenomatous nodules (Fig. 8). Cystic degeneration in nodules may result in a variety of sonographic appearances. These lesions may be entirely anechoic or hypoechoic secondary to hemorrhage. Bright echogenic foci may result from dense colloid material. Degenerating nodules may have variously thick intracystic septations that result in multilobulated lesions. Most patients have a mixture of characteristics (8,13).

Follicular Adenomas

Follicular adenomas are benign tumors of the thyroid that grow in follicular or glandular patterns. They tend to grow within a capsule of surrounding, compressed thyroid tissue. Over time they may develop a dense capsule surrounding the lesion (14). On ultrasound, adenomas are usually solid lesions that may be isoechoic, hypoechoic, or hyperechoic (Fig. 9). Like degenerating adenomatous nodules, they may also have a peripheral hypo-

▶ **TABLE 2 Ultrasound Appearance of Benign Thyroid Lesions**

Lesion	Appearance
Multinodular goiter:	■ Multiple, well-defined nodules
	■ Heterogeneous internal pattern
	■ Areas of hemorrhage, cystic degeneration, coarse calcifications
Adenoma:	■ Well-defined margin
	■ Homogeneous internal pattern
	■ Complete halo
Thyroiditis:	■ Generally diffuse
	■ Heterogeneous pattern in enlarged gland
Graves' disease:	■ Diffuse, hypoechoic
	■ Homogeneous pattern in enlarged gland
Cyst:	■ Solitary, well-defined margins
	■ Anechoic
	■ Posterior enhancement

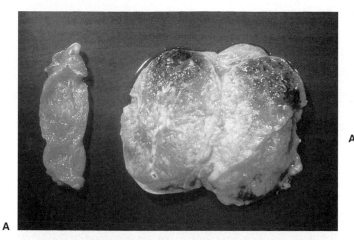

A

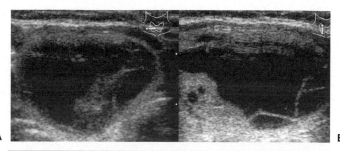

A   B

FIGURE 8. Transverse (**A**) and longitudinal (**B**) views of a large adenomatous nodule with extensive cystic degeneration.

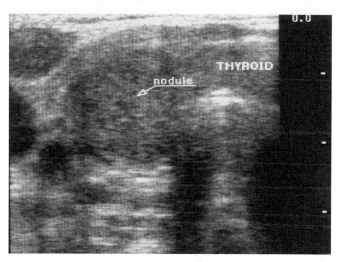

FIGURE 9. Hypoechoic thyroid nodule (arrow) found to be a follicular adenoma.

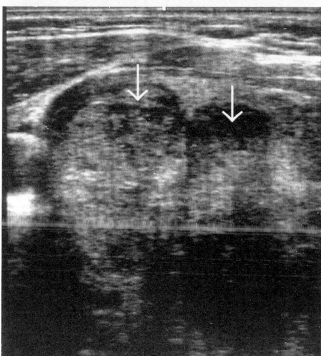

B

FIGURE 6. A: Gross pathology of multinodular goiter demonstrating areas of hemorrhage, fibrosis, and cystic degeneration. **B:** Ultrasound image of well-defined nodules (*arrows*) in multinodular goiter.

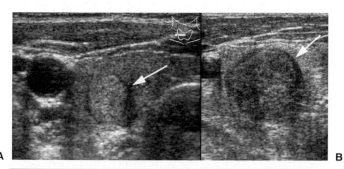

A   B

FIGURE 7. A: A nearly complete halo (*arrow*) around a benign-appearing nodule. **B:** An incomplete halo (*arrow*).

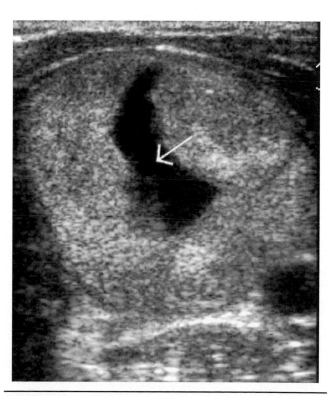

FIGURE 10. Follicular adenoma with central area of cystic degeneration (*arrow*).

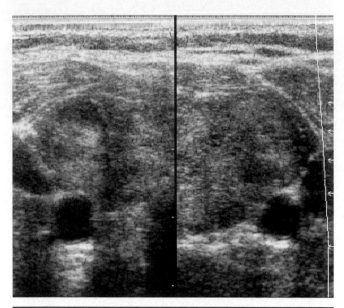

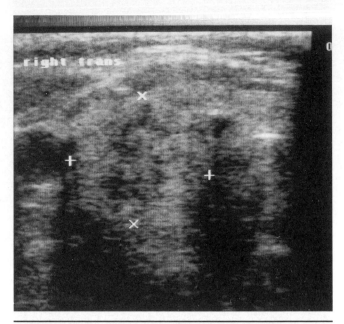

FIGURE 11. Transverse image of the right and left lobes of a patient with Graves' disease. (From Harness JK, Wisher DB, eds. *Ultrasound in surgical practice: basic principles and clinical applications*. New York: Wiley–Liss, 2001, with permission.)

FIGURE 12. Thyroiditis showing a coarse heterogeneous internal echo pattern with diffuse enlargement (cursors).

echoic complete halo secondary to the development of a fibrous capsule.

Cystic degeneration of follicular adenomas may present as single or multiple foci (15) (Fig. 10). Hemorrhagic cysts of the thyroid gland often result from spontaneous hemorrhage into a follicular adenoma (1). A hemorrhagic cyst appears as a sonolucent mass with irregular borders and multiple internal septae (16).

Diffuse Thyroid Enlargement

Graves' disease, Hashimoto's thyroiditis, iodine deficiency, and different types of thyroiditis may cause a diffuse enlargement of the thyroid gland, but with different sonographic appearances. A more or less homogeneous enlargement can be seen with Graves' disease (Fig. 11). Thyroiditis displays a typical but nonspecific sonographic appearance of diffuse enlargement with a coarse echo pattern in low amplitudes (17) (Fig. 12). Multinodular goiters have a generalized distortion of the glandular structure with nodules of various sizes and states of degeneration, as previously described.

Carcinomas

Carcinoma of the thyroid gland is an uncommon malignancy. Most thyroid carcinomas are well-differentiated papillary or papillary–follicular cancers; these account for 75% to 90% of all cases diagnosed (18). Pure follicular, medullary, Hürthle cell, and anaplastic carcinomas combined account for 10% to 25% of all thyroid carcino-

mas in Canada and the United States (8). Thyroid cancer is often characterized by an irregular, infiltrative mass with areas of necrosis; in the case of papillary type, lymph node metastases are a common occurrence.

Papillary

Although the sonographic appearance of papillary thyroid carcinoma varies, it most often displays vague, irregular borders, an incomplete halo, and a hypoechoic interior relative to the thyroid parenchyma (13). The hypoechogenicity is caused by minimal colloid substance and tightly packed cell content (Fig. 13). The interior may be somewhat heterogeneous due to areas of necrosis, hemorrhage, and microcalcifications (psammoma bodies) appearing as punctuate, irregular hyperechoic foci (11) (Fig. 14). These lesions most often demonstrate hypervascularity on duplex scan (19).

Follicular

Pure follicular carcinoma accounts for 5% to 15% of all cases of thyroid carcinoma. These cancers are usually seen in older individuals. There are two variants of pure follicular carcinoma: minimally invasive and invasive. Minimally invasive carcinomas are encapsulated and demonstrate only focal capsular and/or vascular invasion on histologic examination. To differentiate a follicular adenoma from a minimally invasive follicular carcinoma requires close histopathologic examination. By contrast, invasive follicular carcinomas are not well encapsulated,

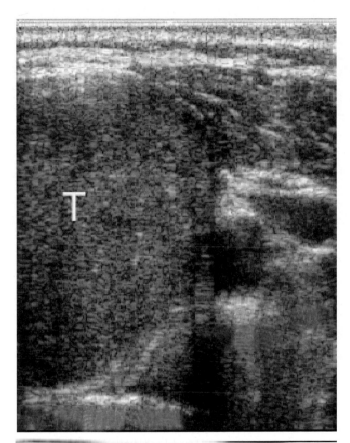

FIGURE 13. Transverse image of a 5.4 cm left thyroid papillary carcinoma (T) that is homogeneous and hypoechoic. (From: Harness JK, Wisher DB, eds. *Ultrasound in surgical practice: basic principles and clinical applications*. New York: Wiley–Liss, 2001, with permission.)

and the invasion of the surrounding thyroid gland and blood vessels is more readily apparent.

The ultrasound appearance of follicular carcinoma depends on the type encountered. There are no unique sonographic features that allow the differentiation of minimally invasive follicular carcinoma from a benign follicular adenoma (Fig. 15). However, invasive follicular carcinomas often show irregular tumor margins and a thick, incomplete halo (20). The vascularity of the invasive form may be seen as tortuous and irregular blood vessels (21).

Medullary

Patients presenting with palpable medullary carcinomas have a higher incidence of local invasion and cervical metastases than do patients with papillary carcinoma. As a result, ultrasound of the neck may be an important adjunct to the physical examination of the thyroid and regions of typical cervical metastases. Ultrasound of the neck may assist the surgeon's operative planning by allowing detection of disease not appreciated on routine physical examination.

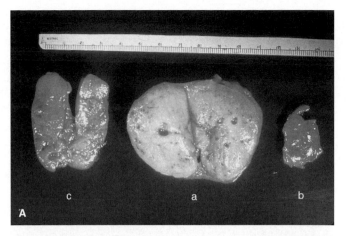

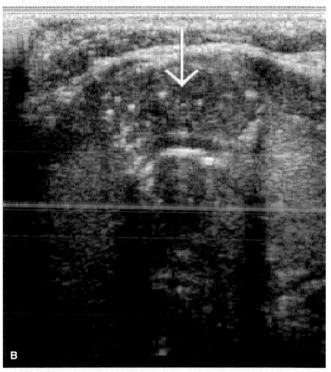

FIGURE 14. **A:** Gross pathology (cut surfaces) of papillary thyroid cancer **(a)** demonstrating necrosis and fibrosis, lymph node metastases **(b),** and normal contralateral thyroid lobe **(c).** **B:** Transverse view of a papillary carcinoma of the thyroid isthmus (*arrow*). Prominent, hyperechoic microcalcifications (psammoma bodies) are seen. (From Harness JK, Wisher DB, eds. *Ultrasound in surgical practice: basic principles and clinical applications*. New York: Wiley–Liss, 2001, with permission.)

The sonographic appearance of medullary carcinoma is similar to that of papillary carcinoma (8). In addition to indistinct or irregular borders and interior, amyloid deposits seen in medullary carcinoma appear as bright, highly echogenic foci similar to calcifications (22) (Fig. 16). As with papillary carcinoma, microcalcifications also may be seen in the primary tumor as well as in metastases to the liver and lymph nodes. Metasta-

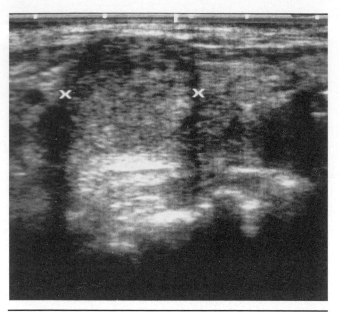

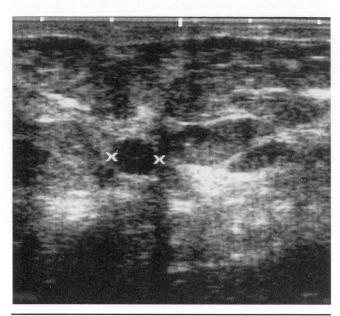

FIGURE 15. Ultrasound image of a hypoechoic, ill-defined thyroid nodule (*cursors*) shown to be a minimally invasive follicular thyroid cancer.

FIGURE 17. Simple cyst (*cursors*) of the thyroid.

ses may also have bright echogenic foci from amyloid deposits.

Anaplastic

Anaplastic thyroid carcinoma is the most aggressive form of thyroid cancer. These carcinomas are found more

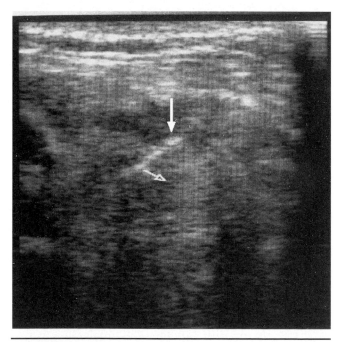

FIGURE 16. Ultrasound-guided fine needle aspiration (*long arrow*) of medullary thyroid cancer; a *short arrow* indicates indistinct border.

commonly in countries with iodine-deficient populations and have been proposed to be the result of dedifferentiation of either papillary or follicular carcinomas (23). Sonographically, these carcinomas are usually hypoechoic with diffuse infiltrative edges that appear indistinct. They are often found encasing cervical blood vessels and invading other neck structures (8).

SONOGRAPHIC CHARACTERISTICS OF THYROID NODULES

Other than the rare simple cysts, which have the same ultrasound appearance as simple cysts in other anatomic locations (i.e., completely anechoic, smoothly marginated, thin-walled, and posterior enhancement) (Fig. 17), no single sonographic criterion distinguishes benign from malignant thyroid nodules. However, a number of characteristics may be used to better categorize a thyroid lesion. The main sonographic characteristics evaluated are internal patterns, echogenicity, margins, microcalcifications, peripheral halo, and blood flow patterns (8) (Table 3).

Internal Pattern

The internal echo pattern of thyroid lesions may be solid, mixed solid and cystic, or purely cystic. Most follicular adenomas have a homogeneous, hypoechoic internal pattern. Benign colloid and adenomatous nodules associated with multinodular goiter usually have a significant cystic component (Fig. 18). Most malignancies, on the other hand, are completely solid. Rarely, papillary carci-

▶ **TABLE 3** Sonographic Features of Thyroid Lesions

Feature	Benign	Malignant
Internal pattern	Homogeneous	Heterogeneous
Echogenicity	Anechoic/hyperechoic	Hypoechoic
Margins	Smooth, well defined	Irregular, vague
Calcifications	Coarse, peripheral	Fine, punctate
Halo	Thin, complete	Thick, incomplete
Vascularity	Peripheral, hypovascular	Intratumoral, hypervascular

nomas may exhibit cystic changes in the primary lesion; this is often seen in metastatic lymph nodes. In such cases, the primary papillary carcinoma may appear similar to a benign cystic nodule (24).

Echogenicity

Most benign and malignant thyroid nodules are hypoechoic relative to normal thyroid parenchyma (8) (Fig. 19). However, hyperechoic nodules are more likely to be benign (13). Isoechoic nodules are uncommon and have an intermediate risk for malignancy.

Margins

As is the case with breast lesions, benign thyroid nodules tend to have sharp, well-defined margins whereas malignant nodules tend to have poorly defined or irregular margins (8) (Fig. 20).

Microcalcifications

Microcalcifications in the thyroid gland are an uncommon finding. Fine and punctuate microcalcifications

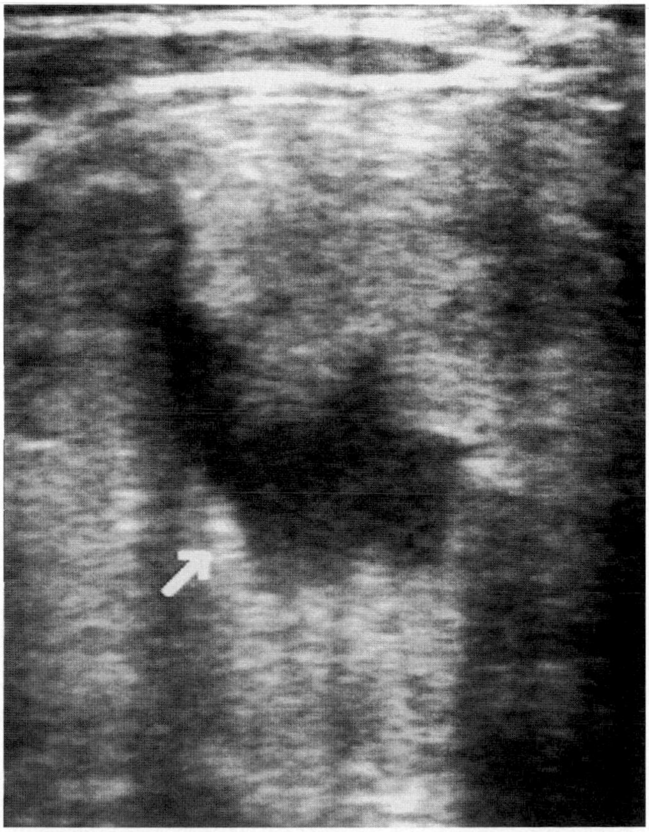

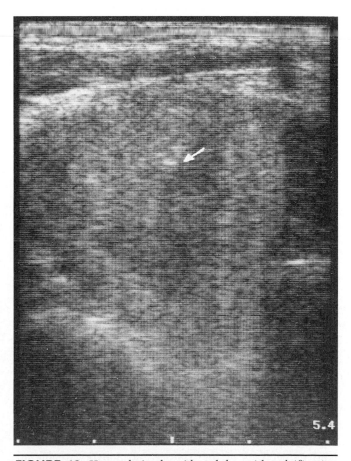

FIGURE 18. Colloid nodule demonstrating cystic degeneration (*arrow*).

FIGURE 19. Hypoechoic thyroid nodules with calcification (*arrow*) shown to be a papillary thyroid cancer.

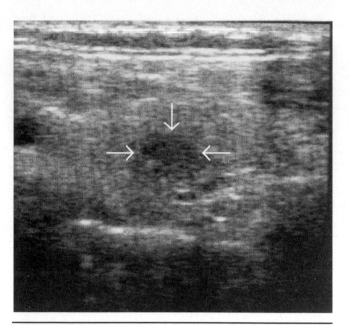

FIGURE 20. Poorly defined borders (*arrows*) in ultrasound image of a small papillary thyroid cancer.

found in the parenchyma of nodules are more likely to indicate a malignant lesion. Psammoma bodies are fine microcalcifications commonly seen with papillary carcinomas (13) (Figs. 14B and 19). Peripheral or coarse calcifications are more likely to be benign.

Peripheral Halos

Peripheral halos are found in approximately 60% to 80% of benign thyroid nodules (Fig. 7) and 15% of thyroid malignancies (14,25). Halos may represent compressed normal thyroid parenchyma. The combination of an absent or thick, incomplete halo, irregular margins, hypoechogenicity, and fine microcalcifications in a thyroid nodule is worrisome for malignancy. Benign nodules most often demonstrate thin, complete halos.

Blood Flow Pattern

Doppler ultrasound may be useful in differentiating benign from malignant nodules. Most hyperplastic thyroid nodules are less vascular than normal thyroid parenchyma whereas most well-differentiated carcinomas are hypervascular. Furthermore, benign thyroid nodules tend to display peripheral vascularity whereas most malignancies show internal vascularity, with or without a peripheral component (8,21). Anaplastic and poorly differentiated carcinomas are usually rapidly growing, which can lead to necrosis of the tumors and a hypovascular appearance with Doppler ultrasound.

THYROID INCIDENTALOMAS

The increased use of diagnostic imaging studies such as carotid duplex and transesophageal echocardiography has led to a corresponding increase in the identification of "incidentalomas" (occult nodules) in organs such as the adrenal glands and the thyroid. The issue becomes what to do with these occult, incidental lesions.

Most incidental thyroid nodules are small, nonpalpable, and lack malignant features. They may rarely be malignant. However, lesions 1.5 cm or greater in diameter require further evaluation, regardless of their ultrasound appearance (26). Lesions smaller than 1.5 cm may be followed, provided they are not associated with palpable cervical adenopathy and have no malignant sonographic features. They should be followed on a regular basis to ensure stability.

ULTRASOUND-GUIDED BIOPSY

FNA biopsy is widely considered the diagnostic technique of choice in the assessment of nodular disease of the thyroid gland. The advantages of this technique are that it is minimally invasive, safe, highly accurate, and can be performed as an outpatient procedure. A false-negative FNA result may occur as the result of a sampling error (tip of the needle in the wrong place) or when insufficient material is obtained. The interpretation of FNA cytologic material requires an experienced cytopathologist.

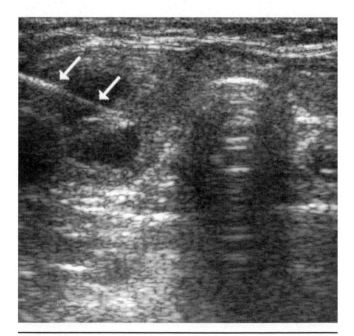

FIGURE 21. Transverse image of a 25-gauge needle (*arrows*) in a hypoechoic lesion in the right lobe of the thyroid.

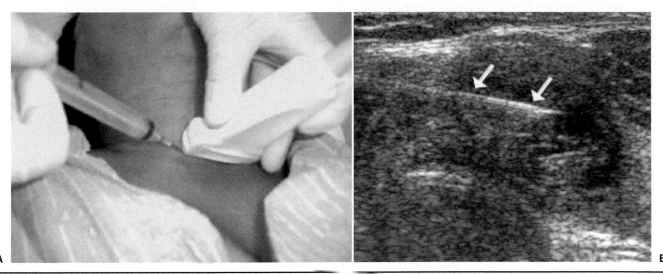

FIGURE 22. A: Use of a transverse scanning approach to perform a fine needle aspiration biopsy of a hypoechoic lesion in the lower pole of the left thyroid lobe in a 45-year-old woman. **B:** Proper placement of the 25-gauge needle (*arrows*). The lesion lies anterior and slightly to the left of the patient's trachea.

Ultrasound-guided FNAs are appropriate for vaguely palpable and nonpalpable thyroid nodules and cervical lymph nodes and for initially "insufficient" specimens. The main advantage of ultrasound guidance is the ability of the clinician to view the needle in real time and to ensure that the tip of the needle is in the correct position in the lesion of interest (Fig. 21). It is recommended that neophytes at ultrasound-guided biopsies initially begin by using ultrasound while they biopsy palpable thyroid nodules and cervical lymph nodes. Only after becoming comfortable with ultrasound guidance for palpable lesions should the clinician move on to nonpalpable thyroid nodules and cervical lymph nodes. Informal feedback from clinicians comfortable with ultrasound-guided biopsies suggests that the number of procedures needed for a clinician to feel confident ranges from 25 to 30 biopsies.

Our technique for performing ultrasound-guided freehand FNAs of the thyroid requires a preliminary scan to determine the safest and most comfortable approach to a thyroid (or other cervical) lesion. Care must be taken to avoid important structures such as the carotid arteries, jugular veins, and trachea. If possible, we prefer to approach most thyroid nodules while scanning transversely. Often we take a medial-to-lateral approach (Fig. 22), although the reverse may be appropriate if this minimizes the distance from the skin surface to the lesion. We prefer a 25-gauge needle mounted on a syringe. We pass the needle (without suction) back and forth in the target lesion while slightly changing the angle of each stroke. Usually six to eight strokes are done for each sample, with a total of three different samples. Each sample is checked for its quantity as it is sprayed onto a glass slide.

With this technique, samples are usually quite adequate and bleeding is minimal.

Most clinicians are reluctant to perform core needle biopsies of the thyroid gland because of fears of injuring surrounding structures and bleeding complications. This approach may warrant reevaluation based on a recent report from the United Kingdom suggesting that core needle biopsies of the thyroid can be performed safely and with greater accuracy than FNA biopsy (27). By using a freehand technique, the specimen notch of either a 16- or 18-gauge single-action spring-loaded biopsy needle is advanced into optimal position in the thyroid lesion. The spring-activated blade is then fired. Overall accuracy in differentiating benign from malignant lesions was 96% (27). Only 3 of 198 patients developed small hematomas, and there were no injuries to any surrounding neck structures. (See Chapter 4 for more description of ultrasound-guided needle biopsy.)

ULTRASOUND OF THE PARATHYROID GLANDS

Primary hyperparathyroidism (pHPT) is a disorder of excessive secretion of parathyroid hormone that results from hyperplasia or neoplasia of the parathyroid glands. The incidence is reported to be 4 per 100,000 person-years or about 100,000 new cases per year in the United States with a 3:1 female-to-male ratio (28). In outpatient settings, pHPT is the most common cause of hypercalcemia. Surgical resection of dysfunctional parathyroid gland or glands has been the treatment of choice for pHPT.

▶ **TABLE 4** Application of Parathyroid Ultrasound

1. Preoperative localization (with or without sestamibi scintigraphy)
   ■ Initial operation: debatable
   ■ Reoperation: indicated
2. Intraoperative localization: during operative exploration (particularly reoperation)
3. Guidance of fine needle aspiration of parathyroid adenoma
4. Guidance of percutaneous ablation of parathyroid adenoma

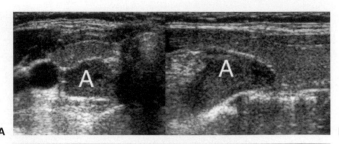

FIGURE 23. **A:** Transverse view of a hypoechoic, inferior parathyroid adenoma (A). **B:** The same adenoma (A) in the longitudinal view. The adenoma is attached to the lower pole of the right lobe of the thyroid gland.

Traditionally, bilateral neck exploration, without any preoperative studies, has been the standard in the surgical management of pHPT. Approximately 95% of patients are treated successfully at initial exploration when performed by experienced surgeons (29). However, surgeons with less experience perform most parathyroid operations (30). Graduates of general surgery residency programs have been reported to have inadequate experience in parathyroid surgery (31). As a result, the actual success rate by less experienced surgeons may be as low as 70% (30). The use of preoperative localization studies has been advocated as a means to lessen the extent of surgical explorations, maximize success rates, and decrease costs. The clinical applications of ultrasound of the parathyroid glands are summarized in Table 4.

Preoperative Localization

The use of noninvasive imaging techniques as preoperative localization for detection of abnormal parathyroid glands in pHPT has remained a subject of debate. These imaging techniques include ultrasound, technetium ^{99m}Tc sestamibi scintigraphy, computed tomography, and magnetic resonance imaging. The main reason for debate over the use of noninvasive imaging techniques prior to initial parathyroidectomy has been questionable cost effectiveness. There is, however, current consensus in the need for preoperative imaging of the putative gland in reoperative cases.

Reports on the use of ultrasound to image parathyroid adenomas started to appear in the late 1970s (32). Over the past decade, sonography and parathyroid scintigraphy have been studied extensively. Recent studies have shown ultrasound, in conjunction with sestamibi parathyroid scintigraphy, to be a cost-effective preoperative test prior to initial pHPT surgical exploration (33,34). Since sonography is operator and equipment dependent, the sensitivity reported in the literature ranges from 27% to 95%, with a recent figure of 65% (33). Interestingly, ultrasound sensitivity is comparable for patients having either an initial operation or reoperation. Sestamibi parathyroid scintigraphy has been reported to have a sensitivity ranging from 50% to 91%, with a recent figure of 80%

(33). Combination of sonography and sestamibi localization may raise this sensitivity to 95% (29). Ultrasound is more sensitive for parathyroid tumors located immediately adjacent to the thyroid gland or within the thyroid gland as well as large adenomas elsewhere in the neck (Figs. 2, 23). The test is less sensitive in a background of nodular thyroid disease, thyroiditis, and lymphadenopathy. Furthermore, parathyroid adenomas in retrotracheal, retroesophageal, and mediastinal locations are difficult to detect using ultrasound. These locations are more amenable to sestamibi localization.

Some authors suggest that the sensitivity of sonography and specificity of parathyroid scintigraphy make this combination ideal for noninvasive preoperative testing (35). When both the ultrasound and sestamibi scans localize the same parathyroid tumor in patients with sporadic pHPT, that gland is the only abnormal parathyroid gland in 96% of patients (33). However, there has been a wide range of success reported in the literature (43% to 96%) when these studies are used in combination (5,33, 34,36,37). This combined approach may lower the rate of postoperative hypoparathyroidism, improve recovery times, enhance cosmesis, and reduce hospital stays (38). In cases of discordant imaging, hyperplasia or double adenoma is often encountered. Bilateral neck exploration is recommended with discordant imaging results.

Most patients with persistent pHPT after surgical exploration have a missed adenoma or multiple-gland hyperplasia. Missed adenomas are often ectopic in location. Adequate preoperative localization is indicated in these cases, as success rates without preoperative localization studies for reoperation for pHPT approach only 60% (39). Image-directed exploration in a scarred reoperative field and disrupted anatomy can be invaluable. The localization of thoracic adenomas requires preoperative localization before more invasive approaches are utilized, including sternotomy, thoracoscopy, or thoracotomy. Sestamibi localization is particularly sensitive and specific in these ectopic locations; however, such scans usually do not provide information on size and position

⟩ **TABLE 5** Ultrasound Appearance
of Parathyroid Adenoma

- Well-defined margins
- Oval shape of 8 to 15 mm
- Homogeneous, hypoechoic internal pattern
- Separated from posteromedial aspect of thyroid by hyperechoic line

relative to other structures, making ultrasound an important adjunct. In technically challenging cases, intraoperative sonography has been reported to be "essential" for identifying the adenomas (33).

Ultrasound of Abnormal Parathyroid Glands

Certain characteristics of the parathyroid gland may aid in optimal sensitivity to ultrasound imaging (Table 5). Normal parathyroid glands are generally not seen by ultrasound. Most parathyroid adenomas are oval, measure between 8 and 15 mm, and weigh 500 to 1000 mg (4) (Fig. 24). Pathologic parathyroid adenomas tend to be hypercellular and solid, projecting a uniform signal cross sectionally. Their internal echoes are homogenous and hypoechoic in comparison with the thyroid gland (Fig. 23). Cystic degeneration is noted in less than 5% of parathyroid adenomas (40). They may be separated from the thyroid by a fine, hyperechoic line. False-negative results are generally due to small adenomas, multinodular goiters, and ectopic locations of adenomas. False-positive results can be caused by a prominent blood vessel, protrusion of the esophagus, location of the longus colli muscle in the transverse plane, thyroid nodules, and cervical lymph nodes (41).

Interventional Ultrasound and Minimally Invasive Parathyroidectomy

When noninvasive methods fail to provide conclusive results, or if two imaging modalities (e.g., ultrasound and sestamibi scan) do not have concordant results, ultrasound-guided biopsy has been advocated as a minimally invasive method to confirm or reject the localization of an apparent parathyroid adenoma (42,43). In comparison with other invasive tests, including angiography and selective venous sampling, ultrasound-guided FNA does not require sophisticated hospital resources or expertise. Reports indicate a sensitivity of 70% and specificity of 100% with ultrasound-guided FNA (44). With a 100% positive predictive value, no other tests are needed before surgery when the PTH immunoassay result is positive for parathyroid tissue. If the aspirate is negative, further invasive tests are recommended. Tissue implantation or parathyromatosis concern during FNA of parathyroid gland is mostly theoretical (42).

Ultrasound-guided percutaneous laser ablation (45) and ethanol injection (46) into the parathyroid adenoma is a minimally invasive alternative to conventional surgery for selected patients with high operative and anesthetic risks. A low success rate of 70% to 80% for curing pHPT and an unfavorable side effect profile, including vocal cord paralysis, make these approaches unsuitable for all but a very small group of patients.

Intraoperative ultrasound has been used to decrease the length of operative time. However, the ultimate out-

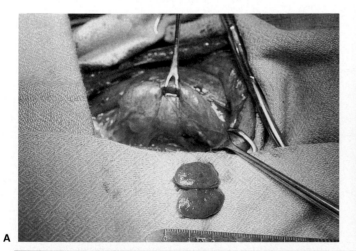

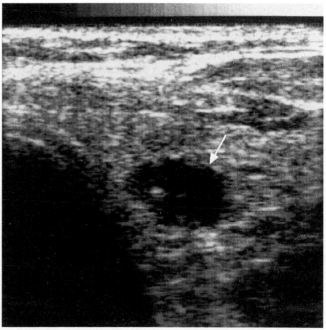

FIGURE 24. **A:** Intraoperative image of large (2 cm) transected parathyroid adenoma found in tracheoesophageal groove. **B:** Ultrasound image of parathyroid adenoma (*arrow*) shown grossly in **(A)**.

oome of the surgery is unchanged in comparison with preoperative ultrasound (47).

Since the first endoscopic parathyroidectomy performed by Gagner in 1996, interest in this method of management of pPHT has been increasing (48). Preoperative imaging is a prerequisite for this surgical approach (49). Supposed advantages include improved cosmetic result and decreased postoperative pain.

CONCLUSIONS

The use of ultrasound for thyroid and parathyroid diseases is described in this chapter. Head and neck ultrasound is an important adjunct to the physical examination and the clinical decision making process. Using ultrasound, the surgeon becomes a sonographic clinician who synthesizes the patient's history, physical examination, and laboratory data into a probable diagnosis and/or a further diagnostic workup. Not only should surgeons be capable of performing and interpreting their own ultrasound examinations, but they should also perform their own ultrasound-guided biopsies. Once surgeons become comfortable with these tasks, they will find that this technology becomes a fundamental component of their practice of head and neck surgery, particularly surgery of the thyroid and parathyroid glands.

REFERENCES

1. Butch, RJ, Simeone JF, Mueller PR. Thyroid and parathyroid ultrasonography. *Radiol Clin North Am* 1985;23:57–71.
2. Clark OH, Okerlund MD, Moss AA, et al. Localization studies in patients with persistent or recurrent hyperparathyroidism. *Surgery* 1985;98:1083–1094.
3. Sample WF, Mitchell SP, Bledsoe RC. Parathyroid ultrasonography. *Radiology* 1978;127:485–490.
4. Herrera MF, Gamoba-Dominguez A. Parathyroid embryology, anatomy, and pathology. In: Clark OH, Duh Q-Y, eds. *Textbook of endocrine surgery*. Philadelphia: WB Saunders, 1997:277–283.
5. Wang CH. The anatomic basis of parathyroid surgery. *Ann Surg* 1976;183:271–275.
6. Thompson NW, Eckhauser FE, Harness JK. The anatomy of primary hyperparathyroidism. *Surgery* 1982;92:814–821.
7. Akerström G, Malmaeus J, Bergström R. Surgical anatomy of human parathyroid glands. *Surgery* 1984;95:14–21.
8. Solbiati L, Charboneau JW, James EM, et al. The thyroid gland. In: Rumack CM, Wilson SR, Charboneau JW, eds. *Diagnostic ultrasound*. St. Louis: Mosby, 1998:703–729.
9. Vander JB, Gaston EA, Dawber TR. The significance of nontoxic thyroid nodules. Final report of a 15-year study of the incidence of thyroid malignancy. *Ann Intern Med* 1968;69: 537–540.
10. Hennemann G. Non-toxic goitre. *Clin Endocrinol Metab* 1979;8:167–179.
11. Solbiati L, Cioffi V, Ballarati E. Ultrasonography of the neck. *Radiol Clin North Am* 1992;30:941–954.
12. Muller HW, Schroder S, Schneider C, et al. Sonographic tissue characterization in thyroid gland diagnosis. *Klin Wschr* 1985;63:706–710.
13. Solbiati L, Volterrani L, Rizzatto G, et al. The thyroid gland with low uptake lesions: evaluation by ultrasound. *Radiology* 1985;155:187–191.
14. Smeds S, Heldin N-E. Growth factor, thyroid hyperplasia, and neoplasia. In: Clark OH, Duh Q-Y, eds. *Textbook of endocrine surgery*. Philadelphia: WB Saunders, 1997:205–213.
15. Noyek AM, Greyson ND, Steinhardt MI, et al. Thyroid tumor imaging. *Arch Otolaryngol* 1983;109:205–224.
16. Katz JF, Kane RA, Reyes J, et al. Thyroid nodules: sonographic–pathologic correlation. *Radiology* 1984;151:741–745.
17. Blum M, Passalaqua AM, Sackler JP, et al. Thyroid echography of subacute thyroiditis. *Radiology* 1977;125:795–798.
18. Hay ID. Thyroid cancer. *Curr Ther Intern Med* 1991;3:931–935.
19. Solbiati L, Ierace T, Lagalla R, et al. Reliability of high frequency US and color Doppler US of thyroid nodules: Italian multicenter study of 1,042 pathologically confirmed cases with role of scintigraphy and biopsy. [Abstract] Presented at Radiological Society of North America meeting, 1995.
20. Solbiati L, Livragh T, Ballarati E, et al. Thyroid gland. In: Solbiati L, Rizzatto G, eds. *Ultrasound of superficial structures: high frequencies, Doppler and interventional procedures*. Edinburgh: Churchill Livingstone, 1995:49–85.
21. Lagalla R, Caruso G, Midiri M, et al. Echo Doppler-couleur et pathologic thyroidienne. *JEMU* 1992;13:44–47.
22. Gorman B, Charboneau JW, James EM, et al. Medullary thyroid carcinoma: role of high-resolution ultrasound. *Radiology* 1987;162:147–150.
23. van der Laan F, Freeman JL, Tsang RW, et al. The association of well-differentiated thyroid carcinoma with insular or anaplastic thyroid carcinoma: evidence for dedifferentiation in tumor progression. *Endocr Pathol* 1993;4:215–219.
24. Hammer M, Wortsman J, Folse R. Cancer in cystic lesions of the thyroid. *Arch Surg* 1982; 17:1020–1023.
25. Propper RA, Skolnick ML, Weinstein BJ, et al. The nonspecificity of the thyroid halo sign. *J Clin Ultrasound* 1980;8:129–132.
26. Giuffrida D, Gharib H. Controversies in the management of cold, hot, and occult thyroid nodules. *Am J Med* 1995;99: 642–650.
27. Screaton NJ, Berman LH, Grant JW. US-guided core-needle biopsy of the thyroid gland. *Radiology* 2003;226:827–832.
28. Wermers RA, Khosla S, Atkinson EJ, et al. The rise and fall of primary hyperparathyroidism: a population-based study in Rochester, Minnesota, 1965–1992. *Ann Intern Med* 1997; 126:433–440.
29. NIH Conference. Diagnosis and management of asymptomatic primary hyperparathyroidism: Consensus Development Conference statement. *Ann Intern Med* 1991;114:593–597.
30. Shen W, Duren M, Morita E, et al. Reoperation for persistent or recurrent primary hyperparathyroidism. *Arch Surg* 1996; 131:861–869.
31. Harness JK, Organ CH Jr, Thompson NW. Operative experience of U.S. general surgery residents in thyroid and parathyroid disease. *Surgery* 1995;118:1063–1070.
32. Edis AJ, Evans TC. High-resolution, real-time ultrasonography in the preoperative location of parathyroid tumors. Pilot study. *N Engl J Med* 1979;301:532–534.
33. Arici C, Cheah K, Ituarte PH, et al. Can localization studies be used to direct focused parathyroid operations? *Surgery* 2001;129:720–729.
34. Purcell GP, Dirbas FM, Jeffrey RB, et al. Parathyroid localization with high-resolution ultrasound and technetium Tc 99m sestamibi. *Arch Surg* 1999;134:824–830.
35. Feingold DL, Alexander R, Chen CC, et al. Ultrasound and sestamibi scan as the only preoperative imaging tests in reoperation for parathyroid adenomas. *Surgery* 2000;128: 1103–1110.
36. Casara D, Rubello D, Piotto A, et al. 99mTc-MIBI radioguided minimally invasive parathyroid surgery planned on the basis of a preoperative combined 99mTc-pertechnetate/99mTc-MIBI and ultrasound imaging protocol. *Eur J Nucl Med* 2000;27:1300–1304.

37. Ryan JA, Eisenberg B, Pado KM, et al. Efficacy of selective unilateral exploration in hyperparathyroidism based on localization tests. *Arch Surg* 1997;132: 886–891.
38. Smit PC, Borel Rinkes IHM, van Dalen A, et al. Direct, minimally invasive adenomectomy for primary hyperparathyroidism: an alternative to conventional neck exploration? *Ann Surg* 2000;231:559–565.
39. Satava RM Jr, Beahrs OH, Scholz DA. Success rate of cervical exploration for hyperparathyroidism. *Arch Surg* 1975; 110:625–628.
40. Krudy AG, Doppman JL, Shawker TH, et al. Hyperfunctioning cystic parathyroid glands: CT and sonographic findings. *AJR Am J Roentgenol* 1984;142:175–178.
41. Hopkins CR, Reading CC. The parathyroid glands. In: Rumack CM, Wilson SR, Charboneau JW, eds. *Diagnostic ultrasound*. St. Louis: Mosby, 1998:731–750.
42. Kendrick ML, Charboneau JW, Curlee KJ, et al. Risk of parathyromatosis after fine-needle aspiration. *Am Surg* 2001;67:290–294.
43. Sardi A, Bolton JS, Mitchell WT Jr, et al. Immunoperoxidase confirmation of ultrasonically guided fine needle aspirates for patients with recurrent hyperparathyroidism. *Surg Gynecol Obstet* 1992;175:563–568.
44. MacFarlane MP, Fraker DL, Shawker TH., et al. Use of preoperative fine-needle aspiration in patients undergoing reoperation for primary hyperparathyroidism. *Surgery* 1994; 116:959–965.
45. Bennedbaek FN, Karstrup S, Hegedus L. Ultrasound guided laser ablation of a parathyroid adenoma. *Br J Radiol* 2001; 74:905–907.
46. Karstrup S, Hegedus L, Holm HH. Ultrasonically guided chemical parathyroidectomy in patients with primary hyperparathyroidism: a follow-up study. *Clin Endocrinol (Oxf)* 1993;38:523–530.
47. Norton JA, Shawker TH, Jones BL, et al. Intraoperative ultrasound and reoperative parathyroid surgery: an initial evaluation. *World J Surg* 1986;10:631–639.
48. Gagner M. Endoscopic subtotal parathyroidectomy in patients with primary hyperparathyroidism. [Letter] *Br J Surg* 1996;83:875.
49. Miccoli P. Minimally invasive surgery for thyroid and parathyroid diseases. *Surg Endosc* 2002;16:3–6.

Chapter 7

Head and Neck Ultrasound

Alex Senchenkov and Edgar D. Staren

This chapter is a general introduction to the application of modern ultrasound (US) in the diagnosis of head and neck conditions that are common in surgical practice. While the use of US in the investigation of pathologic lesions of the thyroid and parathyroid glands and the vascular system will be the subject of separate sections (see Chapters 6 and 8), this chapter will focus primarily on the general head and neck sonographic examination and the use of US in the evaluation of lymph node pathologic processes and the imaging of salivary glands, oral cavity, larynx, and hypopharynx. In addition, a brief overview of US use in common congenital conditions of the head and neck is included.

EQUIPMENT AND TECHNIQUE OF HEAD AND NECK ULTRASOUND

Optimal sonographic imaging of head and neck structures requires high-frequency real-time specific transducers ranging from 7.5 megahertz (MHz) to 15 MHZ, and on occasion as high as 20 MHz. Focused on the near field, these small-part transducers can achieve an axial resolution of 0.5 mm and a lateral resolution of 1 mm that allows appreciation of even subtle differences in acoustic impedance of the tissues. Axial resolution is directly proportional to the frequency of the transducer, but higher frequency waves are attenuated more rapidly by the tissues and result in lower penetration. As such, a more powerful impulse is required to achieve adequate levels of acoustic energy in the deep tissues. Lateral resolution is mostly determined by the width of the US beam. Narrower high-frequency beams provide a superior quality of sonographic image that is essential for diagnostic studies of the head and neck region.

In performing US of the head and neck, the transducer is typically applied to the skin directly with an acoustic coupling medium such as a gel. On occasion a standoff pad of silicon gel may be used for optimal contact and visualization of near-field images. *Systematic sonographic examination* of the head and neck begins with the thyroid gland, followed by examination of the carotid sheath, floor of the mouth, tongue, salivary glands, and tonsils. If clinically indicated, lymph nodes of the neck, larynx, and cervical esophagus are evaluated (1) (Fig. 1).

Ultrasound-guided percutaneous needle biopsy has emerged as an important diagnostic modality in head and neck practice. Several techniques are utilized for US-guided needle biopsies (see Chapter 4). Vertical and lateral insertions are most common (Fig. 2). Most often the lesion is positioned in the middle aspect of the screen and the needle is advanced in the plane of the scan. Therefore, this approach is safer in close proximity to vital structures as it allows the needle to be visualized throughout its entire tract (2) (Fig. 2A, B). Some interventional US probes with a central biopsy channel allow for a very precise *perpendicular* percutaneous needle insertion, but the needle depth must be determined prior to insertion and the difficulty in cleansing have precluded their general use (3). *Fine needle aspiration (FNA), medium-size needle biopsy (MNB),* and *large-core needle biopsy* can be used in conjunction with sonographic guidance; however, FNA using a 20- or 22-gauge hypodermic needle is a preferred biopsy technique in the head and neck because of the proximity of vital structures.

CERVICAL LYMPH NODES

The normal adult has more than 300 cervical lymph nodes that are located along lymphatic vessels. Cervical nodes can be classified according to anatomic location as well as American Joint Commission for Cancer (AJCC) topographic classification (4) (Tables 1 and 2; Fig. 3).

Sonographic examination of cervical lymph nodes usually begins with visualization of the common carotid artery and internal jugular vein at the base of the neck. Axial scans, transverse to the vessels, are performed in a cephalad direction. Nodes are viewed in relation to the carotid artery and jugular vein. Level IV, III, and II nodes are sequentially visualized anterior to, and level V posterior to, the vessels. Nodes with recurrency may be im-

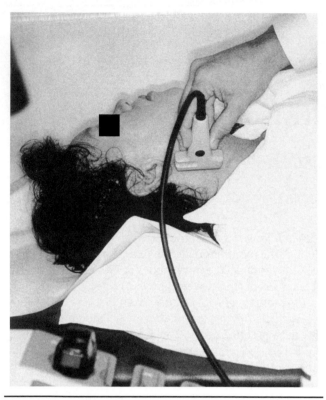

FIGURE 1. Sonographic examination of the mid-jugular cervical lymph nodes utilizing a high-frequency (7 to 10 MHz), linear array transducer.

> ▎**TABLE 1** **American Joint Commission for Cancer Topographic and Anatomic Classification of Cervical Lymph Nodes**[a]

Level 1	Submental and submandibular nodes
Level 2	High jugular nodes
Level 3	Midjugular nodes
Level 4	Low jugular nodes
Level 5	Spinal accessory and transverse cervical nodes
Level 6	Anterior cervical nodes

[a]Parotid and retropharyngeal nodes are not included.

aged during swallowing or significant hyperextension of the neck.

Most normal cervical lymph nodes in an adult person have an axial diameter of 2 to 5 mm, whereas jugulodigastric and juguloomohyoid lymph nodes can be as large as 15 to 20 mm longitudinally and 8 to 10 mm axially. Normal cervical lymph nodes are generally difficult to visualize because of their echogenicity, which is similar to that of surrounding fat. They consist of an outer cortex formed with lymphoid follicles and an inner medulla that contains lymphatic sinuses, blood vessels, and connective tissue. Numerous converging lymphatic sinuses in the central portion of the medulla form a hilum. Pathologic

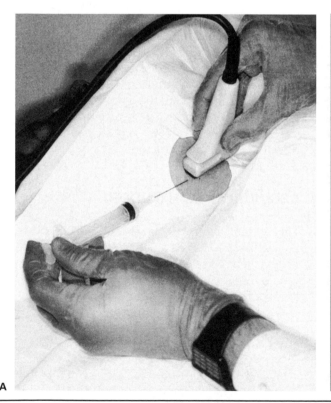

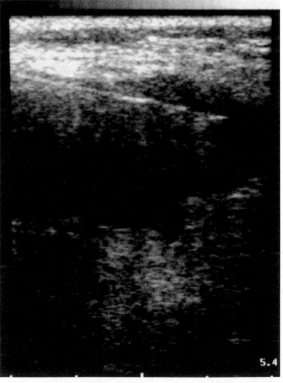

FIGURE 2. **A:** Ultrasound-guided fine needle aspiration biopsy of a cervical mass. **B:** Ultrasound image demonstrating entire needle pathway (*white line*) into perijugular, midneck mass.

▶ TABLE 2 Drainage Pattern

Level 1
- Submandibular nodes located along the inferior aspect of the mandible, lateral to the anterior belly of the digastric muscle
- Submental nodes located between the anterior bellies of the digastric muscles, superficial to the mylohyoid muscle
- Drainage region of lower lip, anterior chin, tip of the tongue, floor of the mouth, gingiva, and internal facial structures

Level 2
- Base of the skull to hyoid bone
- First station for tumor of nasopharynx, oropharynx, posterior oral cavity, supraglottic larynx, and the parotid gland are common primaries. Second station for hypopharynx, glottis, and anterior oral cavity can also metastasize

Level 3
- Between hyoid bone and cricoid cartilage
- It is the first station for hypopharyngeal, glottic, and subglottic cancers

Level 4
- Between cricoid cartilage and clavicle

Level 5
- Posterior cervical triangle: behind the sternocleidomastoid muscle

Level 6
- Nodes of the juxtavisceral area. Superficial nodes beneath platysma. Prelaryngeal nodes located anterior to the cricothyroid membrane. Pretracheal nodes. Paratracheal nodes in the visceral space. Intertracheoesophageal and recurrent nodes located in the groove between the trachea and esophagus

Parotid nodes
- Located around and within parotid gland
- Drainage includes area of skin between line over temporozygomatic arch to labial attachment of the nose inferiorly, sagittal line from the base of the nose to the vertex medially, and imaginary line from the vertex to the temporozygomatic arch posteriorly. In addition, it drains the external auditory canal, posterior oral cavity, and the parotid gland

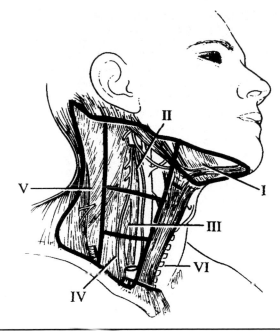

FIGURE 3. The level system for describing the location of lymph nodes in the neck. (From Robbins KT. Classification of neck dissection: current concepts and future considerations. *Otolaryngol Clin North Am* 1998;31:639–655, with permission.)

underlying inflammation in up to 50% of cases (6,7). Furthermore, 20% to 40% of normal-size nodes may be demonstrated to contain metastatic disease in the head and neck cancer patient (8). US has emerged as an accurate modality for identifying suspicious nodes that will require further study.

Size is typically regarded as the maximal transverse diameter (Fig. 5). Although large size is more commonly associated with malignancy, 33% to 71% of nodal metastases were found to have a maximal transverse diameter of

changes in lymph nodes due to inflammation or metastatic growth lead to enlargement of the node and reduction of its echogenicity (Fig. 4). When evaluating cervical adenopathy by US, eight parameters are important to assess: size; shape; echogenic hilum; level of echogenicity; presence of necrosis; extracapsular extension; calcifications; and characteristics of vascularity (5) (Table 3).

Identification of metastatic adenopathy is the main objective of lymph node imaging studies, including US. Preoperative assessment of cervical lymph nodes is important in staging and often determines optimal treatment approaches to cancers in the head and neck region. For example, the decision to proceed with node dissection or radiation therapy is based on clinical assessment of the cervical lymph nodes. However, the presence of adenopathy in the head and neck cancer patient can be a result of

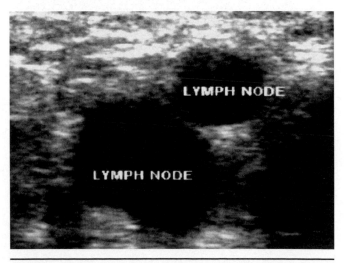

FIGURE 4. Enlarged and irregularly shaped level III cervical lymph nodes.

▶ **TABLE 3 Sonographic Criteria of Lymph Node Metastases**

1. Size (maximal transverse diameter): nodes are larger
2. Shape: round and long/short ratio usually less than 2.0[a]
3. Appearance of hilum: eccentric, thinned, or absent[a]
4. Echogenicity of the nodal parenchyma: heterogeneous echogenic cortex (metastatic carcinoma) or uniformly enlarged hypoechoic cortex (lymphoma)
5. Necrosis strongly suggestive of malignancy; can lead to cystic appearance of the involved nodes (cystic necrosis)
6. Nodal margins: extracapsular extension is sign of advanced malignancy (grave sign)
7. Calcifications: microcalcifications (metastatic thyroid cancer), coarse calcifications (lymph node treated with chemoradiation)
8. Characteristics of vascularity: displacement of intranodal vessels, focal absence of flow, and aberrant or subcapsular vessels that do not originate from the hilar or longitudinal vessels

[a]Decreased long/short ratio and absence of the hilar echoes are the most significant ultrasound indications of malignancy.

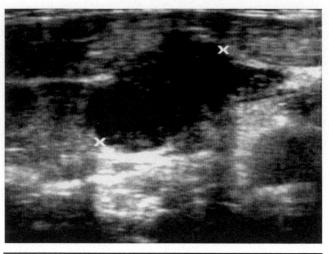

FIGURE 6. Malignant cervical lymph node (*cursors*) demonstrating irregular shape with jagged margins.

less than 1 cm; therefore, the size criterion alone will misrepresent a substantial number of nodal metastases (9).

Shape is an important feature of metastatic involvement (Fig. 6). Malignant infiltration commonly begins in the cortex of the lymph node. Therefore, metastatic nodes tend to have an irregular, rounded shape that is reflected by the decreased ratio between the longitudinal and transverse diameters of the node. This ratio, also known as long/short (L/S) axis, can be measured on long-axis scan of the lymph node as the largest and smallest diameter. An L/S ratio greater than 2 is predictive of inflammatory disease in 84%, whereas a ratio less than 1.5 indicates metastatic disease in 71% (10). The capability for multiplanar analysis of the node makes sonography superior to computed tomography (CT) or magnetic resonance imaging (MRI) for determining the L/S ratio. An L/S ratio of 2.0 is 81% to 95% sensitive and 67% to 96% specific in determining metastatic involvement of the lymph node (11). Chang et al. determined that mean L/S ratio for benign and malignant nodes was 1.9 and 1.4, respectively (12). Furthermore, the optimal cutoff L/S values for different cervical lymph node stations have been calculated: submental (2.0), submandibular (1.4), parotid (2.0), upper cervical (2.5), middle cervical (3.3), and posterior triangle (2.5) (13).

The *hilum* of the lymph node is a centrally located, thick, and echogenic structure. As the cortical parenchyma of the node undergoes malignant invasion, the hilum becomes eccentric, thinned, or frequently completely lacking (14).

Level of echogenicity of the node is a formal part of the sonographic evaluation. A normal lymph node consists of a thin, homogeneous, hypoechoic cortex and prominent, hyperechoic hilum. A uniformly enlarged hypoechoic cortex is suggestive of lymphoma as opposed to metastatic nodes that have heterogeneous and more echogenic cortices. By itself, echogenicity is a weak parameter in the differentiation of benign and malignant processes. In one study, 11% reactively enlarged nodes were heterogeneous, whereas 38% of metastatic nodes were homogeneous (7). Thickness of the cortex parenchyma can be

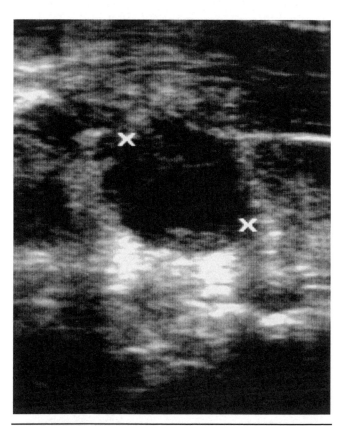

FIGURE 5. Maximum transverse diameter (*cursors*) of a suspicious 18-mm lymph node.

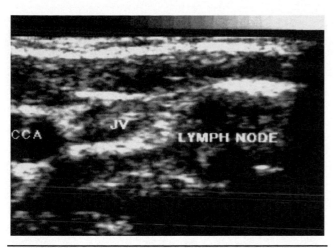

FIGURE 7. Enlarged midneck lymph node with involvement by metastatic squamous cell carcinoma showing indistinct margins adjacent to jugular vein (JV) and carotid artery (CCA).

evaluated if the hilum is present. If the cortex is less than half of the transverse diameter of the node and a normal-appearing hilum is present, the probability of malignancy is less than 9%, whereas eccentric cortical thickening is suggestive of nodal metastatic involvement (15).

Necrosis in the node of a cancer patient is strongly suggestive of metastatic disease. When it presents in the form of coagulation, necrosis appears as a hyperechoic area. Liquefaction (cystic) necrosis is usually imaged as an anechoic area with an irregular surface. Apart from metastases, necrosis is seen in granulomatous diseases of the nodes, especially tuberculosis. If an area of cystic necrosis is identified in the node, image-guided aspiration biopsy and microbiologic studies should be performed (5).

Nodal margins are commonly evaluated as a component of the study. The normal lymph node has smooth, well-delineated margins. In the case of metastatic involvement, margins of the node may remain smooth until the advanced stages of the disease when extracapsular extension occurs (Fig. 7). Moritz et al. noted that 46% of nodular metastases had well-delineated margins, whereas 14% of inflammatory nodes had ill-defined margins (7). Therefore, nodal margin imaging frequently does not permit differentiation between benign nodal disease and malignant involvement.

The presence of *microcalcifications* has been associated with metastases of papillary and medullary cancers of the thyroid. Large *coarse calcifications* in the cortex are encountered in lymph nodes treated with chemoradiation as well as in nodes involved with granulomatous disease.

Doppler and color Doppler sonography have come into use for evaluation of the *vascularity* of cervical lymph nodes (16). The addition of the contrast (D-galactose) has been reported to yield an even higher diagnostic

accuracy (7). However, many metastatic lymph nodes do not have hemodynamic and vascular abnormalities. Furthermore, the techniques are very operator dependent and the published results are quite variable. The value of these techniques in the evaluation of metastatic lymph nodes remains to be determined.

Multivariate analysis of US findings suggests that the criteria most predictive of metastatic cervical lymph node involvement were absent hilar echoes and increases in short axis length, as assessed by logistic regression analysis. When compared with gray scale criteria, color flow criteria had fewer predictive advantages. Although multivariate analysis did not support any significant contribution of the color flow criteria in predicting nodal metastases, these criteria appear to improve the overall diagnostic accuracy for the less experienced sonographer (17).

Advances in US-guided FNA have rendered it a superior technique for the evaluation of metastatic squamous cell carcinoma of the cervical lymph nodes. CT and MRI provide information regarding the size of suspicious nodes; by itself, this is an unreliable criterion for malignancy. If systematic sonographic examination of the nodal basin identifies any node suspicious for metastatic disease (e.g., enlarged, rounded shape with absence of the hilum), US-guided FNA biopsy should be performed to obtain targeted histologic confirmation of the lymph node status. This technique demonstrated a 24.3% higher accuracy rate and reduced the number of inadequate samples by 84% as compared with palpation-guided FNA (18). Sensitivity and specificity of 98% and 95%, respectively, have been reported (19).

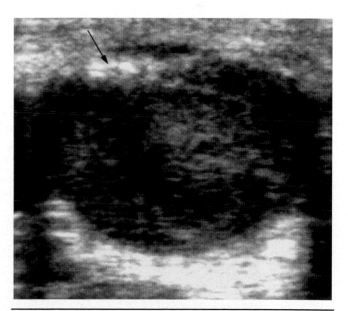

FIGURE 8. Zoom ultrasound image of a reactive lymph node demonstrating enlarged size but normal homogeneous, hypoechoic echotexture with smooth margins and a distinct, hyperechoic linear hilum (*arrow*).

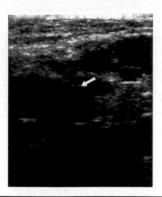

FIGURE 9. Cervical lymph node involved by tuberculosis demonstrating caseous necrosis and intranodal cystic degeneration (*arrow*) adjacent to carotid sheath.

Reactive lymphadenopathy is a common sonographic finding in otherwise healthy individuals. It is more common in submandibular and posterior cervical nodes. In acute lymphadenitis the nodes are tender and enlarged. Reactive enlargement of the lymph node and increased vascularity are typically results of inflammation in response to antigenic stimulation. Both lymphoid follicles and sinusoids are enlarged but are structurally identical to normal nodes. Reactive lymph nodes preserve normal sonographic appearance (i.e., elongated or oval shape with smooth and rounded borders) (Fig. 8). They have a homogeneous echo texture with a distinct, hyperechoic, linear hilum extending less than one third of the longitudinal axis of the node.

Specific lymphadenitis (granulomatous disease) of cervical nodes is a common manifestation of tuberculosis or sarcoidosis (Fig. 9). Tuberculosis of the cervical nodes is a common form of granulomatous disease in developing countries. Their appearance is sometimes indistinguishable from that of metastases. Sonographically, the in-

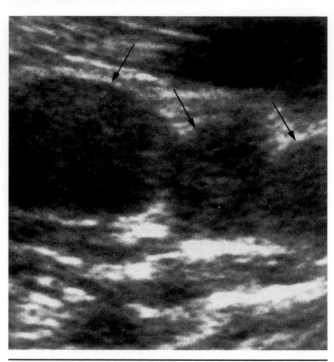

FIGURE 10. Well-demarcated, homogeneous, and hypoechoic lymph nodes (*arrows*) involved with non-Hodgkin's lymphoma.

volved nodes appear sharply delineated, rounded, and hypoechoic. They typically demonstrate homogeneity, matting, edema of surrounding soft tissue, and posterior enhancement. Multiple nodes are typically affected. Involvement of the posterior triangle is very typical, occurring in as many as 70% of cases (20). Caseous (intranodal cystic) necrosis is common. It is typically visualized as a hypoechoic node with ill-defined, irregular margins. Occasionally, a central intranodal area of caseous necrosis can present as a pseudohilum (21). When an abscess

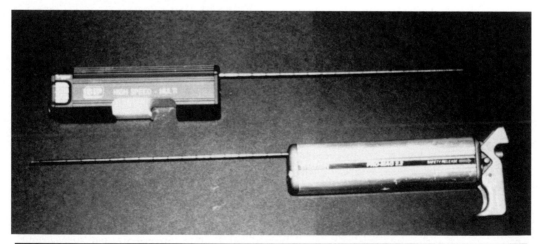

FIGURE 11. Medium-sized (18-gauge) spring-loaded, core biopsy needle guns amenable to ultrasound-guided biopsy of the cervical lymph node masses.

▶ **TABLE 4** **Sonographic Features of Lymph Node Pathologic Lesions**

Reactive lymphadenopathy
- Clinical enlargement and tenderness
- Enlarged lymph node with homogeneous parenchyma that has a normal structure

Specific adenopathy
- Clinical presence of tuberculosis, sarcoidosis, or other granulomatous disease; posterior triangle (level V), multiple lymph node involvement
- Sharply delineated, rounded, homogeneous, and hypoechoic lymph nodes with matting, edema of the surrounding tissues, and posterior enhancement; caseous necrosis can be present
- Difficult to differentiate from malignancy sonographically

Lymphomas
- Well-delineated, homogeneous, and hypoechoic lymph node with posterior enhancement that is very typical for lymphoma
- Medium-size needle biopsy with ultrasound guidance

forms, it appears as an area of irregular echogenicity with inhomogeneous acoustic shadowing. Fistula formation is common and has a sonographic appearance of hypoechoic linear stripes contrasting with the echogenic surrounding soft tissues. Except for known cases of cervical tuberculous lymphadenitis, a finding of multiple oval or round lymph nodes mandates biopsy with histologic and microbiologic study.

Sarcoidosis is another common granulomatous disease. Typically, the disease presents with lymphadenopathy that has mediastinal and pulmonary involvement with little or no associated necrosis. The clinical and sonographic picture can be quite similar to that of lymphoma. US is used to locate a suitable biopsy target in the supraclavicular lymph node station (level V) that is often involved.

Lymphomas are a heterogeneous group of lymphoproliferative disorders that are broadly divided into the Hodgkin's and non-Hodgkin's lymphomas. These diseases commonly present with lymphadenopathy that often involves cervical lymph nodes. The head and neck region is second only to the gastrointestinal tract as a site of extranodal lymphoma. Involved lymph nodes appear as well-delineated, homogeneous, and hypoechoic nodal masses with posterior enhancement (Fig. 10). Posterior enhancement is usually not present in normal lymph nodes but is demonstrated in 95% of nodes afflicted with lymphoma (22). Cytologic FNA is sufficient in squamous cell carcinoma but has a limited role in the diagnosis of lymphoma. Open biopsy of the involved lymph node is considered the gold standard. However, *medium-size (18-gauge) needle biopsy (MNB)*, utilizing spring-loaded, core biopsy needles, has been advocated for diagnosing lymphomas (Fig. 11). The use of MNB has decreased the nondiagnostic sampling rate from 25% to 3% in comparison to FNA (23) (Table 4).

MAJOR SALIVARY GLANDS

Parotid, submandibular, and sublingual glands form a distinct system of glandular tissue and extensively branched excretory ducts. Because of their superficial location, US can achieve superior high-resolution imaging. High-frequency, small-part transducers (7.5 to 15 MHz), commonly utilized for imaging most superficial structures, are used in salivary gland US. The availability of Doppler capability has facilitated identification of vascular landmarks (24).

Anatomy and Imaging

The *parotid* is the largest of the major salivary glands. It occupies almost the entire retromandibular fossa. The superficial layer of the deep cervical fascia splits to invest the trapezius and sternomastoid muscles as well as to form a tough capsule for the parotid and submandibular glands. Laterally, the parotid gland is covered by skin, subcutaneous connective tissue, and superficial cervical fascia. The anterior boundary of the parotid space includes the ramus of the mandible with the masseter and pterygoid muscles. Posteriorly and medially, it is bordered by the sternomastoid and the posterior belly of the digastric muscle, the styloid process and its muscles, and the retrostyloid space containing the internal jugular vein, carotid artery, and cranial nerves IX, X, and XI. Medially, the deep lobe extends into the parapharyngeal space. Inferiorly, the lower pole of the parotid gland is separated from the submandibular gland by the stylomandibular ligament. This structure is a thickening of the superficial layer of the deep cervical fascia that fuses before splitting again to form a capsule over the submandibular gland.

Adequate knowledge of the parotid gland's relation to nerves and vessels is critical to performance of high-quality head and neck US. The facial nerve traverses the tissue of the gland from the base of the skull where it exits via the stylomastoid foramen. In the gland, it divides into zygomatic, buccal, marginal mandibular, and cervical branches. The course of the facial nerve serves as the artificial division of the parotid into the deep and superficial lobes; however, there is in fact no true anatomic plane.

The parotid (Stensen's) duct is about 4 to 7 cm long. It originates from the anterior border of the superficial lobe and passes over the masseter. Anterior to the masseter, the parotid duct penetrates the buccinator muscle and opens into the mouth opposite to the second upper molar.

The external carotid enters the parotid from the posteromedial surface. It traverses cephalad through the gland and bifurcates into maxillary and superficial temporal arteries. A distinctive feature of the parotid gland

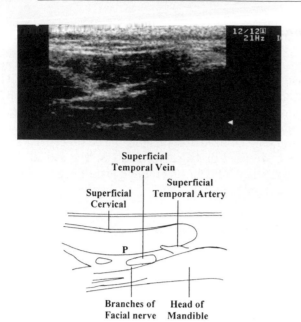

FIGURE 12. Longitudinal orientation ultrasound image of normal parotid gland (P) adjacent to mandible and the superficial cervical fascia. Note superficial temporal artery and vein and facial nerve branches.

anatomy is the presence of a large amount of lymphoid tissue in the gland parenchyma. Late formation of the parotid capsule during embryogenesis allows development of an extensive lymphatic network prior to the completion of encapsulation. Parotid lymphatic plexus includes intra- and extraglandular lymph nodes. It drains lymph from the area of skin between the border over the temporozygomatic arch extending to the labial attachment of the nose inferiorly, the sagittal line from the base of the nose to the vertex medially, and an imaginary line from the vertex to the temporozygomatic arch posteriorly (25). In addition, it drains the external auditory canal, orbital content, posterior oral cavity, and parotid gland.

US examination of the parotid is performed in a longitudinal and transverse direction at right angles to the ramus of the mandible. Tissue structures surrounding the parotid gland are readily visualized sonographically. These include the skin, subcutaneous tissue with fat and extracapsular lymph nodes, superficial cervical fascia, and capsule of the parotid gland. The superficial cervical fascia is seen as a highly echogenic structure between the masseter and sternomastoid muscles, adjacent to the parotid capsule (Fig. 12). In transverse view, acoustic shadows are typically formed by the ramus of the mandible and the mastoid process. The normal parotid gland has a homogeneous appearance sonographically. Similar to the thyroid gland, it is slightly hyperechoic as compared with adjacent musculature. The superficial parotid is readily accessible to sonographic evaluation. Imaging of the portion of the deep lobe located between

the external carotid artery and the venous plane may be improved with the use of a lower frequency transducer. This does, however, sacrifice some resolution quality. The pharyngeal and retrostyloid portions of the parotid are usually not accessible for sonographic examination (26). The extraglandular course of the facial nerve is not visualized by US, and the intraglandular portion can be imaged in only 30% of normal subjects (24). The venous plane that is located just superficial to the facial nerve can be visualized in the majority (70%) of people. The use of the Valsalva maneuver and especially color Doppler raises this yield to 93% (27). Intraparotid ducts are not visible sonographically, although Stensen's duct can sometimes be found on transverse view in front of the masseter muscle. Intraglandular lymph nodes are visualized as small hypoechoic nodules in a number of subjects. The presence of an eccentric echogenic hilum is suggestive of parotid lymphadenopathy (28).

The *submandibular gland* lies in the submandibular triangle between the internal surface of the mandible, the base of the tongue, the pharynx, and the suprahyoid muscles. Posteriorly, the gland extends to the inferior part of the paratonsillar space almost at the angle of the jaw. It is separated from the lower part of the parotid gland by a fibrous septum. The superior digastric lymph node (Kuttner's node) is often interposed between the parotid and the submandibular glands (24). The anterior and superior aspects are adjacent and intimately related to the mylohyoid muscle. Inferiorly, the submandibular gland extends just below the inferior border of the body of the mandible where it reaches the subcutaneous tissue.

The submandibular (Wharton's) duct is the main structure draining the submandibular gland. The duct originates from the deep portion of the gland and passes above the mylohyoid muscle between the inner surface of the mandible and the lateral aspect of the hyoglossus and genioglossus muscle, lateral to the hypoglossal nerve. It is located initially below and subsequently medial to the lingual nerve. The duct ends in the anterior floor of the mouth. It drains through the sublingual papilla that is adjacent to the frenulum of the tongue.

The facial artery passes across the superior aspect of the gland before reaching the inferior border of the mandible. The facial vein is located inferior to the artery. The marginal mandibular nerve is superficial to these vessels. The lingual nerve passes over the superior aspect of the gland in the anterior direction. It crosses Wharton's duct and assumes a position lateral to the duct. In this area, indentation of the duct caused by the lingual nerve may be visible on a sialogram. The hypoglossal nerve is located on the medial aspect of the gland and its duct.

The entire submandibular gland is amenable to visualization by US by placement of a small probe under the border of the mandible. High-frequency transducers allow for superior sonographic resolution of the gland.

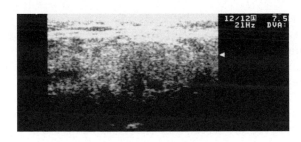

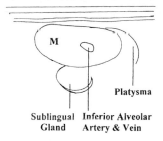

FIGURE 13. Image of longitudinal ultrasound over the mandible (M) demonstrating underlying sublingual gland which is obscured by shadowing.

Echo structure of the parotid and submandibular glands is similar although the smaller size of the submandibular gland allows for somewhat better resolution.

The mylohyoid muscle serves as an important landmark. It allows imaging of the anterior portion of the gland that rests superior to the mylohyoid. Facial and lingual arteries and their branches can be imaged with color Doppler study. Wharton's duct is visualized in 53% of normal individuals as it crosses through the sublingual space (29).

The *sublingual gland* is located under the mucosa on the floor of the mouth. It is surrounded by the mylohyoid muscle inferiorly, the mandible laterally, the genioglossus muscle anteriorly, and the hyoglossus and styloglossus muscles medially. Posteriorly, the sublingual gland is in contact with submandibular gland (Fig. 13). The gland drains through more than 12 sublingual (Rivinus's) ducts opening directly into the oral cavity in the sublingual fold. Anterior sublingual ducts can fuse to form the major sublingual duct of Bartholin. This duct can open directly into the oral cavity or into Wharton's duct. The sublingual gland receives its blood supply from the lingual artery. Lymphatic drainage of the gland is into the ipsilateral submental and submandibular lymph nodes (27).

Sonographically, the sublingual gland is best visualized in transverse and longitudinal planes obtained from the submental position. The average size of the normal gland is 32 × 12 mm (29). It has an echogenic structure similar to that of other major salivary glands. The gland is covered by the mandible, which may obscure the anterior part of the gland. The mylohyoid and genioglossus muscles are readily identified. Normally the sublingual ductal system cannot be visualized with US.

Sonographic Pathology

Acute bacterial sialoadenitis is an infection of the salivary gland that occurs mainly in debilitated, immunocompromised, and elderly individuals with poor oral hygiene and infection in adjacent head and neck structures. Salivary stasis secondary to stones and decreased saliva production leads to sialoadenitis in nearly half of the patients. Bacterial sialoadenitis more commonly involves the parotid. It rarely involves the submandibular gland; it is thought that its mucinous secretion may serve a protective function. *Staphylococcus aureus* is the most common offender; others involved are *Streptococcus viridans* and *pyogenes, Haemophilus influenzae, Escherichia coli,* and *Streptococcus pneumoniae* (30). The diagnosis is made clinically. The patient often appears septic with a gland that is painful, tender, and swollen. If the duct is not completely obstructed, purulent drainage can be present from the papilla. US is the diagnostic study of choice because sialography is contraindicated in the presence of an acute purulent process in the ductal system. Sonographically, the gland is enlarged with inhomogeneous parenchyma and decreased echogenicity secondary to edema (28). Abscesses appear as primarily anechoic structures with irregular borders and posterior enhancement (Fig. 14). Marked thickening of the surrounding tissues is common. Debris within the abscess cavity can make it appear multiechoic. Cervical adenopathy may be present (27). US-guided aspiration can be performed for sizable abscesses for both diagnostic and therapeutic purposes (24,31) (Fig. 15). One of the most important objectives in evaluation of acute sialoadenitis is to exclude sialectasia, which is secondary to sialolithiasis in 90% of the cases. When the intraglandular ductal system is dilated, the ducts become visible as tubular hypoechoic structures (26).

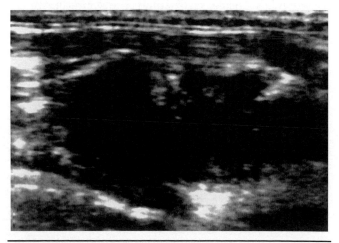

FIGURE 14. Parotid abscess demonstrating inhomogeneous parenchyma and cavitation with debris, irregular borders, and posterior enhancement.

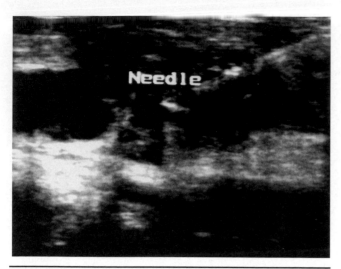

FIGURE 15. Ultrasound-guided fine needle aspiration of parotid abscess.

Viral sialoadenitis is frequently caused by mumps virus and is the most common cause of parotitis. Influenza, parainfluenza, Ebstein–Barr, Coxsackie A, echovirus, and cytomegalovirus have also been implicated. It is commonly bilateral but can be unilateral. Viral and bacterial sialoadenitis have a similar local manifestation, but abscess and pus are uncommon. Generalized symptoms are those of acute viral infection. The diagnosis is clinical and does not require imaging. US is the first-line study in documenting recurrences and monitoring their resolution with therapy (32), whereas sialography is recommended for an atypical form or when US is not informative (27).

Chronic recurrent sialoadenitis is characterized by periacinar lymphocytic infiltration and microcystic ductal dilatation (27). Acinar ectasia is a diagnostic finding on sialogram. Sonographically, it typically appears as multiple, round, hypoechoic structures 2 to 4 mm in size (1). However, sonographic abnormalities are present in only 18% of patients with chronic sialoadenitis, and therefore a normal US study does not rule out the diagnosis. *Sjögren's disease* is a variant of chronic sialoadenitis that presents as a classic triad of keratoconjunctivitis sicca, dryness of mucous membranes, and rheumatoid arthritis. US can be unrevealing even in the presence of documented sialographic abnormalities. Irregularity of the parenchyma secondary to fibrosis and ductal ectasia is also an important diagnostic feature (1). A typical sonographic feature of Sjögren's disease is the presence of multiple cystic areas throughout the parenchyma due to nonobstructive sialectasia. In cases of a longstanding process, ectasia of the intraglandular ducts can be very substantial with multiple complex cystic masses (up to 3 cm) with well-defined margins (33). Progressive fibrotic changes in the gland lead to more pronounced hetero-geneity of the parenchyma. Marked hypervascularity of the parenchyma has been demonstrated in up to 50% of patients (1). A few reactive lymph nodes that appear as hypoechoic lesions with eccentric, echogenic hila are frequently present.

Sialography is a very sensitive study for early diagnosis of both chronic recurrent sialoadenitis and Sjögren's disease (26). However, the role of the sialogram as a primary diagnostic modality has recently been challenged, as good correlation between US and digital sialography has been reported (34,35). These studies recommend US as the initial screening examination of patients with symptoms suggesting an inflammatory process involving the salivary glands. If US yields a normal result or reveals a solid mass, sialography is not indicated. If, however, US examination demonstrates the presence of calculi, duct dilatation, cystic elements, or an enlarged gland, sialography should be performed to identify lesions in the main duct such as strictures or calculi.

Sialolithiasis is the formation or presence of salivary stones. This process is limited to the gland and is not associated with stone formation in the renal and biliary system. Sialolithiasis is associated with recurrent painful swelling and pain during eating. Salivary stones are found in 1.2 % of the population, and two-thirds of patients with chronic sialoadenitis have at least one sialolith (30). The submandibular gland is the most common site of stone formation (80% to 92%), followed by the parotid (10% to 20%) and sublingual glands (2% to 7%). This distribution of the disease is related to the concentration of mucin in the saliva produced by different salivary glands. Mucin increases the viscosity of saliva and slows salivary flow, which predisposes to precipitation of calcium and stone formation. The majority of stones are solitary and measure less than 1 cm; only 25% of patients have multiple sialoliths (30). Multiglandular involvement is unusual (less than 3%) (27). Eighty percent of submandibular and 60% of parotid stones are radiopaque because they contain calcium carbonate and calcium phosphate. Radiolucent stones are typically composed of urates (24).

Physical examination is important because submandibular stones are frequently palpable. Plain radiograms, including oral films, have been the traditional imaging study for sialolithiasis and are helpful in localizing radiopaque stones. Sialogram has been used in identifying radiolucent stones. US has emerged as a highly sensitive modality in the diagnosis of sialolithiasis. It has a superior ability to detect both radiopaque and radiolucent concrements, with sensitivities reported from 80% to 94% (1,26,36). The stone typically appears as a highly echogenic image with posterior acoustic shadow. Stones smaller than 2 mm often do not have a shadow. Exact location of the stone in relation to the salivary ducts, as well as concomitant ductal ectasia, can also be defined.

Differentiation of the stone as intraductal versus intraglandular has an important therapeutic implication. Distally located intraductal stones are amenable to ductal incision or dilatation and extraction of the stone, whereas symptomatic intraglandular stones may require surgical extirpation of the gland. Extracorporeal shock wave lithotripsy is a new, rapidly evolving treatment for salivary gland stones that is becoming an alternative to surgical treatment and a primary treatment modality in some centers (37). US can be effectively used as an adjunct to extracorporeal lithotripsy by allowing delineation of ductal structures and in monitoring progress of the treatment (38).

The general approach to the patient with suspected sialolithiasis includes obtaining initial plain radiographs. If the stone is not seen or its position is not certain, US is performed. If the latter still does not provide a satisfactory image and clinical suspicion remains, a sialogram should be obtained (26). Because 40% of parotid sialoliths are radiolucent and radiographic imaging of the gland is compromised by superposition of osseous structures, US is the first-line diagnostic study for suspected parotid sialolithiasis.

Simple hypertrophy is diffuse, bilateral, symmetric, chronic, or recurrent enlargement of the salivary gland with preservation of the normal shape and echo structure (30). The parotid is usually involved; however, submandibular, sublingual, and minor salivary glands can also be affected. It is more common in certain populations (Egyptians and North Africans) and often is associated with obesity, alcoholism, diabetes, thyroid disease, and uremia. Diagnosis is made based on the clinical presentation (24). Sialography reveals paucity of the ductal system with the typical "dead tree" appearance due to the markedly increased gland volume. CT, MRI, and US findings are nonspecific. Sonography reveals a homogeneous, hypertrophic gland with fatty pathologic changes.

Cystic lesions (sialoceles) constitute up to 5% of salivary gland masses. The majority of cysts are in the parotid gland. They are due to accumulation of saliva secondary to obstruction of the ductal system that can be congenital or acquired (traumatic, calculous, or inflammatory stricture). In the case of complete ductal obstruction, atrophy of the corresponding area of the gland follows, and such a cyst can reach a considerable size. This retention cyst is known as a mucocele of a major salivary gland. Such cysts generally occur in the submandibular gland, but the same process in the sublingual gland is referred to as a ranula. Sonographic evaluation of the walls of the cyst is critical for accurate diagnosis. A typical cyst appears as a solitary, well-delineated, echo-free mass with smooth, thin, and regular walls. Irregularity in thickness and nodularity of the wall should be investigated to exclude Warthin's tumor (solitary or multiple) and the lymphoepithelial cysts often associated with human immu-

▶ **TABLE 5 Ultrasound of Benign Pathologic Processes of Salivary Glands**

Acute bacterial sialoadenitis
- Debilitated, dehydrated patient with salivary stasis often secondary to stones
- Parotid is the most common site
- Ultrasound is the study of choice; sialogram is contraindicated
- Enlarged gland with inhomogeneous parenchyma and decreased echogenicity due to edema. Abscess will appear as an anechoic structure with irregular borders; ultrasound assists the drainage
- Rule out sialolithiasis by ultrasound

Viral sialoadenitis
- Generalized symptoms of viral infection
- Often bilateral
- Ultrasound is the first-line study; sialogram is reserved for atypical cases

Chronic recurrent sialoadenitis
- Pathologic landmark is acinar (nonobstructive) sialectasia
- Multiple round hypoechoic structures 2–4 mm in size
- Sialogram is indicated if ultrasound reveals calculi, ductal dilatation, cystic elements, or an enlarged gland to identify strictures or calculi of the main duct

Sialolithiasis
- Submandibular gland is the most common site; multiglandular involvement is rare
- Initial plane radiograph: if stone is not seen or its position is undetermined, ultrasound should be performed
- Stones appear as a highly echogenic image with posterior acoustic shadow
- Location of the stone and concomitant ductal ectasia can be defined

Simple hypertrophy
- Diffuse bilateral, symmetric, chronic enlargement
- Homogeneous hypertrophic gland with fatty pathologic changes (nonspecific)
- Sialogram reveals paucity of ductal system ("dead tree" appearance)

Cystic lesions
- Obstruction of the ductal system leads to atrophy and cyst formation (sialoceles)
- Cyst appears as a solitary, well-defined, echo-free mass with smooth and thin walls

nodeficiency virus (HIV) infection. A parotid cyst with extraglandular fistulous connection to the area of the external auditory canal may represent remnants of the first branchial cleft system (30) (Table 5).

Neoplasms of salivary glands account for less than 3% of tumors and are responsible for 750 deaths annually (30,36). They are more common in Eskimos. A history of head and neck irradiation is another significant risk factor. A palpable nodule is the most common presentation of a salivary gland tumor. US has an important role in the management of salivary gland neoplasms as a highly sensitive and accurate technique. Sonographic examination

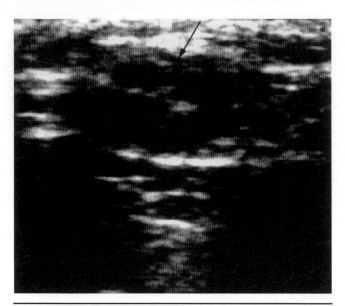

FIGURE 16. Fine needle aspiration of a pleomorphic adenoma (*arrow*) appearing as a hypoechoic mass with posterior enhancement. Note a hyperechoic needle in the center of the tumor.

allows confirmation of the intraglandular location of the tumor and delineation of the relation of the mass to the surrounding structures (e.g., facial nerve). US can facilitate FNA biopsy of nonpalpable, small, or vaguely palpable salivary masses (39) and can be used to perform a local staging (24).

Between 70% and 85% of salivary gland tumors originate from the parotid gland, and for every 100 parotid tumors there are 10 submandibular tumors, 10 minor salivary gland tumors, and 1 sublingual tumor. Approximately 80% of parotid tumors are benign. Pleomorphic adenomas (benign mixed tumors) are the most common benign parotid (85% to 90%) and overall major salivary gland (70% to 80%) neoplasm. They are composed of epithelial, myoepithelial, and mesenchymal tissues; calcifications and ossifications within the tumor matrix are a remarkable pathologic feature of these tumors (30). The rate of developing malignancy in the pleomorphic adenoma, so-called *carcinoma ex pleomorphic adenoma*, is believed to be 2% to 5%, but if left untreated as many as 25% may undergo malignant transformation (40). Sudden changes in a longstanding parotid lesion are suggestive of malignant transformation. Ninety percent of these tumors are located in the superficial lobe of the parotid gland, making them amenable to US examination. Sonographically, pleomorphic adenoma appears as a superficial, well-demarcated, hypoechoic mass with distinct posterior enhancement (Fig. 16). Large tumors may appear lobular with heterogeneous areas of necrosis or hemorrhage, calcification, or ossification (30). Malignant transformation manifests sonographically by irregular

borders and heterogeneous, hypoechoic appearance of the lesion. MRI is the most important complementary study and is indicated for atypical lesions, large pleomorphic adenomas (greater than 3 cm), or extension of the tumor to the deep lobe or parapharyngeal space. Treatment is resection with an adequate margin that typically requires a formal parotidectomy or en bloc removal of the entire involved salivary gland. US or MRI should be used for follow-up since a recurrence rate as high as 13% at 10 years has been reported (27).

Warthin's tumor (adenolymphoma or papillary cystadenoma lymphomatosum) is the second most common parotid tumor, representing 6% to 10% of all parotid neoplasms. It occurs almost exclusively in the parotid gland. Warthin's tumors are bilateral and multicentric in 10% of patients and have a higher propensity for recurrence (24). These tumors consist of papillary epithelial projections into the cystic spaces surrounded by the lymphoid stroma. Sonographically, Warthin's tumors have a hypoechoic, homogeneous appearance with smooth borders. Cystic areas of variable size with multiple septae can appear heterogeneous and may produce a prominent posterior acoustic enhancement.

Malignant salivary gland tumors are uncommon. Similar to their benign counterpart, salivary malignancies present as a slowly growing mass. Pain is present in association with the mass in 5% of benign and 6% of malignant tumors. Parotid mass with facial nerve paralysis occurs in 12% to 14% of patients with parotid malignancies and is a grave prognostic sign. These patients carry a 66% to 77% chance of cervical lymph node metastases and a 5-year survival of 9% to 14% (30).

Approximately 20% of parotid, 60% of submandibular, and 80% of sublingual and minor salivary gland tumors are malignant (30). Although the majority of parotid neoplasms are benign, the parotid gland is still the most common site of salivary gland malignancies because 70% and 85% of all salivary gland tumors originate from the parotid.

Mucoepidermoid carcinoma is the most common malignant neoplasm of the parotid and the second most common cancer of the submandibular and minor salivary glands. It is overall the most common salivary gland malignancy in both adults and children (30,41).

Adenoid cystic carcinoma (cylindroma) is a relatively uncommon tumor in the parotids but is the most common neoplasm in the other salivary glands, particularly the minor salivary glands about the mouth. Bilateral tumors are encountered 3% of the time (41). An important biologic feature of this tumor, seen in 50% to 60% of cases, is its high propensity for perineural invasion. The tumor can spread in both an antegrade and a retrograde direction to the skull base. The facial and the mandibular nerves are commonly involved.

Acinic cell carcinoma is a rare salivary gland malignancy that almost exclusively originates in the parotid.

This is the second most common pediatric salivary gland malignancy. Acinic cell carcinoma tends to have hematogenous rather than lymphatic spread. This slow-growing tumor often has a relentless course, and multiple long-term recurrences beyond 5 years are not uncommon. Grossly the tumor is unencapsulated but circumscribed, and it may be solid or cystic.

Metastases into the parotid are common. Rapid growth of the tumor is clinically suggestive of its metastatic nature. Metastases outnumbered primary salivary gland malignancies in some series. Parotid lymph nodes drain lymph from the extensive area of skin of the face and scalp, external auditory canal, orbital content, posterior oral cavity, pharynx, and the parotid gland (25). Metastatic squamous cell carcinoma and melanoma constitute, in equal proportions, 80% of these metastases (42). Hematogenous metastases of breast, lung, kidney, and gastrointestinal primaries to the parotid gland have also been described (30). Primary lymphoma of the salivary gland is very rare. Secondary involvement has been reported in 1% to 8% of lymphoma patients. Large cell lymphoma is the most common histologic type, and the parotid is the most common salivary gland involved.

Evaluation of the patient with suspected salivary gland mass must include a thorough clinical examination. Diagnosis of malignancy is obvious in 22% of patients with parotid carcinoma due to the presence of complete or partial facial nerve paralysis, cervical lymph node metastases, or invasion of the tumor into skin or

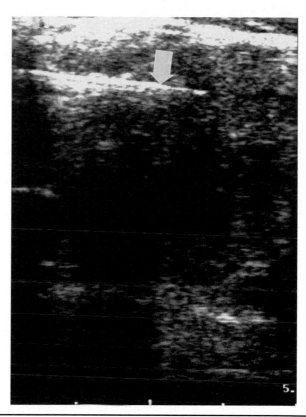

FIGURE 18. Fine needle (arrow) aspiration biopsy of parotid neoplasm.

adjacent structures (43). US is used as a first-line study of masses that are thought to originate from the salivary glands. Sonographic examination can confirm intraglandular as opposed to perisalivary lymph node location of the mass. It is also helpful in screening the contralateral parotid gland in patients with tumors known to be bilateral (Warthin's tumor and adenoid cystic carcinoma). Sonographic imaging of salivary gland tumors does not allow delincation of the malignant nature of the neoplasm. US typically does not demonstrate features that are suspicious for malignancy in tumors smaller than 2 cm. Larger and more locally advanced malignancies may have irregular borders as a result of their invasive property and heterogeneous areas of necrosis and hemorrhage (1) (Fig. 17). Using sharp as opposed to ill-defined borders as the criterion to distinguish benign from malignant tumors, Gritzmann reported that 28% of malignant masses were misclassified as benign (26). The majority of salivary gland cancers have no specific imaging features; therefore, a definitive histopathologic diagnosis is imperative before proceeding with treatment.

Preoperative tissue diagnosis is best established by FNA biopsy (FNAB) (Fig. 18). The accuracy of this procedure has been well established in numerous studies. Overall sensitivity has been from 85% to 99% and specificity from 93% to 100% (44). In a classic study of 101

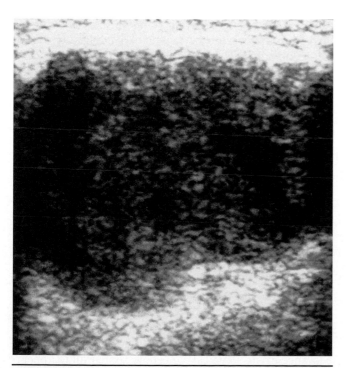

FIGURE 17. Metastatic squamous cancer involving the parotid demonstrating irregular borders and heterogeneous interior.

consecutive patients with major salivary gland tumors, Heller et al. showed that FNAB changed the clinical approach in 35% of patients (45). However, sampling error remains the major limitation of the technique. Sonographic guidance assures that the needle tip is correctly placed in the solid portion of the tumor, avoiding the pitfall of nondiagnostic aspiration of the cystic component of the mass. It improves the yield of FNAB for poorly palpable or nonpalpable masses where the tumor can only be seen on CT or MRI and for multiple palpable masses where localization is critical. Cytology is particularly helpful in the diagnosis of metastatic disease in the parotid gland and can change the management approach to this group of patients. FNAB can be indeterminate in tumors such as pleomorphic adenomas and hemangiomas; therefore, it may be necessary to proceed with excisional biopsy when cytologic findings do not correlate with clinical impression (39).

Cervical node metastases are present in 18% of parotid, 28% of submandibular, and 15% of minor salivary gland malignancies on initial presentation (43). Sonography with an option of US-guided FNAB is the best diagnostic technique for evaluation of cervical lymph node involvement (27). Lymphoma is usually suggested by history and the presence of cervical adenopathy. US allows an examination of the involvement of the regional lymph nodes with lymphoma. US-guided core needle biopsy has a lower nondiagnostic sampling rate than does FNAB (23) (Table 6).

▶ **TABLE 6 Ultrasound of Tumors of Salivary Glands**

Salivary gland neoplasms
- Lesion with irregular borders and heterogeneous, hypoechoic appearance
- Confirm intraglandular position of the tumor and assess relation to the surrounding anatomic structures
- Ultrasound-guided fine needle aspiration biopsy for morphologic verification of the diagnosis
- Regional staging of the tumor: sonographic evaluation of the lymph nodes
- Evaluation of the contralateral gland for tumors with known bilaterality (Warthin's tumor, cylindroma, etc.)
- Surveillance
- Magnetic resonance imaging is indicated for benign or malignant lesions greater than 3 cm and for suspected extraglandular extension into parapharyngeal and retrostyloid spaces or parapharyngeal and retromandibular adenopathy

Parotid lymph node metastases
- Malignancy location with predominant drainage to the parotid nodes
- Evaluation of the of the cervical lymph nodes
- Ultrasound-guided fine needle aspiration biopsy for morphologic verification of the diagnosis

SOFT-TISSUE LESIONS AND CONGENITAL ANOMALIES OF THE NECK

Masses of the neck are a diverse group of acquired and congenital conditions. Differential diagnosis is dependent on the clinical presentation and the age of the patient. Although congenital malformations are more common in children, a painless firm node in the neck of an adult patient is a malignancy until proven otherwise. This section will discuss the role of US in the diagnosis of neck masses not originating from the lymph nodes (Table 7).

Cystic Lesions

Cystic lesions are relatively common in the head and neck region. Most of the cystic lesions originate from the thyroglossal duct, thyroid gland, branchial clefts, and developing lymphatic channels. Less common cystic masses include laryngocele, pharyngocele, and sublingual and odontogenic cysts. Occasionally, an abscess or cavitation of a lymph node metastasis can present as a cystic mass in the neck (46).

Thyroglossal duct cysts are these most common congenital mass in the neck. They are three times as common as branchial cleft cysts (47). The thyroid gland originates initially as a thickening and later as a thyroglossal duct growing from the ventral pharyngeal wall, beginning in the fourth week of embryogenesis. The normal remnants of the thyroglossal duct are the foramen cecum and the pyramidal lobe of the thyroid. Cysts of the thyroglossal duct can be anywhere along the course of the duct from the base of the tongue to as low as the suprasternal area; however, 60% are located between the hyoid bone and the thyroid cartilage. Multiple tracts or "lateral branches" may exist so that as many as 38% may present away from the midline (48), and 10% to 25% of the cysts were found in the lateral neck (47).

The combination of history, physical examination, and US is sufficient for the diagnosis. Clinically the thyroglossal cyst presents as a soft or hard, mobile, and sometimes fluctuating swelling in the midline of the neck. The overlying skin is nontender and movable. The cyst moves with swallowing and tongue protrusion. If a thyroglossal cyst becomes inflamed, pain, tenderness, and skin swelling with attachment are common findings. Fistulization is the result of infection, trauma, and inadequate previous operations seen in one third of patients with this condition. Sonographically, the thyroglossal duct cyst has the cystic appearance of a well-delineated, hypoechoic, or anechoic cystic lesion with posterior acoustic enhancement (Fig. 19). Significant variation of sonographic appearance exists. "Typical" anechoic sonographic appearance is reported in 42% to 68.2% of children, but in only

▶ **TABLE 7 Ultrasound of Soft-Tissue Lesions and Congenital Anomalies of the Head and Neck**

Thyroglossal duct cyst
- Cysts are located anywhere from the base of the tongue to suprasternal area (most commonly between the hyoid bone and the thyroid cartilage). Entire duct should be visualized
- Most are at the midline, but branching and fistulization are common and 25% of cysts are in the lateral neck
- Noninflamed cyst has anechoic, thin-walled appearance with posterior enhancement. Inflamed cyst is hypoechoic with accumulation of low-amplitude free-floating debris and has a thickened wall
- Routine preoperative ^{131}I scan is important for the evaluation of ectopic thyroid

Branchial cleft anomalies
- Most pathologic lesions originate from the second branchial cleft; cysts are the most common. Children and young adults are the typical age groups
- Inflammation is common manifestation
- Noninflamed cyst is thin-walled, hypoechoic structure with posterior acoustic enhancement; inflamed cyst appears more heterogeneous, and echogenic walls become thickened and internal debris are more prominent
- In older age group, cystic metastasis in the neck should be suspected

Congenital cystic lesions
- Epidermal cyst (does not contain skin appendages), dermoid cyst (contains skin appendages), and teratoid cyst (contains connective tissue elements)
- They have well-defined borders and hypoechoic or hyperechoic content with some internal echogenicity. Significant internal echoes can be present in teratoid cyst if it contains bony elements

Lymphatic malformations (cystic hygroma)
- Anomalous development of lymphatic vessels that fail to establish communication with developing veins; posterior cervical triangle and cervicothoracic region are common sites
- Ultrasound reveals thin-walled, multicystic compressible mass with regular borders
- Does not respect anatomic boundaries, and encasement of neurovascular structure is common

Lipoma
- Well-defined, compressible, elliptical mass; its longest dinmeter is parallel to the skin. It is more commonly hyperechoic but can be iso- or hypoechoic; heterogeneous internal echoes are common

Neurogenic tumors
- Originate in the vicinity of nerve trunks; vagus involvement is the most common
- Solid, hypoechoic mass with posterior enhancement; it is difficult to distinguish from the lymph node

Soft tissue sarcoma
- Ultrasound assists with initial evaluation; use of computed tomography or magnetic resonance imaging is important for resection planning

Carotid body tumor
- Slow-growing, painless mass in the area of the carotid sheath that is mobile in the horizontal direction
- Selective angiogram is the gold standard. However, Doppler ultrasound is sufficient
- Heterogeneous, hypoechoic lesion located at the carotid bifurcation
- Fine needle aspiration or biopsy is contraindicated

28% of adults, which may be secondary to frequent inflammatory episodes with increasing age (49). On sonography in adults, 50% of the lesions are thin walled and 88% have posterior enhancement. The thyroglossal duct cyst is always hypoechoic compared to surrounding tissues. Different degrees of echogenicity, heterogeneity, and thickness and structure of the wall can be present. The homogeneous, hypoechoic appearance of some thyroglossal cysts is a result of accumulation of low-amplitude, free-floating debris and accounts for 18% of all presenting cysts in adults (48). The presence of multiple, small anechoic spaces or dense internal echoes and a thick (greater than 5 mm) cystic wall are other common manifestations of inflammatory changes in the thyroglossal duct cysts (50).

It is routine to sonographically visualize the entire course of the thyroglossal duct and demonstrate any additional cysts or extension of the fistula to the skin and tongue, as well as the relationship with the hyoid bone (48). Thyroglossal duct cysts may present as complex cysts with a solid component due to the presence of thyroid tissue in the lesion or malignant transformation of the inner lining that may occur in 1% of the cysts (51). When a complex cyst is found or associated lymphadenopathy is present, FNA biopsy of both the cystic duct remnant and sonographically or physically abnormal lymph nodes is prudent to confirm the presence of normal thyroid tissue and to rule out a papillary adenocarcinoma. Infection is a common complication. Sonographic examination of an infected cyst reveals inhomogeneous echoes from pus.

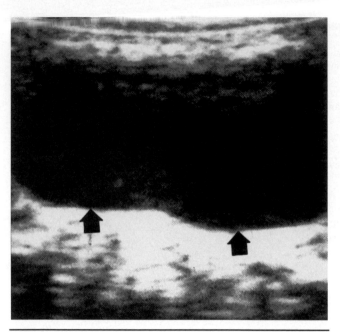

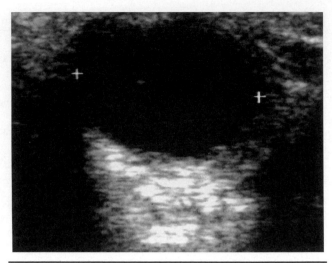

FIGURE 20. A superficially located branchial cleft cyst (*cursors*) with posterior enhancement, which had become infected.

FIGURE 19. A typical thyroglossal duct cyst (*arrows*) demonstrating anechoic interior, smooth margins, and posterior enhancement.

It is believed that 1% to 2% of thyroglossal duct anomalies are associated with ectopic thyroid gland. Multiple cases of inadvertent removal of the only functional thyroid tissue from ectopic locations have been reported. Therefore, routine thyroid US should be performed to identify a normal position of the thyroid gland if thyroglossal duct remnants are discovered and an operative procedure is planned (52). Thyroid scan may yield further information if ectopic thyroid is suspected on US (53).

Branchial cleft anomalies are commonly encountered in the lateral neck. The majority of these lesions (90% to 95%) originate from the second branchial cleft and occur in young individuals. Obliteration of the second branchial cleft normally takes place during the sixth and seventh weeks of development. Complete failure of obliterating the branchial cleft leads to formation of a *branchial cleft fistula* that typically has its external opening in the lower third of the neck anterior to the sternomastoid muscle. The fistula traverses posterior to the caudal aspect of the platysma and through the deep cervical fascia and reaches the carotid sheath. It turns medially coming underneath the stylohyoid muscle and the posterior belly of the digastric muscle. The fistula passes through the carotid bifurcation, where it is located in front of the hypoglossal nerve. It finally enters the pharynx in the anterior aspect of the posterior faucial tonsil or occasionally into the tonsil itself. Variable degree of persistence of the second branchial cleft can be present into the adult life. Failure to obliterate the distal part of the branchial cleft tract results in formation of the *external sinus*. Likewise,

the *internal sinus* forms when the most proximal part of the tract persists. Failure to obliterate a segment of the branchial cleft results in a *branchial cleft cyst* (47). Four locations of the cysts are recognized: (a) superficial cysts anterior to the sternomastoid muscle, (b) cysts under the deep cervical fascia and anterior to the carotid sheath (the most common variant), (c) cysts with branchial extension toward the pharynx, and (d) cysts between the carotid sheath and the pharyngeal wall (54) (Fig. 20).

The most common presentation of the lesion is a cystic mass without sinus or fistula located behind the angle of the mandible in a child or a young adult. Of these second branchial cleft remnants, 97% contain lymphoid tissue that can become hypertrophic during upper respiratory tract infection when the condition often manifests for the first time.

First branchial cleft anomalies are rare and account for 8% to 10% of all branchiogenic pathologic processes. Fistulas or tracts are half as common as the cysts and more common in younger patients (55). The internal tract of the complete first branchial cleft fistula opens into the external auditory canal, commonly at the anteroinferior aspect of the bony–cartilaginous junction. It may be associated with anomalies of the temporal bone. The external opening is commonly located in the periauricular region or in the upper neck, anterior to the sternocleidomastoid muscle. Common presentation in these patients includes periauricular swelling or sinus, mass in the external auricular canal, or drainage from the ear. The parotid gland, external auditory canal, and the angle of the mandible are usual locations of the first branchial cleft cyst. Multiple attempts to drain the "parotid abscess" and antibiotic treatments are common in the history of these patients. If the lesion communicates with the external auditory canal, ear drainage may be a presenting complaint. US reveals a well-demarcated cystic lesion with posterior enhancement in the inferior pole of the parotid, with extraglandular fistulous connection to the area of external auditory canal (30). Variable amounts of debris are typically present in the cyst.

Third and fourth branchial cleft anomalies are extremely rare. A piriform sinus fistula or a lateral neck mass associated with a recurrent inflammatory process in a young person should raise suspicion of this entity. Cystic hygroma, laryngocele, adenopathy, epidermoid cyst, or salivary gland tumors can present in a similar manner and should be excluded before the diagnosis of third and fourth branchial cleft pathology is entertained. If diagnosis is strongly suspected, barium swallow with or without CT scan is the preferred imaging study (56).

Malignant transformation of remnants of the branchial cleft (malignant branchioma) has been hypothesized, but evidence of its existence is lacking. In one large retrospective study, all 136 cystic squamous cell carcinomas of the neck were cavitating metastases most commonly from lingual and faucial tonsil (64%) and nasopharyngeal tonsillar tissue (8%) (46).

Sonographically, remnants of branchial clefts have variable echogenicity (Fig. 20). When not inflamed, they have a typical cystic appearance. They can be completely anechoic, but are more commonly hypoechoic with a very fine granular pattern due to accumulation of cellular debris within the cyst or sinus. Walls of the cyst are well defined, and posterior acoustic enhancement is typically present. If the cyst becomes infected, it appears more echogenic and heterogeneous (57). The walls of the cyst become thickened and ill defined; internal debris and septation is commonly present. This lesion is difficult to differentiate from cystic metastasis; therefore, if diagnosis is in doubt, US-guided FNA should be performed. Discovery of malignancy requires a formal staging workup.

Congenital cystic lesions include three different types. *Epidermal cysts* are the most common in the head and neck region (Fig. 21). The cyst is formed by epithelial lining in the fibrous capsule and does not contain skin appendages, in contrast to the *dermoid cyst*, which has a similar structure but contains skin appendages. *Teratoid cysts* are also similar to epidermoid cysts but have connective tissue elements. Sonographically, these cysts have well-defined borders and hypoechoic content with some internal echogenicity as a result of accumulation of cellular debris. Dermoid cysts may have mixed heterogeneous internal echoes due to the presence of fat and bony or dental elements that could be noted by dense echogenic foci and shadowing. Sonographic differentiation between epidermoid and dermoid cysts is only possible in the presence of osseodental elements.

Lymphatic malformations are congenital malformations that are most commonly discovered during the first

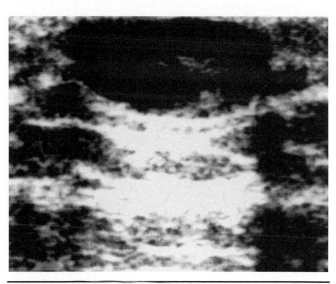

FIGURE 21. Epidermal inclusion cyst of the neck which demonstrates heterogeneous interior, superficial location, and posterior enhancement.

2 years of life (Fig. 22). They represent anomalous development of lymphatic vessels (rather than true neoplasms) that arise when lymphatic channels fail to establish communication with developing veins. *Cystic hygromas* have large lymphatic spaces; cavernous lymphangiomas have smaller spaces and result from the anomaly of terminal lymphatics; and capillary lymphangiomas have the smallest spaces. They are soft, subfascial masses adherent to the deep cervical structures located in the lateral neck or, less commonly, in the axilla, floor of the mouth, and parotid region. When they present in children, the posterior cervical triangle and cervicothoracic region are common sites. In adults, they are typically located in the submandibular, submental, and parotid regions. Physical examination is generally diagnostic because cystic hygromas are large soft masses that often transilluminate. Hemorrhage and infection can obscure clinical presentation and alter imaging. US examination reveals thin-walled multicystic compressible mass with regular borders. Significant hypervascularity of the septae can be appreciated on color flow Doppler study (Fig. 23). US is important for assessment of the extent of the lesion because cystic hygromas may extend into multiple cervical spaces and do not respect anatomic boundaries (58). Infection or hemorrhage in the cystic hygroma may mimic a solid lesion.

Solid Masses of the Neck

Solid masses of the neck are often metastatic. Primary solid cervical masses can be of neurogenic, muscular, vascular, or other soft-tissue origin.

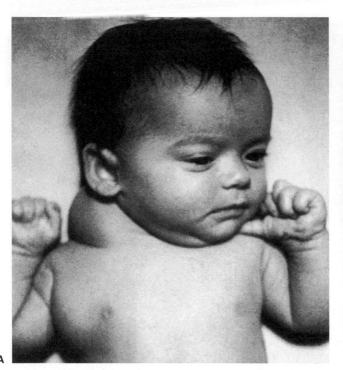
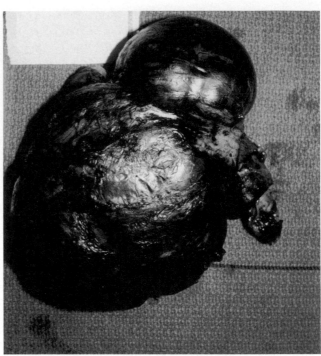

A   B

FIGURE 22. In situ (**A**) and gross pathology (**B**) of a cystic hygroma of the neck in an infant. (Courtesy of Abid Khan, M.D.)

Lipomas are the most common benign mesenchymal tumors. They commonly grow on the head and neck region (13%) and are multiple in 5% patients (59). Head and neck lipomas are commonly encapsulated lesions located adjacent to the clavicle in females and in the posterior cervical triangle in males. Most lipomas have an innocuous clinical course, are rarely infiltrating, and intramuscular head and neck lipomas lack a capsule and have a local recurrence rate as high as 50% to 65% (58). Clinical impression is supported by finding a well-defined, compressible, elliptical mass on US examination, with its

longest diameter parallel to the skin surface. The lesion is most commonly hyperechoic compared to the adjacent muscles (76%), but it can be isoechoic (8%) or hypoechoic (16%). Lipomas have heterogeneous, internal echoes and contain linear echogenic lines at a right angle to the US beam (Fig. 24). There is no posterior enhancement or significant vascularity (58).

Benign neurogenic tumors include schwannoma, neurofibroma, and ganglioneuroma, of which schwannoma is the most common in the head and neck region. Schwannoma describes two of the most common benign

FIGURE 23. **A:** B-mode ultrasound of a cystic hygroma. **B:** Color Doppler image of the same lesion with localization of major vascular structures (posterior to the cystic lesion).

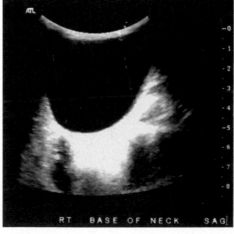
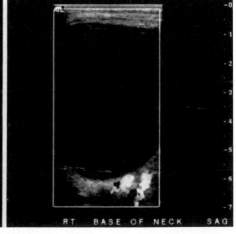

A   B

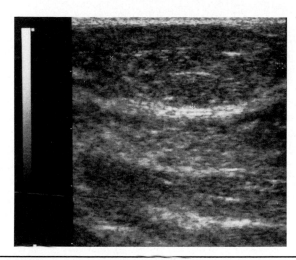

FIGURE 24. A 3 × 1.5 cm lipoma (*cursors*) in the right lateral neck. Note heterogeneous internal echoes with linear echogenic lines.

tumors of the peripheral nerve: neurilemomas and neurofibromas that originate from the Schwann cells of the peripheral nerves. The head and neck region is the most common location of the solitary benign schwannoma (42%), with the remainder being extremities, trunk, and mediastinum.

Neurilemoma is a benign, encapsulated neoplasm in which the fundamental component is structurally identical to a syncytium of Schwann cells, but axonal elements are usually not found. In contrast, neurofibroma is a moderately firm, benign, encapsulated tumor resulting from proliferation of Schwann cells in the endoneurium in a disorderly pattern that includes portions of nerve fibers. Neurofibromas are common in patients with neurofibromatosis type 1 (von Recklinghausen's disease).

Most schwannomas are painless and do not cause neurologic deficits. These tumors are slow-growing masses originating from the nerve trunks, but they usually do not initially affect nerve function. Schwannomas can reach a large size before neurologic dysfunction develops. In the neck, the vagus nerve is involved most commonly, followed by the cervical sympathetic nerve. Cervical nerve roots and the brachial plexus spinal accessory, glossopharyngeal, and hypoglossal nerves are affected less frequently.

The location of the tumor suggests its origin. Tumors arising from the vagus are typically located in the anterior cervical triangle, whereas tumors from cervical nerve roots are in the posterior triangle. Solitary schwannomas rarely undergo malignant transformation; however, in the presence of von Recklinghausen's disease, this risk is substantial.

Sonographically, these tumors appear as solid, hypoechoic masses with posterior enhancement. Cavitation is common and is not a sign of malignant transformation. A pseudocystic appearance with posterior enhancement is common. A well-defined cystic component is especially typical for neurilemomas, whereas neurofibromas may appear lobulated (60). Borders of the tumor are usually well defined. Thickening of the adjacent nerve may signify the origin of the tumor.

Sonographic differentiation of schwannomas from lymph nodes is difficult. Normal lymph nodes usually have an oval shape, well-defined borders, and do not have posterior enhancement. Lymph nodes afflicted with lymphoma typically reveal posterior enhancement (22). Metastatic nodes are round, frequently do not demonstrate a hilum, and may have areas of necrosis. They are more difficult to differentiate from schwannomas. FNA with sonographic guidance demonstrating benign-appearing spindle cells may significantly facilitate the diagnosis of schwannoma, but FNA is rarely conclusive and provides preoperative diagnosis in only one of eight cases (61). CT or MRI will clearly define the anatomic extent of the tumor to facilitate a safe excision.

Soft-tissue sarcomas of the head and neck are rare. They encompass a diverse group of pathologic entities. Von Recklinghausen's disease is a well-known predisposing condition, but otherwise the etiology is poorly understood. Soft-tissue sarcomas in the head and neck, especially rhabdomyosarcoma, are more common in children. US can have a role in the initial evaluation of the lesion and is more helpful in initial staging of superficial lesions. These tumors typically present as hypoechoic, heterogeneous masses with poorly defined margins. High-resolution CT or MRI is frequently necessary for detailed delineation of the invaded structures prior to the resection.

Carotid body tumor (chemodectoma) is the most common cervical paraganglioma originating from the chemoreceptor tissue of the carotid body that has a neural crest origin. The vagal, tympanic, and jugular are other common sites of chemodectomas in decreasing order of frequency (61). In general, carotid body tumors are found at the bifurcation of the common carotid as a 5- to 6-mm mass adherent to the adventitia of the medial aspect of the vessel. One third of paragangliomas of the neck originate from the glomus jugulare, aortic bodies, and adrenal gland (62). Approximately 10% of these tumors are bilateral and 10% are familial. Fewer than 10% are malignant. Carotid body tumors are rarely functional, but they may occur along with other paragangliomas or pheochromocytomas. Despite their low malignant propensity, chemodectomas tend to invade surrounding neurovascular and bony structures.

Physical examination classically reveals a slowly growing, painless neck mass in the area of the carotid sheath located underneath the anterior edge of the sternocleidomastoid muscle just lateral to the tip of the hyoid bone. The mass is mobile in the horizontal but not in the vertical direction and may transmit an arterial pulse (63). Auscultation may reveal bruits over the mass due to very high vascularity of the tumor.

Selective angiogram has been the gold standard for preoperative diagnosis of carotid body tumors (63). US and color Doppler have emerged as other important modalities in the diagnosis of these tumors. The tumor is usually a solid, heterogeneous, hypoechoic lesion located at the bifurcation of the common carotid artery (64). Color Doppler assists in identifying this vascular lesion and the adjacent vascular structures. Because of the unique Doppler features, sonographic diagnosis is sufficient. Neither FNA nor open biopsy of the carotid body tumor is recommended. MRI is another commonly used diagnostic modality and may be especially helpful in defining the extent of large tumors prior to resection (Table 7).

ORAL CAVITY AND TONGUE

Sonographic evaluation of the oral cavity is performed with the use of low- and high-frequency transducers. Submental and/or intraoral examinations are performed depending on the nature of the pathology. *Submental technique* is useful in evaluation of the floor of the mouth and the base of the tongue. If tumor is suspected, the patient is asked to swallow so as to displace the mass from the acoustic shadow of the hyoid bone (65). With this technique, a low-frequency (5-MHz) probe is needed for imaging of the bulk of the entire tongue from the apex to the base (66). *Intraoral examination* is carried out with a high-frequency intraoperative or endoscopic probe providing high-quality, detailed imaging of the superficial structures. Very-high-frequency intraoral probes demonstrate mucosa that has a mean thickness of 2.1 mm, the lamina propria, and the lingual musculature (67). High-frequency sonography of the floor of the mouth allows delineating the anterior bellies of the digastric and mylohyoid muscles as well as the septum and tongue muscles. Dynamic sonography of the tongue is also utilized but is not commonly used in surgical diagnosis.

Dermoid cysts are typically located close to the midline of the tongue, on the floor of the mouth, and in the upper neck at the level of the hyoid bone. Embryologically, they are epidermoid inclusions that occur in the process of fusion of the branchial clefts during early gestation. Dermoid cysts often have high echogenicity because of the fluid, hair, or sebum that has accumulated inside the cyst. The appearance of dermoid cysts is similar to that of their cutaneous counterparts.

Retention cysts containing mucous (*mucoceles*) often occur as a result of obstruction of the ductal system in the minor salivary glands in the buccal and lingual regions. When this affects the sublingual gland, it is known as a ranula. *Simple ranulae* are confined to floor of the mouth above the level of mylohyoid muscle and are typically located on the floor of the mouth or the undersurface of the tongue. They are true cysts that are surrounded by a complete epithelial lining. *Deep (plunging) ranulae* are the result of rupture of the wall of a simple ranula that leads to leakage of saliva into the surrounding tissues. They typically extend below the level of mylohyoid muscle and clinically present as a painless mass in the submental or submandibular triangle without a mass in the floor of the mouth. Histologically, a deep ranula is a pseudocyst because inflammatory tissue forms a part of the wall (30). US reveals a solitary, well-delineated, echofree mass (26). In deep ranulae most of the cystic collection is in the submandibular space and a small amount can be present in the sublingual space. The lesion may contain fine internal echoes and debris.

Cancer of the floor of the mouth is responsible for about 10% of aerodigestive cancers. Although these cancers are readily amenable to physical examination, US allows evaluation of the tumor volume invasion of mylohyoid muscles and the extension of the tumor between sublingual and lingual spaces. Flexible endosonography has demonstrated high accuracy in the detection of bone involvement by tumors of the floor of the mouth and tonsils. Transcutaneous US was found to be accurate only in assessment of bony involvement by the cancers of the floor of the mouth. Moreover, in the reported study the sonographer was able to distinguish cortical involvement from cancellous bone involvement in many cases but failed to diagnose periosteal invasion (68).

Carcinoma of the tongue represents 20% of upper aerodigestive malignancies. It is classified according to its location. Two thirds of these cancers arise from the mobile tongue and the remaining third from the base of the tongue. More posterior lesions carry a worse prognosis due to more advanced stage on presentation with frequent metastatic nodal involvement that is as high as 60% unilaterally and 15% bilaterally.

Clinical examination of the patient with cancer of mobile part of the tongue emphasizes several important points, such as invasion of the midline and extension to the floor of the mouth, mandible, base of the tongue, and tonsils. These findings will influence staging as well as the extent of the ablative operation. When the patient with cancer of the base of the tongue is evaluated, extension to the mobile portion of tongue, valleculae, suprahyoid epiglottis, glossotonsillar sulcus, tonsils, and pharyngoepiglottic folds is important (69). Lymph node evaluation is a routine part of the staging.

Sonographically, cancer of the tongue appears as a space-occupying lesion with blurred borders within the echogenic intrinsic tongue muscles. The tumor is less echogenic than adjacent normal muscles. Small cancers usually are homogeneous, but larger tumors may demonstrate some internal heterogeneity. Fluid and debris in the area of ulceration are seen as zones of hyperechogenicity. Evaluation of the extension of the tumor is a primary objective of US imaging. Depth of tumor invasion can be accurately assessed with intraoral US (70) that also allows more accurately visualized borders of the tumor and healthy tissues. Tumor invasion of the cancer of the mobile tongue to the base of the tongue, floor of the mouth, and tonsillar region can be adequately evaluated by US (71). The extent of the process is viewed in relation to the septum, which is typically seen as a hyperechoic midline structure. Hypoechoic infiltration into the extrinsic muscles of the tongue and across the midline is highly suggestive of a malignant invasion (65). Limitations of US for the evaluation of tongue cancer include inability to differentiate residual disease from postirradiation fibrotic changes and difficulty in staging large lesions, especially with retropharyngeal and parapharyngeal extension. As such, CT and MRI are considered to have better diagnostic capability in these cases (72,73).

Cancer of the tonsil is a common head and neck malignancy. Tumor extension toward the base of the tongue, pharyngeal wall, soft palate, and oral cavity is common. US may assist in delineation of the borders of invasion of the base of the tongue, but detection of posterior and superior extension is problematic. Management of the tonsillar primaries as well as those of the base of the tongue is nonsurgical, but management of the cervical lymph nodes may require node dissection. US of the cervical nodes is an important adjunct in the staging of these tumors (Table 8).

VISCERAL NECK: LARYNX, HYPOPHARYNX, AND CERVICAL ESOPHAGUS

High-resolution spiral CT and MRI have been established as diagnostic modalities in the evaluation of laryngeal and pharyngeal pathologic processes. Percutaneous and endoscopic US still has limited applications because of anatomic obstacles, technical difficulties, and unfamiliarity with the technique.

On US examination, the patient is in the supine position with head slightly hyperextended to stretch the base of the tongue and the floor of the mouth. A high-frequency transducer is used. Midline and lateral axial and transverse scanning is performed from the hyoid bone to the cricoid cartilage while the patient breathes quietly. The pyriform sinuses are examined in the coronal plane during Valsalva maneuver. The cricoid, thyroid cartilages, the entire subglottic region, epiglottis, preepiglottic space, and the base of the tongue are usually imaged. Tumor invasion usually presents as hypoechoic infiltration. The main focus of percutaneous laryngeal US is in evaluation of erosion of the cartilage and extralaryngeal spread to the surrounding soft tissues. US is felt to be superior to CT in the evaluation of carotid artery invasion because both the tumor and the vascular wall can have the same attenuation in CT, whereas in US sonographic impedance between the tumor and vascular wall can be appreciated. Examination of the cervical lymph nodes is also an important part of sonographic staging (65).

The major impediments of percutaneous laryngeal US are ossification and calcification of the laryngeal framework. Calcification of the laryngeal cartilages is a normal phenomenon that increases with age. Mineralization is asymmetric and has inhomogeneous distribution. Both calcification and ossification increase differences in sonographic impedance and alter acoustic reflection. They are seen as hyperechoic nodular structures with strong posterior shadowing, often create an impression of pseudotumoral nodules or invasion, and prevent one from obtaining a clear US image of the endolaryngeal structures.

Endolaryngeal US can be performed during microlaryngoscopy using a small-caliber, high-frequency transducer similar to the one used for endovascular US. A cuffed endotracheal tube is placed just above the carina, and the larynx is visualized through a laryngoscope. Then the larynx is filled with saline to prevent the retention of air in the anterior commissure and to improve sound transmission, and a sonographic image of the larynx is

---

▶ **TABLE 8** Ultrasound of Pathologic Lesions of the Oral Cavity and Tongue

Dermoid cyst
- Midline cysts (floor of the mouth, tongue, upper neck at the level of hyoid bone)
- High echogenicity from the hair and sebum accumulated in the cyst

Retention cyst
- Results from occlusion of the minor or major (ranula) salivary gland
- Simple ranula is a true located on the undersurface of the tongue above mylohyoid muscle
- Deep (plunging) ranulae result from the rupture of the simple ranula with extension below the mylohyoid muscle and present as a submental/submandibular mass
- Ultrasound reveals anechoic mass in sublingual space (simple) that extends into submandibular space (deep ranula)

Cancer of the floor of the mouth and the tongue
- Invasion of midline and extension to the floor of the mouth, mandible, base of the tongue, and tonsils as well as lymph node assessment are important parts of clinical and ultrasound examination
- Tumor appears as a space-occupying lesion with blurred borders and is less echogenic than surrounding muscles

obtained through a high-frequency US catheter connected to a 30-degree laryngoscopy endoscope and recorded on the videotape. Good resolution is achieved in the radius of 2.5 cm (74). The major drawback of the technique is its complexity (75).

The majority of masses discovered in the neck are normal or abnormal lymph nodes or cysts. The presence of the air in these locations raises concern of an abscess containing gas-producing flora or an abnormal communication with the sacculus of a laryngocele or piriform sinus for pharyngocele. Air is recognized sonographically as a hyperechoic area with scattered artifacts (76).

A *laryngocele* is a dilatation of the saccule of the laryngeal ventricle of Morgagni. The ventricle of the larynx is a lateral extension of mucosa between the true and false vocal cords. The laryngeal saccule, or appendix of the ventricle, is a diverticulum located on the anterior end that extends upward between the vestibular fold and the inner surface of the thyroid cartilage. Thin thyroarytenoid muscle forms the wall of the ventricle and facilitates its drainage. Three variants of laryngocele exist: internal, external, and mixed. An internal laryngocele remains strictly inside the larynx. In the external variant (exolaryngeal type), the saccule herniates through the thyrohyoid membrane at the weak point created by passage of the upper branch of the superior laryngeal nerve and blood vessels, protruding outward into the tissue of the lateral neck. A thin channel connects the external laryngocele with nondilated ventricle. The mixed type is defined as the presence of both external and internal components on the same side. This is the most common type and is responsible for almost half of all cases. The saccule typically contains mucus, saliva, or air. Clinical diagnosis is straightforward. Patients most commonly present with hoarseness, stridor, dysphagia, and fluctuating neck swelling that are commonly related to the mass effect of the laryngocele. Laryngoceles readily distend in response to Valsalva's maneuver and collapse on palpation with a gurgling and hissing sound (77).

Sonographically, a fluid-containing laryngocele appears as a well-delineated, hypoechoic cyst located within the thyroid cartilage, adjacent to the thyrohyoid membrane. If a solid or complex cystic structure is discovered, it is imperative that FNAB be carried out to evaluate the histologic origin of the lesion and exclude tumor, which may be present in 20% of the reported cases (78). An air-filled laryngocele is more difficult to evaluate sonographically because it can mimic air contained in the larynx. On laryngoscopy, internal and mixed laryngoceles appear as smooth supraglottic swellings. In confusing cases, a high-resolution neck CT provides detailed information. An internal laryngocele is treated with simple endoscopic uncapping. External laryngoceles are surgically excised.

Laryngeal cysts include retention and saccular cysts. Retention or mucous cysts comprise three fourths of the laryngeal cystic lesions (79). They develop as a result of obstruction of the glandular duct that leads to accumulation of mucus. These cysts are small in size and often multiple. They occur anywhere in the larynx except the mucosa of the free border of the vocal cords, which does not contain any glands. Saccular cysts are commonly acquired as a result of stenosis of the neck of the laryngeal saccule or its herniation into the ventricle. In contrast to a laryngocele, in which the saccule contains air, a saccular cyst is filled with mucus (79). Congenital saccular cysts are extremely rare and represent a congenital fourth branchial arch remnant. Experience with laryngeal cyst US is very limited. Mucus-containing cysts appear hypoechoic with well-defined hyperechoic border and posterior acoustic enhancement (75).

A *pharyngocele* is a protrusion of the mucosa into one of the two weak areas of the pharyngeal wall. The superior area is at the junction of the superior and middle pharyngeal constrictor muscles. An entrance point is located at the inferior pole of the tonsil at the lateral side of vallecula. The inferior area is between the middle and inferior pharyngeal constrictor muscles and the thyrohyoid membrane. The entrance point is on the base of the pyriform fossa (80). In contrast, a Zenker (pharyngoesophageal) diverticulum is a mucosal herniation in the Killian triangle, which is the space bordered by oblique fibers of the inferior constrictor muscle of the pharynx and the transverse fibers of the cricopharyngeus muscle. A pharyngocele is a hypopharyngeal false diverticulum that is most commonly located at the junction of hypopharynx and esophagus. Clinical symptoms include dysphagia, dysphonia, cervical pain, and mass, and sometimes regurgitation and weight loss (80). Under normal circumstances, air in the piriform sinuses appears symmetric (75). The presence of air in a cervical mass and asymmetry of the piriform sinuses is diagnostic (76). For sonographic examination, calcifications of the thyroid cartilage remain a major obstacle. Transverse axial scans are the most useful in overcoming this problem. Valsalva's maneuver may facilitate the diagnosis (76).

Laryngeal cancer is the most common head and neck malignancy. Early laryngeal cancer is managed with radiation therapy, whereas locally advanced disease requires partial, total, or sometimes extended ("wide field") laryngectomy. The degree of laryngeal involvement with tumor determines whether or not a conservative procedure is possible. The patient is usually evaluated with indirect laryngoscopy and direct microlaryngoscopy for the tumor extension; however, the depth of invasion is often difficult to assess, and the pretreatment accuracy of endoscopic staging alone was approximately 60%. Invasion of pre- and paraepiglottic spaces, cartilaginous skeleton, and extralaryngeal soft tissues can often be missed with endoscopy (81,82). For this reason, gadolinium-enhanced MRI or high-resolution contrast-enhanced CT is often performed as an additional imaging technique for determining local invasion of the tumor (83). The combination of laryngeal endoscopy with either CT or MRI imaging in the staging of laryngeal cancer has a superior accuracy rate of 80% and 88%, respectively, and is the standard of care at this time (81).

Percutaneous US is limited to evaluation of pre-, sub-, and supraglottic extension of the tumor and to the detection of direct penetration of the tumor in the laryngeal cartilages. However, calcification of the laryngeal skeleton may mimic invasion of the tumor into cartilage (65). High-frequency (10 to 20 MHz) endolaryngeal US can be used as a supplemental technique during microlaryngoscopy. Invasion of the bright echogenic inner perichondrium with a hypoechoic infiltrate serves as an important landmark of invasiveness. T2–4 glottic cancers and invasion into the preepiglottic space and ventricular folds by supraglottic carcinoma have been accurately detected by the combination of percutaneous and endolaryngeal US (74). The major technical difficulty is imaging of lesions of the anterior commissure. The oncologic importance of the anterior commissure has been repeatedly emphasized in the literature as a preferential pathway of cancer extension to the anterior angle of the thyroid cartilage and to the subcommissural area and cricothyroid membrane (84). Therefore, laryngeal US remains an experimental technique in the staging of laryngeal cancer and at this time cannot substitute for MRI or CT.

The *cervical esophagus* is amenable to both percutaneous and endoscopic US. Major conditions affecting the cervical esophagus are tumors and Zenker's diverticula. Endoscopic US has proven to be a superior adjunct in the assessment of local invasion of esophageal cancer and is the subject of detailed discussion in a separate chapter (see Chapter 20). Percutaneous US is helpful in the evaluation of metastatic involvement of the cervical lymph nodes, especially in patients with supracarinal esophageal cancers (Fig. 25). The sensitivity of this study reaches 75% and the specificity 94% (85).

Pharyngoesophageal or Zenker's diverticulum is a pulsion diverticulum developing between the oblique fibers of the inferior constrictor muscle of the pharynx and the transverse fibers of the cricopharyngeus muscle (socalled Killian triangle). It is the most common type of esophageal diverticulum. Suggestive clinical findings include dysphagia, regurgitation, noisy deglutition, and compression of the esophagus in the cases of large diverticulum. The diverticulum often contains air and fluid with retained food debris. Anatomically, this diverticulum is present at the level of the thyroid and as such it raises the possibility of diagnostic confusion during thy-

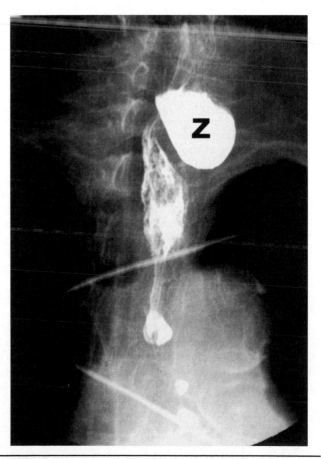

FIGURE 26. Barium swallow image of Zenker's diverticulum (Z).

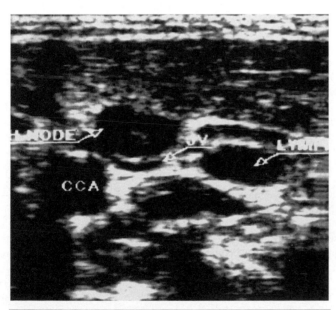

FIGURE 25. Cervical lymph nodes involved by metastatic cancer. Note compressed jugular vein (JV) and carotid artery (CCA).

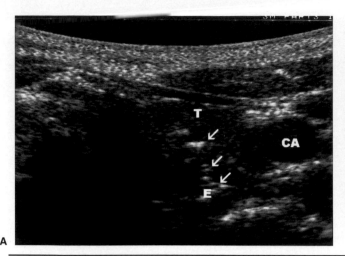 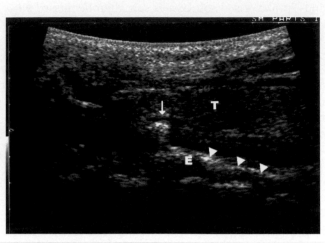

A

B

FIGURE 27. A: Zenker's diverticulum. A transverse view of cervical ultrasound. On real-time imaging, the motion of hyperechoic air (*arrows*) between the lesion and the esophagus (E) was visualized. T, thyroid gland, CA, carotid artery. **B:** Zenker's diverticulum. A sagittal view of cervical ultrasound showing the connection of the lesion (*arrow*) and the esophagus (E). *Arrowheads* indicate the lumen of the esophagus with air. T, thyroid gland.

roid US, when it can be perceived as a thyroid nodule (86–89). Diagnosis of Zenker's diverticulum is routinely established and confirmed by a barium swallow study (Fig. 26). It typically reveals a wide-necked diverticulum filling with barium. US diagnosis of Zenker's diverticulum is important for differentiating this condition from a thyroid nodule during sonographic evaluation of the thy-

roid gland. The diverticulum may be mistaken for an intrathyroidal structure, especially in the presence of cystic changes in the thyroid gland. An important diagnostic feature is the presence of air, demonstrated as echogenic lines and foci with or without dirty shadowing (87) (Fig. 27). Changeable internal echoes of the air must be differentiated from strong echogenic foci caused by calcifica-

▶ **TABLE 9 Ultrasound of Pathologic Lesions of the Visceral Neck**

Laryngocele
- Dilatation of the laryngeal ventricle of Morgagni
- Presents with hoarseness, stridor, dysphagia, and fluctuating neck swelling. Distends with Valsalva's maneuver and collapses on palpation with gurgling and hissing sound
- Sonographically, fluid-filled laryngocele appears as a well-delineated, hypoechoic cyst, located inside the thyroid cartilage, adjacent to the thyroid membrane. Air-filled laryngocele is difficult to evaluate. Computed tomography can be useful in difficult cases

Laryngeal cyst
- Retention (mucous) cysts develop as result of obstruction of the glandular duct
- Saccular cyst is acquired as a result of stenosis of the neck of the laryngeal saccule. In contrast to laryngocele, it does not contain air
- Cysts appear hypoechoic with well-defined hyperechoic walls and posterior acoustic enhancement

Laryngeal cancer
- Magnetic resonance imaging and high-resolution computed tomography are the imaging modalities of choice. Endolaryngeal ultrasound remains an experimental technique. Main limitation is its inability to visualize extent of the invasion of the anterior commissure

Pharyngocele and pharyngoesophageal (Zenker's) diverticulum
- Protrusion of the mucosa into weak points of pharyngeal wall: between pharyngeal constrictor muscles; Zenker's diverticulum protrudes through the Killian triangle located between inferior constrictor and cricopharyngeus muscle
- Present with dysphagia, dysphonia, cervical pain, and regurgitation of undigested food from the diverticula
- Barium swallow study is diagnostic; ultrasound is important for differentiating Zenker's diverticulum from thyroid nodule. Compression maneuver and ingestion by the patient are important in ultrasound diagnosis

tions in a thyroid nodule (88). A gas-producing thyroid abscess can have a very similar appearance, but the condition is typically symptomatic with high fever, chills, and dysphagia. In addition, compression of the diverticulum during a real-time US study allows movement of the air and fluid into the esophagus (87). Ingestion of water by the patient also enables the ultrasonographer to confirm communication of the diverticulum with the esophagus (89) (Table 9).

CONCLUSIONS

US is an important and rapidly evolving diagnostic adjunct in the modern head and neck surgery practice. Recent advances in high-frequency transducer technology allow the sonographer to achieve high-quality imaging of important head and neck structures. US is a portable and noninvasive study that is widely available in the office setting. In experienced hands, it confirms an initial clinical impression and further refines findings of the physical examination. US-guided biopsy technique enhances safety and accuracy of the tissue diagnosis that is critical in the head and neck region, which is rich in important neurovascular structures. Intraoperative US may provide additional assistance in assessing the local extent of head and neck malignancies during tumor resections. Due to its harmless nature and low cost, US is a superior technique for repeated follow-up examinations of postoperative patients treated for head and neck tumors, where physical examination is obscured by postoperative and postirradiation changes. Proficiency in the use of US is becoming imperative for every step of diagnosis and treatment of head and neck surgical patients.

REFERENCES

1. Koischwitz D, Gritzmann N. Ultrasound of the neck. *Radiol Clin North Am* 2000;38:1029–1045.
2. Fornage BD, Coan JD, David CL. Ultrasound-guided needle biopsy of the breast and other interventional procedures. *Radiol Clin North Am* 1992;30:167–185.
3. Rizzatto G, Solbiati L, Croce F, et al. Aspiration biopsy of superficial lesions: ultrasonic guidance with a linear-array probe. *AJR Am J Roentgenol* 1987;148:623–665.
4. Robbins KT. Classification of neck dissection: current concepts and future considerations. *Otolaryngol Clin North Am* 1998;31:639–655.
5. Solbiati L, Osti V, Cova L, et al. Ultrasound of thyroid, parathyroid glands and neck lymph nodes. *Eur Radiol* 2001; 11:2411–2424.
6. van den Brekel MW, Stel HV, Castelijns JA, et al. Cervical lymph node metastasis: assessment of radiologic criteria. *Radiology* 1990;177:379–384.
7. Moritz JD, Ludwig A, Oestmann JW. Contrast-enhanced color Doppler sonography for evaluation of enlarged cervical lymph nodes in head and neck tumors. *AJR Am J Roentgenol* 2000;174:1279–1284.
8. Dillon WP. Cervical nodal metastases: another look at size criteria. *AJNR Am J Neuroradiol* 1998;19:796–797.
9. van den Brekel MW, Castelijns JA, Snow GB. The size of lymph nodes in the neck on sonograms as a radiologic criterion for metastasis: how reliable is it? *AJNR Am J Neuroradiol* 1998;19:695–700.
10. Solbiati L, Rizzatto G, Bellotti E. High-resolution sonography of cervical lymph nodes in head and neck cancers: criteria for differentiation of reactive versus malignant nodes. *Radiology* 1988;169(P):113.
11. Bruneton JN, Matter D, Lassau N, et al. Lymph nodes. In: Bruneton JN, ed. *Applications of sonography in head and neck pathology*. Berlin: Springer-Verlag, 2002;137–164.
12. Chang DB, Yuan A, Yu CJ, et al. Differentiation of benign and malignant cervical lymph nodes with color Doppler sonography. *AJR Am J Roentgenol* 1994;162:965–968.
13. Ying M, Ahuja A, Brook F, et al. Nodal shape (S/L) and its combination with size for assessment of cervical lymphadenopathy: which cut-off should be used? *Ultrasound Med Biol* 1999;25:1169–1175.
14. Rubaltelli L, Proto E, Salmaso R, et al. Sonography of abnormal lymph nodes in vitro: correlation of sonographic and histologic findings. *AJR Am J Roentgenol* 1990;155:1241–1244.
15. Vassallo P, Wernecke K, Roos N, et al. Differentiation of benign from malignant superficial lymphadenopathy: the role of high-resolution US. *Radiology* 1992;183:215–220.
16. Wu CH, Hsu MM, Chang YL, et al. Vascular pathology of malignant cervical lymphadenopathy: qualitative and quantitative assessment with power Doppler ultrasound. *Cancer* 1998;83:1189–1196.
17. Chikui T, Yonetsu K, Nakamura T. Multivariate feature analysis of sonographic findings of metastatic cervical lymph nodes: contribution of blood flow features revealed by power Doppler sonography for predicting metastasis. *AJNR Am J Neuroradiol* 2000;21:561–567.
18. Robinson IA, Cozens NJ. Does a joint ultrasound guided cytology clinic optimize the cytological evaluation of head and neck masses? *Clin Radiol* 1999;54:312–316.
19. Baatenburg de Jong RJ, Rongen RJ, Verwoerd CD, et al. Ultrasound-guided fine-needle aspiration biopsy of neck nodes. *Arch Otolaryngol Head Neck Surg* 1991;117:402–404.
20. Ying M, Ahuja AT, Evans R, et al. Cervical lymphadenopathy: sonographic differentiation between tuberculous nodes and nodal metastases from non-head and neck carcinomas. *J Clin Ultrasound* 1998;26:383–389.
21. Evans RM, Ahuja A, Metreweli C. The linear echogenic hilus in cervical lymphadenopathy—a sign of benignity or malignancy? *Clin Radiol* 1993;47:262–264.
22. Ahuja A, Ying M, Yang WT, et al. The use of sonography in differentiating cervical lymphomatous lymph nodes from cervical metastatic lymph nodes. *Clin Radiol* 1996;51:186–190.
23. Elvin A, Sundstrom C, Larsson SG, et al. Ultrasound-guided 1.2-mm cutting needle biopsies of head and neck tumours. *Acta Radiol* 1997;38:376–380.
24. Candiani F, Martinoli C. Salivary glands. In: Solbiati L, Rizzatto G, eds. *Ultrasound of superficial structures*. Edinburgh: Churchill Livingstone, 1995.
25. Batsakis JG. *Tumors of the head and neck: clinical and pathological considerations*, 2nd ed. Baltimore: Williams & Wilkins, 1979.
26. Gritzmann N. Sonography of the salivary glands. *AJR Am J Roentgenol* 1989;153:161–166.
27. Raffaelli C, Amoretti N, Carlotti B. Salivary glands. In: Bruneton JN, ed. *Applications of sonography in head and neck pathology*. Berlin: Springer-Verlag, 2002;91–136.
28. Derchi LE, Solbiati L. Salivary glands. In: Cosgrove D, Meire H, Dewbury K, eds. *Abdominal and general ultrasound*. Edinburgh: Churchill Livingstone, 1993;677–681.
29. Yasumoto M, Nakagawa T, Shibuya H, et al. Ultrasonography of the sublingual space. *J Ultrasound Med* 1993;12:723–729.
30. Silvers AR, Som PM. Salivary glands. *Radiol Clin North Am* 1998;36:941–966, vi.

31. Magaram D, Gooding GA. Ultrasonic guided aspiration of parotid abscess. *Arch Otolaryngol* 1981;107:549.

32. Rubaltelli L, Sponga T, Candiani F, et al. Infantile recurrent sialectatic parotitis: the role of sonography and sialography in diagnosis and follow-up. *Br J Radiol* 1987;60:1211–1214.

33. Bradus RJ, Hybarger P, Gooding GA. Parotid gland: US findings in Sjogren syndrome. Work in progress. *Radiology* 1988; 169:749–751.

34. Murray ME, Buckenham TM, Joseph AE. The role of ultrasound in screening patients referred for sialography: a possible protocol. *Clin Otolaryngol* 1996;21:21–23.

35. Yoshiura K, Yuasa K, Tabata O, et al. Reliability of ultrasonography and sialography in the diagnosis of Sjogren's syndrome. *Oral Surg Oral Med Oral Pathol Oral Radiol Endod* 1997;83:400–407.

36. Wittich GR, Scheible WF, Hajek PC. Ultrasonography of the salivary glands. *Radiol Clin North Am* 1985;23:29–37.

37. Iro H, Schneider HT, Fodra C, et al. Shockwave lithotripsy of salivary duct stones. *Lancet* 1992;339:1333–1336.

38. Ottaviani F, Capaccio P, Rivolta R, et al. Salivary gland stones: US evaluation in shock wave lithotripsy. *Radiology* 1997;204:437–441.

39. Feld R, Nazarian LN, Needleman L, et al. Clinical impact of sonographically guided biopsy of salivary gland masses and surrounding lymph nodes. *Ear Nose Throat J* 1999;78:905, 908–12.

40. Som PM, Shugar JM, Sacher M, et al. Benign and malignant parotid pleomorphic adenomas: CT and MR studies. *J Comput Assist Tomogr* 1988;12:65–69.

41. Rabinov JD. Imaging of salivary gland pathology. *Radiol Clin North Am* 2000;38:1047–1057, x–xi.

42. Pope TH, Jr., Lehmann WB. Regional metastasis to parotid nodes. *Arch Otolaryngol* 1967;86:673–675.

43. Spiro RH. Salivary neoplasms: overview of a 35-year experience with 2,807 patients. *Head Neck Surg* 1986;8:177–184.

44. Rice DH. Malignant salivary gland neoplasms. *Otolaryngol Clin North Am* 1999;32:875–886.

45. Heller KS, Dubner S, Chess Q, et al. Value of fine needle aspiration biopsy of salivary gland masses in clinical decision-making. *Am J Surg* 1992;164:667–670.

46. Thompson LD, Heffner DK. The clinical importance of cystic squamous cell carcinomas in the neck: a study of 136 cases. *Cancer* 1998;82:944–956.

47. Skandalakis JE, Gary SW, Todd NW. The pharynx and its derivatives. In: Skandalakis JE, Gary SW, eds. *Embryology for surgeons: the embryological basis for the treatment of congenital anomalies*, 2nd ed. Baltimore: Williams &Wilkins, 1994: 17–64.

48. Ahuja AT, King AD, King W, et al. Thyroglossal duct cysts: sonographic appearances in adults. *AJNR Am J Neuroradiol* 1999;20:579–582.

49. Bruneton JN. *Applications of sonography in head and neck pathology*. Berlin: Springer-Verlag, 2002.

50. Wadsworth DT, Siegel MJ. Thyroglossal duct cysts: variability of sonographic findings. *AJR Am J Roentgenol* 1994;163: 1475–1477.

51. Jaques DA, Chambers RG, Oertel JE. Thyroglossal tract carcinoma. A review of the literature and addition of eighteen cases. *Am J Surg* 1970;120:439–446.

52. Gupta P, Maddalozzo J. Preoperative sonography in presumed thyroglossal duct cysts. *Arch Otolaryngol Head Neck Surg* 2001;127:200–202.

53. al-Dousary S. Current management of thyroglossal-duct remnant. *J Otolaryngol* 1997;26:259–265.

54. Bruneton JN, Tranquart F, Brunner PP, et al. Congenital cervical anomalies. In: Bruneton JN, ed. *Applications of sonography in head and neck pathology*. Berlin: Springer-Verlag, 2002:253–260.

55. Mandell DL. Head and neck anomalies related to the branchial apparatus. *Otolaryngol Clin North Am* 2000;33:1309–1332.

56. Yang C, Cohen J, Everts E, et al. Fourth branchial arch sinus: clinical presentation, diagnostic workup, and surgical treatment. *Laryngoscope* 1999;109:442–446.

57. Baatenburg de Jong RJ, Rongen RJ, Lameris JS, et al. Evaluation of branchiogenic cysts by ultrasound. *ORL J Otorhinolaryngol Relat Spec* 1993;55:294–298.

58. Ahuja AT. Lumps and bumps in the head and neck. In: Ahuja AT, Evans RM, eds. *Practical head and neck ultrasound*. London: Greenwich Medical Media, 2000:85–119.

59. Fornage BD, Tassin GB. Sonographic appearances of superficial soft tissue lipomas. *J Clin Ultrasound* 1991;19:215–220.

60. Fornage BD. Soft tissue masses. In: Fornage BD, ed. *Musculoskeletal ultrasound*. Edinburgh: Churchill Livingstone, 1995:21–42.

61. Bruneton JN, Tranquart F, Brunner PP, et al. Neurogenic tumors. In: Bruneton JN, ed. *Applications of sonography in head and neck pathology*. Berlin: Springer-Verlag, 2002:264–268.

62. Irons GB, Weiland LH, Brown WL. Paragangliomas of the neck: clinical and pathologic analysis of 116 cases. *Surg Clin North Am* 1977;57:575–583.

63. Lees CD, Levine HL, Beven EG, et al. Tumors of the carotid body. Experience with 41 operative cases. *Am J Surg* 1981; 142:362–365.

64. Derchi LE, Serafini G, Rabbia C, et al. Carotid body tumors: US evaluation. *Radiology* 1992;182:457–459.

65. Gritzmann N, Traxler M, Grasl M, et al. Advanced laryngeal cancer: sonographic assessment. *Radiology* 1989;171:171–175.

66. Maniere-Ezvan A, Duval JM, Darnault P. Ultrasonic assessment of the anatomy and function of the tongue. *Surg Radiol Anat* 1993;15:55–61.

67. Bruneton JN, Tranquart F, Brunner PP, et al. Oropharynx and esophagus. In: Bruneton JN, ed. *Applications of sonography in head and neck pathology*. Berlin: Springer-Verlag, 2002:268–276.

68. Heppt WJ, Issing WJ. Assessment of tumorous mandibular involvement by transcutaneous ultrasound and flexible endosonography. *J Craniomaxillofac Surg* 1993;21:107–112.

69. Bruneton JN, Geoffray A. Masses of the neck and oral cavity. In: Solbaiti L, Rizzatto G, eds. *Ultrasound of superficial structures*. Edinburgh: Churchill Livingstone, 1995:115–124.

70. Shintani S, Nakayama B, Matsuura H, et al. Intraoral ultrasonography is useful to evaluate tumor thickness in tongue carcinoma. *Am J Surg* 1997;173:345–347.

71. Ikezoe J, Nakanishi K, Morimoto S, et al. Sonographic staging of cancer of the mobile tongue. *Acta Radiol* 1991;32:6–8.

72. Fruehwald FX. Clinical examination, CT and US in tongue cancer staging. *Eur J Radiol* 1988;8:236–241.

73. Crecco M, Vidiri A, Palma O, et al. T stages of tumors of the tongue and floor of the mouth: correlation between MR with gadopentetate dimeglumine and pathologic data. *AJNR Am J Neuroradiol* 1994;15:1695–1702.

74. Arens C, Glanz H. Endoscopic high-frequency ultrasound of the larynx. *Eur Arch Otorhinolaryngol* 1999;256:316–322.

75. Chevallier P, Marcy PY, Arens C, et al. Larynx and hypopharynx. In: Bruneton JN, ed. *Applications of Sonography in head and neck pathology*. Berlin: Springer-Verlag, 2002:165–191.

76. Chevallier P, Motamedi JP, Marcy PY, et al. Sonographic discovery of a pharyngocele. *J Clin Ultrasound* 2000;28:101–103.

77. Thawley SE, Bone RC. Laryngopyocele. *Laryngoscope* 1973; 83:362–368.

78. Canalis RF, Maxwell DS, Hemenway WG. Laryngocele: an updated review. *J Otolaryngol* 1977;6:191–199.

79. DeSanto LW, Devine KD, Weiland LH. Cysts of the larynx: classification. *Laryngoscope* 1970;80:145–176.

80. van de Ven PM, Schutte HK. The pharyngocele: infrequently encountered and easily misdiagnosed. *J Laryngol Otol* 1995; 109:247–249.

81. Zbaren P, Becker M, Lang H. Pretherapeutic staging of laryngeal carcinoma. Clinical findings, computed tomogra-

phy, and magnetic resonance imaging compared with histopathology. *Cancer* 1996;77:1263–1273.

82. Sulfaro S, Barzan L, Querin F, et al. T staging of the laryngohypopharyngeal carcinoma. A 7-year multidisciplinary experience. *Arch Otolaryngol Head Neck Surg* 1989;115:613–620.

83. Medina JE. *Clinical practice guidelines for the diagnosis and management of cancer of the head and neck*. American Head and Neck Society, 2002.

84. Bagatella F, Bignardi L. Behavior of cancer at the anterior commissure of the larynx. *Laryngoscope* 1983;93:353–356.

85. Natsugoe S, Yoshinaka H, Shimada M, et al. Assessment of cervical lymph node metastasis in esophageal carcinoma using ultrasonography. *Ann Surg* 1999;229:62–66.

86. Biggi E, Derchi LE, Cicio GR, et al. Sonographic findings of Zenker's diverticulum. *J Clin Ultrasound* 1982;10:395–396.

87. Kumar A, Aggarwal S, Pham DH. Pharyngoesophageal (Zenker's) diverticulum mimicking thyroid nodule on ultrasonography: report of two cases. *J Ultrasound Med* 1994;13:319–322.

88. Komatsu M, Komatsu T, Inove K. Ultrasonography of Zenker's diverticulum: special reference to differential diagnosis from thyroid nodules. *Eur J Ultrasound* 2000;11:123–125.

89. DeFriend DE, Dubbins PA. Sonographic demonstration of a pharyngoesophageal diverticulum. *J Clin Ultrasound* 2000;28:485–487.

Chapter 8

Vascular Ultrasound

David B. Pilcher

VASCULAR ULTRASOUND IS DIFFERENT

Most surgical ultrasound is B-mode ultrasound with color or Doppler used adjunctively to determine whether a structure is a blood vessel and if it is well vascularized. In vascular applications, much of the diagnostic information comes from Doppler shift, the acquisition and interpretation of which requires sophistication and accuracy.

Vascular ultrasound is usually performed by a registered vascular technologist (RVT) with physician direction and interpretation. Certified RVTs have special skills in vascular applications and frequently devote all their professional time to such applications. This requires additional training, supervision, and ongoing continuing medical education requirements and quality assurance. Vascular ultrasound laboratories are certified to meet volume and quality assurance requirements by the Intersocietal Commission for the Accreditation of Vascular Laboratories (ICAVL). The physician frequently interprets video and still images instead of being present for the real-time study.

This chapter discusses pertinent ultrasound applications of interest to vascular surgeons, although the author recognizes that no such brief article can encompass the large field of vascular ultrasound.

CONTINUOUS WAVE DOPPLER AND PULSED WAVE DOPPLER (TABLE 1)

A continuous wave (CW) transducer contains two crystals; one crystal transmits constant sound waves and the other receives sound waves. Doppler shifts occur when sound is echoed from a moving reflector and the returned sound has a different frequency than the transmitted sound. Police departments use radar Doppler to measure vehicle velocity. Changes in received sounds versus transmitted frequencies are characteristically displayed audibly (the shifts are within the audible frequency range). CW Doppler transducers receive sound reflected from various levels simultaneously and are mainly used to detect the motion of red cells in a vessel qualitatively. If an artery and a vein, or two arteries are both in the path of a CW Doppler probe, reflected sounds will be heard from both vessels at the same time.

A pulsed wave (PW) Doppler uses the same crystal to send and receive. However, it sends only a brief pulse of sound, then listens selectively for sound coming from a given distance away (depth). The fraction of time spent transmitting sound is referred to as the duty factor. The sound is on characteristically 0.1% to 1% of the time. The fact that so much time is spent listening limits the number of pulses per time segment. The number of pulses per time is referred to as the pulse repetition frequency (PRF). One can increase the PRF by not listening so deeply, decreasing sample size (the area in which one listens), or decreasing the frequency (lower frequency = longer wavelength). If the frequency shift (Nyquist limit) exceeds one half of the PRF, measuring frequency shifts cannot be achieved (1).

DUPLEX ULTRASOUND AND COLOR DOPPLER

Duplex ultrasound encompasses B-mode ultrasound and PW Doppler. The B-mode information is optimally acquired with normal incidence at about 90 degrees. PW Doppler at 90 degrees would theoretically be zero velocity. This is according to the Doppler equation, which can be expressed:

$$V = \frac{\Delta f \, c}{2f \cos \theta}$$

where *V* is velocity of moving target (red cells)

c is speed of sound in soft tissue (approximately 1,540 m/sec on average)

Δf is the change in frequency of reflected versus transmitted sound

f is frequency of transmitted sound

▶ TABLE 1 Continuous Wave Doppler and Pulsed
              Wave Doppler

1. Continuous wave Doppler:
   Sending and receiving crystals lack depth discrimination
2. Pulsed wave Doppler:
   Sending occurs only 0.1% –1% of the time
3. Duplex ultrasound:
   Includes simultaneous B-mode ultrasound and pulsed wave
      Doppler
   Doppler shifts are to be measured at 60 degrees
4. Color Doppler
   Duplex is usually performed with color (but color is not
      necessary)
5. Aliasing occurs with high frequencies more frequently with
      color flow
6. Power Doppler useful in determining if a structure is vascular

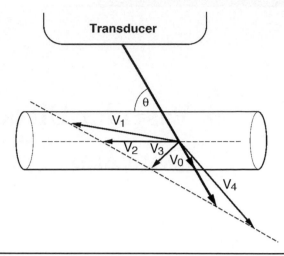

FIGURE 1. If all red cells were traveling parallel to the vessel wall, V2 would be the correct velocity vector and θ would be the Doppler angle. Since this assumption is incorrect for individual vessels, vectors V1, V3, and V4 also exist and would make the Doppler formula for cos θ incorrect.

The constant "2" is included because the sound makes a round trip to and from the transducer.

Cos θ = the angle between the ultrasound beam and the direction of red cell motion (1).

The change in frequency (the sound reflected from the moving red blood cells) = Δf is the frequency difference between the transmitted sound and the reflected sound. The cosine of 0 degree is 1 and, therefore, if you were measuring this reflecting from a red cell coming straight at you, the frequency shift would not necessitate angle correction. This is not often possible.

To utilize the Doppler formula and obtain velocity of moving red cells requires a number of assumptions, which may build in error. For example, we assume that all red blood cells are traveling parallel to the vessel wall. Although this may be true on average, many cells are traveling in varied directions at the same time (Fig. 1). The errors in this type of calculation with the Doppler formula can be decreased in amount by always using the same angle. By convention, we try to use an angle of 60 degrees, which is an angle we can usually utilize in clinical situations, by angling the probe or electronically steering the Doppler sound beam. Situations arise in which we do not know the direction of the blood vessel, as with renal arteries or transcranial Doppler. That is when we use an angle of 0 degree (cos 0 = 1). The errors become unacceptable when exceeding the 60 degree limit. The assumption that red cells travel in a straight line is incorrect. At 90 degrees, some Doppler shifting is still detectable.

Color is Doppler. Within the color box window, Doppler average flows are superimposed on the B-mode image. This is an alternative to spectral analysis for display of Doppler information. The amount of Doppler data for each specific site on the B-mode image is less than with spectral display, but it shows Doppler information over a wider area. The Doppler color averaging window can be steered electronically to get away from the 90 degree no-flow problem, but not as precisely as the PW Doppler for the spectral analysis.

A color bar near the image shows the color assignment and scale being used. The color is usually set up so that arterial flow is red and venous is blue (Fig. 2). Since not all red cells are traveling parallel to the vessel wall, the assumption that flow away from the probe is always red

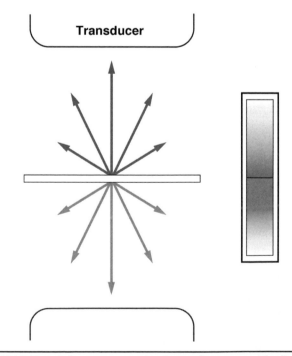

FIGURE 2. Color representation is usually set up with all vectors toward the transducer red and away from the transducer blue (except with venous imaging). (See Color Plate 2.)

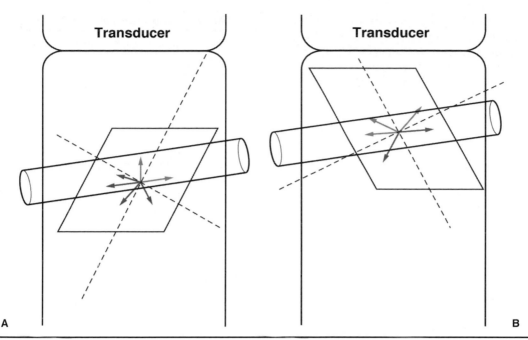

FIGURE 3. A: With the usual color representation vectors toward the head (conventionally set up to the left of the image if this was a carotid artery) are red. (See Color Plate 3.) B: With steering of the color box to the right most vectors toward the head would now be blue. (See Color Plate 4.)

does not hold up, with some vectors of cells traveling in a nonlinear fashion (Fig. 3). Color flow is Doppler averaging and, therefore, not as accurate as PW Doppler small-sample-size spectral analysis.

Doppler frequency shifts do not show such high velocities (frequency shifts) with color as with spectral analysis. The color changes are most useful in detecting the specific areas that will be most informative to query with the PW Doppler spectral analysis.

ALIASING

With spectral analysis display, Doppler frequency shifts that are too high go off the top of the display and are artifactually displayed again at the bottom so as to wrap

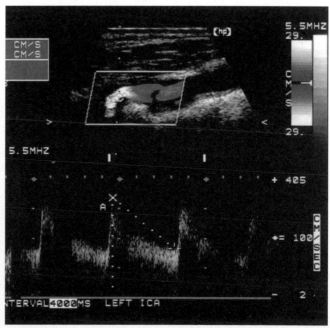

FIGURE 4. A: Blood cells are traveling from right to left, but they have different color representations because their color vectors are different. This is not reversal of flow nor aliasing. (See Color Plate 5.) B: Blood is traveling left to right, but color aliasing is evident when red changes to blue with intervening white or yellow (high velocities). (See Color Plate 6.)

around on top of the original display. Since color flow images are imaged at low shift frequencies (low PRF), aliasing is more common in color flow images than in spectral display images (Fig. 4). Color flow aliasing is a shift from red to blue with intervening white or yellow. This is distinguished from tortuosity angle changes, which are displayed as red to blue without intervening white or yellow.

POWER DOPPLER

Power Doppler assigns brighter color to an area from amplitude changes of the Doppler shift (strength changes of the Doppler shift), which does not rely on the interpretation of angle vectors. It shows moving blood in arteries and veins as the same color and does not give speed, direction, or flow character information. This modality is useful in determining where a vessel is and therefore in directing sample acquisition from a vessel for Doppler spectral analysis. It is also useful in determining if a structure is vascular or not. Since there is no aliasing, power Doppler can show slow flows at deeper and smaller vessels with improved sensitivity.

ABDOMINAL AORTIC ANEURYSM DETECTION (TABLE 2)

Emergency room physicians and critical care physicians frequently perform their own "focused" examinations with B-mode ultrasound for aortic aneurysms for the purpose of determining the presence or absence of an aneurysm. They then may request a vascular consultation. Responding to such a request to have the emergency

> **TABLE 2 Abdominal Aortic Aneurysm Detection**
>
> 1. This is a focused B-mode examination to determine aneurysm diameter
> 2. Normal aortic diameter = 1.7 cm in men
> 3. Aneurysm: more than 50% increase over the normal proximal vessel

department physician "run" the ultrasound imaging and transducer manipulation is very different from having an RVT acquire images and accurately document aortic size. Focused B-mode results should be accurate and reproducible in the hands of a vascular surgeon.

Technique

With the patient supine and hopefully fasting, a low-frequency probe is selected for the aorta usually with a setting depth of about 13 cm. Usually a curved linear array transducer set at 2 to 4 MHz is used, but phased array or straight linear array transducers are possible. The scan begins in the transverse plane above the umbilicus, proceeding down to the umbilicus. The aorta is usually easily identified anterior and to the left of the vertebral column. The largest diameter image is frozen, measured, and annotated appropriately. The transducer is then rotated to a longitudinal plane and the largest anteroposterior diameter frozen, measured, and recorded (Fig. 5). Alternatively, the scan may begin in the longitudinal plane and transverse images after rotation. A normal aortic diameter is 1.7 cm in men and 1.5 cm in women (2). An aneurysm is defined as more than a 50% increase over the normal proximal vessel.

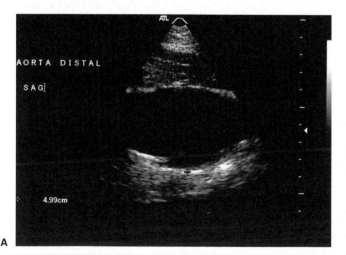
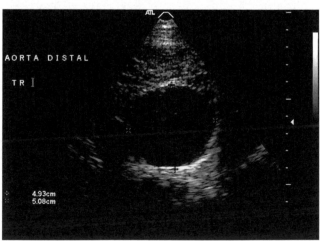

A   B

FIGURE 5. A: Measurement in the longitudinal anteroposterior view is usually more accurate than transverse measurement. B: Transverse anteroposterior measurement is better than transverse measurement because lateral walls are not as well defined with B-mode ultrasound.

Surgeon/Technologist Involvement

A focused exam determines the presence and size of an aneurysm and can be performed by a vascular surgeon accurately and with little practice. Examining the relation of an aneurysm to the mesenteric and renal veins and scanning the iliac arteries for aneurysms is more demanding. Intraabdominal Doppler information should be reserved for experienced RVTs and not confused with a scan to detect and measure aortic aneurysm by B-mode examination.

EXTRACRANIAL CEREBROVASCULAR DUPLEX (TABLE 3)

The most common area of severe plaque buildup in the carotid arteries is at the origin in the first centimeter above the bifurcation. The localization of this plaque is what has allowed carotid endarterectomy to be so highly successful. Both the North American Symptomatic Carotid Endarterectomy Trial (NASCET) study (3) and the Asymptomatic Carotid Atherosclerosis Study (ACAS) study (4) showed that angiography was associated with a more than 1% incidence of cerebral complications. This and the improvement of duplex imaging have led to the frequent use of diagnostic duplex as the sole imaging modality for determining the appropriateness and feasibility of carotid endarterectomy.

The percentage of carotid stenosis is usually compared with the angiographic criteria of the NASCET and ACAS studies; the angiographic diameter of the stenosis is divided by the angiographic diameter of the normal distal vessel × 100. The percentage of stenosis is determined by the peak systolic velocity (PSV), the end-diastolic velocity (EDV), and the systolic velocity ratios (Fig. 6). Each laboratory must validate its criteria repetitively as new equipment is added. Different duplex machines may have different criteria as, suggested by Fillinger et al. (5). Criteria based on Zierler's study (6) are listed in Table 4. Moneta et al. (7) looked at the 70% NASCET criteria and suggested that a PSV ratio greater than 4.0 corre-

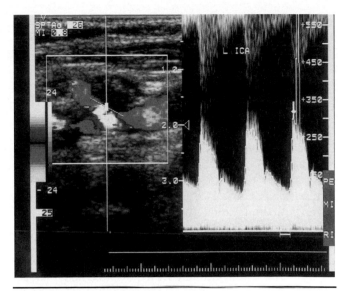

FIGURE 6. Internal carotid artery stenosis is defined by the peak systolic velocity (310 cm/sec here) and the end-diastolic velocity (113 cm/sec here) placing this stenosis in the 80% to 99% range. (See Color Plate 7.)

lated best with 70%. A PSV velocity greater than 260 cm/sec and an EDV greater than 70 cm/sec gave the greatest accuracy to correlate with a 60% stenosis (ACAS criteria) (8).

If the contralateral internal carotid artery (ICA) is occluded, it is logical that the velocity in the patent ICA may be increased to compensate as a collateral. AbuRahma et

▶ TABLE 3 Extracranial Cerebrovascular Duplex

1. Stenosis is determined by:
   - Peak systolic velocity of the internal carotid artery
   - End diastolic velocity of the internal carotid artery
   - Systolic velocity ratios (peak systolic velocity ratio)
2. Accessibility of plaque anatomy to surgical approach can be defined by ultrasound.
   - Beyond determining extent of internal carotid artery stenosis, features relevant to surgical endarterectomy should be assessed (e.g., distal extent of plaque, tortuosity, and possibility of proximal or distal stenosis)

▶ TABLE 4 Internal Carotid Artery Classification

Class	Percent Stenosis	Duplex Findings
A	Normal	*Normal* PSV <125 cm/sec No spectral broadening ICA/CCA velocity (PSV, EDV) ratio <2.0
B	1%–49%	*Minimal Disease* PSV <125 cm/sec Minimal spectral broadening ICA/CCA velocity (PSV) ratio <2.0
C	50%–79%	*Moderate Disease* PSV >125 cm/sec EDV >50 cm/sec Marked Spectral Broadening ICA/CCA systolic velocity ratio 2–4
D	80%–99%	*Severe Disease* PSV >125 cm/sec EDV >105 cm/sec
E	100%	*Occluded* Low CCA velocity (to zero in diastole) No flow in ICA

PSV, peak systolic velocity; ICA, internal carotid artery; CCA, common carotid artery; EDV, end-diastolic velocity.

al. (9) has suggested that in this circumstance stenosis in excess of 50% is associated with a more than 140 cm/sec PSV and that stenosis in excess of 80% is associated with an EDV of more than 140 cm/sec.

Wain et al. (10) attempted to quantify and document the amenability of carotid artery stenosis to surgical correction by measuring the distance of the bifurcation below the angle of the mandible, the length of the ICA plaque cephalad to the bifurcation, and the diameter of the distal ICA. All of these measures correlated with the surgical specimen at endarterectomy. In practice, if the bifurcation and distal extent of the plaque are easily visualized with duplex, then the lesion is low enough to be accessible for endarterectomy.

Studies continue to differentiate lesions likely to produce symptoms in the carotid arteries. A recent study by Tegos et al. (11) suggested that hypoechoic and homogeneous echo pattern were associated with symptomatic carotid plaques.

Vertebral arteries usually have stenosis at their origin. When scanning carotid with ultrasound, most studies report vertebral velocities between vertebrae where the vertebral artery is easily identified. Detection of vertebral artery origin stenosis requires different techniques, which may be more difficult. We usually look distally and inferiorly rather than directly at the stenotic area.

Technique

Much has been written about diagnostic carotid scanning, which cannot be duplicated here. Special considerations regarding preoperative imaging require some modifications of usual protocol. Scanning is frequently started with B-mode in a transverse and then longitudinal view to visualize plaque, plaque characteristics, arterial diameter, and residual lumen. It is especially important to visualize the transverse distal ICA to confirm that the image extends above the end of the plaque. This should be combined with longitudinal scanning, which may be more revealing with or without the color on. Conventional diagnostic carotid scanning permits identification of the maximal stenotic area; it focuses on determining the percentage of stenosis by searching carefully for maximal velocity changes. Once this has been accomplished, the preoperative duplex scanning should focus on plaque extent and confirmation that no proximal or distal stenosis exists.

If one of the two branches of the common carotid artery (CCA) is stenotic or occluded, it is usually the ICA. It is essential that these vessels be accurately differentiated. Confusion can arise if only one vessel is patent. The external carotid artery (ECA) has a high resistance pattern and the ICA a low resistance pattern. The ECA has branches, and occasionally a large branch may be mistaken for the ICA. A temporal artery tap has some usefulness. Extreme ICA tortuosity may be relevant to operability, and confusion as to vessel identification here can be ameliorated with the use of high-quality, high-velocity scanners. Low or absent diastolic flow in the distal ICA may raise concern about distal stenosis. Turbulent or low flow in the CCA may suggest proximal stenosis of the CCA, particularly if it is very different from the opposite CCA.

Many sonographers image the vertebral arteries only at midneck, which misses the area usually associated with stenosis. It will, however, show occlusion or reversal of flow and may show low flow or inequality with the other side, prompting further evaluation. To visualize the vertebral artery origin, the sonographer should begin the scan longitudinally in the low midline and angle laterally passing the CCA to identify the prevertebral subcla-

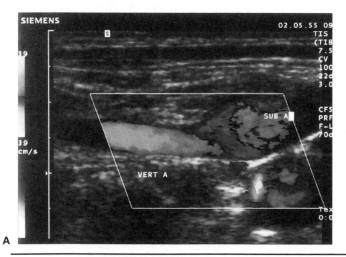

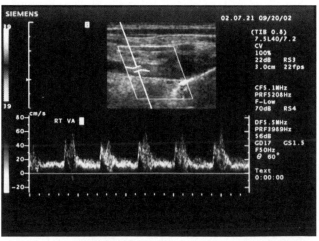

A

B

FIGURE 7. **A:** The right vertebral origin from the subclavian can frequently be visualized. In this patient a 7.5-MHz linear probe is used (See Color Plate 8). **B:** Vertebral origin velocities can be determined. Although normal values are not well established, inferences from other vessel norms can be utilized.

▶ **TABLE 5** Carotid Completion Duplex
(Intraoperative)

1. Peak systolic velocity <150 cm/sec and peak systolic velocity >50 cm/sec with no diastolic flow unacceptable
2. Low "volume flow" may be predictive of risk
3. Mobile flaps >3 mm in length are at risk
4. A clamp may be applied to the external carotid artery while sonographer is performing duplex ultrasound distally to ensure that the internal carotid artery is being heard

vian. The vertebral comes off at a very acute angle, which appears inferolateral on the duplex image (Fig. 7).

CAROTID COMPLETION DUPLEX (INTRAOPERATIVE) (TABLE 5)

Palpation of an ICA pulse without a thrill and/or CW Doppler assessment of carotid flow following endarterectomy has been supplanted by completion angiography or completion duplex by many practitioners (12–20). Bandyk (13,14) has emphasized that an elevated PSV of more than 150 cm /sec or a low flow of less than 50 cm/sec and no diastolic flow indicates the need for further evaluation or correction. Ascher (12) has emphasized low volume flow as being indicative of residual stenosis/defects of significance. Bandyk's "low flow" and

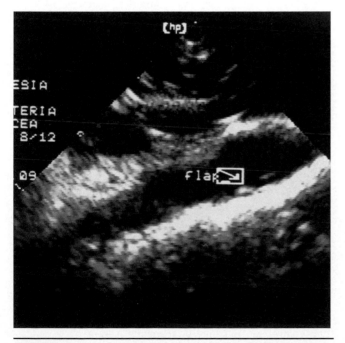

FIGURE 8. B-mode image of an internal carotid artery showing a 2-mm mobile flap. (From Pilcher DB, Ricci MA. Vascular ultrasound. *Surg Clin North Am* 1998;78:273–293, with permission.)

Ascher's "low volume flow" may differ with large patches and spasm in the immediate postoperative period. In addition, B-mode imaging (with or without color) may demonstrate flaps and platelet aggregates that may be significant. Turbulence may also be a poor prognosticator of thrombosis/embolus. Archie (20) has suggested that the proximal step is a harbinger of late stenosis, but prospective studies are lacking.

Bandyk in 1988 (13) showed no recurrent stenosis in 175 patients with normal arterial flow after carotid endarterectomy. Using Duplex as the prime modality, 5–10% of patients may be re-explored after carotid endarterectomy (15,17,18). Those who have used Duplex routinely have adopted it as the primary modality, resorting to the use of digital subtraction angiography to resolve equivocal findings or to confirm duplex findings (17,19). Angiography gives complementary information of anatomic information to the duplex findings.

Ascher (12) has suggested that a B-mode–detected mobile flap longer than 2 mm in the ICA or 3 mm in the CCA or any defect that caused more than 30% luminal diameter reduction would be an indication for reintervention (Fig. 8).

Technique

Intraoperative completion duplex ultrasound is performed with a 7- to 12-MHz linear array probe, usually sheathed in a sterile sleeve. Sterile gel (or saline) is used to interface the transducer surface with the sleeve. Saline is usually placed in the wound as an acoustic coupler. Sterile gel will *not* cause irritation or reaction in the open wound and is usually irrigated and washed out after duplex ultrasound if used.

Usually the CCA and ICA are first visualized in a longitudinal direction with color on. It is convenient at this time to obtain the PSV in the most distal ICA and then to transverse the distal patch end point with the PW Doppler and listen through the ICA to the bulb to find any elevated velocities (Fig. 9). Especially if there is tortuosity of the ICA, it is helpful to repeat the distal ICA velocities with a clamp on the ECA to be 100% sure that velocities are not being measured from the ECA in error.

It is usually helpful to visualize the endarterectomy site in B mode without color to assess for flaps and platelet thrombi or a proximal shelf. This is usually satisfactory in longitudinal view. If a polytetrafluoroethylene patch is used, it may be necessary to insonate from the side because the patch may not transmit sound if it contains microscopic air bubbles.

Surgeon/Technologist Involvement

This is a focused examination with the area of interest directly exposed in the wound. The surgeon should be able

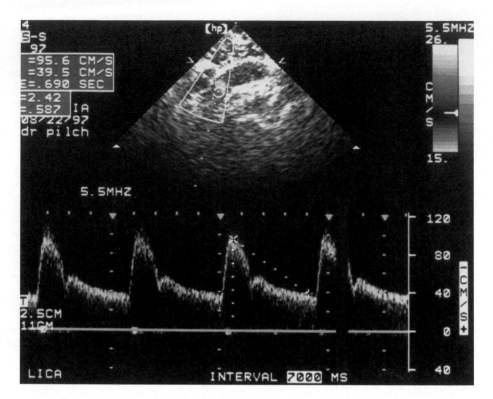

FIGURE 9. Normal carotid completion duplex with measurement of velocities just beyond distal patch. (From Pilcher DB, Ricci MA. Vascular ultrasound. *Surg Clin North Am* 1998; 78: 273–293, with permission.)

to manipulate the probe in the operative field. An RVT will usually bring the ultrasound machine to the operating room and manage the imaging without being scrubbed. Experienced surgeons can perform the tech-nologist's role to help another surgeon, or the surgeon can obtain adequate information by controlling the ultrasound machine in a sterile drape or with a nonsterile gloved hand (Fig. 10).

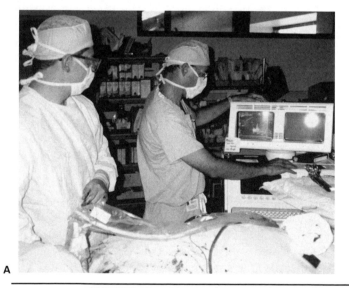

A

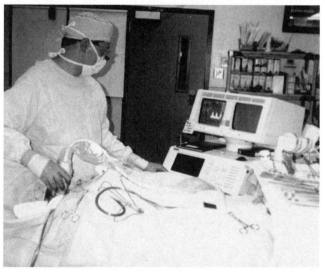

B

FIGURE 10. **A:** The usual scenario for completion carotid duplex is for the surgeon to manipulate the transducer and the registered vascular technologist to control the machine adjustments. (From Pilcher DB, Ricci MA. Vascular ultrasound. *Surg Clin North Am* 1998;78:273–293, with permission.) **B:** An experienced surgeon can manage both roles for transducer and machine manipulation with a nonsterile glove, as shown here, or with a sterile cover over the controls.

DUPLEX ARTERIAL MAPPING (PREOPERATIVE) (TABLE 6)

With skilled technologists and high-quality duplex ultrasound machines, accurate arterial mapping can be performed from the aortic bifurcation to the pedal vessels (21–24). Ascher et al. (21) have shown that this study takes an average of 66 minutes. Ascher has more recently suggested a short protocol to lessen this time (25).

Duplex monitoring alone was considered satisfactory without angiography in 74% to 78% of cases (21,23). Accurate correlation with angiography was documented by Ascher et al. (21) in 95% of 210 patients. Half of the miscalls were runoff and half inflow. The inflow miscalls were all corrected by iliac stenting intraoperatively at the time of infrainguinal bypass. Bostrom et al. (24) had 90% correlation with outflow in 123 patients.

Excellent 1- to 2-year patency results have been reported and compared with historical controls (22,23) showing no differences from bypasses based on contrast angiography.

Technique

Arterial segments are imaged from the aorta to the pedal vessels. Multiple transducers of 7–4, 10–5, 12–5, 5–2, and 3–2 MHz are needed to obtain high-quality B-mode, color, and power Doppler images as well as velocity spectra. In general, color and power Doppler were used primarily, and B-mode images and velocity spectra were used to supplement these data. At the completion of the test, a color-coded map of the entire arterial tree was drawn to help develop a revascularization strategy (21).

The short protocol (25) for femoral–popliteal or femoral distal bypass scans the common, superficial, and profunda femoral arteries as well as the popliteal artery; and then switches to the perimalleolar level. The technologist can scan the peroneal artery proximally until significant stenosis is found, then immediately shift to the anterior tibial. If significant stenosis is found in the anterior tibial, the technologist should shift immediately to the posterior tibial artery. The test is completed with the scan of one disease-free infrapopliteal artery or a scan of all three if all three have proximal occlusions.

Surgeon/Technologist Involvement

The surgeon and technologist should work closely so that the scanning protocol and resultant arterial map provide accurate data for the purpose required. On rare occasion a focal area in question may be required to show a surgeon real time, but the technologist should be able to do this time-consuming, technically demanding duplex study on his or her own time. It may be appropriate to

▶ TABLE 6 Duplex Arterial Mapping

1. Can be highly accurate but time consuming
2. 95% accurate correlation with angiography

have only selected RVTs perform this test in any given laboratory.

INTRAOPERATIVE DUPLEX MONITORING OF BYPASS GRAFTS (TABLE 7)

Duplex assessment of technical graft success has been successfully demonstrated for many years by Bandyk and others (14,26–28). In a recent article, Johnson et al. (27) reported 626 infrainguinal vein bypass grafts with a 15% initial revision rate and a secondary graft patency of 99% at 90 days. These results are better than any reported using other modalities for intraoperative assessment.

Duplex scanning can be used to assess synthetic graft outflow at the distal anastomosis even though imaging through the graft itself is largely thwarted by air in the graft wall. The criteria proposed by Mills and Bandyk in 1995 (29) have not changed in their recent studies, as presented in Table 8.

Technique

Grafting is completed and flow established before scanning is necessary. With in situ grafts, preoperative duplex mapping is helpful in identifying branches.

With a CW Doppler and a gas-sterilized probe, the Doppler can easily be placed in a sterile bag to be brought onto the field. Alternatively, the sterilized probe can be on the field and the box off the field. This requires a nurse to respond to "Doppler on" and "Doppler off" requests. After the proximal anastomosis is completed and flow is proceeding to the fistulas (before distal anastomosis), the CW Doppler is placed on the proximal flowing graft. Dig-

▶ TABLE 7 Intraoperative Duplex Monitoring of Bypass Grafts

1. There is a 15% revision rate, with vein grafts
2. Synthetic grafts can be assessed by looking distal to distal anastomosis
3. Continuous wave Doppler can be used to detect fistula location
4. Papaverine injected into distal vein graft increases duplex sensitivity
5. Velocity ratios accurately detect stenosis
6. Low-flow grafts are particularly problematic

▶ **TABLE 8 Duplex Intraoperative Criteria**

Peak Systolic Velocity (cm/sec)	Velocity Ratio (V_r)	Management
< 45	NA	Rescan after papaverine. Consider angiogram. If no diastolic and flow remains low: augment outflow.[a]
45–125 with diastolic component	<2	NORMAL
>125 and <180	2–3	Rescan after papaverine. Consider angiography.
>180 and <300	3–5	Repair defect. Before accepting these readings, perform angiography.
>300	>5	Critically unacceptable. Repair/revision mandatory, especially if low-flow graft

[a]Augment outflow by considering changing the outflow vessel, jump graft to another outflow vessel, or arteriovenous fistula construction.
Modified from Johnson BL, Bandyk DF, Back MR, et al. Intraoperative duplex monitoring of infrainguinal vein bypass procedures. *J Vasc Surg* 2000;31:678–690.

ital compression walking down the vein graft easily and precisely identifies the location of branches with flow. These can be marked and ligated through small incisions (Fig. 11). The Doppler is a thump when no fistulas exist between the finger compression and the probe, and has flow present when the finger compresses distal to a fistula. We frequently leave one distal fistula to allow graft flow with a clamp just distal to the fistula until the distal anastomosis is completed and open.

Once the distal anastomosis is completed and there is flow through the graft, duplex graft scanning is commenced. A high-frequency probe of 5 to 12 MHz (usually 10 MHz) with a sequenced linear array is used in a sterile

sleeve with sterile gel coupling in the sleeve (Fig. 12). Saline is usually placed in the wound for acoustic coupling, but sterile gel can be used and will not produce a recognizable inflammatory reaction.

Bandyk et al. (26) emphasized the importance of injecting 30 to 60 mg of papaverine into the distal vein graft to augment graft flow and increase the sensitivity of duplex scanning in detection of stenosis using velocity criteria (Fig. 13).

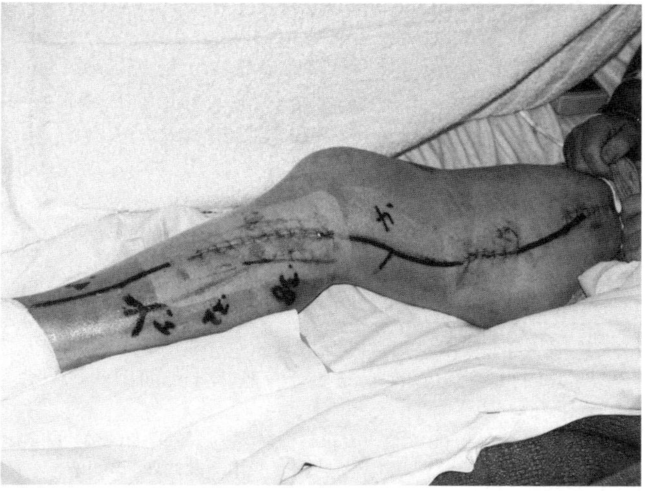

FIGURE 11. Preoperative mapping and continuous wave detection of fistulas allows multiple small incisions for arteriovenous fistula ligation after in situ vein grafting.

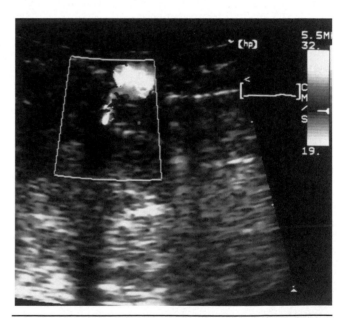

FIGURE 12. Transverse scan easily identifies residual fistulas after graft flow established. (From Pilcher DB, Ricci MA. Vascular ultrasound. *Surg Clin North Am* 1998;78:273–293, with permission.)

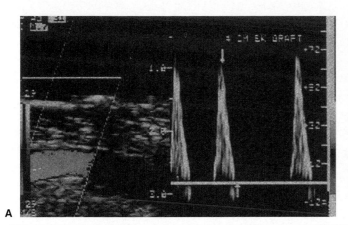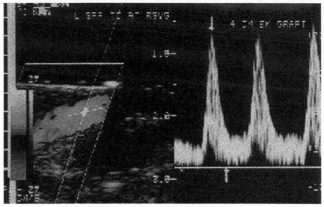

A   B

FIGURE 13. Intraoperative graft velocity spectra before **(A)** (See Color Plate 9) and after **(B)** (See Color Plate 10) papaverine injection. (From Johnson BL, Bandyk DF, Back MR, et al. Intraoperative duplex monitoring of infrainguinal vein bypass procedures. *J Vasc Surg* 2000;31:678–690, with permission.)

Longitudinal scanning with color flow is started at the distal anastomosis and proceeds proximally to image the entire graft and proximal anastomosis. Transverse imaging may be helpful in looking for residual branches or evaluating B-mode imaging of narrow or suspect areas. Velocity determinations of spectral analysis are made with θ = 60 degrees at distal vessel, distal graft, proximal graft, proximal artery, and any place where there is disturbed flow with color Doppler or a questionable abnormality such as a valve area or a caliber change in vein diameter.

Any stenotic area is assessed by determining PSV proximal and PSV maximal at the area of stenosis to allow calculation of the velocity ratio V_r (V_r = PSV at lesion/PSV proximal).

Low-flow grafts pose a particularly challenging problem (Table 8). If no stenotic lesion can be found and corrected, augmentation of flow by jump graft, arteriovenous fistula, or revision of anastomotic site should be considered. If low flow cannot be remedied, anticoagulation may be the only option.

Surgeon/Technologist Involvement

A vascular technologist is not needed until the duplex scanning portion of the procedure. Interrogation of the bypass graft is a technically demanding exercise, and quality will be best assured with an RVT running the ultrasound machine. A surgeon experienced in duplex ultrasonography can effectively handle the probe so that the technologist need not be scrubbed in the sterile field.

For the less complex interrogation of non–in situ vein grafts, the surgeon may direct an assistant in obtaining duplex images, or cover the controls of the duplex machine with a sterile cover, or use an unsterile gloved hand to control the duplex machine. This also applies to checking outflow with synthetic grafts.

VEIN GRAFT SURVEILLANCE (TABLE 9)

The practice guidelines for lower extremity revascularization (30), published in 1993, quoted the parameters by Bandyk et al. (31) from 1985 as the standard that "autogenous vein bypass grafts should be examined by duplex scanning with determination of graft flow velocity." This parameter has been demonstrated to be a sensitive indicator of impending graft failure. Numerous authors have since documented this (32–36), emphasizing that the best criterion for a failing graft is a PSV ratio greater than 2.5 to 3.5 from the proximal artery to stenosis. Ryan et al. (37) suggested that this velocity ratio criterion may not be valid at the proximal anastomosis because PSV increases at this location may regress and not predict graft failure. Calligaro et al. (38) suggested this was also true of distal anastomotic or outflow vessel stenoses, and that both inflow and outflow increased PSV were significant when associated with graft flows of less than 45 cm/sec.

Darling et al. (39) showed that in a 5-year follow up 9% to 10% of vein grafts required revision. The 5-year patencies were 78% to 81% for unrevised excised and in situ grafts and 68% to 69% for revised grafts.

▶ **TABLE 9 Vein Graft Surveillance**

1. 9%–10% of vein grafts require revision
2. Failing graft identified by:
   a. Peak systolic velocity ratio >2.5
   b. Graft flow of <45 cm/sec

Technique

This is a time consuming and demanding duplex examination. The surgeon can be most helpful in assisting the RVT to find the distal anastomosis and defining the anatomy of the graft, particularly when the course is deep or in an unusual location. With an excellent map of velocities accompanying the report, there is usually little need for the surgeon to also review the images.

The high-frequency "intraoperative " transducers have been useful in vein grafts in the superficial areas such as in situ or subcutaneous grafts.

DUPLEX IMAGING AFTER ANGIOPLASTY/STENT (TABLE 10)

Mewissen et al. (40) showed that angiographically successful percutaneous transluminal angioplasty could be shown to have duplex residual stenosis of more than 50% diameter reduction. Such residual stenosis was predictive of subsequent clinical deterioration and percutaneous transluminal dilation failure. A residual PSV greater than180 cm/sec or velocity ratio greater than 2.5 was associated with a 15% 1-year clinical success rate as opposed to an 84% success when the residual stenosis was less than 50% by these criteria. These results have been confirmed by Spijkerboer et al. (41).

Technique

This is especially applicable to femoral–popliteal angioplasty of native arteries or vein graft stenoses. Since the interventional radiologist is usually scrubbed, the high-frequency ultrasound probe can be placed in a sterile sheath and the area of stenosis draped into the sterile field.

Angioplasty/stent is performed until radiographic success is achieved (less than 30% residual stenosis). Duplex ultrasound can then be used to confirm or refute this success. Redilation with a larger balloon, if judged safe, is done until duplex ultrasound confirms 30% residual stenosis. If duplex-documented success is not achievable, the patient should be followed with consideration for surgical intervention.

Use of ultrasound guidance for angioplasty without fluoroscopy/digital subtraction angiography has been shown to be feasible (42) but has not found widespread use because the patient is usually in the angiography suite for access to angiography.

SURVEILLANCE OF PROSTHETIC GRAFTS

Calligaro et al. (43) have shown, as have others, that duplex surveillance of femoral–popliteal synthetic grafts offers no advantage over noninvasive testing with pulse volume recordings and segmental pressure studies in detecting failing grafts appropriate for revision. Their study suggests that PSVs greater than 300 cm/sec at inflow outflow with graft velocity of less than 45 cm/sec, or stenoses with velocity ratios of in excess of 3 are predictive of failing femorotibial grafts.

DEEP VENOUS THROMBOSIS (TABLE 11)

Duplex ultrasound has become the gold standard for the diagnosis of deep venous thrombosis (DVT) (44,45). Controversy regarding whether a bilateral study is necessary with unilateral symptoms remains. Garcia et al. (46) suggested that it might not be necessary in all patients. They found 2% bilaterality of unilateral symptoms in 276 outpatients. They also found a 10% incidence in the asymptomatic leg in 159 inpatients.

Improved ultrasound equipment and techniques have allowed reliable detection of calf vein thrombi. The controversy regarding significance of isolated calf vein thrombi is summarized by Meissner et al. (47) as showing persistent symptoms in 25% and pulmonary embolism in 11% of cases.

In the review of Mustafa et al. (48), the value of ultrasound in detecting upper extremity acute venous thrombosis has been summarized as a specificity of 94% to 100% but a sensitivity of 56% to 100%.

Technique

The highest frequency transducer capable of imaging the venous segment under study should be used for B-mode imaging (5 to 10 MHz). Low gain and color settings (and low wall filter setting) are appropriate to visualize venous flow velocities.

Transverse imaging for compressibility is followed by longitudinal imaging for augmentation and phasicity

▶ **TABLE 10 Duplex Imaging After Angioplasty/Stenting**

1. Angiographic success and duplex >50% stenosis at risk for failure
2. Seek peak systolic velocity <180 cm/sec or velocity ratio <2.5

▶ **TABLE 11 Deep Venous Thrombosis**

1. Now accepted as the "gold standard"
2. Reliable detection of calf vein thrombi should now be standard

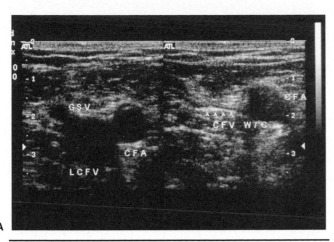

A   **B**

FIGURE 14. **A:** The normal left common femoral vein (LCFV) before compression. GSV, greater saphenous vein. **B:** After compression, no hypoechoic lumen was visible [*four arrows*, common femoral vein (CFV), with compression (W/C)]. Compression should be enough to minimally distort the common femoral artery (CFA) but not to collapse the artery.

with color and Doppler imaging (Figs. 14 and 15). Convention shows flow toward the heart below the baseline in venous duplex ultrasound scans. Absence of reflux demonstrated using the Valsalva maneuver is also associated with venous occlusion. Adequate venous compression is associated with minimal deformity of the adjacent artery. Compressibility is usually not possible as a criterion in iliac veins. The character of the thrombus and dilation of the vein are associated with acute thrombus.

Surgeon/Technologist Involvement

This is a time consuming test whose accuracy is contingent on complete visualization of the entire limb. The value of screening a portion of the venous system has

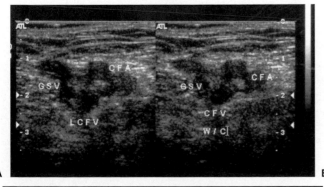

A   **B**

FIGURE 15. **A:** Before compression. **B:** After compression. The common femoral vein and greater saphenous vein do not collapse with compression (W/C), indicating that the vein lumen is full of clot.

not been evaluated, but it appears at this time that partial screening is not efficacious. The physician can rely on the RVT performance of a deep venous thrombosis study with review of static images in reliable vascular laboratories.

CHRONIC VENOUS INSUFFICIENCY (TABLE 12)

Varicose Veins

Traditionally, saphenous reflux has been identified by the Trendelenburg test and confirmed by CW Doppler, sometimes supplemented by plethysmographic testing. Reliance on these modalities will cause the clinician to miss significant reflux 30% of the time and result in unnecessary removal of the greater saphenous vein in 10% of cases (49).

Labropoulous et al. (50) showed that patients with primary varicose veins had reflux at various levels and in the saphenofemoral junction alone in only 40% of patients. Bergan (51) has suggested that in the case of recurrent varicose veins about two of three arise from a retained saphenous segment. Other causes were midthigh perforation or inadequate operation at the saphenofemoral junction. It would seem that Duplex evaluation should have a role in such recurrent varicose vein patient evaluations.

Meissner (52) suggested that appropriate therapy of chronic venous insufficiency should identify any component of deep venous obstruction, level of valvular reflux, or nonsaphenous sources of reflux; and identify all significant sources of deep to superficial reflux. Such studies can decrease greater saphenous operations by 10% and increase lesser saphenous operations from 6% to 21%.

Technique

In evaluating reflux, the patient should stand with leg slightly bent and weight supported by the opposite limb (52). Sequential segmental imaging with rapid proximal cuff inflation and deflation documents valve closure in less than 0.5 second. Perforators can also be identified in the standing position with high accuracy (i.e., more than 80%) (53).

▶ **TABLE 12 Chronic Venous Insufficiency**

1. Only 40% of primary varicose vein patients have saphenofemoral reflux by duplex ultrasound
2. Retained saphenous segments are common with recurrent varicose veins

▶ **TABLE 13** Endovenous Saphenous Vein Obliteration
1. Percutaneous vein puncture usually is possible
2. Saphenous obliteration is achieved more than 95% of the time

Surgeon/Technologist Involvement

The physician should be familiar with these techniques if he or she needs to validate and identify incompetent perforators intraoperatively. Otherwise, a map drawn on the leg is usually performed for communication.

ENDOVENOUS SAPHENOUS VEIN OBLITERATION (TABLE 13)

Numerous investigators have reported success with duplex guidance of a radiofrequency catheter to ablate the saphenous vein of varicose veins replacing conventional vein stripping (54–58). A catheter is inserted in the saphenous vein below the knee, and a radiofrequency catheter delivers heat to 85°C within the vein. The heat disrupts the intima, causing collagen in the vein wall to shrink. Disrupted intima and lumen obliteration lead to thrombosis. This prevents a groin incision, and the catheter can usually be inserted into the saphenous vein at the knee with ultrasound guidance through a percutaneous puncture or small stab wound. Chandler et al. (55) showed that acute occlusion was achieved in 96% of 290 limbs. Weiss (58) showed that at 1 week 98% of 140 patients had absent saphenous flow, and at 24 months 19 of 21 patients had complete disappearance of the saphenous vein.

Technique

An ultrasound vein map of the greater saphenous vein from the saphenofemoral junction to below the knee is performed with attention to abnormalities (such as duplication) of the saphenous vein and location of large varicosities where the catheter can get diverted from the greater saphenous vein. Depth of the vein from the skin surface is measured (Fig. 16). This mapping can be performed in the office before surgery. It can also be performed or repeated in the operating room before patient preparation. A vein located less than 10 mm from the skin surface requires subcutaneous saline injection to prevent skin thermal injury.

After preparing the leg, the ultrasound transducer in a sterile sheath is placed over the saphenous vein just below the knee to allow ultrasound-guided vein puncture (Fig. 17), wire insertion, and blind catheter advancement to the groin. Using B-mode ultrasound, the saphenofemoral junction is visualized and the inferior epigas-

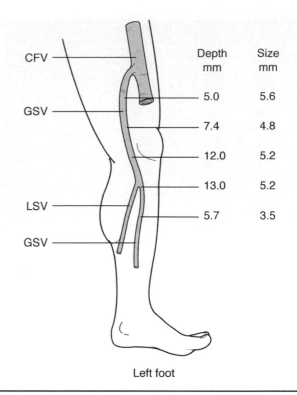

	Depth mm	Size mm
	5.0	5.6
	7.4	4.8
	12.0	5.2
	13.0	5.2
	5.7	3.5

Left foot

FIGURE 16. Scanning the greater saphenous vein with B-mode ultrasound before prepping is mapped out as to vein depth and size. This allows saline injection if the vein is too superficial to prevent skin thermal injury (less than 10 mm).

tric vein is identified (Fig. 18). The catheter tip is placed at the inferior epigastric junction distal to the level of the first valve. Radiofrequency ablation then proceeds without ultrasound guidance, and the catheter is slowly withdrawn while ablation continues. Once the ablation proce-

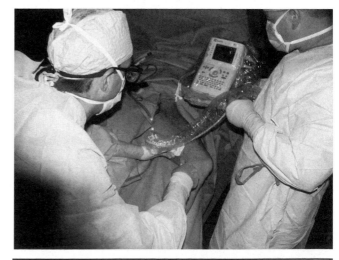

FIGURE 17. The surgeon holds the transducer with one hand to enable greater saphenous vein puncture with the other hand. The registered vascular technologist adjusts B-mode for optimal image with this duplex machine in a sterile cover.

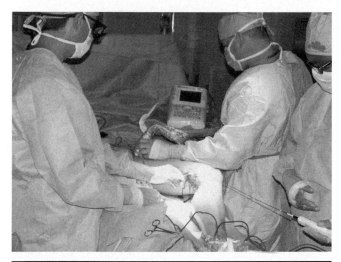

FIGURE 18. With the B-mode demonstrating the sapheno-femoral junction, the catheter is carefully threaded and the tip visualized just distal to the saphenofemoral junction. (Note the radiofrequency ablation instrument.)

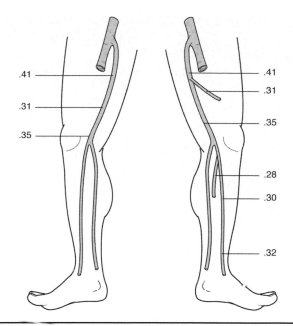

FIGURE 19. In addition to drawing the vein map on the leg as in Figure 11, a map is kept for reference as a report best done as a sketch. The numbers are vein sizes in centimeters.

dure is completed, imaging of the greater saphenous vein is performed to assess for the presence or absence of flow, reduced vein size, or thrombosis of the vein.

Surgeon/Technologist Involvement

The vein map is performed by the technologist before preparing the leg. The surgeon may hold the probe for saphenous vein puncture. The technologist, who usually is scrubbed, identifies the saphenofemoral junction while the surgeon manipulates the probe.

VEIN MAPPING (TABLE 14)

Mapping of the saphenous vein preoperatively to determine vein anatomy as well as vein size and suitability has become common practice. A map is usually drawn on the leg with sizes noted as well as location of branches. This is especially important for in situ bypass where limited skin incisions may be used (Fig. 19). A vein size greater than 2.5 mm is associated with success in vein bypass.

Technique

Mapping usually begins in the thigh and is performed with high-frequency transducers generally in the transverse orientation. Any thick wall or narrow area is marked in the lab with a dotted line and a comment on the leg as well as on the report.

Communication between surgeon and technologist is critically important to determining how much usable vein must be identified with the vein map.

ULTRASOUND-GUIDED PSEUDOANEURYSM THROMBIN INJECTION (TABLE 15)

Use of ultrasound guidance to inject thrombin into pseudoaneurysms, which occur mostly after groin catheterizations, is associated with a greater than 90% success rate in recent series (59–64). Early recurrence occurs in as many as 8% of cases (61). Intraarterial injection leading to limb-threatening ischemia requiring surgical

▶ **TABLE 14 Vein Mapping**

1. Preoperative vein mapping to determine vein anatomy and vein size
2. Veins of >2.5 mm and flexible walls are usually adequate for bypass
3. Important for in situ bypass

▶ **TABLE 15 Pseudoaneurysm Treatment**

1. Ultrasound-guided thrombin injection: ■ Is over 90% successful ■ Can be used even in anticoagulated patients 2. Ultrasound-guided compression of pseudoaneurysm ■ Has been largely replaced by thrombin because the former is painful and less effective

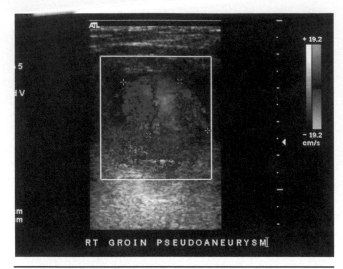

FIGURE 20. Pseudoaneurysm of the common femoral artery shows back-and-forth color distinctive from arterial flow seen beneath the pseudoaneurysm. (See Color Plate 11.)

thrombectomy has been reported by Kang et al. (61) and Khoury et al. (62). The latter authors also reported a rupture 1 day after injection, leading to death of the patient. There appears to be success with no discontinuation of anticoagulant drugs, which many of these patients require.

Technique

Usually 4- to 10-MHz linear transducers are used, although for some deep pseudoaneurysms curved linear or phased arrays have been used. First a scan is performed using color flow to determine if there is a narrow neck and if there is associated arteriovenous communication. Many authors (61–63) use a 1-ml³ syringe with bovine thrombin at a concentration of 1,000 U/ml³. Others (64) and I use a 10-ml³ syringe with 1,000 U (100 U/ml³).

The pseudoaneurysm is imaged and measured (Fig. 20). With the color turned off, using B mode alone allows optimal visualization of the needle entering the pseudoaneurysm. The needle should enter obliquely in the plane of the transducer (Fig. 21). The 21-gauge, 8-cm-long Echotip needle (Cook Inc., Bloomington, IN) is especially easy to see. It is important not to aspirate blood into the syringe, as it will immediately clot.

Once the needle tip is visualized appropriately in the pseudoaneurysm, the color is turned on, and 200 to 1,000 U of thrombin is injected. (We routinely inject 5 ml³, which is 500 U). The surgeon should be looking at the ultrasound screen and not at his or her hand while injecting the thrombin solution. Injection should produce a kaleidoscope of color throughout the pseudoaneurysm briefly. Then almost immediately, thrombosis should be demonstrated by the absence of color flow (Fig. 22),

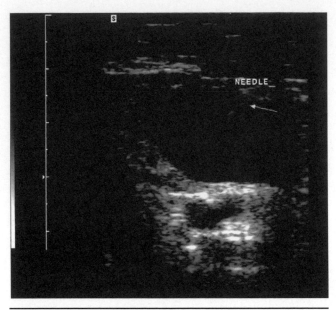

FIGURE 21. The needle tip can be seen on B-mode scan, well positioned in the pseudoaneurysm chamber.

which can be confirmed by PW Doppler ultrasound. A minimal dressing is all that is needed after a successful injection.

Some authors have recommended bed rest for 1 to 4 hours (61,62), but no data exist to confirm that this is necessary. We have not had problems with postinjection immediate ambulation.

Surgeon/Technologist Involvement

The technologist can hold the probe with a sterile glove (or sheath) and, using sterile gel, prepare and drape the area to be treated. The surgeon should use two hands to

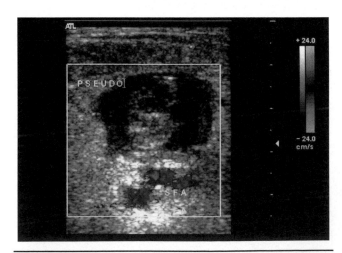

FIGURE 22. After thrombin injection, there is no flow in the pseudoaneurysm cavity on color Doppler imaging. An echogenic thrombus is seen. (See Color Plate 12.)

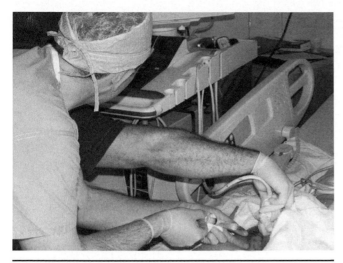

FIGURE 23. Pseudoaneurysm injection is best performed with the registered vascular technologist holding the transducer and optimizing the images, and the surgeon stabilizing and advancing the needle for optimal accuracy of thrombin injection.

manipulate and steady the needle. Although some surgeons like to hold the transducer in one hand and the syringe in the other, this procedure does not give optimal needle stability, which is important (Fig. 23).

ULTRASOUND-GUIDED COMPRESSION REPAIR OF PSEUDOANEURYSMS

In contrast to the greater than 90% success rate of thrombin injection for pseudoaneurysms, ultrasound-guided compression repair is associated with a 63% to 74% success rate (64,65). The discomfort patients experience and the difficulty in exerting pressure for the required time have led to a marked decrease in the use of this procedure in favor of thrombin injection. In addition, there is a strong negative correlation with the success and use of anticoagulation (65).

Technique

Using a 4- to 10-MHz linear transducer, the technologist locates the neck of the pseudoaneurysm with color Doppler. With the color turned on, the physician or technologist applies sufficient pressure over the neck of the pseudoaneurysm to eliminate all flow from the pseudoaneurysm. This pressure is held with the color on for 20 minutes. The pressure is then released, and if there is still flow in the pseudoaneurysm the pressure obliteration of flow is repeated for another 20 minutes. Sonographer and patient rarely tolerate a third 20-minute session.

Surgeon/Technologist Involvement

It would be ideal for a surgeon to hold the transducer during this compression, but technologists do this in many institutions. From the patient's point of view, enough anxiety and discomfort accompanies this procedure that there is merit in having the surgeon physically present even if he or she is not holding the transducer.

VEIN CATHETERIZATION WITH ULTRASOUND GUIDANCE (TABLE 16)

Subclavian vein catheterization is associated with failure to access the vein, inadvertent arterial puncture, pneumothorax or hemothorax, and nerve injury. Internal jugular vein (IJV) puncture has a lower incidence of pneumothorax or hemothorax. Subclavian vein catheterization has been shown to be much more successful for inexperienced operators using ultrasound guidance than without, with a 92% as opposed to a 44% success rate (66). Gordon et al. reported a 99.9% success rate in 868 IJV catheterization cases using ultrasound guidance (67). In this series, arterial puncture occurred in 1.5% of cases. Percutaneous intravenous central line access via peripheral veins with ultrasound guidance may also aid in difficult cases.

Technique

For subclavian puncture, a high-frequency transducer identifies the artery and vein below the clavicle. The physician should select a high-frequency linear probe greater than 7 MHz and cover it with a sterile sheath. The high-frequency intraoperative probe seems less stable when held on the skin for this application, although visualization is good. B-mode ultrasound is all that is required for adequate artery and vein identification using compressibility and pulsatility. If Doppler ultrasound with color flow is available, look for respiratory variability within the vein. Its absence may suggest central vein stenosis and should prompt immediate consideration of going to the other side before cannulating the vein and having problems inserting the wire.

▶ **TABLE 16 Vein Catheterization with Ultrasound Guidance**

1. Ultrasound guidance decreases complications:
   - Inadvertent arterial puncture
   - Hemo- or pneumothorax
   - Nerve injury
2. Can be used for internal jugular, subclavian, and other peripheral veins

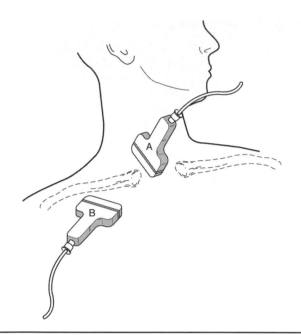

FIGURE 24. Transducer positions for longitudinal scanning when inserting internal jugular **(A)** or subclavian **(B)** central venous lines.

Transverse scanning is useful in identifying the relationship between the carotid artery and the jugular vein. Gordon et al. showed the usual anatomic relationship between the carotid artery and the IJV, with the IJV anterolateral in only 50% of cases (67). During transverse scanning for IJV venipuncture, the needle denting into the anterior vein wall can be seen. Rebound of the anterior wall will assure the operator that the needle is in the vein lumen. Visualization of the needle tip in the lumen is usually possible with this technique. The advantage of this technique is that it allows simultaneous visualization of artery and vein to help avoid arterial puncture. It also allows lower insertion in the vein, which is advisable especially for dialysis access central lines. Longitudinal scanning of the jugular and subclavian veins as originally advocated by Machi et al. (Fig. 24) allows visualization of the needle tip in the vein as well as the guidewire and sheath (Fig. 25) (68).

Special needles are designed for better visualization with ultrasound, but the needle supplied in the central venous kit allows good visualization and is usually well seen. The distal needle can be scraped with a clamp or a scalpel to roughen the outer wall in order to increase the reflection of the sound waves. Ultrasound-guided needle placement is detailed in Chapter 4.

Surgeon/Technologist Involvement

The technique is simpler if one person holds the transducer while another person performs the puncture, with two hands to aspirate and advance the wire and sheath. The B-mode image can be obtained and optimized by the physician. A relatively inexperienced steady-handed person can hold the probe while needle insertion is accomplished. With experience, one person can hold the probe and insert the needle. It is important to hold the probe at 90 degrees without angulation because angulation will thwart orientation. This may improve orientation and

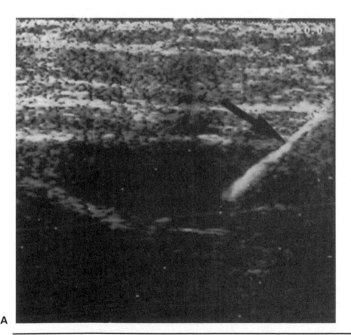

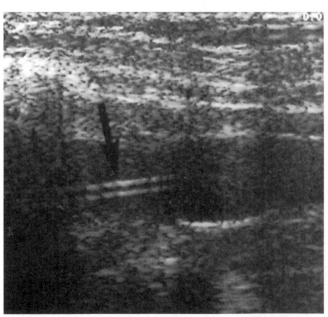

FIGURE 25. A: Visualization of the hyperechoic needle (*arrow*) within the vein lumen in longitudinal scan. **B:** Visualization of the catheter (*arrow*) within the lumen.

visibility of the vein lumen in difficult cases. The expertise of an RVT is helpful but usually not necessary. Inexpensive portable B-mode ultrasound devices are available that are suitable for this application.

INFERIOR VENA CAVA FILTER PLACEMENT WITH ULTRASOUND GUIDANCE (TABLE 17)

Placement of inferior vena cava (IVC) filter devices has been accomplished using duplex ultrasound instead of x-ray (69–73), allowing its placement in the intensive care unit, patient's room, or treatment room. This avoids operating room or radiology interventional suite requirements, as well as exposure to ionizing radiation. Conners et al. (69) showed that this saves $2,388 per patient in hospital charges.

In Conners's series (69) of 325 patients, 35 were unsuitable for filter placement due to visualization difficulties, 4 due to IVC thrombus, and 2 patients had IVC diameters too large for the planned filter. Sato et al. (71) achieved placement in 85% of intensive care unit patients.

Stainless steel Greenfield vena cava filters and Venatech filters have been used with good B-mode ultrasound visualization.

Technique

Low-frequency 2- to 3-MHz curved linear array probes are usually used to image the iliac veins and IVC for patency and size. The renal veins are identified and their location relative to the right renal artery determined. In longitudinal scan, the right renal artery is a prominent landmark as it passes behind the IVC. The anatomy of the IVC bifurcation is also identified.

The J tip of the guidewire and sheath are visualized in the longitudinal scan and placement coordinated with the right renal artery as a cephalad landmark (Fig. 26). The filter is deployed using this longitudinal scan. Position is verified after deployment by B-mode ultrasound and can be confirmed by a flat plate x-ray film of the abdomen.

> ▶ TABLE 17 Inferior Vena Cava Filter Placement with Ultrasound Guidance

1. Possible with over 85% success rate and precludes the need for fluoroscopy
2. Can be performed at bedside (e.g., in an intensive care unit) and is much less costly

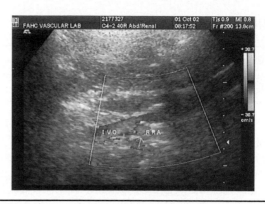

FIGURE 26. The right renal artery (RRA) passing beneath the inferior vena cava (IVC) serves as a landmark for inferior vena cava filter placement. (See Color Plate 13.)

Surgeon/Technologist Involvement

The technologist should first perform a surface scan to ensure adequate visualization of femoral and iliac veins, IVC, renal veins, and IVC bifurcation; adequate size of the IVC for the planned filter; and absence of clot in access veins and IVC.

During filter insertion, the technologist need not be sterile and should handle the transducer. The surgeon should be sterile working in the groin, with direct visualization of the ultrasound screen. If the surgeon encounters difficulty in cannulating the femoral vein in the groin, duplex using a sterile transducer sheath can be implemented for ultrasound-guided cannulation; however, this is rarely necessary.

INFERIOR VENA CAVA FILTER PLACEMENT USING INTRAVASCULAR ULTRASOUND

Intravascular ultrasound (IVUS) has been used for bedside IVC filter placement (73). This technique gives excellent measurement of IVC size and level of renal veins, but the actual deployment is not visualized. The distance from the groin puncture site to the "landing zone" is measured with IVUS, and then the filter is deployed blindly at that same level. Ebaugh et al. (73) had one deployment in the iliac vein because of a measurement error in their series of 24 patients.

ENDOLEAK DETECTION BY DUPLEX ULTRASOUND AFTER AORTIC ENDOGRAFT (TABLE 18)

Although computed tomography (CT) scanning has been the imaging modality of choice for detection of endoleaks after aortic aneurysm endografting, numerous studies

▌**TABLE 18 Endoleak Detection
by Duplex Ultrasound**

1. Highly sensitive and specific, but a technically demanding study
2. To and fro color pattern possibly predictive of spontaneous endoleak closure

▌**TABLE 19 Intravascular Ultrasound**

1. A new ultrasound technology, originally used for coronary artery stenting
2. May prove useful in aortic and peripheral endografting.

have shown the effectiveness of color flow duplex for this purpose (74–77). McLafferty et al. (74) summarized nine reports comparing duplex to CT scanning for detection of endoleak and showed 95% sensitivity, 97% specificity, and 93% accuracy of all reports, along with 99% accuracy in their own series of 79 patients.

Parent et al. (75) suggested that the duplex study showing a "to/fro Doppler scan waveform pattern . . . similar to signals observed in the neck of a femoral false aneurysm" (Fig. 27) preceded spontaneous endoleak closure in most cases. They contrasted this with intra-endoleak monophasic or biphasic flow patterns. Comparing duplex examination to CT scanning for identification of the source vessel in type 2 endoleaks, Parent et al. (75) identified all of 36 feeding vessels by duplex and only 7 of 18 (39%) by CT scan.

CT scan and duplex may be complementary in this application as in many others in showing different information. Duplex clearly has been shown to be useful.

Technique

As outlined by Sato et al. (76) using low-frequency probes, a B-mode imaging study is performed followed by color Doppler scan imaging with appropriate gain settings. It is

necessary to scan the entire aortic aneurysm sac outside the graft in both longitudinal and transverse views with color Doppler scanning. Spectral analysis outside the graft and within the endograft is also required. Search for feeding vessels is performed if an endoleak is detected.

Sato et al. (76) in reviewing videotaped studies found that adequate studies were present in only 19% of studies. On the other hand, Parent et al. (75) in a prospective study of patients in a single vascular laboratory, had only 6% (of 141 studies) suboptimal studies using similar criteria.

Surgeon/Technologist Involvement

This is an extremely time consuming and demanding study that will usually be performed without surgeon involvement and reviewed with static and recorded video images. Surgeon involvement in defining protocol and assuring quality is essential.

INTRAVASCULAR ULTRASOUND (TABLE 19)

IVUS has been used to assess adequacy of endovascular stent deployment and angioplasty (78,79) for stenoses and for aneurysm endografts (Fig. 28). This development

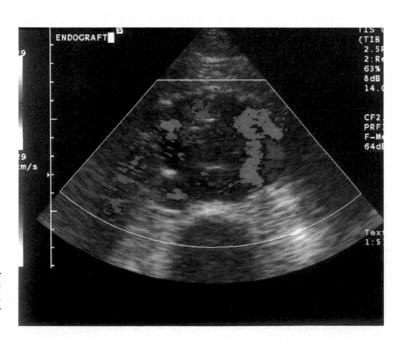

FIGURE 27. Type I endoleak after aortic endograft has back-and-forth pattern similar to that in femoral catheterization–related pseudoaneurysms. (See Color Plate 14.)

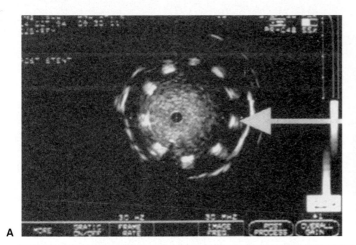
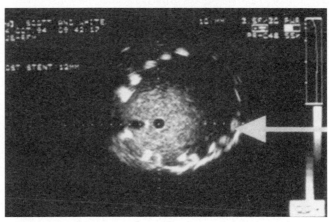

A   B

FIGURE 28. **A:** Underdeployed stent demonstrated by intravascular ultrasound. **B:** Underdeployment was corrected by dilation with a larger balloon. (From Arko F, Mettauer M, McCollough R, et al. Use of intravascular ultrasound improves long-term clinical outcome in the endovascular management of atherosclerotic aortoiliac occlusive disease. *J Vasc Surg* 1998;27:614–623, with permission.)

has followed the widespread use for coronary artery stenting using IVUS. Arko et al. (78) showed no restenosis or occlusions in 36 patients where stent deployment was assisted by IVUS and 25% restenosis or occlusion when IVUS was not used.

The expense of disposable IVUS probes and the requirement for a specialized ultrasound machine for this use only have limited more widespread applicability of this technology. The information does seem useful, and since the probes must be placed within the vessels, the interventionist/surgeon necessarily manipulates the probe.

CONCLUSION

Duplex ultrasound has become the primary modality for determining aneurysm size as well as for evaluating extracranial cerebrovascular arteries, vein graft surveillance, deep venous thrombosis, and preoperative vein mapping. These studies are usually performed by RVTs with supervision by physicians (frequently surgeons).

As surgeons have gained experience with ultrasound, they have had success using the technology to aid in preoperative evaluation, such as with arterial mapping and chronic venous insufficiency; intraoperatively with carotid endarterectomy and arterial bypass and stent/angioplasties; and for interventions in the case of pseudoaneurysms, subclavian/IJV catheterizations, endovenous saphenous vein obliteration, and IVC filter placement.

As improvements both in ultrasound technology and in surgeons' (and physicians') competence in using it occur, the applications of ultrasound along with its accuracy and reliability will increase. The challenge is to have uncompromised quality in patient care.

REFERENCES

1. Kremkau FW. *Diagnostic ultrasound: principles and instruments*, 6th ed. Philadelphia: WB Saunders, 2002.
2. Ricci MA, Kleeman M, Case T, et al. Normal aortic diameter by ultrasound. *J Vasc Tech* 1995;19:17–19.
3. North American Symptomatic Carotid Endarterectomy Trial (NASCET) Collaborators. Beneficial effect of carotid endarterectomy in symptomatic patients with high-grade stenosis. *N Engl J Med* 1991;325:445–453.
4. Executive Committee for the Asymptomatic Carotid Atherosclerosis Study. Endarterectomy for asymptomatic carotid stenosis. *JAMA* 1995;273:1421–1428.
5. Fillinger MF, Baker RJ, Zwolak RM, et al. Carotid duplex criteria for a 60% or greater angiographic stenosis: variation according to equipment. *J Vasc Surg* 1996; 24:856–864.
6. Zierler RE. Basic and practical aspects of cerebrovascular testing. In: Bernstein, ed. *Vascular diagnosis*, 1995.
7. Moneta GL, Edwards JM, Chitwood RW , et al. Correlation of North American Symptomatic Carotid Endarterectomy Trial (NASCET) angiographic definition of 70% to 90% internal carotid artery stenosis with duplex scanning. *J Vasc Surg* 1993;17:152–159.
8. Moneta GL, Edwards JM, Papanicolaou G , et al. Screening for asymptomatic internal carotid artery stenosis: duplex criteria for discriminating 60–99% stenosis. *J Vasc Surg* 1995;21:989–994.
9. AbuRahma AF, Richmond BK, Robinson PA, et al. Effect of contralateral severe stenosis or carotid occlusion on duplex criteria of ipsilateral stenoses: comparative study of duplex parameters. *J Vasc Surg* 1995;22:751–761.
10. Wain RA, Lyon RT, Veith FJ, et al. Accuracy of duplex ultrasound in evaluating carotid artery anatomy before endarterectomy. *J Vasc Surg* 1998;27:235–244.
11. Tegos TJ, Stavropoulos P, Sabetai MM, et al. Determinants of carotid plaque instability: echoicity versus heterogeneity. *Eur J Vasc Endovasc Surg* 2001;22:22–30.
12. Ascher E, Markevich N, Hingorani AP, et al. Internal carotid artery flow volume measurement and other intraoperative duplex scanning parameters as predictors of stroke after carotid endarterectomy. *J Vasc Surg* 2002;35:439–444.
13. Bandyk DF. Postoperative surveillance of infrainguinal bypass. *Surg Clin North Am* 1990;70:71–85.
14. Bandyk DF, Mills JL, Gahtan V, et al. Intraoperative duplex scanning of arterial reconstructions: fate of repaired and unrepaired defects. *J Vasc Surg* 1994 ;20:426–432.

15. Kinney EV, Seabrook GR, Kinney LY, et al. The importance of intraoperative detection of residual flow abnormalities after carotid artery endarterectomy. *J Vasc Surg* 1993;17: 912–922.

16. Lingenfelter KA, Fuller BC, Sullivan TM. Intraoperative assessment of carotid endarterectomy: a comparison of techniques. *Ann Vasc Surg* 1995;9:235–240.

17. Papanicolaou G, Toms C, Yellin AE, et al. Relationship between intraoperative color-flow duplex findings and early restenosis after carotid endarterectomy: a preliminary report. *J Vasc Surg* 1996;24:588–595.

18. Pilcher DB, Ricci MA. Vascular ultrasound. *Surg Clin North Am* 1998;78:273–293.

19. Seelig MH, Oldenburg WA, Chowla A, et al. Use of intraoperative duplex ultrasonography and routine patch angioplasty in patients undergoing carotid endarterectomy. *Mayo Clin Proc* 1999;74:870–876.

20. Archie JP. The endarterectomy-produced common carotid artery step: a harbinger of early emboli and late restenosis. *J Vasc Surg* 1996;23:932–939.

21. Ascher E, Hingorani A, Markevich N, et al. Lower extremity revascularization without preoperative contrast arteriography: experience with duplex ultrasound arterial mapping in 485 cases. *Ann Vasc Surg* 2002;16:108–114.

22. Proia RR, Walsh DB, Nelson PR, et al. Early results of infragenicular revascularization based solely on duplex arteriography. *J Vasc Surg* 2001;33:1165–1170.

23. Koelemay MJ, Legemate DA, de Vos H, et al. Duplex scanning allows selective use of arteriography in the management of patients with severe lower leg arterial disease. *J Vasc Surg* 2001;34:661–667.

24. Bostrom A, Ljungman C, Hellberg A, et al. Duplex scanning as the sole preoperative imaging method for infrainguinal arterial surgery. *Eur J Vasc Endovasc Surg* 2002;23:140–145.

25. Ascher E. Ultrasound arterial mapping prior to femoral popliteal reconstruction in claudicants: a proposal for a new shortened protocol. Presented at the Society of Clinical Vascular Surgery, Las Vegas, Nevada, March 14, 2002.

26. Bandyk DF, Johnson BL, Gupta AK, et al. Nature and management of duplex abnormalities encountered during infrainguinal vein bypass grafting. *J Vasc Surg* 1996;24:430–438.

27. Johnson BL, Bandyk DF, Back MR, et al. Intraoperative duplex monitoring of infrainguinal vein bypass procedures. *J Vasc Surg* 2000;31:678–690.

28. Mackenzie KS, Hill AB, Steinmetz OK. The predictive value of intraoperative duplex for early vein graft patency in lower extremity revascularization. *Ann Vasc Surg* 1999;13:275–283.

29. Mills JL, Bandyk DF, Gahtan V, et al. The origin of infrainguinal vein graft stenosis: a prospective study based on duplex surveillance. *J Vasc Surg* 1995;21:16–25.

30. DeWeese JA, Leather R, Porter J. Practice guidelines: lower extremity revascularization. *J Vasc Surg* 1993;18:280–294.

31. Bandyk DF, Cato RF, Towne JB. A low flow velocity predicts failure of femoro-popliteal and femoro-tibial bypass grafts. *Surgery* 1985;98:799–809.

32. Bandyk DF, Bergamini TM, Towne JB, et al. Durability of vein graft revisions: the outcome of secondary procedures. *J Vasc Surg* 1991;13:200–210.

33. Bandyk DF. Essentials of graft surveillance. *Semin Vasc Surg* 1993;6:92–102.

34. Bandyk DF, Schmitt DD, Seabrook GR, et al. Monitoring functional patency of in situ saphenous vein bypasses: the impact of a surveillance protocol and elective revision. *J Vasc Surg* 1989;9:286–296.

35. Landry GJ, Moneta GL, Taylor LM Jr., et al. Patency and characteristics of lower extremity vein grafts requiring multiple revisions. *J Vasc Surg* 2000;32:23–31.

36. Visser K, Idu MM, Buth J, et al. Duplex scan surveillance during the first year after infrainguinal autologous vein bypass grafting surgery: costs and clinical outcomes compared with other surveillance programs. *J Vasc Surg* 2001;33:123–130.

37. Ryan SV, Dougherty MJ, Chang M, et al. Abnormal duplex findings at the proximal anastomosis of infrainguinal bypass grafts: does revision enhance patency? *Ann Vasc Surg* 2001;15:98–103.

38. Calligaro KD, Syrek J, Rua I, et al. Use of duplex ultrasonography to replace preoperative arteriography for failing arterial grafts. *J Vasc Surg* 1998;27:89–95.

39. Darling RC III, Roddy SP, Chang BB, et al. Long-term results of revised infrainguinal arterial reconstructions. *J Vasc Surg* 2002;35:773–778.

40. Mewissen MW, Kinney EV, Bandyk DF, et al. The role of duplex scanning versus angiography in predicting outcome after balloon angioplasty in the femoropopliteal artery. *J Vasc Surg* 1992;15:860–864.

41. Spijkerboer AM, Nass PC, de Valois JC, et al. Evaluation of femoropopliteal arteries with duplex ultrasound after angioplasty. Can we predict results at one year? *Eur J Vasc Endovasc Surg* 1996;12:418–423.

42. Katzenschlager R, Ahmadi A, Minar E, et al. Femoropopliteal artery: initial and 6 month results of color duplex US-guided percutaneous transluminal angioplasty. *Radiology* 1996;199:331–334.

43. Calligaro KD, Doerr K, McAffee-Bennett S, et al. Should duplex ultrasonography be performed for surveillance of femoropopliteal and femorotibial arterial prosthetic bypasses? *Ann Vasc Surg* 2001;15:520–524.

44. Comerota AJ, Katz ML, Greenwald LL. Venous duplex imaging: should it replace hemodynamic tests for deep venous thrombosis? *J Vasc Surg* 1990;11:53–61.

45. Heijboer H, Buller HR, Lensing AW, et al. A comparison of real-time compression ultrasonography with impedance plethysmography for the diagnosis of deep-vein thrombosis in symptomatic outpatients. *N Engl J Med* 1993;329:1365–1369.

46. Garcia ND, Morasch MD, Ebaugh JL, et al. Is bilateral ultrasound scanning of the legs necessary for patients with unilateral symptoms of deep venous thrombosis? *J Vasc Surg* 2001;34:792–797.

47. Meissner MH, Caps MT, Bergelin RO, et al. Early outcome after isolated calf vein thrombosis. *J Vasc Surg* 1997;26:749–756.

48. Mustafa BO, Rathbun SW, Whitsett TL, et al. Sensitivity and specificity of ultrasonography in the diagnosis of upper extremity deep vein thrombosis: a systematic review. *Arch Intern Med* 2002;162:401–404.

49. Wills V, Moylan D, Chambers J. The use of routine duplex scanning in the assessment of varicose veins. *Aust NZ J Surg* 1998;68:41–44.

50. Labropoulous N, Athanasios DG, Kostas D, et al. Where does venous reflux start? *J Vasc Surg* 1997;26:736–742.

51. Bergan JJ. Surgical management of primary and recurrent varicose veins. In: Gloviczki P, Yao JST, eds. *Handbook of venous disorders. Guidelines of the American Venous Forum.* London: Chapman and Hall, 1996:394–415.

52. Meissner MH. Venous evaluation: vein mapping, perforator identification, and venous access. American College of Surgeons Postgraduate course 28 syllabus. 2001;34–37.

53. Pierik E, Toonder IM, vanUrk H, et al. Validation of duplex ultrasonography in detecting competent and incompetent perforating veins in patients with venous ulceration of the lower leg. *J Vasc Surg* 1997;26:49–52.

54. Kabnick LS, Merchant RF. Twelve and twenty four month follow up after endovascular obliteration of saphenous vein reflux after endovascular obliteration of saphenous vein reflux: a report from the Multi-Center Registry. *J Phleb* 2001:1:17–24

55. Pichot O, Sessa C, Chandler JG, et al. Role of Duplex imaging in endovenous obliteration for primary venous insufficiency. *J Endovasc Ther* 2000;7:451–459.

56. Chandler JG, Pichot O, Sessa C, et al. Defining the role of extended saphenofemoral junction ligation: a prospective comparative study. *J Vasc Surg* 2000;32:941–953.

57. Chandler JG, Pichot O, Sessa C, et al. Treatment of primary venous insufficiency by endovenous saphenous vein obliteration. *Vasc Surg* 2000;34:201–214.

58. Weiss, RA, Weiss, MA. Controlled radiofrequency endovenous occlusion using a unique radiofrequency catheter under duplex guidance to eliminate saphenous venous reflux: a 2 year follow up. *Dermatol Surg* 2002;28:38–42.

59. Calton WC, Franklin DP, Elmore JR, et al. Ultrasound-guided thrombin injection is a safe and durable treatment for femoral pseudoaneurysms. *Vasc Surg* 2001;35:379–383.
60. Friedman SG, Pellerito JS, Scher L, et al. Ultrasound-guided thrombin injection is the treatment of choice for femoral pseudoaneurysms. *Arch Surg* 2002;137:462–464.
61. Kang SS, Labropoulos N, Mansour MA, et al. Expanded indications for ultrasound-guided thrombin injection of pseudoaneurysms. *J Vasc Surg* 2000;31:289–298.
62. Khoury M, Rebecca A, Greene K, et al. Duplex scanning–guided thrombin injection for the treatment of iatrogenic pseudoaneurysms. *J Vasc Surg* 2002;35:517–521.
63. Sackett WR, Taylor SM, Coffey CB, et al. Ultrasound-guided thrombin injection of iatrogenic femoral pseudoaneurysms: a prospective analysis. *Am Surg* 2000;66:937–940.
64. Taylor BS, Rhee RY, Muluk S, et al. Thrombin injection versus compression of femoral artery pseudoaneurysms. *J Vasc Surg* 1999;30:1052–1059.
65. Eisenberg L, Paulson EK, Kliewer MA, et al. Sonographically guided compression repair of pseudoaneurysms: further experience from a single institution. *AJR Am J Roentgenol* 1999;173:1567–1573.
66. Thompson DR, Gualtiere E, Deppe S, et al. Greater success in subclavian vein cannulation using ultrasound for inexperienced operators. *Crit Care Med* 1995;23:692–697.
67. Gordon AC, Saliken JC, Johns D, et al. US-guided puncture of the internal jugular vein: complications and anatomic considerations. *J Vasc Intervent Radiol* 1998;9:333–338.
68. Machi J, Takeda J, Kakegawa T. Safe jugular and subclavian venipuncture under ultrasonographic guidance. *Am J Surg* 1987;153:321–323.
69. Conners MS, Becher S, Guzman RJ et al. Duplex scan-directed placement of inferior vena cava filters: a five year institutional experience. *J Vasc Surg* 2002;35:286–291.
70. Han DC. Vena cava filter placement and evaluation by ultrasound. American College of Surgeons Postgraduate course no. 27 manual, 2001.
71. Sato DT, Robinson KD, Gregory RT, et al. Duplex directed caval filter insertion in multitrauma and critically ill patients. *Ann Vasc Surg* 1999;13:365–371.
72. Nunn CR, Neuzil D, Naslund T, et al. Cost effective method for bedside insertion of vena caval filters in trauma patients. *J Trauma* 1997;43:752–758.
73. Ebaugh JL, Chiou AC, Morasch MD, et al. Bedside vena caval filter placement guided with intravascular ultrasound. *J Vasc Surg* 2001; 34:21–26.
74. McLafferty RB, McCrary BS, Mattos MA, et al. The use of color-flow duplex scan for the detection of endoleaks. *J Vasc Surg* 2002;36:100–104.
75. Parent EN, Meier GH, Godziachvili V, et al. The incidence and natural history of type I and type II endoleak: a 5-year follow up assessment with color duplex ultrasound scan. *J Vasc Surg* 2002;35:474–481.
76. Sato DT, Goff CD, Gregory RT, et al. Endoleak after aortic stent graft repair: diagnosis by color duplex ultrasound scan versus computed tomography scan. *J Vasc Surg* 1998;28:657–663.
77. Wolf, YG, Johnson BL, Hill BB, et al. Duplex ultrasound scanning versus computed tomographic angiography for postoperative evaluation of endovascular abdominal aortic aneurysm repair. *J Vasc Surg* 2000;32:1142–1148.
78. Arko F, Mettauer M, McCollough R, et al. Use of intravascular ultrasound improves long-term clinical outcome in the endovascular management of atherosclerotic aortoiliac occlusive disease. *J Vasc Surg* 1998;27:614–623.
79. Diethrich EB, Ivens FD, AbuRahma AF. Intravascular ultrasound imaging of iliac stenoses during endovascular surgery. *J Cardiovasc Technol* 1989;8:287–293.

Trauma Ultrasound

Heidi L. Frankel and David L. Coffman

Ultrasound has become an established component of initial evaluation of the injured patient. After two large series were reported in the United States a decade ago, ultrasound has become as important a diagnostic tool as it is in Europe and Asia where experience has accumulated for nearly 20 years (1,2). As the American experience with ultrasound grows and our understanding of its strengths and limitations matures, the indications for its use in trauma will continue to be refined. At present, the primary goal of trauma ultrasound is to identify fluid, presumably blood, as a surrogate for organ damage in blunt-injured patients. More advanced applications allow diagnosis of intraparenchymal organ injury, pneumothoraces, and diaphragmatic, fascial, and vascular injuries; however, they are presently not included in the standard trauma examination. The standard trauma examination has been designated the focused assessment with sonography in trauma (FAST), an appellation that acknowledges the rapid, goal-directed nature of the test (3). The European, Asian, and American literatures are replete with statistics attesting to the ability of surgeons to perform FAST accurately as an extension of the physical examination of the injured patient (1–5).

HISTORY

An American radiologist first described the detection of free intraperitoneal fluid by ultrasound in 1970. Ultrasound was successfully used to detect as little as 100 mL of saline instilled into cadavers in this work by Goldberg (6,7). The significance of this finding in the trauma patient population was not recognized for many years. In fact, the first clinical reports of ultrasound in trauma did not describe the technique of identifying fluid, presumably hemoperitoneum; rather, they related detailed examinations for intraabdominal and retroperitoneal organ injuries (8–10). In both European and U.S. studies, early ultrasound use was dedicated to describing intraparenchymal hematomas and diaphragmatic injury (8–14). It was not until the late 1980s that the primary goal of

trauma ultrasound became fluid detection. The largest series was reported by Kohlberger and colleagues, where ultrasound compared favorably to diagnostic peritoneal lavage (DPL) in more than 2,000 patients studied (15). The first large clinical experience with ultrasound to detect hemoperitoneum in the United States was reported by Tso and colleagues at the University of Maryland in 1992 (1). Rozycki and colleagues reported a two part series in 1993 and 1995, highlighting the fact that trauma surgeons and their trainees can accurately identify fluid with FAST (2,16).

TECHNIQUE

The purpose of FAST is to survey for fluid in the pericardial space and dependent regions of the abdomen in the supine patient (Fig. 1). This limited examination should be completed in 1 to 2 min during the primary survey in an unstable trauma patient (as part of the circulatory evaluation) or during the secondary survey of a hemodynamically stable patient (allowing more time for fluid to collect). It is helpful to have the ultrasound machine turned on, warmed up, and ready prior to patient arrival, if this is feasible with the trauma resuscitation area setup. A convex, curvilinear 2.5- to 5.0-MHz transducer is employed to maximize penetration in trauma patients at the expense of resolution. Water-soluble ultrasound acoustic coupling transmission gel may be stored in the warmer of the trauma bay if such equipment is present (Table 1).

Cardiac Examination

The transducer is first oriented in the sagittal plane in the subxiphoid region for examination of the heart. It is helpful to perform this view first so as to set the gain and time gain compensation pods to a fluid-filled structure for optimization of images. Fluid appears anechoic (black) in comparison with the surrounding structures. Normal

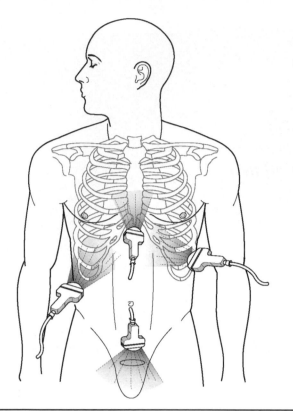

FIGURE 1. Schematic for transducer placement for FAST. Note the position and direction of four transducers.

and pathologic views of the pericardial space are depicted in Figures 2 and 3.

Abdominal Examination

Longitudinal views of the right upper quadrant (Morison's pouch) and the left upper quadrant (splenorenal recess) are obtained next. The right-sided view is obtained at the 10th or 11th intercostal space at the posterior axillary line, although it is our opinion that more anterior visualization (7th to 9th intercostal space) may permit detection of smaller amounts of fluid. The left-sided view must be posterior because gastric or intestinal air obscures proper visualization in a more anterior view. Nor-

▶ **TABLE 1 FAST Techniques**

1. Goal: to detect or exclude fluid in pericardial space and abdomen in the supine patient
2. 1–2 min during the primary survey in unstable patients or during the secondary survey in stable patients
3. 2.5- to 5.0-MHz curvilinear transducer
4. Cardiac examination: sagittal view in the subxiphoid region
5. Abdominal examination: longitudinal views of right and left upper quadrants, and transverse view of the pelvis
6. Thoracic examination: scan upward from upper quadrants for detection of pleural fluid (or pneumothorax)

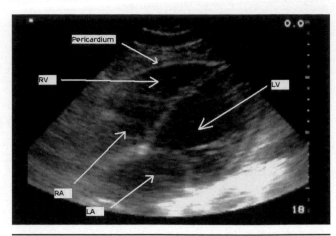

FIGURE 2. Normal FAST view of the pericardium. RA, right atrium; RV, right ventricle; LA, left atrium; LV, left ventricle

mal and abnormal views of the right upper quadrant and left upper quadrant are demonstrated in Figures 4 and 5, and 6 and 7, respectively. Finally, the transducer is oriented transversely over the pelvis for a coronal view of the bladder and surrounding structures (Fig. 8). A multicenter study revealed that, regardless of its cause, hemoperitoneum is more often detected in Morison's pouch than in any other region; hence, this abdominal view is accomplished first (17). There are actually several studies in the literature that advocate this ultrafast FAST (i.e., to view Morison's pouch only); however, the sensitivity of this approach (compared to all four views) is 20% to 67% versus 77% to 100% in one study that compared the two techniques (18).

Thoracic Examination

Although not a part of the FAST as initially conceived, the transducer is moved slightly from the right and left upper quadrant to image the thorax for presence of fluid (Figs. 9 and 10). The transducer is positioned pointed to the cranium rather than in a more inferior location. Sisley and colleagues reported that in the acute trauma setting, the sensitivity and specificity of ultrasound for pleural fluid detection was 97.5% and 99.7%, respectively, as compared with 92.5% and 99.7% for conventional chest radiographs (19). Time for performance of the examination was about a minute and a half. In the intensive care setting, this thoracic view may be used to detect, and potentially manage, pleural effusions with reasonable accuracy and speed. Rozycki and colleagues report 84% sensitivity, 100% specificity, and 94% accuracy in this setting (20). Finally, thoracic ultrasound may be utilized to diagnose a pneumothorax, which would be typified by absence of the comet tail artifact (Fig. 11) or defect in lung sliding, a motion artifact, which can only be visualized on a real-time video image. The comet tail artifact is pro-

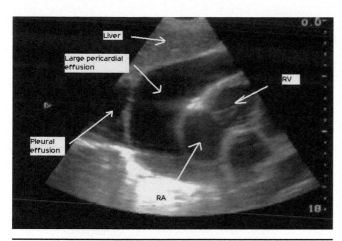

FIGURE 3. Pericardial fluid in a patient with tamponade. RA, right atrium; RV, right ventricle.

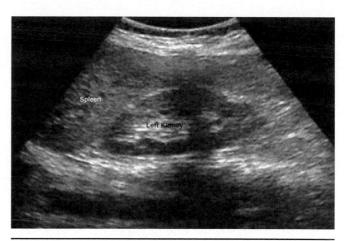

FIGURE 6. Normal longitudinal left upper quadrant FAST view.

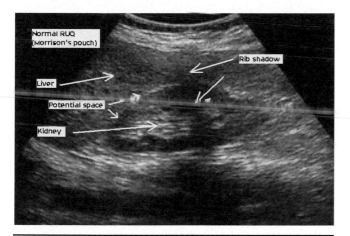

FIGURE 4. Normal longitudinal right upper quadrant FAST view.

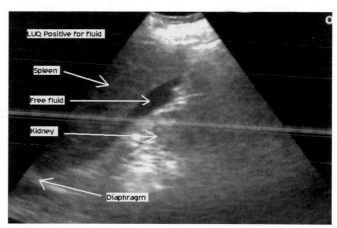

FIGURE 7. Left upper quadrant FAST view with fluid.

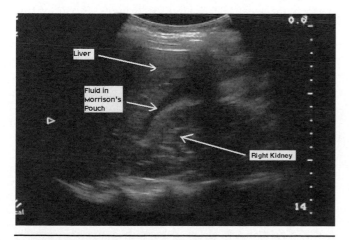

FIGURE 5. Right upper quadrant FAST view with fluid.

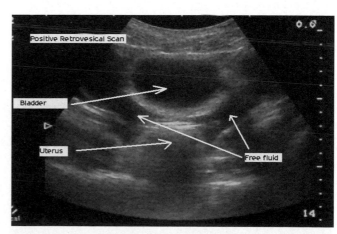

FIGURE 8. Transverse views of bladder with free peritoneal fluid.

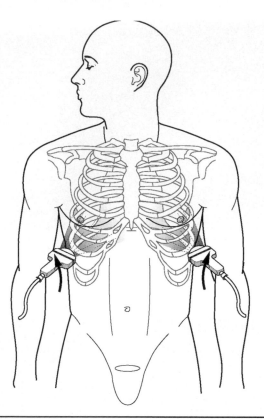

FIGURE 9. Schematic of transducer placement for thoracic views. Note the position and direction of two transducers that are moved and angled upwardly (*curved arrows*), as compared with those in Figure 1.

duced by the visceral pleura; therefore, its presence excludes a pneumothorax. Dulchavsky reported 95% sensitivity and 100% specificity in 382 patients, including 22% of patients with penetrating injury mechanisms. Pneumothoraces that could not be successfully detected occurred in the presence of large amounts of subcutaneous

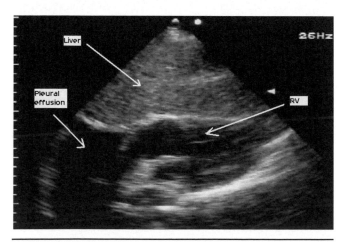

FIGURE 10. FAST with pleural fluid. RV, right ventricle.

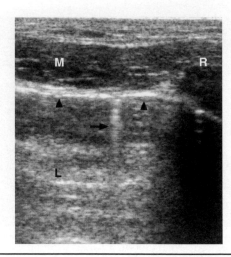

FIGURE 11. Comet tail artifact (*arrow*) indicating the absence of pneumothorax. *Arrowheads* indicate the pleura. L, lung; M, pectoral muscle; R, rib.

emphysema (21). Optimally, this examination is performed with a high-frequency (e.g., 7.5 or 10 MHz) linear transducer; thus, its effectiveness might be limited with a portable low-frequency ultrasound unit that may be ideal for emergency department trauma bay deployment. (See Chapter 10 for further discussion of thoracic ultrasound in the acute setting.)

INDICATIONS

Hemodynamically Unstable Patients for the Diagnosis of Hemoperitoneum (Fig. 12)

FAST is most helpful for diagnosing hemoperitoneum in blunt-injured patients with hypotension. For this reason, performance of FAST during the primary survey in this setting is preferred to expedite care. Hypotensive patients with fluid in the abdomen on FAST should proceed directly to laparotomy while resuscitation is ongoing. If the FAST result is negative or indeterminate in this setting, it suggests that abdominal injury is not the primary cause of hypotension; however, this does not exclude the presence of abdominal injury. These patients should undergo repeat FAST studies with continued resuscitation, computed tomography (CT) scanning of the torso if stability is achieved, or DPL. However, the latter is unlikely to be positive with abdominal trauma causing hypotension in the face of an appropriately performed and interpreted FAST that is negative. As a result, centers that routinely use FAST in the workup of hemodynamically unstable trauma patients rarely use DPL for this reason. In many centers, DPL has been relegated to the sampling of in-

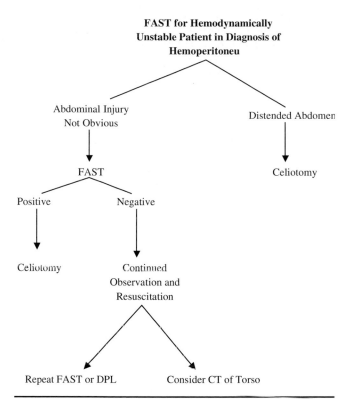

FAST for Hemodynamically Unstable Patient in Diagnosis of Hemoperitoneu

Abdominal Injury Not Obvious

Distended Abdomen

FAST

Celiotomy

Positive

Negative

Celiotomy

Continued Observation and Resuscitation

Repeat FAST or DPL

Consider CT of Torso

FIGURE 12. Hemodynamically unstable FAST algorithm.

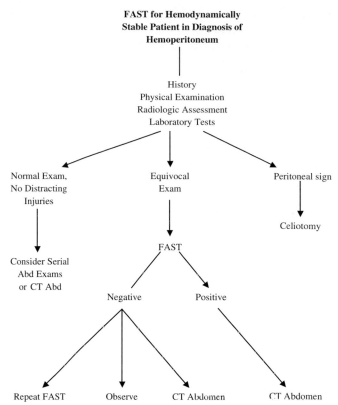

FAST for Hemodynamically Stable Patient in Diagnosis of Hemoperitoneum

History
Physical Examination
Radiologic Assessment
Laboratory Tests

Normal Exam, No Distracting Injuries

Equivocal Exam

Peritoneal sign

Celiotomy

Consider Serial Abd Exams or CT Abd

FAST

Negative

Positive

Repeat FAST

Observe

CT Abdomen

CT Abdomen

FIGURE 13. Hemodynamically stable FAST algorithm.

traperitoneal fluid to determine its characteristics (i.e., succus versus blood; the former would mandate a laparotomy even if the patient became hemodynamically stable). In one series, the number of annual DPLs per resident per year decreased from 22 to 3 (22). In our institution with a similar volume of trauma patients, the current number of annual DPLs is less than five institution-wide.

Hemodynamically Stable Patients for the Diagnosis of Hemoperitoneum (Fig. 13)

In hemodynamically stable patients, a positive FAST should be followed up with a CT scan to identify the site of organ injury so as to guide therapy further. Controversy exists as to the treatment of a patient with a negative FAST result. Some advocate follow-up with a repeat FAST. However, since approximately one third of patients with abdominal injuries do not have associated hemoperitoneum according to several studies, the most conservative approach is to perform a CT scan on everyone so as to miss no injuries (23–25). This feature is not affected by the skill level of the sonographer but rather is inherent to the strengths and weaknesses of the FAST examination. Whereas most patients with such an injury

pattern do not require operative treatment, in some series up to 10% do. Furthermore, although these patients may not require surgery, they may warrant close observation, counseling, and lifestyle modification as treatment for their solid visceral injuries to ensure adequate healing. There have been studies that address which patients are likely to have visceral trauma without hemoperitoneum. They include patients with hematuria as well as those with lower rib and pelvic ring fractures. For example, Ballard and colleagues noted that 18.5% of patients with pelvic ring fractures had false-negative FAST results (26). Thus, one might follow up a negative FAST outcome with a CT scan in this patient population. However, wishing to miss no injuries and to simplify trauma diagnosis, we perform CT scans on all hemodynamically stable patients requiring abdominal evaluation. We find it disturbing to read studies that promote the use of FAST as a means to diminish the number of CT scans performed in hemodynamically stable patients (27). Why, then, should this patient population undergo FAST at all if both positive and negative studies will be supplemented with a CT scan? First, performing FAST examinations on all injured patients improves examiner comfort level with the technique at no risk to the patient. More importantly, FAST may be effective in the diagnosis of a large hemoperitoneum in the absence of hemodynamic instability that may become clinically significant and necessitate patient resuscitation. It is better to travel to CT scan well prepared in these patients!

Patients with Penetrating Precordial Wounds (Figs. 14 and 15)

The "kill zone" or "box" describes an area bounded by the nipples laterally, sternal notch superiorly and xiphoid inferiorly. Stab wounds to this area or gunshot wounds that traverse this region can potentially violate the heart. FAST is a rapid, accurate method for diagnosing cardiac injury by detecting fluid in the pericardial sac. In a multicenter trial, the mean time from positive ultrasound for penetrating cardiac injury to operation was 12 ± 5 minutes (28). The sensitivity, specificity, and accuracy of FAST approaches 100% for this indication, and thus a positive study in a patient with a penetrating precordial wound should result in sternotomy and repair. Negative studies are also diagnostic with the exception of those involving a concomitant hemothorax into which pericardial blood can theoretically decompress. In these patients and in those with indeterminate studies, a surgical subxiphoid pericardial window should be considered. Blaivas and colleagues also caution that epicardial fat pads may be mistaken for pericardial fluid by an inexperienced examiner and recommend obtaining secondary views to increase accuracy (29). In fact, a second intercostal space transverse view can be obtained (Fig. 16) not only in these patients but in those in whom the traditional view is difficult to obtain (i.e., obese individuals or those with sternal trauma for whom the subxiphoid scanning is too painful) (30).

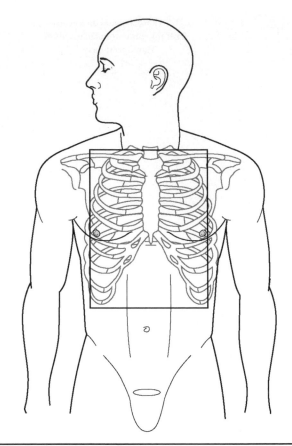

FIGURE 15. Kill zone schematic.

ACCURACY OF FAST

FAST is a rapid, noninvasive screening test of reasonable accuracy. The issue of organ injury without hemoperitoneum has already been addressed. However, interpretation errors may also occur due to improper machine set-

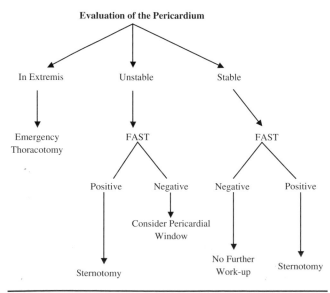

FIGURE 14. Pericardial evaluation algorithm.

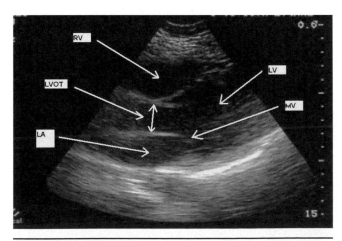

FIGURE 16. Transthoracic view of heart. RV, right ventricle; LA, left atrium; LV, left ventricle; MV, mitral valve; LVOT, left ventricular outflow tract.

▶ **TABLE 2** **Large Ultrasound Series: FAST Accuracy in Fluid Detection in Blunt Abdominal Trauma in the Literature 1992–2001**

Authors	Year	No. of Patients	Sensitivity	Specificity
Tso and colleagues (1)	1992	163	69	99
Bode et al. (72)	1993	353	92.8	100
Rozycki et al. (2)	1993	476	84	95.6
Glaser et al. (73)	1994	1151	99	98
Golletti et al. (74)	1994	250	98	99
McKenney et al. (75)	1994	200	83	100
Ma et al. (34)	1995	245	90	99
Rozycki et al. (16)	1995	371	81.5	99.7
McKenney et al. (4)	1996	1000	88	99
Dolich et al. (31)	2001	2576	86	98

ting, suboptimal image quality, or misinterpretation of structures (i.e., bowel loops, clotted blood, or the bladder). Sensitivity and specificity for various large ultrasound series are reported in Table 2. A current series from Ryder Trauma Center, a facility with nearly a decade's experience in trauma surgeon–performed ultrasound, revealed a sensitivity of FAST for detection of intraabdominal injuries of 86%, a specificity of 98%, and an accuracy of 97% (31).

SCORING SYSTEMS

Two investigators have developed scoring systems to quantitate the amount of hemoperitoneum and estimate the need for operative intervention. Huang and colleagues established a scoring system in an experimental setting with a range of 0 to 8 (32). A patient with a score of 3 or higher, which corresponded to 1 liter or more of hemoperitoneum, had a 96% probability of needing a therapeutic laparotomy compared with 37% for patients with a score of less than 3. McKenney and colleagues have developed a hemoperitoneum score that adds the anterior to posterior depth (in centimeters) of the region containing the largest collection of fluid (e.g., Morison's pouch) to the total additional regions that fluid is found (above and below the liver and spleen and in the pelvis) (33). Eighty-seven percent of patients with an ultrasound score of 3 or higher required therapeutic laparotomy, whereas 85% of those with a score of less than 3 did not. A third investigator has developed a "scoring system" whereby fluid accumulation is rated as small (less than 1.0 cm fluid stripe), moderate (1 to 3.0 cm stripe), or large (more than 3.0 cm stripe). The sensitivity for detecting a large fluid accumulation on FAST in this series was 89%, 100% if accompanied by hemodynamic instability; and 60% for a moderate accumulation; 67% if accompanied by instability (although in our hands hemodynamic

instability with any degree of hemoperitoneum by FAST would likely prompt laparotomy) (34). The simplicity of this system may render it more user friendly. All three scoring systems highlight the fact that hemodynamically stable patients with what we term "ragingly positive" FAST examinations will likely progress to instability and eventually require laparotomy.

CHALLENGES

There are features of the FAST examination that render accurate diagnosis challenging. These are summarized in Table 3. Some patients are difficult to image, including those who are morbidly obese or those with marked amounts of subcutaneous emphysema. As discussed before, intraabdominal injuries may not be associated with free fluid and thus can be missed by FAST or pericardial fluid may have decompressed into a hemothorax. Finally, FAST cannot distinguish fluid of other types (e.g., succus, urine, ascites) from blood. Experienced trauma surgeons have taken patients to the operating room with a "kill

▶ **TABLE 3** **FAST: Challenges to Optimal Use**

Patient factors
1. Body habitus: obese or narrow xiphoid angle
2. Subcutaneous emphysema

Sonographer factors
1. Training level
2. Bowel loops may be mistaken for fluid
3. Artifacts may be misinterpreted

FAST factors
1. Fluid is not necessarily blood
2. Visceral injury may not be associated with blood or fluid collection
3. Hemopericardium may decompress into thorax instead

zone" wound whose pericardial fluid was secondary to a chronic effusion and not blood or whose "hemoperitoneum" was, in fact, longstanding ascites. It is important to consider the setting in which a positive FAST occurs.

SPECIAL USES (TABLE 4)

Pediatrics

Is FAST as valuable a diagnostic examination tool in the pediatric trauma patient as it is in the adult given differences in size, organ structure, and the rate with which hemodynamic instability occurs? Moreover, how common is the use of FAST in the pediatric age population? Several studies have attempted to address this issue (35–40). Baka and colleagues described in a 2002 report that only 14% of pediatric emergency medicine physicians routinely used FAST in the evaluation of injured patients, in comparison with 74% of adult emergency medicine physicians. Ninety-two percent of adult emergency physicians and trauma surgeons felt that FAST was "extremely useful" for assessing adult trauma patients. Seventy-two percent of these physicians held the same opinion for the assessment of the injured pediatric patient by FAST. On the other hand, 57% of pediatric emergency physicians felt that FAST was extremely useful in trauma evaluation. Moreover, of the 39 pediatric trauma centers surveyed where FAST was not available for diagnosis, only 13% planned to institute ultrasound evaluation of injured patients (35). Sensitivity of the FAST examination in the pediatric population for the detection of free fluid has been somewhat lower than that reported in adult studies (83% to 87% for adults versus 71% to 91% for children) as has specificity (97% to 100% for adults ver-

sus 84% to 100% for children) (37). Furthermore, the incidence of intraabdominal injury without free fluid is about the same in children as it is in adults; one study reported a rate of 23% (36). Nonetheless, the most appropriate use of FAST in the pediatric population with the highest accuracy appears to be in the hemodynamically unstable patient (36, 38). Finally, FAST is advantageous in children because it is often better tolerated than abdominal CT scanning with ingestion of contrast and the need to remain still for several minutes.

Pregnancy

FAST may be used to diagnose incidental pregnancy as described in a study by Bochicchio and colleagues (41). FAST was successful in establishing a diagnosis of pregnancy in 8 of 12 patients imaged. Three of the four patients whose pregnancy was not diagnosed had gestation times of less than 8 weeks. Goodwin and associates reported 83% sensitivity and 97% specificity of FAST for detecting fluid in the pregnant trauma population (42). FAST during pregnancy is advantageous because of its lack of ionizing radiation. In addition, a FAST examination can be performed rapidly; the pregnant patient can be transported to the labor and delivery suite where fetal monitoring may be instituted immediately.

Triage

FAST can be used to triage patients to CT scanning or the operating room, and can help the surgeon decide which body cavity to address first in the multiply injured patient. Ultrasound has been successfully used to triage patients injured in the 1988 Armenian earthquake (43). Multiple injured patients arriving simultaneously to the hospital who are hemodynamically stable can be triaged to CT scanning or the operating room based on the amount of free fluid detected on FAST or the hemoperitoneum score. Although not widely used for penetrating injured patients, FAST can be used in this triage scenario. Finally, a penetrating injured patient with wounds of multiple body cavities (e.g., pericardium, thorax, and abdomen) can have these regions assessed by FAST for the presence or absence and the amount of fluid. Comparison of the amount of fluid present in each body cavity can determine which should be entered first in the operating room or if simultaneous approach by multiple teams is necessary.

Prehospital

The miniaturization of ultrasound technology has allowed consideration of use of FAST in the prehospital setting. Hand-held ultrasound units, originally conceived as portable devices that surgeons and veterinarians could

▶ **TABLE 4 Special Uses of FAST or Ultrasound in Trauma**

1. *Pediatric:* FAST used less than for adult, sensitivity and specificity somewhat lower, most useful in the unstable patient, better tolerated than CT
2. *Pregnancy:* FAST can diagnose pregnancy, no ionizing radiation, rapid
3. *Triage:* FAST can be used to triage patients to CT or the operating room, and to determine which body cavity to address first
4. *Prehospital:* potentially able to triage patients to appropriate trauma facilities
5. *Follow-up:* repeat FAST valuable in the inpatient setting if a patient's condition changes
6. *Penetrating torso trauma:* FAST not as accurate as blunt trauma, "positive" for free fluid by FAST indicates the need for exploration, but "negative" does not preclude it
7. *Intraparenchymal injury, diaphragmatic injury, fracture, fascial injury, vascular injury:* ultrasound use limited or need for future studies

transport easily to various offices, have appeared in many trauma resuscitation areas. The 2.4-kg SonoSite unit was compared head to head with a more conventional ultrasound machine and was found to have a FAST sensitivity, specificity, and accuracy of 75%, 98%, and 96% compared with 78%, 100% and 97% for conventional ultrasound (44). A feasibility study performed in-flight on 14 patients revealed that FAST with a portable machine was accomplished easily with no interference by helicopter avionics (45). However, a study published a year later questioned the practicality of helicopter nonphysician trauma teams performing FAST. Nearly half of 71 trauma patients enrolled in the study could not be imaged, mostly due to insufficient time, inadequate patient access, or patient combativeness. Approximately 20% were not imaged due to technical difficulties such as difficult screen visualization caused by ambient lighting, battery failure, and machine malfunction (46). Nonetheless, the concept of prehospital FAST, which might allow triage of patients to appropriate facilities if much free fluid is found or if associated with hemodynamic instability, is a potentially attractive one.

Follow-up Studies

If it is deemed necessary to perform repeat imaging studies of healing liver or splenic injuries, it may be appropriate to use ultrasound to diminish the cost of CT scanning. In our practice, we limit follow-up outpatient imaging to very active patients and athletes in whom we wish to document complete splenic or liver healing prior to return to full activities. In this circumstance, because we wish to provide complete intraparenchymal evaluation, we prefer to use CT scanning rather than ultrasound. On the other hand, repeat FAST evaluation is valuable in the inpatient setting if a previously stable patient becomes unstable or if there is a drop in hematocrit in a patient with a known abdominal injury source. For example, if a patient with a known splenic laceration experiences a drop in hematocrit after an orthopedic procedure, a FAST examination may provide information as to the likely source of blood loss (i.e., intraabdominal versus orthopedic).

Penetrating Torso Trauma

The success of FAST in the rapid and accurate diagnosis of cardiac tamponade has been discussed previously. There are other indications to consider FAST in the evaluation of penetrating torso-injured patients. FAST may be helpful in a multiple penetrating injured patient scenario as occurs not too infrequently in urban trauma centers. FAST will help answer the question "on whom do I operate first?" which may not be readily apparent if patients are not hemodynamically unstable. In addition, in patients with penetrating injuries of multiple body cavi-

ties (thorax, pericardium, and abdomen), the presence or absence of fluid in these regions as indicated by FAST results may determine which areas should be explored first or if simultaneous exploration with multiple teams is necessary. Two research groups reported their experience with FAST in civilian penetrating trauma. Udobi and colleagues from the University of Maryland reported a 46% sensitivity and 94% specificity for FAST in this setting (47). Boulanger and associates at the University of Kentucky at Lexington reported sensitivity and specificity of 67% and 98%, respectively (48). This variability in numbers may reflect a difference in transport time and thus the degree of fluid accumulation or a difference in demographics between the two groups; the Lexington study had a higher proportion of gunshot wound patients. Nonetheless, both highlight that FAST is not as accurate in the evaluation of penetrating injury to the abdomen as it is in blunt trauma. The salient question in patients with penetrating abdominal injury is not "Is there free fluid in the abdomen?" as may be answered by FAST, but rather "Is there visceral injury?" The consequences of missing a small intraparenchymal injury in blunt trauma if one evaluates the abdomen by FAST alone are not as devastating as those of missing a small colonic perforation or blast injury with penetrating trauma assessed by FAST. Most abdominal gunshot wounds should be managed by exploratory laparotomy. Selective management can be considered in the small subset of patients in whom the trajectory can be determined to be clearly extraperitoneal or intrahepatic (49–51). This diagnosis requires CT scanning with careful assessment of the trajectory. FAST probably cannot accomplish this task. On the other hand, victims of stab wounds are more often treated nonoperatively. Once again, CT scanning is successful in appreciating the trajectory in posterior stab wounds and less so in anterior and lateral wounds where laparoscopy may be more helpful (52). In summary, the presence of free fluid by FAST in penetrating abdominal trauma provides a clear indication for laparotomy; however, a "negative" FAST result does not preclude the need for operative exploration.

Intraparenchymal Evaluation

Ultrasound is not routinely used to describe the nature of solid organ injury in its current iteration, although FAST may detect specific organ injures such as liver or splenic injuries. Because of the rapidity and availability of high-speed CT scanning, the need for ultrasound to assume the role of specific organ imaging may be limited.

Diaphragmatic Injury Evaluation

As described previously, the purpose of ultrasound evaluation of the injured patient in earlier series was careful description of actual organ injury, which included diaphragm evaluation (53). Ammann described the first case of ultrasound diagnosis of diaphragm injury in 1983 (8). Other studies document the use of ultrasound for the same reason (53,54). In rare series, ultrasound is the most effective modality in establishing its diagnosis. Nonetheless, the accurate diagnosis of diaphragmatic injury is difficult, and ultrasound should be viewed as one of several modalities available with none ideal (55).

Fracture Evaluation

There are several reported series, mostly in the European literature, of the successful use of ultrasound in the evaluation of fractures of the elbow, shoulder, knee, wrist, mandible, and sternum (56–60). The use of this modality decreases the amount of ionizing radiation needed for the diagnosis of fractures; this is beneficial, particularly in children. Hubner and colleagues noted, "Sonographic assessment of the skeleton requires time, patience and practice. The quality of our results improved with experience. Ultrasound examination may become a satisfactory substitute for radiography in certain well-defined circumstances, thus saving time and money" (56). These statements can certainly apply to the use of ultrasound for any reason.

Fascial Evaluation

Ultrasound may be used to diagnose fascial dehiscence, herniation, and the presence of hematomas or abscesses (61–64).

Vascular Injury Evaluation

The use of ultrasound with high-frequency, high-resolution transducers to diagnose penetrating and blunt vascular injury has been well described. Additional studies are needed to clarify the niche of ultrasound in vascular injury (see "The Future").

TRAINING AND CREDENTIALING

The issue of training and credentialing is further addressed in subsequent chapters. The challenge in attaining proficiency in FAST arises from the fact that the vast majority of study results are negative. In most series, the positive FAST rate is not higher than 10% or 20%. Thus, one's learning curve in terms of the ability to correctly identify a positive result is limited by its relative infrequency and the unfamiliarity of the examiner with recognizing it. There are significant opportunities to gain familiarity with FAST. The American College of Surgeons has taught the technique to surgeons in ultrasound courses since 1996. Presently, instruction in FAST is a key

component of the Acute Setting modular course. This module can be completed after basic competency with and training in ultrasound principles is demonstrated to the College, as can be done by completion of the Basic course. The concept of whether a learning curve exists for the performance of FAST, and if so how steep, is controversial. Thomas and colleagues suggested that the institutional learning curve for FAST appeared to plateau around 100 examinations (65). Shackford and associates suggested that the error rate dropped precipitously after 10 examinations (66). Gracias and Frankel reported that their individual examiner's learning curve, which included surgical trainees and staff, was somewhere between these numbers but could be reduced if exposure to positive studies was included as a part of training. This can be accomplished by utilizing peritoneal dialysis patients to mimic a positive FAST as the American College of Surgeons does for its course (67,68). On the other hand, Smith and colleagues were not able to demonstrate a learning curve among its trainees, nor were McCarter and colleagues for attending trauma surgeons (69,70).

THE FUTURE

Authors of Chapter 21 will discuss new innovations in ultrasound technology. One modality that may someday have utility in the evaluation of injured patients is the use of ultrasound contrast agents such as a galactose-based agent (Levovist). For example, these agents are viewed with

▶ **TABLE 5 Comparison of Ultrasound, Computed Tomography, and Diagnostic Peritoneal Lavage**

Category	US	CT	DPL
Cost	++		+
Integration in resuscitation	++		+
Ease of interpretation	+		++
Ease of repetition	++	+	
Evaluation of pericardium	++	+	
Evaluation of retroperitoneum		++	
Injury localization	+	++	
Patient acceptance	++	+	
Noninvasive	++	++	
Portable	++		+
Radiation exposure	++		++
Rapidity	++		+
Sensitivity	+	++	+
Specificity	+	++	+
Quantitative	+	++	

++ is significant advantage.
CT, computed tomography; DPL, diagnostic peritoneal lavage; US, ultrasound.
From Ng A. www.trauma.org; December 2001.

a wide-band harmonic ultrasound and allow for the visualization not just of free intraperitoneal fluid but of intraparenchymal hematomas as well. Use of wide-band harmonic ultrasound allowed visualization all lesions greater than 1.0 mm in an animal model of renal trauma (71). How this ultrasound technology as well as three-dimensional imaging will fare in comparison with the work being done on portable CT scans in the resuscitation area remains to be seen.

CONCLUSIONS

FAST is a rapid, noninvasive method for evaluating the torso of injured patients. Although it does not provide accurate organ-specific information as does CT, FAST can rapidly exclude life-threatening injury in hemodynamically unstable patients. These features of ultrasound as compared with CT and DPL are highlighted in Table 5.

ACKNOWLEDGMENTS

The authors thank Drs. Chris Moore and S. Jamal Bokhari for their assistance with image acquisition and Mr. John Plessner with manuscript preparation.

REFERENCES

1. Tso P, Rodriguez A, Cooper C, et al. Sonography in blunt abdominal trauma: a preliminary progress report. *J Trauma* 1992;33:39–44.
2. Rozycki GS, Ochsner MG, Jaffin JH, et al. Prospective evaluation of surgeons' use of ultrasound in the evaluation of trauma patients. *J Trauma* 1993;34:516–527.
3. FAST. Consensus Conference Committee. Focused assessment with sonography for trauma (FAST): results from an international consensus conference. *J Trauma* 1999;46:466–472.
4. McKenney MG, Martin L, Lentz K, et al. 1000 consecutive ultrasounds for blunt abdominal trauma. *J Trauma* 1996;40: 607–611.
5. Kimura A, Otsuka T. Emergency center ultrasonography in the evaluation of hemoperitoneum: a prospective study. *J Trauma* 1991;31:20–26.
6. Goldberg BB, Goodman GA, Clearfield HR. Evaluation of ascites by ultrasound. *Radiology* 1970;96:15–22.
7. Goldberg BB, Clearfield HR, Goodman GA. Ultrasonic determination of ascites. *Arch Intern Med* 1973;131:217–221.
8. Ammann A, Brewer WH, Maull KI, et al. Traumatic rupture of the diaphragm: real-time sonographic diagnosis. *Am J Radiol* 1988;140:915–918.
9. Kristensen JK, Buemann B, Kuehl E. Ultrasonic scanning in the diagnosis of splenic hematomas. *Acta Chem Scand* 1971; 137:653–657.
10. Asher WM, Parvin S, Virgilia RW, et al. Echographic evaluation of splenic injury after blunt trauma. *Radiology* 1976; 118:411–417.
11. Chambers JA, Pilbrow WJ. Ultrasound in abdominal trauma: an alternative to peritoneal lavage. *Arch Emerg Med* 1988;5:26–31.
12. Tiling T, Boulton B, Schmid A, et al. Ultrasound in blunt abdomino-thoracic trauma. In: Border JF, et al., eds. *Blunt multiple trauma: comprehensive pathophysiology and care.* New York: Marcel Dekker, 1990:415–430.
13. Hoffman R, Nerlich D, Muggia-Sullam M, et al. Blunt abdominal trauma in cases of multiple trauma evaluated by ultrasonography: a prospective analysis of 291 patients. *J Trauma* 1992;32:452–460.
14. Viscomi GN, Gonzalez R, Taylor KJ, et al. Ultrasonic evaluation of hepatic and splenic trauma. *Arch Surg* 1980;115:320–324.
15. Kohlberger EJ, Strittmatter B, Waninger J. Ultrasound diagnosis following blunt abdominal trauma. Sonography in acute and follow-up diagnosis. *Rev Fortschr Med* 1989;107: 244–260.
16. Rozycki GS, Ochsner MG, Schmidt JA, et al. A prospective study of surgeon-performed ultrasound as the primary adjuvant modality for injured patient assessment. *J Trauma* 1995;39:492–500.
17. Rozycki GS, Oschner MG, Feliciano DV, et al. Early detection of hemoperitoneum by ultrasound examination of the right upper quadrant: a multicenter study. *J Trauma* 1998; 45:557–567.
18. Ma OJ, Kefer MP, Mateer JR, et al. Evaluation of hemoperitoneum using a single-vs. multiple-view ultrasonographic examination. *Acad Emerg Med* 1995;2:581–586.
19. Sisley AC, Rozycki GS, Ballard RB, et al. Rapid detection of traumatic effusion using surgeon-performed ultrasonography. *J Trauma* 1998;44:291–297.
20. Rozycki GS, Pennington SD, Feliciano DV. Surgeon-performed ultrasound in the critical care setting: its use as an extension of the physical examination to detect pleural effusion. *J Trauma* 2001;50:636–642.
21. Dulchavsky SA, Schwarz KL, Kirkpatrick AW, et al. Prospective evaluation of thoracic ultrasound in the detection of pneumothorax. *J Trauma* 2001;50:201–205.
22. Davis JR, Morrison AL, Perkins GE, et al. Ultrasound: impact on diagnostic peritoneal lavage, abdominal computed tomography and resident training. *Am Surg* 1999;65:555–559.
23. Ochsner MG, Knudson MM, Pachter HL, et al. Significance of minimal or no intraperitoneal fluid visible on CT scan associated with blunt liver and splenic injuries: a multicenter analysis. *J Trauma* 2000;49:505–510.
24. Shanmuganathan K, Mirvis SE, Sherbourne CD, et al. Hemoperitoneum as the sole indicator of abdominal visceral injuries: a potential limitation of screening abdominal US for trauma. *Radiology* 1999;212:423–430.
25. Chiu WC, Cushing BM, Rodriguez A, et al. Abdominal injuries without hemoperitoneum: a potential limitation of focused abdominal sonography for trauma (FAST). *J Trauma* 1997;42:617–623.
26. Ballard RD, Rozycki GS, Newman PG, et al. An algorithm to reduce the incidence of false-negative FAST examinations in patients at high risk for occult injury. Focused assessment for the sonographic assessment of the trauma patient. *J Am Coll Surg* 1999;189:145–150.
27. Rose JS, Levitt M, Porter J, et al. Does the presence of ultrasound really affect computed tomographic scan use? A prospective randomized trial of ultrasound in trauma. *J Trauma* 2001;51:545–550.
28. Rozycki GS, Feliciano DV, Ochsner MG, et al. The role of ultrasound in patients with possible penetrating cardiac wounds: a prospective multicenter study. *J Trauma* 1998;46:543–552.
29. Blaivas M, DeBehnke D, Phelan MB. Potential errors in the diagnosis of pericardial effusion on trauma ultrasound for penetrating injuries. *Acad Emerg Med* 2000;7:1261–1266.
30. Carrillo EH, Guinn BJ, Ali AT, et al. Transthoracic ultrasonography is an alternative to subxiphoid ultrasonography for the diagnosis of hemopericardium in penetrating precordial trauma. *Am J Surg* 2000;179:34–36.
31. Dolich MO, McKenney MG, Varela JE, et al. 2,576 ultrasounds for blunt abdominal trauma. *J Trauma* 2001;50:108–112.
32. Huang M, Liu M, Wu J, et al. Ultrasonography for the evaluation of hemoperitoneum during resuscitation: a simple scoring system. *J Trauma* 1994;36:173–177.

33. McKenney KL, McKenney MG, Cohn SM, et al. Hemoperitoneum score helps determine need for therapeutic laparotomy. *J Trauma* 2001;50:650–656.

34. Ma OJ, Mateer JR, Ogata M, et al. Prospective analysis of a rapid trauma ultrasound examination performed by emergency physicians. *J Trauma* 1995;38:879–885.

35. Baka AG, Delgado CA, Simon HK. Current use and perceived utility of ultrasound for evaluation of pediatric compared with adult trauma patients. *Pediatr Emerg Care* 2002; 18:163–167.

36. Holmes JF, Brant WE, Bond WF, et al. Emergency department ultrasonography in the evaluation of hypotensive and normotensive children with blunt abdominal trauma. *J Pediatr Surg* 2001;36:968–973.

37. Yen K, Gorelick MH. Ultrasound applications for the pediatric emergency department: a review of the current literature. *Pediatr Emerg Care* 2002;18:226–234.

38. Patrick DA, Bensard DD, Moore EE, et al. Ultrasound is an effective triage tool to evaluate blunt abdominal trauma in the pediatric population. *J Trauma* 1998;45:57–61.

39. Chambers JA, Ratcliffe JF, Doig CM. Ultrasound in abdominal injury in children. *Injury* 1986;17:399–405.

40. Filiatrault D, Longpre D, Patriquin G, et al. Investigation of childhood blunt abdominal trauma: a practical approach using ultrasound as the initial diagnostic modality. *Pediatr Radiol* 1987;17:373–379.

41. Bochicchio GV, Hahn J, Scalea TM. Surgeon-performed focused assessment with sonography for trauma as an early screening tool for pregnancy after trauma. *J Trauma* 2002; 52:1125–1128.

42. Goodwin H, Holmes JF, Wisner DH. Abdominal ultrasound examination in pregnant blunt trauma patients. *J Trauma* 2001;50:689–694.

43. Sarkisian AE, Khondkarian RA, Amirbekian NM, et al. Sonographic screening of mass casualties for abdominal and renal injuries following the 1988 Armenian earthquake. *J Trauma* 1991;31:247–250.

44. Kirkpatrick AW, Simons RK, Brown R, et al. The hand-held FAST: experience with hand-held trauma sonography in a level-I urban trauma center. *Injury* 2002;33:303–308.

45. Price DD, Wilson SR, Murphy TG. Trauma ultrasound feasibility during helicopter transport. *Air Med J* 2000;19:144–146.

46. Melanson SW, McCarthy J, Stromski CJ, et al. Aeromedical trauma sonography by flight crews with a miniature ultrasound unit. *Prehosp Emerg Care* 2001;5:399–402.

47. Udobi KF, Rodriguez A, Chiu WC, et al. Role of ultrasonography in penetrating abdominal trauma: a prospective clinical study. *J Trauma* 2001;50:475–479.

48. Boulanger BR, Kearney PA, Tsuei B, et al. The routine use of sonography in penetrating torso injury is beneficial. *J Trauma* 2001;51:320–325.

49. Grossman MD, May AK, Schwab CW, et al. Determining anatomic injury with computed tomography in selected torso gunshot wounds. *J Trauma* 1998;45:446–456.

50. Ginzburg E, Carrillo EH, Kopelman T, et al. The role of computed tomography in selective management of gunshot wounds to the abdomen and flank. *J Trauma* 1998;45:1005–1009.

51. Renz BM, Feliciano DV. Gunshot wounds to the right thoracoabdomen: a prospective study of nonoperative management. *J Trauma* 1994;37:737–744.

52. Hallfeldt KK, Trupka AW, Ehard J, et al. Emergency laparoscopy for abdominal stab wounds. *Surg Endosc* 1998; 12:907–910.

53. Fung HM, Vickar DB. Traumatic rupture of the right hemidiaphragm with hepatic herniation. Real-time ultrasound demonstration. *J Ultrasound Med* 1991;10:295–298.

54. Somers JM, Gleeson FV, Flower CD. Rupture of the right hemidiaphragm following blunt trauma: the use of ultrasound in diagnosis. *Clin Radiol* 1990;42:97–101.

55. Guth AA, Pachter HL, Kim U. Pitfalls in the diagnosis of blunt diaphragmatic injury. *Am J Surg* 1995;170:5–9.

56. Hubner U, Schlicht W, Outzen S. Ultrasound in the diagnosis of fracture in children. *J Bone Joint Surg Br* 2000;82:1–7.

57. Martinoli C, Bianchi S, Zamorani MP, et al. Ultrasound of the elbow. *Eur J Ultrasound* 2001;14:21–27.

58. Vocke-Hell AK, Schmid A. Sonographic differentiation of stable and unstable lateral condyle fractures of the humerus in children. *J Pediatr Orthop* 2001:10:138–141.

59. Landes C, Walendzik H, Klein C. Sonography of the temporomandibular joint from 60 examinations and comparison with MRI and axiography. *J Craniomaxillofac Surg* 2000; 28:352–361.

60. Munk B, Bolvig L, Kroner K, et al. Ultrasound for diagnosis of scaphoid fractures. *J Hand Surg Br* 2000;25:369–371.

61. Wiener MD, Bowie JD, Baker ME, et al. Sonography of subfascial hematomas after cesarean delivery. *AJR Am J Roentgenol* 1987;148:907–910.

62. Greenberg RN, Poepsel PR, Reynaud SP, et al. Staphylococcal infection of fascial space diagnosed by ultrasonography. *South Med Assoc J* 1983;76:814–816.

63. Nelson RL, Renigers SA, Nyhus LM, et al. Ultrasonography of the abdominal wall in the diagnosis of spigelian hernia. *Am Surg* 1980;46:373–376.

64. Spangen L. Ultrasound as a diagnostic aid in ventral abdominal hernia. *J Clin Ultrasound* 1975;3:211–213.

65. Thomas B, Falcone RE, Vasquez D, et al. Ultrasound evaluation of blunt abdominal trauma: program implementation, initial experience, and learning curve. *J Trauma* 1997;42: 384–390.

66. Shackford SR, Rogers FB, Osler TM, et al. Focused abdominal sonogram for trauma: the learning curve of nonradiologist clinicians in detecting hemoperitoneum. *J Trauma* 1999; 228:557–567.

67. Gracias VH, Gupta R, Schwab CW, et al. Defining the learning curve for the focused abdominal sonogram for trauma (FAST) examination: implications for credentialing. *Am Surg* 2001;67:364–367.

68. Gracias VH, Frankel H, Gupta R, et al. The role of positive examinations in training for the focused assessment sonogram in trauma (FAST) examination. *Am Surg* 2001;68: 1008–1011.

69. Smith RS, Kern SJ, Fry WR, et al. Institutional learning curve of surgeon-performed trauma ultrasound. *Arch Surg* 1998;133:530–535.

70. McCarter FD, Luchette FA, Molloy M, et al. Institutional and individual learning curves for focused abdominal ultrasound for trauma. *Ann Surg* 2000;231:689–700.

71. Hochmuth A, Fleck M, Hauff P, et al. First experiences in using a new ultrasound mode and ultrasound contrast agent in the diagnosis of blunt renal trauma: a feasibility study in an animal model. *Invest Radiol* 2000;35:205–211.

72. Bode PJ, Niezen RA, vanVugt AB, et al. Abdominal ultrasound as a reliable indicator for conclusive laparotomy in blunt abdominal trauma. *J Trauma* 1993;34:27–31.

73. Glaser K, Tschmelitsch J, Klinger B, et al. Ultrasonography in the management of blunt abdominal and thoracic trauma. *Arch Surg* 1994;129:743–748.

74. Golletti O, Ghiselli G, Lippolis PV, et al. The role of ultrasonography in blunt abdominal trauma: results in 250 consecutive cases. *J Trauma* 1994;36:178–182.

75. McKenney M, Lentz K, Nunez D, et al. Can ultrasound replace DPL in the assessment of blunt trauma? *J Trauma* 1995;38:379–383.

76. Ng A. www.trauma.org; December 2001.

Chapter 10

Ultrasound in the Acute Setting

Amy C. Sisley and James P. Bonar

The surgeon's use of ultrasound (US) in acute settings, such as in the intensive care unit (ICU) and the emergency department (ED), has occurred largely as an outgrowth of the popularity of sonography in evaluating trauma patients (1–3). As surgeons have become more comfortable and competent with sonography, applications of US in acute settings have been extended to include non-trauma patients as well as trauma patients.

The same features that make US a useful adjunct in evaluating acutely injured patients (rapidity, portability, noninvasiveness) apply to the evaluation of critically ill patients (Table 1). An additional quality of this modality that enhances its value to clinicians is that it can be used as both a diagnostic and a therapeutic tool. The consequence has been a proliferation of reports in the surgical literature on the use of US, which addresses a wide range of clinical problems encountered in the acutely ill patient (4–7).

Several characteristics of critically ill patients in the ICU and ED make the inclusion of US in the surgeon's clinical armamentarium particularly useful. Critically ill patients present the challenge of a continuously changing clinical picture in which the ability to frequently reassess the patient's condition is highly advantageous. Moreover, physical examination may be difficult in this patient population due to altered or depressed mental status. Thus, a portable and noninvasive technique such as US provides a means of garnering important clinical information rapidly and repetitively. Also, US enables the clinician to examine both superficial structures, such as soft tissue and superficial vessels, as well as deeper intraperitoneal and intrathoracic structures. Finally, bedside sonography may obviate the necessity of transporting critically ill patients to the radiology suite for evaluation. Such transport requires significant allocation of resources, such as nursing personnel and respiratory therapists, and is not without risk to the patient (8).

EVALUATION OF THE THORAX

In the acute setting, the principal applications of bedside US in the thorax are identification of pleural fluid (hemothorax, effusion, empyema) and air (pneumothorax).

Pleural Effusion

The portable supine chest roentgenogram (CXR) is the most common tool used to evaluate critically ill patients for the presence of pleural fluid. However, the technique for obtaining CXRs is limited because pleural fluid may "layer out" posteriorly making it difficult to detect. Furthermore, obtaining an upright or lateral decubitus chest roentgenogram in the ICU patient may be difficult in the presence of multiple monitoring devices, catheters, and intravenous lines. Gryminski first demonstrated the superiority of US scanning over chest radiography in the detection of pleural fluid (9). The use of US in the routine screening of ICU patients for pleural fluid has been reported to have an overall accuracy of 93.6% (6). Another advantage over chest radiography is that US can be used to guide therapeutic interventions such as thoracentesis. It should be emphasized the US evaluation does not replace chest radiography because it does not detect other important pulmonary pathologic conditions, such as atelectasis, infiltrates, or acute respiratory distress syndrome (ARDS).

Technique for Pleural Effusion

The US examination of the thorax is performed with the patient supine. A 3.5-MHz convex array transducer, oriented for longitudinal (coronal) sections, is placed in the midaxillary line (Table 2). It is generally easiest to start at the 9th or 10th rib, visualize the kidney and liver (or spleen) interface, and then move the transducer slowly cephalad until the diaphragm is seen (Fig. 1). The diaphragm is readily apparent as a strongly echogenic (white) curved band which moves in concert with the patient's breathing. In the absence of pleural fluid, the lung is poorly visualized because air-filled structures, such as alveoli, do not transmit US well (Fig. 2). Hence, when visualizing the supradiaphragmatic space, the normal lung appears as an indistinct gray shadow. However, when pleural

▶ **TABLE 1** **Advantages of Ultrasound in the**
Intensive Care and Emergency Setting

1. No patient transportation is needed; ultrasound is portable.
2. Examinations are easily repeated; can reassess patients frequently.
3. Ultrasound can be both diagnostic and therapeutic.
4. Ultrasound can be used to evaluate both superficial soft tissues and deeper intraperitoneal and intrathoracic structures.

fluid is present, it is readily identifiable as an anechoic (black) collection superior to the diaphragm (Fig. 3).

Intervention (US-Guided Thoracentesis)

When thoracentesis is indicated, US may be used to guide drainage of the pleural cavity (Table 3). If the patient's condition permits, the head of the bed is elevated to 45 degrees. Alternatively, the bed may be placed in the reverse Trendelenburg position. The pleural fluid collection is identified as previously described. Generally, the indirect US guidance method can be performed for thoracentesis (see Chapter 4 for details). The skin where the needle puncture will be performed is marked with a pen, and the direction and angle of needle insertion are determined. The chest wall is prepared and draped sterilely, and the skin and subcutaneous tissues are infiltrated with a local anesthetic. Aspiration of a small fluid collection or sampling for Gram stain and culture is accomplished with an 18-gauge needle or angiocatheter and syringe. Larger fluid collections may be drained with a standard thoracentesis kit or with a central line kit. As the 18-gauge needle is inserted into the pleural space, correct positioning is confirmed by the aspiration of fluid. A guidewire is subsequently passed through the needle into the pleural space. A stiff dilator is passed over the guidewire. The dilator should not be passed completely into the pleural cavity as it may increase the risk of iatrogenic pneumothorax. A standard central line catheter is the passed over the guidewire into the pleural cavity. This is followed by aspiration of the fluid using a syringe and collection bag attached to the catheter by means of a three-way stopcock. Complete aspiration of the fluid is confirmed using US. Lastly, the catheter is withdrawn while the clinician places continuous negative

▶ **TABLE 2** **Ultrasound Evaluation**
of Pleural Effusions

1. Use a 3.5-MHz convex array transducer.
2. Place transducer in the midaxillary line at 9th or 10th rib and move cephalad.
3. Diaphragm appears as a strongly echogenic (white) curved line.
4. Pleural fluid appears as an anechoic (black) collection.

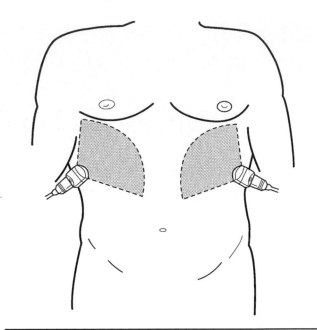

FIGURE 1. Transducer position for the evaluation of the chest for pleural effusion.

suction on the attached syringe. Alternatively, the entire thoracentesis may be viewed in real-time using US (direct US guidance method). While not usually necessary for the evacuation of simple effusions, real-time US visualization and guidance is desirable in situations where the fluid is loculated, the amount of fluid is relatively small, or when attempting to place a drain in a collection surrounded by a thick fibrous peel often present in empyema. When performing a thoracentesis using real-time US guidance, the US transducer should be prepared in a sterile manner (see Chapter 4); for example, it is placed inside a sterile sleeve or a sterile glove.

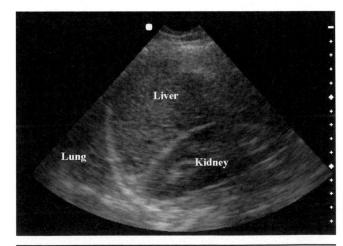

FIGURE 2. Longitudinal view of the normal right hemithorax. Note the hyperechoic diaphragm between the liver and lung.

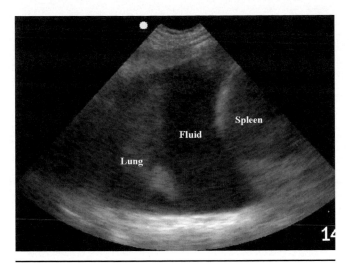

FIGURE 3. Longitudinal view of the left hemithorax demonstrating pleural fluid.

Pneumothorax

While pneumothorax is commonly associated with chest trauma, it can also occur spontaneously, as a consequence of barotrauma in mechanically ventilated patients, or as a complication of biopsy, thoracentesis, or central line placement. As a result of the high acoustic impedance of air-filled structures such as alveoli, US does not transmit well through lung tissue (10). In fact, until recently the use of US to detect intrapleural pathologic processes was very limited. The use of US to detect a pneumothorax was first reported in a horse in 1986 in the veterinary literature (11). Subsequently, US detection of a pneumothorax in humans has been widely reported (12–17). A recent prospective evaluation of the detection of a pneumothorax by US showed a sensitivity of 95% and a specificity of 100% (15). In the acute setting, prompt diagnosis or exclusion of pneumothorax with a bedside US is valuable, particularly when the patient's respiratory condition changes suddenly. The detection of a pneumothorax by US has been described as "paradoxical" in that a pneumothorax is not visualized on US; rather it is excluded (Table 4). As such, the exclusion of a pneumothorax is based on visualizing normal artifacts

TABLE 3 Ultrasound-Guided Thoracentesis and Drainage of Pleural Fluid

1. Elevate head of bed 45 degrees or use reverse Trendelenberg position.
2. Generally, indirect ultrasound guidance method can be used.
3. Use 18-gauge needle or larger.
4. If using Seldinger technique, do not pass the dilator completely into the pleural cavity (increased risk for iatrogenic pneumothorax).

TABLE 4 Ultrasound Evaluation of Pneumothorax

1. Use a 7.5-MHz transducer.
2. Ultrasound detection of pneumothorax is "paradoxical."
3. Pneumothorax is not visualized with ultrasound; it is excluded.
4. Pneumothorax is present when there is absence of two artifacts.
5. Sliding lung is absent in pneumothorax.
6. Comet tail artifact is absent in pneumothorax.

that occur *only* when the lung–chest wall interface is intact. In essence, sonographic evidence of a pneumothorax is based on the *absence* of two artifacts: lung sliding and the comet tail artifact (16). During US evaluation of the normal thorax, the lung–chest wall interface is seen as an echogenic band called the pleural line (Fig. 4). Lung sliding refers to the "to and fro" sliding motion of the pleural line in concert with the patient's respiration (15, 16,18). Lung sliding is noticeably absent when a pneumothorax is present. Furthermore, the comet tail, a reverberation artifact, occurs just distal to a strong reflector and appears as a dense, raylike trail of echoes (see Figure 11 in Chapter 9) (19). In the normal lung, the comet tail artifact is a consequence of an acoustic impedance mismatch between the lung and the intact pleura. The absence of the comet tail is sonographic evidence for the presence of a pneumothorax.

Technique for Pneumothorax

The US examination is performed with the patient supine. Acoustic coupling gel is placed across the anterior chest wall in the 3rd or 4th intercostal space. A 7.5-MHz linear array transducer, oriented for longitudinal (sagittal) sections, is placed on the chest wall. If only one

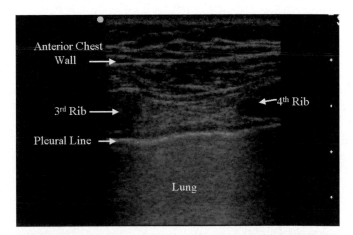

FIGURE 4. Longitudinal view of the anterior chest wall demonstrating the pleural line. In a normal lung, the hyperechoic pleural line moves to and fro in concert with the respiratory cycle (lung sliding). The absence of lung sliding implies pneumothorax.

side of the chest cavity is suspected of having pathology, the unaffected hemithorax should be examined first to establish a baseline. The pleural line is identified as a straight hyperechoic band lying between and slightly deep to the rib shadows. The pleural line is observed over several respirations for evidence of lung sliding in concert with the breathing cycle and for comet tail artifact. The examination is then repeated on the opposite hemithorax.

EVALUATION OF THE ABDOMEN

The surgeon is frequently called on to assess patients in the ICU and ED who present with signs or symptoms of an intraabdominal pathologic process. These patients may be evaluated with a thorough history and physical examination followed by sensitive diagnostic tests, such as computerized axial tomography (CT), in order to delineate the precise nature and extent of their disease. However, in acutely ill patients, altered sensorium with depressed mental status may significantly hamper the physician's ability to obtain a reliable history or physical examination. In addition, the patient may be too unstable hemodynamically to undergo transport to the radiology suite for evaluation. In this clinical scenario, the surgeon's ability to use US to evaluate the abdominal cavity is of paramount importance. US provides a rapid and reliable means of assessing a patient with unexplained hypotension (Table 5). Emergent clinical entities, which may be assessed with US, include intraabdominal bleeding (postoperative), perforated viscus with peritonitis and septic shock, or rupturing abdominal aortic aneurysm (AAA). Furthermore, bedside abdominal US is useful in evaluating patients with acute or chronic ascites who develop peritonitis or those in whom abdominal compartment syndrome (ACS) is suspected.

Intraabdominal Bleeding

In any postoperative patient with hypotension, oliguria, persistent tachycardia, or ongoing intravenous fluid requirements, the diagnosis of postoperative bleeding must

▶ **TABLE 5   Role of Abdominal Ultrasound in Unexplained Hypotension**

1. FAST examination for intraabdominal bleeding (postoperatively)
2. Evaluation for fluid and pneumoperitoneum when perforated viscus is suspected
3. Evaluation for abdominal aortic aneurysm if rupture suspected
4. Confirming significant ascites fluid when abdominal compartment syndrome is suspected

▶ **TABLE 6   Ultrasound Evaluation of Intraabdominal Bleeding or Fluid**

1. Identical to the FAST examination for evaluation of trauma patients.
2. Use a 3.5-MHz convex array transducer.
3. Start with a longitudinal (sagittal) view of the subxiphoid region to visualize the cardiac–hepatic interface; use this view to set the overall gain.
4. Obtain longitudinal views of the hepatorenal fossa and right subdiaphragmatic space.
5. Obtain longitudinal views of the splenorenal fossa and left subdiaphragmatic space.
6. Obtain a transverse view over the bladder to assess for pelvic fluid.

be entertained. US has been clearly shown to be a sensitive diagnostic modality in the detection of hemoperitoneum (1,2,20). Abdominal US, due to the portability of equipment, can be readily performed in the recovery room or the ICU at the first sign of hemodynamic compromise. On average, the US examination takes only 2 to 3 minutes to complete, and the results are available immediately. US provides a means of early detection of postoperative bleeding, enabling timely return to the operating room, which may result in decreased morbidity and mortality.

Technique for Intraabdominal Bleeding

The examination of the abdomen for hemoperitoneum was initially developed for patients with suspected abdominal trauma and is known as focused assessment with sonography for trauma (FAST) (Table 6) (21). The FAST examination is a survey of the dependent regions of the abdominal cavity and pericardium for fluid. It is performed with the patient supine using a 3.5-MHz convex array transducer. Acoustic coupling gel is placed in the subxiphoid region, the right and left upper quadrants, and the suprapubic region. The transducer is first placed in the subxiphoid region, oriented for longitudinal (sagittal) sections, to allow visualization of the heart and the interface of the liver with the diaphragm and pericardium. In trauma patients, this view is obtained to detect pericardial effusion. Although this may not be a consideration in the evaluation of postoperative bleeding, the pericardial view also serves the important function of providing a structure known to be fluid filled (the heart) so that the overall gain may be correctly set on the US machine. An alternative would be to image a full bladder first in order to adjust the gain. Next, the transducer is placed in the right midaxillary line at approximately the 10th rib space to image the longitudinal section of the he-

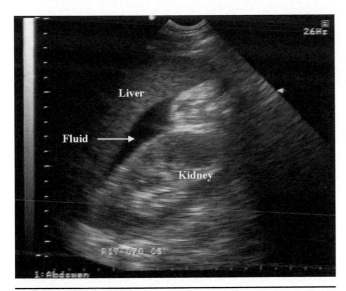

FIGURE 5. Longitudinal view of the right upper quadrant demonstrating fluid in Morison's pouch between the liver and the right kidney.

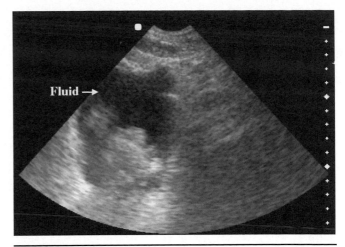

FIGURE 6. Subhepatic fluid collection in a patient with sepsis. The fluid is heterogeneous, suggestive of early abscess formation.

patorenal fossa and is then angled cephalad to view the right subdiaphragmatic space. A similar technique is used on the left side to view the splenorenal fossa and left subdiaphragmatic space. The positioning of the transducer is slightly more cephalad and more posterior on the left. The final view is obtained by orienting the transducer for transverse sections over the bladder. The transducer is positioned slightly superior to the symphysis pubis to image the bladder and pouch of Douglas. Intraabdominal fluid in the right upper quadrant is shown in Figure 5.

Intraabdominal Sepsis

In patients presenting with signs and symptoms of sepsis, an intraabdominal disorder is frequently part of the differential diagnosis. However, the evaluation of patients with an altered sensorium or hemodynamic instability is complicated by an inability to obtain a reliable history and physical examination. US is useful in this situation as an extension of the physical examination, enabling the surgeon to detect free fluid and, in some instances, free air within the patients abdomen (22,23). The dependent regions of the abdomen, as well as the epigastrium, are surveyed for free fluid and bowel edema—both indirect signs of peritonitis (Fig. 6). Recent reports indicate US may be useful for evaluating the abdomen for pneumoperitoneum (7,24). In this situation, US is used to evaluate the epigastrium and right upper quadrant for reverberation artifacts (such as comet tails), which are caused by free air.

Technique for Intraabdominal Sepsis

The US examination for peritonitis is similar to the FAST examination described previously, which surveys the dependent portions of the abdomen for fluid. Evaluation of the right upper quadrant is modified to include US examination of the subhepatic and epigastric regions by sweeping the 3.5-MHz transducer medially. Fluid from a perforated viscus, which can occur in the absence of free air, may collect in these areas. In addition, edema of the bowel wall may be noted. Free fluid and bowel wall thickening constitute *indirect* signs of perforated viscus. Clearly, a *direct* sign of a perforated viscus is pneumoperitoneum. US examination for free air is performed with the head of the bed elevated. With the transducer oriented for longitudinal (sagittal) sections, the epigastrium and right paramedian region of the abdomen are evaluated for a hyperechoic line just under the abdominal wall, associated with reverberation artifacts (see Figure 14 in Chapter 12). The patient is then placed in the left lateral decubitus position and the right upper quadrant examined again for sonographic signs of free intraperitoneal air.

Ascites

The surgeon may be called on to evaluate patients with ascites, often for concern of infection, as in subacute bacterial peritonitis, or because the volume of ascites has resulted in respiratory compromise. US is much more sensitive in detecting intraperitoneal fluid than physical examination, especially when the fluid volume is small. US is also useful to guide paracentesis, which may be warranted either to obtain a sample of ascitic fluid for

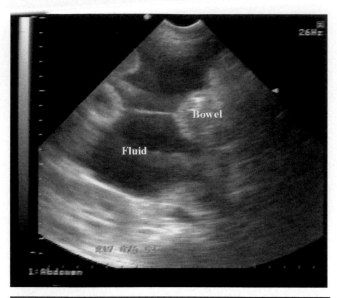

FIGURE 7. Ultrasound image of the midabdomen of a patient with ascites. Loops of bowel, normally obscured by air artifact, are seen clearly.

gram stain and culture, or to reduce the volume of intraperitoneal fluid.

Technique for Detecting Ascites

The examination of the abdomen for ascites is identical to the FAST examination with the addition of an attempt to examine the midabdomen. This is accomplished by sweeping the transducer from the lateral to medial. While the presence of bowel gas can obscure US examination of the midabdomen, the presence of ascitic fluid may provide an acoustic window (Fig. 7). This acoustic window enables the US evaluation of the midabdomen for debris, loculations, bowel thickening, or bowel motility.

Intervention (US-Guided Paracentesis)

Paracentesis is generally performed with the patient supine, although in cases of small fluid volume it may be necessary to place the patient in the right or left lateral decubitus position. As with US-guided thoracentesis, paracentesis can be performed using the indirect US guidance method (see Chapter 4). A "pocket" of fluid is identified using US and the skin is marked with a pen. The area is then prepared and draped sterilely and the skin infiltrated with a local anesthetic. The aspirating needle should be chosen such that it is long enough to penetrate the patient's abdominal wall and reach the fluid collection. This is accomplished by using US to measure the distance from the skin surface to the center of the fluid collection.

A small-bore (22-gauge) aspiration needle or angiocatheter is used if possible. In cases where fluid volume or density requires a larger bore needle or angiocatheter, an 18- or 20-gauge needle may be employed. It should be noted that bowel injury could result from perforation when 18-gauge or larger needles are used.

The aspirating needle is advanced through the abdominal wall while the clinician applies negative suction with a syringe until fluid is encountered. If necessary, the entire paracentesis may be performed under real-time US guidance (directed US guidance method). This is often desirable when the fluid is loculated or if the volume of fluid is small. The US transducer is placed in a sterile sleeve or glove and placed just lateral to the intended aspiration site. The aspirating needle is directed into the abdomen beginning at the edge of the transducer. The needle is readily visualized as a hyperechoic line on the US image as it is guided into the fluid collection. The direct US guidance method is slightly cumbersome because of the need for US transducer preparations; however, this technique can minimize the risk of missed fluid or bowel injury.

Abdominal Compartment Syndrome

ACS is characterized by an increase in intraabdominal pressure resulting in compromise to both renal and respiratory function. The diagnosis can be made clinically based on a distended, tense abdomen with decreasing urine output in conjunction with respiratory compromise and increased central venous pressure. Respiratory compromise occurs as a consequence of decreased lung compliance and may be manifested as tachypnea with shallow breaths or as increasing peak airway pressures in mechanically ventilated patients. Intraabdominal pressure can be measured indirectly by transducing a bladder pressure via a Foley catheter. Generally bladder pressures exceeding 25 mm Hg are considered indicative of ACS (25). Patients with a sudden increase in ascites may also manifest ACS, but it is more commonly seen in patients undergoing large fluid volume resuscitation for shock or sepsis. The treatment for ACS is decompression of the abdomen. Although surgical decompression by wide laparotomy is effective, it is not without problems. The open abdomen created by such a procedure results in both large-volume losses and a wound, which is prone to complications such as bowel fistulization. The increased abdominal pressure causing ACS is a consequence of edema of the tissues (principally bowel wall and mesentery), as is the accumulation of free fluid. The relative contribution of these two factors to abdominal hypertension varies among patients; this can be assessed by US. In patients with a large volume of free fluid associated with

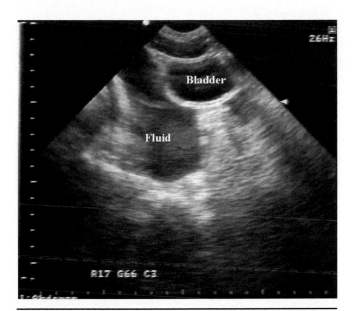

FIGURE 8. FAST examination, pelvic view to evaluate a patient with abdominal compartment syndrome. A large volume of fluid is evident; paracentesis may reduce intraabdominal pressure in such cases.

ACS (Fig. 8), it is possible to decompress the abdomen by draining the fluid by US-guided paracentesis (26). The appeal of this approach is that it avoids the complications associated with decompressive laparotomy and a subsequent open abdomen. Caution must be exercised to ensure that the abdominal decompression is adequate since repeated paracentesis is often required.

Technique for Abdominal Compartment Syndrome

In the patient with ACS, a 3.5-MHz transducer is used to perform the modified FAST examination as previously described for the evaluation of intraabdominal sepsis. If a small amount of fluid is present, paracentesis is unlikely to result in adequate decompression and laparotomy should be performed. If a moderate to large volume of fluid is detected, paracentesis may be effective in reducing intraabdominal pressure. The US-guided procedure is identical to that for paracentesis described for chronic ascites above. Bladder pressures as well as central venous pressure, urine output, and peak airway pressures should be monitored continuously to ensure adequate decompression. It is important to monitor the patient closely in order to anticipate a recurrence of ACS. If the clinical picture deteriorates or the measured bladder pressure begins to rise, repeat US examination, followed by US-guided paracentesis or decompressive laparotomy, should be performed.

Abdominal Aortic Aneurysm

In patients with unexplained abdominal pain, the diagnosis of AAA should be entertained. Unfortunately, physical examination alone has a low sensitivity (50% to 65%) for detecting AAA (27). In cases of rupturing AAA, patients are often too unstable to be transported for evaluation by CT scanning. With bedside US, the surgeon can rapidly evaluate the patient for the presence of AAA and determine whether intraperitoneal rupture has occurred. The sensitivity of US in detecting AAA is close to 100%, and it is as accurate as CT in determining aneurysm size (28–30).

Technique for Abdominal Aortic Aneurysm

The examination is performed with a 3.5-MHz convex transducer and the patient supine. When bowel gas interferes with the examination, a nasogastric tube should be placed in patients with unprepared bowel. The pertinent surface landmarks are the subxiphoid space, where the examination is begun, and the umbilicus, which marks the aortic bifurcation. The transducer is oriented for transverse sections, placed in the subxiphoid space, and the aorta identified. The transducer is then swept slowly toward the umbilicus. Aortic measurements are obtained just above and just below the takeoff of the renal arteries. The transducer is oriented for longitudinal sections and an anteroposterior (AP) measurement obtained. The normal aorta is 3 cm or less in the AP view. In a patient with an aneurysm, the aorta should be evaluated for the extent of dilation, the presence of mural thrombus (Fig. 9), and

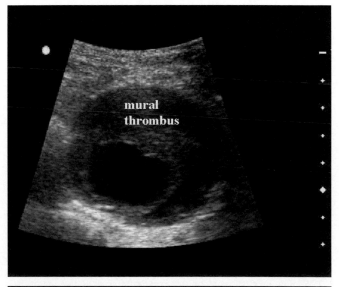

FIGURE 9. Transverse view of abdominal aortic aneurysm with mural thrombus. (Courtesy of SonoSite.)

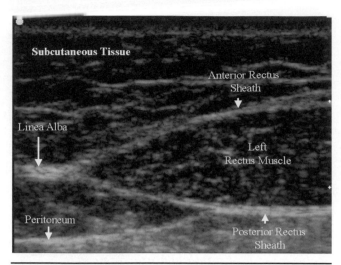

FIGURE 10. Transverse view of the normal anterior abdominal wall obtained with a 7.5-MHz transducer. Tissue and fascial planes are clearly delineated.

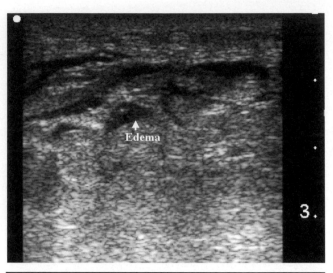

FIGURE 11. Cellulitis characterized by diffuse edema (hypoechoic, mixed echo pattern) in the subcutaneous tissues.

signs of rupture. Rupture of an AAA into the retroperitoneal space may not be evident on US; however, free rupture in the intraperitoneal cavity will be readily detected with the FAST examination.

EVALUATION OF SOFT TISSUE

Visual inspection and palpation may not accurately reflect the extent, character, or depth of soft-tissue pathology. US is an extremely useful adjunct to the physical examination of the soft tissues. Subcutaneous fat, muscle, and fascia are clearly delineated by US, enabling the clinician to determine the precise location of a fluid collection or foreign body (Fig. 10). In addition to detection of soft-tissue pathology, US can guide interventions including aspiration of fluid collections, while also ensuring accurate and complete drainage. The principal applications of US in the evaluation of soft-tissue pathology are (a) assessment of soft tissue infections (cellulitis, abscess, necrotizing fasciitis), (b) evaluation of surgical incisions (wound infection, fascial dehiscence), and (c) detection of foreign bodies (Table 7).

Soft-Tissue Infections

The extent, depth, and character of soft-tissue infections can be assessed at the bedside with US. Appropriate interventions, such as antibiotics, needle aspiration, incision and drainage, or more extensive debridements, can be determined. The signs and symptoms of soft-tissue infection such as warmth, redness, and tenderness to palpation are used to guide the US examination, which can provide more detailed information about the exact nature of the pathologic process. Cellulitis appears on US images as a diffusely edematous process, which is limited to the subcutaneous tissues above the muscle (Fig. 11). Extension of this process into the underlying muscle defines myositis (Fig. 12), whereas extension along fascial planes accompanied by the presence of air in the tissues indicates the far more serious necrotizing fasciitis (Fig. 13). A soft-tissue fluid collection can be readily identified as an anechoic region, which usually has some internal echoes reflecting the heterogeneous character of most abscesses (Fig. 14). The depth of the collection relative to the subcutaneous fat and underlying muscles should be carefully delineated, as this is helpful in guiding therapeutic interventions.

Technique for Soft-Tissue Infections

Examination of the soft tissues is performed with a 7.5-MHz linear transducer oriented alternately in transverse and longitudinal planes. Prior to examining the area of suspected pathology, the transducer should be placed on the patients skin in an area remote from, but similar to, the site of the infection. For example, if the area to be examined is the left thigh, place the probe on the right thigh

▶ **TABLE 7 Role of Ultrasound
in Soft-Tissue Pathology**

1. Assessment of soft tissue infections: differentiating cellulitis, abscess, and necrotizing fasciitis. Guidance of fluid aspiration
2. Evaluation of surgical incisions for infection or dehiscence
3. Detection and removal of foreign bodies

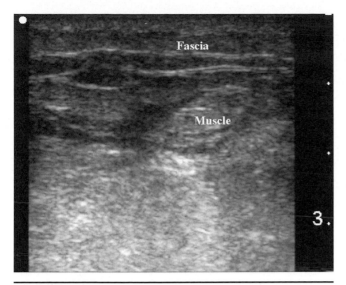

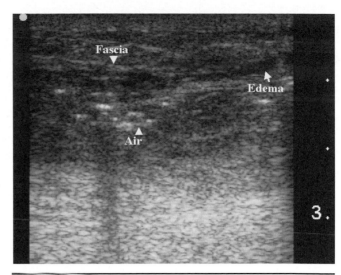

FIGURE 12. Myositis characterized by soft-tissue edema extending deep to the fascia and into the underlying muscle.

FIGURE 13. Necrotizing fasciitis characterized by diffuse edema extending across tissue planes, fluid along fascial borders, and evidence of air in the tissue.

first. This is done because it enables the patient to get used to the feeling of the acoustic coupling gel and the pressure of the transducer (which should be minimal) in an area that is not tender. It also enables the examiner to obtain a baseline "normal" examination of the individual patient in terms of the depth of the subcutaneous tissue and the thickness of the muscle. The US depth should be adjusted and the near and far gain (time gain compensation) and focus set during this portion of the examina-

tion. Acoustic coupling gel is then placed at the site of concern and the probe oriented transversely. The examination should begin at the outer edge of the inflamed area and proceed toward the center, scanning in alternating transverse and longitudinal planes. The sonographer should note the edema in the tissue and its depth relative to the normal soft-tissue architecture. Once the fluid collection is encountered, the size, depth, and character of the fluid should be noted and a decision made as to

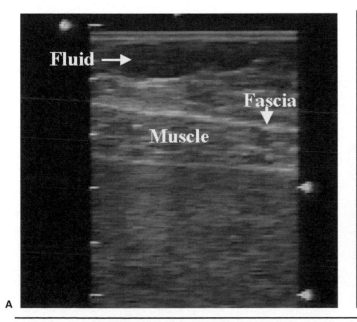

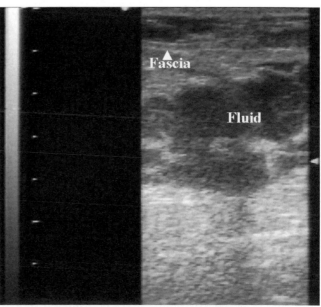

A

B

FIGURE 14. **A:** Fluid collection lying just under the skin. The fluid is relatively homogeneous with few internal echoes. **B:** Heterogeneous fluid collection lying deep to the fascia with overlying edema in the subcutaneous tissues.

▶ TABLE 8 Ultrasound Evaluation of Soft-Tissue Infections

1. Use 7.5-MHz linear array transducer.
2. Measure depth; select long enough aspiration needle.
3. If aspiration unsuccessful, flush needle with 1–2 mL sterile water to clear debris.
4. Cellulitis: uniformly edematous in subcutaneous tissues.
5. Myositis: edema extends into underlying muscle.
6. Necrotizing fasciitis: edema along fascial planes with presence of air.
7. Soft tissue fluid collections: anechoic (black).
8. Abscess: generally anechoic with internal echoes reflecting heterogeneity of most abscesses.

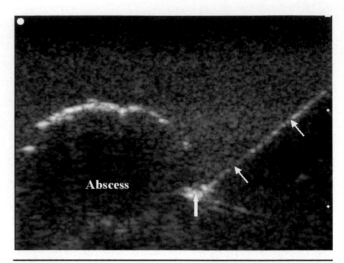

FIGURE 15. Ultrasound-guided needle aspiration of a small abscess. The needle (*thin arrows*) is visible as a strongly echogenic line. The needle tip (*bold arrow*) is at the edge of the abscess.

whether the collection is amenable to percutaneous needle aspiration or if open drainage will be required.

Intervention (US-Guided Aspiration)

A 7.5-MHz transducer is placed over the fluid collection (Table 8). The distance from the surface of the skin at the intended puncture site to the center of the fluid collection is measured. This ensures that the selected aspiration needle is long enough to reach the fluid collection. The character of the fluid may also influence the choice of aspiration needles. Fluid collections with many internal echoes or with loculations are best approached with large-bore aspiration needles (defined as equal to or larger than 18 gauge). An 18-gauge angiocatheter or the 18-gauge needle from a standard central line kit may be used provided it is of sufficient length. The skin is prepared and draped sterilely. The US transducer is prepared in a sterile fashion and held in the nondominant hand. The appropriate skin puncture site is identified and infiltrated with local anesthetic. The aspiration needle, connected to a syringe, is held in the dominant hand and passed into the subcutaneous tissues under direct US guidance until the brightly echogenic line representing the needle echo is visualized (Fig. 15). Failure to see the needle indicates that it is not in the scanning plane. The transducer may be tilted or slid slightly to acquire the needle echo as long as the fluid collection remains in the scanning plane. If the needle is away from the scanning plane demonstrating the fluid, it is pulled back and reinserted appropriately. Once the needle is identified in the correct scanning plane, it is advanced through the tissue until the fluid collection is entered. Suction is then applied via the syringe to aspirate fluid. Loculated fluid collections may require multiple passes of the needle to obtain complete drainage. On occasion, aspiration is unsuccessful despite clear visualization of the needle in the target. This usually occurs when the needle tip is clogged with debris. Instillation of 1 to 2

mL of sterile water or saline via a 3-mL syringe will clear the needle tip.

Evaluation of Surgical Incisions

Postoperative wound complications can be readily evaluated with US. Since US allows both detection and characterization of subcutaneous tissue edema and fluid collections, cellulitis can easily be differentiated from fluid or abscess. This is an important consideration when deciding whether or not to open a surgical incision. Furthermore, wound hematomas and seromas can also be identified using this technique. In conjunction with clinical data such as the white blood cell count and temperature curves, US can guide decision making regarding appropriate treatment. In addition to identifying fluid collections, the capacity of US to precisely delineate tissue planes facilitates the early detection of fascial dehiscence, which may occur while the overlying skin is still intact.

Technique for Surgical Incisions

A 7.5-MHz linear transducer is employed to interrogate the subcutaneous tissues in the region of the incision (Table 9). As with other soft-tissue examinations, the transducer is initially placed a short distance from the affected area. This is done to increase patient comfort with the procedure, as well as to establish a baseline of "normal" for the individual patient. The transducer is then positioned over the incision in the transverse orientation and moved gently along the length of the entire wound. The use of sterile acoustic coupling gel (or K-Y jelly) is

▶ **TABLE 9** **Ultrasound Evaluation of Surgical Incisions and Fascial Dehiscence**

1. Use 7.5-MHz linear array transducer.
2. Initially, start "away" from suspected area to establish "normal" appearance.
3. Examine in both transverse and longitudinal planes.
4. Intact fascia appears as strongly echogenic (white) line.
5. Breaks in fascia indicate dihiscence.

recommended, particularly for relatively fresh postoperative wounds, to avoid any possibility of wound contamination. Povidone-iodine (Betadine) solution can also be used for acoustic coupling for scanning of a short period. Alternatively, it may be convenient to orient the transducer longitudinally and place it at the side of the incision. Angling or tilting the transducer slightly will enable visualization of the tissue directly under the incision. This technique is particularly useful when the wound is very tender or when surgical staples are still in place. The tissues underlying the wound should be evaluated for the presence of tissue edema and fluid collections. Intact fascia appears as a strongly echogenic (white) line; on the other hand, breaks in the fascia are indicative of fascial dehiscence (Fig. 16).

Detection of Foreign Bodies

The detection of foreign bodies embedded in soft tissue is a commonly encountered problem in the ED. Even when history and clinical examination are strongly suspicious for the presence of a foreign body, precise localization

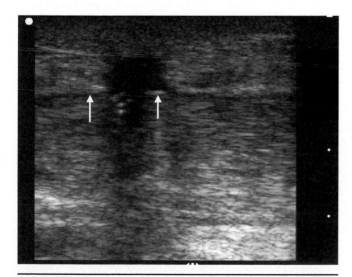

FIGURE 16. Postoperative evaluation of an incision revealing a "gap" (*between arrows*) in the fascia, indicating early wound dehiscence. The overlying skin and soft tissue are still intact.

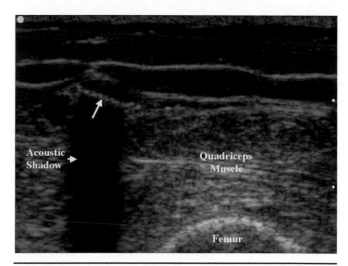

FIGURE 17. Foreign body (wooden splinter) penetrating the thigh muscle. The splinter is strongly hyperechoic with prominent posterior acoustic shadowing. These are sonographic characteristics of many foreign bodies, including wood and plastic.

necessary for removal may be difficult (31). Plastic and wooden foreign bodies are frequently radiolucent, limiting the effectiveness of radiography (32). Fortunately, most foreign bodies, including radiolucent objects, are strongly hyperechoic, enabling the US examination of the soft tissue to detect their presence (33). US is then used to assist or guide extraction of foreign bodies.

Technique for Foreign Bodies

A 7.5-MHz linear transducer is used in both transverse and longitudinal orientations to examine the affected area as identified by history and clinical examination. Acoustic coupling gel is applied and the transducer is swept slowly across the region. If the foreign body has prompted local tissue inflammation, the accompanying tissue edema should be identified with US and provides additional guidance to localization. A foreign body will appear on an US image as a strongly hyperechoic structure with posterior acoustic shadowing (Fig. 17). The size of the foreign body, its depth within the tissues, and the point at which it is closest to the surface of the skin should all be delineated to facilitate extraction. If the foreign body is close to the surface of the skin, it is usually extracted by simply marking the location on the skin and removing it with tweezers. Extraction of foreign bodies, which are deeply embedded in tissue, is facilitated by the real-time direct US guidance method. The transducer is held in the nondominant hand while the dominant hand manipulates the extraction instrument. At times, particularly when a foreign body is small or thin, the use of an exploratory needle is helpful. Under US guidance, a needle is inserted until it

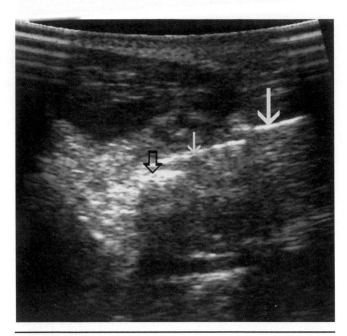

FIGURE 18. Foreign body (15-mm-thin sewing needle) in the soft tissue of the palm. A hyperechoic needle (*short white arrow*) was localized adjacent to the metacarpal bone (*black arrow*) by ultrasound. An exploratory needle (25-gauge spinal needle, *long white arrow*) was inserted toward the foreign body under ultrasound guidance. A 1-cm skin incision was made along the exploratory needle and the foreign body needle was removed.

reaches the foreign body (Fig. 18). The skin and subcutaneous tissues are incised along the needle to facilitate detection and extraction of the foreign body.

SUMMARY

The use of ultrasonography in the acute setting has become extremely valuable as both a diagnostic and therapeutic tool in the surgeon's armamentarium. The portability, rapidity, and noninvasive nature of this technology allows for timely evaluation and often reevaluation of critically ill patients, especially when transport to the radiology suite would place the patient at risk. In the thorax, US has proven to be highly sensitive in the diagnosis of pneumothorax and pleural fluid. In addition, US evaluation of the abdomen in acutely ill patients, who may have an altered sensorium or be hemodynamically unstable, can be of key importance in the rapid diagnosis of emergent clinical entities such as postoperative bleeding, rupturing AAA, or the detection of free air associated with perforated viscus or intraabdominal fluid collection. Finally, the use of US to aid in the diagnosis and management of soft-tissue pathology, including abscesses, necrotizing fasciitis, fascial dehiscence, and detection of foreign bodies has permitted timely bedside decision making and treatment.

REFERENCES

1. Rozycki GS, Ochsner MG, Jaffin JH, et al. Prospective evaluation of surgeons' use of ultrasound in the evaluation of trauma patients. *J Trauma* 1993;34:516–526.
2. Rozycki GS, Ochsner MG, Schmidt JA, et al. A prospective study of surgeon-performed ultrasound as the primary adjuvant modality for injured patient assessment. *J Trauma* 1995; 39:492–498.
3. Shackford SR. Focused ultrasound examinations by surgeons: the time is now. *J Trauma* 1993;35:181–182.
4. Fry WR, Smith RS, Schneider JJ, et al. Ultrasonographic examination of wound tracts. *Arch Surg* 1995;130:605–608.
5. Slasky BS, Auerbach D, Skolnick ML. Value of portable real-time ultrasound in the ICU. *Crit Care Med* 1983;11:160–164.
6. Rozycki GS, Pennington, SD, Feliciano DV. Surgeon-performed ultrasound in the critical care setting: its use as an extension of the physical examination to detect pleural effusion. *J Trauma* 2001;50:636–642.
7. Chen SC, Wang HP, Chen WJ, et al. Selective use of ultrasonography for the detection of pneumoperitoneum. *Acad Emerg Med* 2002;9:643–645.
8. Stevenson VW, Haas CF, Wahl WL. Intrahospital transport of the adult mechanically ventilated patient. *Respir Care Clin* 2002;8:1–35.
9. Gryminski J, Krakowka P, Lypacewicz G. The diagnosis of pleural effusion by ultrasonic and radiologic techniques. *Chest* 1976;70:33–37.
10. Sistrom CL, Reiheld CT, Spencer BG, et al. Detection and estimation of the volume of pneumothorax using real-time sonography. *AJR Am J Roentgenol* 1996;166:317–321.
11. Ratanen NW. Diagnostic ultrasound: diseases of the thorax. *Vet Clin North Am* 1986;2:49–66.
12. Lichtenstein DA, Menu Y. A bedside ultrasound sign ruling out pneumothorax in the critically ill. *Chest* 1995;108:1345–1348.
13. Wernerck K, Lalanski M, Peters PE, et al. Pneumothorax: evaluation by ultrasound—preliminary results. *J Thorac Imaging* 1987;7:76–78.
14. Targhetta R, Bourgeois JM, Chavagneux R, et al. Diagnosis of pneumothorax by ultrasound immediately after ultrasonically guided aspiration biopsy. *Chest* 1992;101:855–856.
15. Dulchavsky SA, Schwarz KL, Kirkpatrick AW, et al. Prospective evaluation of thoracic ultrasound in the detection of pneumothorax. *J Trauma* 2001;50:201–205.
16. Kirkpatrick AW, Alex KT, Dulchavsky SA, et al. Sonographic diagnosis of a pneumothorax inapparent on plain radiography: confirmation by computed tomography. *J Trauma* 2001; 50:750–752.
17. Cunningham J, Kirkpatrick AW, Nicolaou S, et al. Enhanced recognition of "lung sliding" with power color Doppler in the imaging in the diagnosis of pneumothorax. *J Trauma* 2002;52:769–771.
18. Dulchavsky SA, Hamilton DR, Diebel LN, et al. Thoracic ultrasound diagnosis of pneumothorax. *J Trauma* 1999;47: 970–971.
19. Lichtenstein DA, Meziere G, Iderman P, et al. The comet-tail artifact: an ultrasound sign ruling out pneumothorax. *Intensive Care Med* 1999;25:383–388.
20. Rozycki GS, Ballard RB, Feliciano DV, et al: Surgeon-performed ultrasound for the assessment of truncal injuries: lessons learned from 1,540 patients. *Ann Surg* 1998;228:557–567.
21. Scalea TM, Rodriguez, Chiu WC, et al. Focused assessment with sonography for trauma (FAST): results from an international consensus conference. *J Trauma* 1999;46:466–472.
22. Williams RJ, Windsor AC, Rosin RD, et al. Ultrasound scanning of the acute abdomen by surgeons in training. *Ann R Coll Surg Engl* 1994;76:228–233.

23. Chen CH, Yang CC, Yeh YH. Role of upright chest radiography and ultrasonography in demonstrating free air of perforated peptic ulcers. *Hepatogastroenterology* 2001;48:1082–1084.
24. Grecheinig W, Peicha G, Clement HG, et al. Detection of pneumoperitoneum by ultrasound examination: an experimental and clinical study. *Injury* 1999;30:173–178.
25. Ivatury RR, Simon RJ. Intra-abdominal hypertension: the abdominal compartment syndrome. In: Ivatury RR, Cayten GC, eds. *The textbook of penetrating trauma*. Baltimore: Williams & Wilkins, 1996:939–951.
26. Sharpe RP, Pryor JP, Gandhi RR, et al. Abdominal compartment syndrome in the pediatric blunt trauma patient treated with paracentesis: report of two cases. *J Trauma* 2002;53:380–382.
27. Lederle FA, Walker JM, Reinke DB. Selective screening for abdominal aortic aneurysms with physical examination and ultrasound. *Arch Intern Med* 1988;148:1753–1756.
28. Maloney JD, Pairolero PC, Smith BF, et al. Ultrasound evaluation of abdominal aortic aneurysms. *Circulation* 1977;56:80–85.
29. Nusbaum JW, Fremanis AK, Thomford NR. Echography in the diagnosis of abdominal aortic aneurysm. *Arch Surg* 1971;102:385–388.
30. Raskin MM, Cunningham JB. Comparison of computed tomography and ultrasound for abdominal aortic aneurysms: preliminary study. *J Comput Assist Tomogr* 1978;2:21–24.
31. Graham DD. Ultrasound in the emergency department: detection of wooden foreign bodies in the soft tissue. *J Emerg Med* 2002;22:75–79.
32. Boyse TD. US of soft-tissue foreign bodies and associated complications with surgical correlation. *Radiographics* 2001;21:125–126.
33. Hill R, Cornron R, Greissinger P, et al. Ultrasound for the detection of foreign bodies in human tissue. *Ann Emerg Med* 1997;29:353–356.

Chapter 11

Transabdominal Ultrasound: Liver, Biliary Tract, and Pancreas

Daniel J. Deziel and Junji Machi

The basic reason for a surgeon to perform transabdominal ultrasound (TAUS) is to acquire diagnostic information that is not available by physical examination alone. A second important role of TAUS is to guide the surgeon in the performance of specific diagnostic or therapeutic interventions. When surgeons perform TAUS, it does not supplant the need for radiologic expertise or for other imaging studies such as computed tomography (CT) or magnetic resonance imaging (MRI). Rather, it complements these resources by expanding the capability of providing necessary and timely care for patients.

There are prerequisites to the reliable performance of focused sonographic examinations of the abdomen: one must have knowledge of ultrasound physics and instrumentation, one must be thoroughly familiar with the gross and sonographic anatomy of normal and diseased organs and tissues, and one must have the acumen to interpret sonographic findings in the context of a specific clinical situation. For surgeons who are intimately versed in anatomy and pathophysiology and whose clinical judgments are tested daily, the use of real-time ultrasound is a natural extension of the physical examination. Once learned, practiced, and validated, TAUS can be a tremendous tool for improving clinical outcomes from many surgical conditions.

INSTRUMENTS AND SCANNING TECHNIQUES

Transducer Selection

TAUS is performed with a real-time probe at typical frequencies of 2.5 to 5 MHz. The best resolution is obtained using the highest frequency that will provide adequate depth of penetration. A 3.5-MHz transducer is commonly used for TAUS in adults. For children or thin individuals, a 5-MHz probe may be used. Lower frequency probes may be required for the examination of obese patients.

TAUS can be performed with linear, curvilinear, or phased array transducers. Transducer selection depends on the size of the contact surface or "footprint" that will provide the best surface contact at the body site being examined. Linear and curvilinear arrays require a larger, flatter area for optimal contact. Linear arrays produce a rectangular image (Fig. 1) whereas curvilinear transducers produce a truncated sector image (Fig. 2). Phased array transducers typically have smaller footprints so that images can be obtained with smaller contact areas (Fig. 3). This can be advantageous when scanning over irregular body contours or through narrow windows such as the intercostal spaces.

Patient Preparation

Elective TAUS is best performed when the patient has fasted for about 6 hours. Fasting helps to minimize interference from bowel gas and facilitates distention of the gallbladder. The examination is usually started with the patient in the supine position. Variations in position are necessary according to the anatomic region being imaged. Decubitus, semidecubitus, semiupright, erect, or even prone positioning may be useful.

Scanning Planes

The basic scanning planes of TAUS are described in relation to the long axis of the body (Fig. 4). Longitudinal scans include the sagittal plane, which images the body from anterior to posterior, and the coronal plane, which images from one side to the other. The transverse imaging plane is a cross-section perpendicular to the long axis of the body.

The terminology of scanning planes is sometimes confusing because the planes are described differently during TAUS and during intraoperative or laparoscopic ultrasound. During intraoperative ultrasound, the longi-

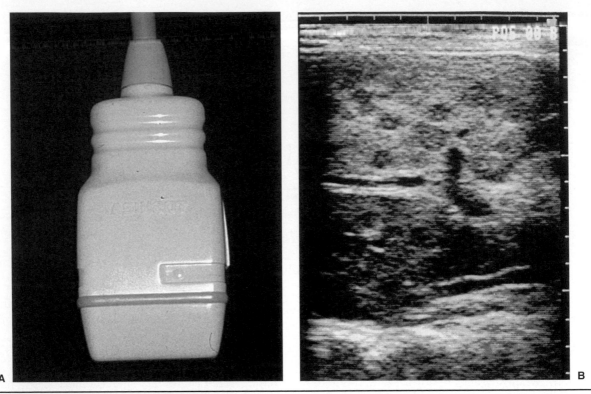

FIGURE 1. Linear array transducer (**A**) and scan (**B**).

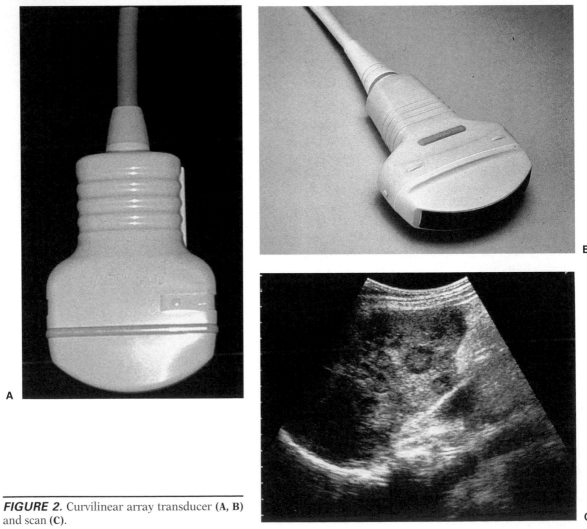

FIGURE 2. Curvilinear array transducer (**A, B**) and scan (**C**).

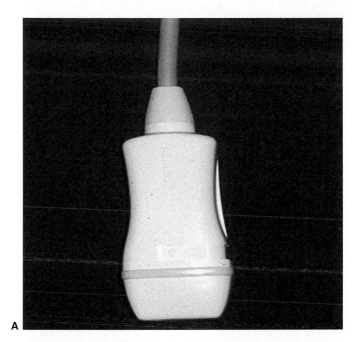

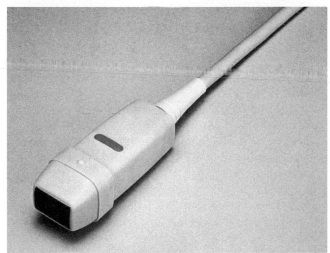

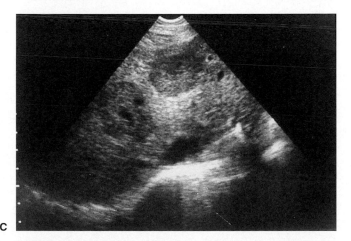

FIGURE 3. Phased array transducer **(A, B)** and scan **(C)**.

tudinal plane refers to the long axis of the particular organ being examined rather than the long axis of the entire body. Thus, an image of the pancreas showing the pancreatic duct in longitudinal section is considered a longitudinal scan using intraoperative terminology but is essentially a transverse scan in the parlance of TAUS.

Multiplanar imaging is a basic tenet of sonographic interpretation. Any structure visualized in one plane should be imaged in a second plane at a 90-degree angle to the first. During real-time sonographic examinations, the structure is imaged in multiple oblique planes between these orientations as the transducer is rotated.

There are established standards for documenting and presenting TAUS images (1,2). The left side of the image display (as viewed by the examiner) should correspond to the right side of the subject when scanning in the transverse plane. In longitudinal planes, the cephalad end of the patient should be at the left side of the image display. The examiner must verify the correct plane or orientation of the transducer and remain orientated to the ultrasound beam during the course of the examination.

Probe Handling

TAUS is a contact scanning technique. Complete surface contact between the probe and the patient's body wall is required for optimal imaging. The probe selected should have a footprint of appropriate size and contour for the body contact site. Acoustic coupling gel should be applied liberally. The transducer is held against the patient's body wall and stabilized preferably by placement of some point of the examining hand on the patient. Probe movements are often slight and subtle; unless the probe is well stabilized, fine control is not possible.

There are four basic probe movements used during TAUS: sliding, rotating, rocking, and tilting. Sliding moves the probe across the body surface without otherwise changing its orientation (Fig. 5). Rotating the probe turns it in a clockwise or counterclockwise direction at a fixed location, thus altering the imaging plane (Fig. 6). During rocking and tilting, the head of the probe remains in a relatively solitary external position while the shaft of the probe is angled to direct the sound beam to different internal positions. Rocking is angulation parallel to the scanning plane (Fig. 7). Tilting is angulation perpendicular to the scanning plane (Fig. 8). In reality, these maneuvers are combined simultaneously to varying degrees to provide optimal sonographic visualization.

Variation in the pressure with which the probe is held against the abdominal wall affects the image obtained. Light contact may improve visualization of more superficial structures in the abdominal wall or in very thin individuals (as will higher frequency transducers and proper

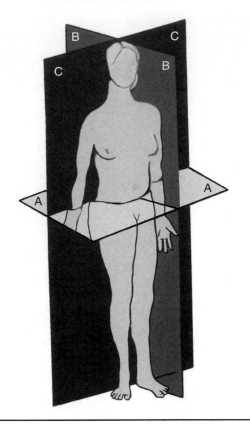

FIGURE 4. Basic scanning planes of transabdominal ultrasound. A, transverse plane; B, longitudinal sagittal plane; C, longitudinal coronal plane.

depth of focus). Deep-pressure or compression scanning can be employed to displace intestinal air between the transducer and the target organ in an effort to improve visualization, as when imaging the distal common bile duct or pancreas.

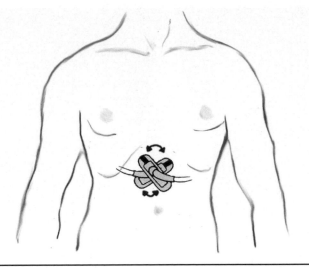

FIGURE 6. Transabdominal ultrasound probe movement: rotating.

Liver Scanning Technique

TAUS of the adult liver is usually performed with a 3.0- or 3.5-MHz transducer. A higher frequency probe (5.0 MHz) may be selected for very thin patients or a lower frequency probe (2.5 MHz) for obese patients or when the liver is hyperechoic. Frequencies of 7 MHz or higher may be useful when evaluating surface structures or nodularity. The patient is positioned supine; different positions may be necessary including left posterior oblique, left lateral decubitus, or erect. A deep, held inspiration will push the liver downward for better visualization. Scans are obtained in both longitudinal (sagittal and coronal) and transverse planes. A systematic evaluation of the hepatic parenchyma is performed, and views are obtained to compare the echogenicity of the liver to the cortex of the right kidney. The dome of the right lobe at the dia-

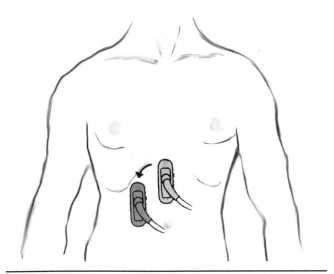

FIGURE 5. Transabdominal ultrasound probe movement: sliding.

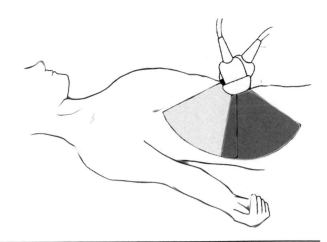

FIGURE 7. Transabdominal ultrasound probe movement: rocking.

subxiphoid position, the probe can be angled or moved to the left and downward to identify the extent of the left lobe. The probe is then moved along the right subcostal margin from anterior to lateral to scan the right lobe. Varying and sometimes sharp subcostal angulation of the probe may be necessary.

The rib cage limits probe contact in the upper abdomen. Attempts to image areas such as the liver, biliary tract, or spleen from a subcostal position are frequently insufficient, even with exaggerated inspiration. Intercostal scanning can access these more difficult areas (Fig. 11). A probe with a small footprint can be used to allow rotation and rocking or tilting without interference from the ribs. Shadowing from the ribs will obscure a segment of the image (Fig. 12). Intercostal scanning can be performed from both anterior and lateral approaches. More complete imaging of the liver may be facilitated by moving the probe upward into successive intercostal spaces.

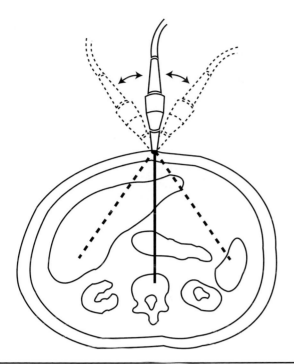

FIGURE 8. Transabdominal ultrasound Probe movement: tilting.

phragm and the right pleural space are imaged. The ligamentum teres, ligamentum venosum, and main lobar fissure are demonstrated. The major vascular structures are imaged including the inferior vena cava (IVC), hepatic veins, portal vein branches, and aorta. The intrahepatic bile ducts are examined for dilatation.

The transducer is first placed in the subxiphoid or subcostal area and then moved (slid) and angled (rocked or tilted) as necessary to provide adequate views (subxiphoid or subcostal scanning) (Figs. 9 and 10). From the

Biliary Tract Scanning Techniques

TAUS of the biliary tract is usually performed with a 3.5-MHz transducer. When possible the patient should be fasted to maximize gallbladder distention. The patient is usually positioned supine, although scanning can be commenced with the patient in the left posterior oblique or left lateral decubitus position. Basic probe positions are depicted in Figure 13 (3). The first step is to locate the gallbladder. The probe is oriented longitudinally below the right costal margin in the midclavicular line and tilted slightly to obtain a long axis view of the gallbladder. A deep, held inspiration may be necessary to bring the gallbladder into view. The gallbladder can then be followed upward during expiration by subcostal angulation

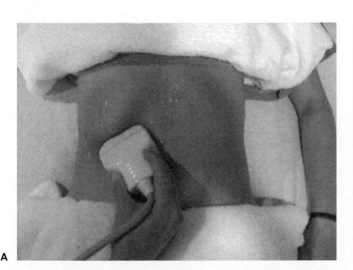
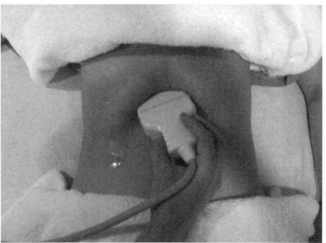

A   B

FIGURE 9. Probe positions for transverse-oblique liver scanning. **A, B:** Right subcostal. *(continued)*

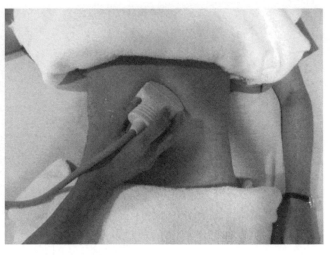

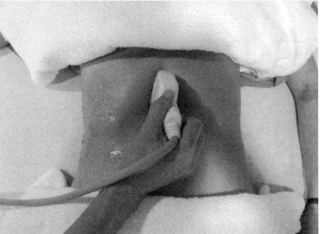

FIGURE 9. *(Continued)* **C:** Subxiphoid. **D:** Left subcostal scanning.

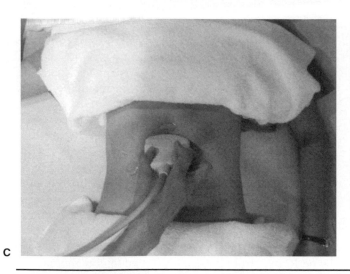

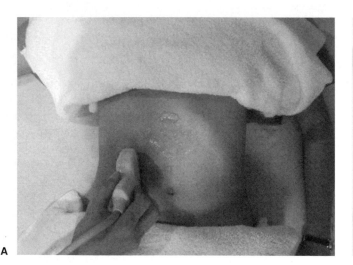

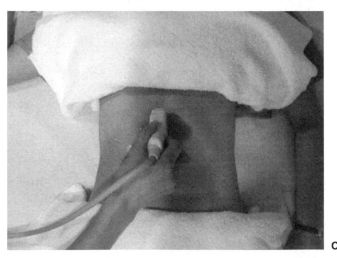

FIGURE 10. Probe positions for sagittal liver scanning. **A:** Right subcostal. **B, C:** Subxiphoid scanning.

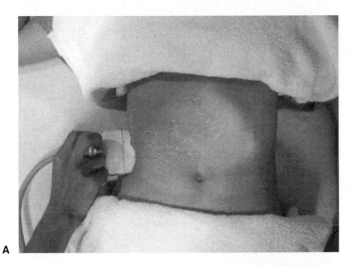

A

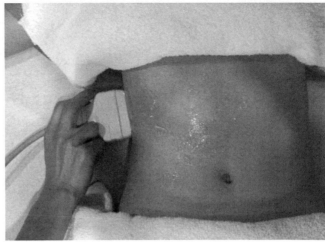

B

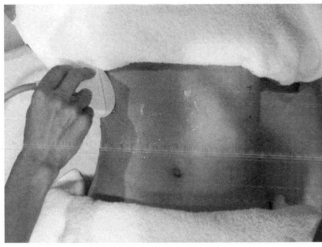

C

FIGURE 11. Probe positions for right intercostal liver scanning. **A–C:** Scanning from different locations and intercostal spaces. Note that the intercostal scanning often shows coronal planes.

of the probe. Rotating the probe parallel to the costal margin will yield oblique and transverse sections. Intercostal scanning may be necessary when the gallbladder is situated higher under the rib cage. The transducer is positioned in the 6th to 9th intercostal spaces and tilted medially. Scanning with the patient in different positions is necessary to diagnose or exclude gallstones. At times the gallbladder is more easily seen when the patient is in the left decubitus position with the transducer in the midclavicular subcostal location (Fig. 14).

The extrahepatic bile duct is identified by its anterior relationship to the portal vein. The left (or right) portal vein can be identified and traced caudally. The proximal extrahepatic duct is seen in longitudinal section with the probe at approximately a right angle to the costal margin in the right epigastric location (Fig. 13B). The best view may be with the patient in a 45-degree left posterior oblique position. The distal duct may be identified with the probe in the epigastrium just right of midline oriented longitudinally or obliquely (Fig. 13E, F). Traditional parasagittal scans of the distal duct have been obtained with the patient in the left lateral decubitus position and the probe parallel to the right midaxillary line (4). The retroduodenal portion of the duct is generally difficult to visualize because of intestinal air. The distal duct may be seen in transverse scans through the head of the pancreas. Improved visualization of distal common duct stones has been reported by transverse scanning in the erect position (4).

Subcostal and intercostal scanning is used for delineation of the hilar duct and intrahepatic ducts on the right side (Fig. 13B, C). The left hepatic duct and its intrahepatic branches are seen as the transducer is slid from the right subcostal area to the subxiphoid region and on epigastric transverse scan (Fig. 13C, D). TAUS does not typically allow good visualization of the smaller intrahepatic ducts unless they are dilated.

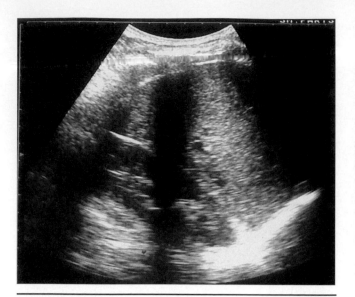

FIGURE 12. Rib shadowing over liver.

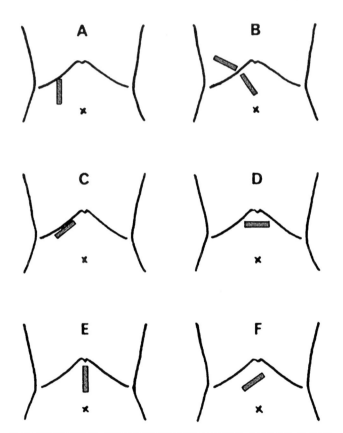

FIGURE 13. Probe positions for the basic biliary tract scanning. **A:** Right subcostal sagittal scan for the delineation of the gallbladder. **B:** Right intercostal (6th to 9th interspace) scan for the gallbladder, right intrahepatic bile ducts, and hilar bile ducts; epigastric right oblique scan for the extrahepatic proximal bile duct. **C:** Right subcostal oblique scan for the left hepatic duct, right hepatic duct, and right intrahepatic duct. **D:** Epigastric transverse scan for the left lateral bile ducts. **E:** Upper abdominal sagittal scan for the distal extrahepatic bile duct. **F:** Upper abdominal left oblique scan for the distal end of the common bile duct. (Reproduced with permission from Okuda K, Tsuchiya Y. Ultrasonic anatomy of the biliary system. *Clin Gastroenterol* 1983,12:50.)

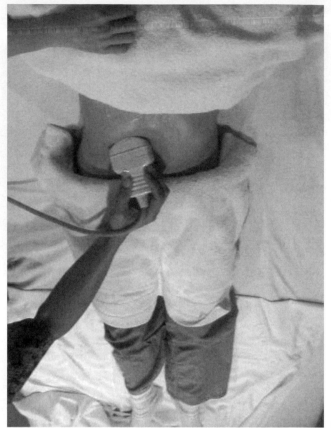

A

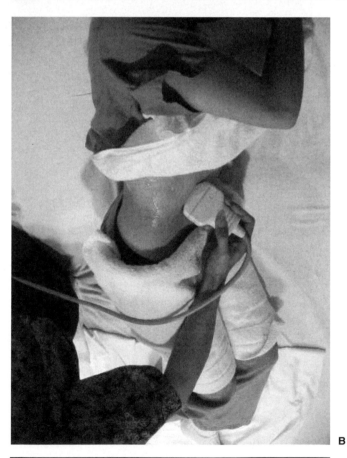

B

FIGURE 14. Change of patient position during gallbladder scanning. **A:** Supine position. **B:** Left lateral decubitus position.

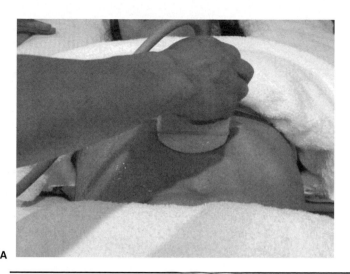
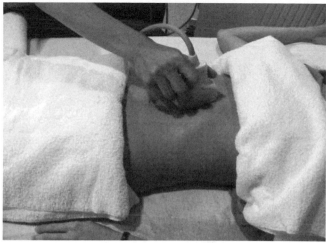

FIGURE 15. Probe positions during pancreas scanning. **A:** Transverse scanning. **B:** Sagittal scanning.

Pancreas Scanning Techniques

TAUS of the pancreas is much more difficult than imaging the liver or biliary tract. Fat and bowel gas are often impediments to successful scanning. Examination is performed with a 3.0- or 3.5-MHz transducer in a fasted patient. The patient is initially positioned supine (Fig. 15). Right lateral decubitus, sitting, or even prone views may be useful (Fig. 16). Techniques to improve imaging of the pancreas include the patient's breathing with held inspi-

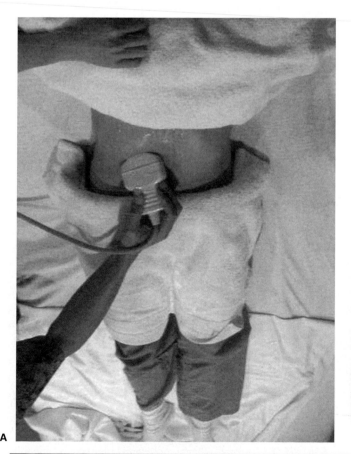
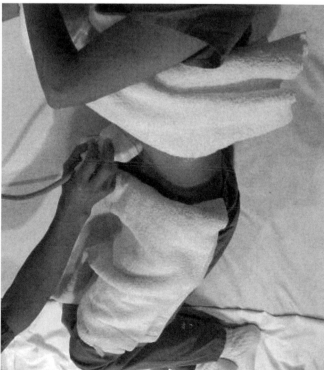

FIGURE 16. Change of patient position during pancreas scanning. **A:** Supine position. **B:** Right lateral decubitus position.

ratiuns (deep or normal), compression scanning with deep pressure on the transducer, or having the patient "push out" against the transducer (5). The stomach can be used as an acoustic window by having the patient drink 500 mL of fluid and then assuming an upright position. Scans can be obtained through both longitudinal and transverse planes to the long axis of the gland. The long axis of the pancreas may be best seen with an oblique orientation of the transducer. The distal tail may be scanned from the left flank through the spleen. The pancreas is identified in relation to its neighboring vascular landmarks.

LIVER

Indications

Some of the indications for liver ultrasound are listed in Table 1. A primary reason to implement TAUS of the liver is to detect the presence of mass lesions, especially malignant neoplasms, but also benign solid neoplasms, cysts, hemangiomas, and abscesses. The clinical presentation prompting sonographic investigation may be pain, fever, abnormal liver chemistry, or routine surveillance for patients who demonstrate no symptoms but have had a previous primary malignancy elsewhere or who may be at higher risk for the development of primary hepatocellular carcinoma.

TAUS is indicated for localization of hepatic masses. The geographic location can be determined according to the involved hepatic segment(s) and the proximity to the hepatic veins and portal vein branches. These features can be crucial to decisions about resectability, to preoperative planning for the potential extent of resection, and to the identification of tumor thrombus in hepatic vessels.

Some hepatic conditions can be characterized by their sonographic features. Simple hepatic cysts and hemangiomas are examples of mass lesions that can often be diagnosed by their appearance on TAUS without the need for further imaging or intervention. TAUS can also be useful for identifying diffuse parenchymal abnormalities such as cirrhosis or fatty infiltration.

TAUS is a convenient method for following the size and number of focal hepatic lesions. This method can be used to assess the response of malignant tumors to therapy or to monitor the status of benign lesions that may not initially warrant intervention, such as cysts, hemangiomas, or abscesses.

TAUS is indicated in the postoperative assessment of patients who have undergone hepatic surgery. After liver resection or transplantation, TAUS can be used to identify bile duct dilatation or fluid collections. Doppler capability allows evaluation of portal venous and hepatic arterial blood flow.

TAUS can be used to guide percutaneous hepatic interventions. Typical procedures that are guided by TAUS include needle biopsy, aspiration, and ablation of tumors by radiofrequency thermal probes or chemical injection.

Normal Ultrasound Anatomy of the Liver

Echogenicity and Size

The normal liver parenchyma has a uniform, medium level echogenic pattern (5). It is usually more echogenic than the adjacent renal cortex, which is useful for comparison (Fig. 17). The liver is normally less echogenic than the spleen and, depending on the age of the patient, less echogenic than or as echogenic as the pancreas.

Liver enlargement can be difficult to accurately diagnose with TAUS. The most commonly used measurement is the sagittal length of the liver (dome to tip of right lobe) in the midclavicular line; a length of more than 15 cm probably represents hepatomegaly.

▶ **TABLE 1 Indications for Transabdominal Ultrasound of the Liver**

- Detection of mass lesions of the liver
- Localization of liver masses
- Characterization of liver conditions
    Parenchymal abnormalities
    Mass lesions
- Serial follow-up of mass lesions
- Assessment for postoperative complications
- Guidance for percutaneous interventions

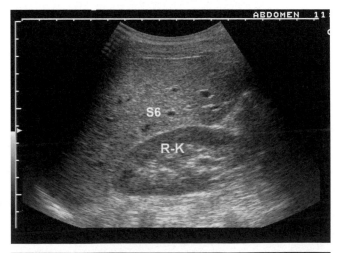

FIGURE 17. Normal liver parenchyma is more echogenic than renal cortex. S6, segment 6 of the liver; R-K, right kidney.

Surgical and Segmental Anatomy

The surgical anatomy of the liver is based on the distribution of the portal structures and the hepatic veins (6). The three main hepatic veins define three vertical scissura. The liver is divided into right and left lobes based on a vertical, angled plane extending from the gallbladder fossa to the left of the IVC. This is the middle scissura or the main lobar fissure and, in its cephalad portion, it contains the middle hepatic vein. The main lobar fissure may be visible on ultrasound as an echogenic structure located just below and anterior to the right portal vein and extending to the gallbladder neck (7,8). Since the fissure itself may be difficult to identify by ultrasound, the middle hepatic vein is a more distinct landmark for separating the right and left lobes. The right lobe is divided into anteromedial (or anterior) and posterolateral (or posterior) segments by the right scissura or intersegmental fissure, which contains the right hepatic vein. The left lobe is divided into medial and lateral segments by the left

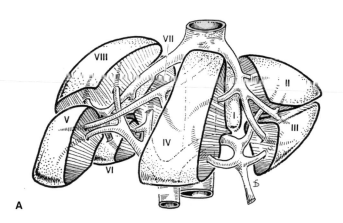

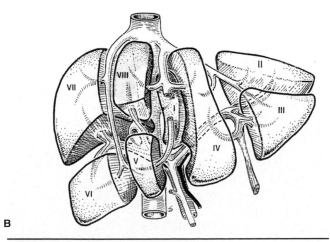

FIGURE 18. The liver segments according to the nomenclature of Couinaud. **A:** As seen in the patient. **B:** In the ex vivo position. (Reproduced with permission from Blumgart LH. *Surgery of the liver and biliary tract.* Edinburgh: Churchill Livingstone, 1988:5).

> **TABLE 2 Hepatic Segments**

Segment 1:	Caudate lobe
Segment 2:	Left lateral superior
Segment 3:	Left lateral inferior
Segment 4a:	Left medial inferior
Segment 4b:	Left medial superior
Segment 5:	Right anterior inferior
Segment 6:	Right posterior inferior
Segment 7:	Right posterior superior
Segment 8:	Right anterior superior

scissura or left intersegmental fissure. Sonographically, the left hepatic vein, the ascending (umbilical) portion of the left portal vein, and the ligamentum teres separate the cephalad, middle, and caudal portions of the lateral and medial segments, respectively. The caudate lobe is demarcated by the transverse portion of the left portal vein and the ligamentum venosum ventrally and by the IVC dorsally.

The liver is divided into eight functional segments (subsegments, actually) as described by Couinaud based on the branches of the portal structures (9) (Fig. 18). These segments are listed in Table 2. Couinaud's segments are identified sonographically by following the portal vein branches peripherally. (See also Chapter 15)

Vascular Structures

The normal homogeneous echo pattern of the liver parenchyma is interrupted by sonolucent tubular structures, which are the hepatic and portal veins. Usually the hepatic and portal veins can be readily differentiated from each other by their sonographic characteristics (Table 3) (5,10).

The hepatic veins do not have very reflective walls and appear simply as anechoic structures within the liver parenchyma. However, the larger hepatic veins may have more reflective walls, especially near the IVC. The hepatic veins are located between the lobes and segments (intersegmental) and are vertically oriented so they are

> **TABLE 3 Sonographic Characteristics of Hepatic Vessels**

Characteristic	Hepatic Vein	Portal Vein
Location	Intersegmental	Intrasegmental
Orientation	Vertical	Horizontal
Caliber	Larger near inferior vena cava	Larger centrally
Vessel wall	Less reflective (less echogenic)	Reflective (echogenic)

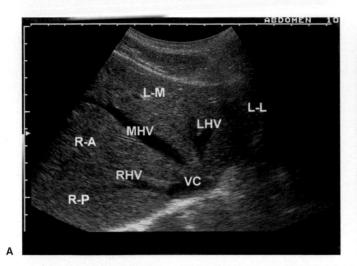
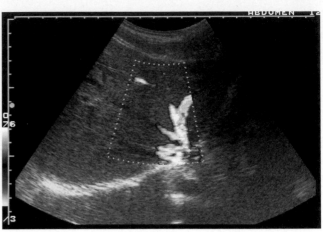

FIGURE 19. **A:** Transverse scan of right (RHV), middle (MHV), and left (LHV) hepatic veins at junction with vena cava (VC). R-P, right posterior segment; R-A, right anterior segment; L-M, left medial segment; L-L, left lateral segment. **B:** The same hepatic veins with color Doppler flow. (See Color Plate 15.)

seen along their long axis with longitudinal scans and in cross-sections with transverse scans. The hepatic veins increase in caliber as they course upward toward their junction with the IVC, which can be clearly demonstrated (Fig. 19).

There are usually three major hepatic veins: right, middle, and left. The middle hepatic vein may enter the IVC separately but most commonly joins the left hepatic vein. Variations in hepatic venous anatomy are relatively common. Up to one third of patients may have more than three major hepatic veins. One variation of surgical significance is the presence of the inferior right hepatic vein, which exists in 10% to 15% of patients. This vein

drains from segment 6, the right posterior inferior segment, and enters the IVC caudad to the main right hepatic vein (see Figure 23C in Chapter 13). At times, it may be larger than the main right hepatic vein.

The portal vein branches have more reflective, hyperechoic walls than the hepatic veins. This appearance has been attributed to the fibrofatty connective tissue in the portal triad and to the accompanying branches of the hepatic artery and bile ducts, which themselves may not be seen by TAUS. Unlike the hepatic veins, the portal vein branches are intrasegmental. One exception is the ascending portion of the left portal vein, which is intersegmental. The portal vein branches are primarily oriented transversely, so that bifurcation of the main portal vein is

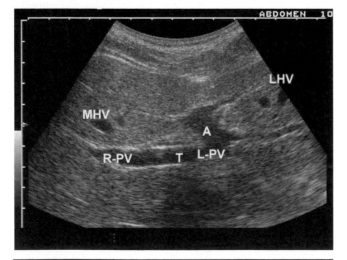

FIGURE 20. Transverse scan at bifurcation of portal vein. R-PV, right portal vein; T, transverse portion of the left portal vein, L-PV; A, ascending portion of the left portal vein; MHV, middle hepatic vein; LHV, left hepatic vein.

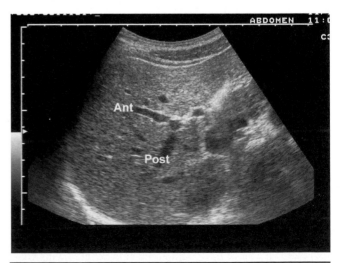

FIGURE 21. Anterior (Ant) and posterior (Post) branches of right portal vein.

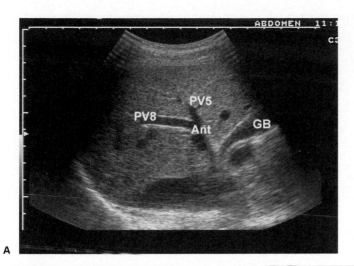
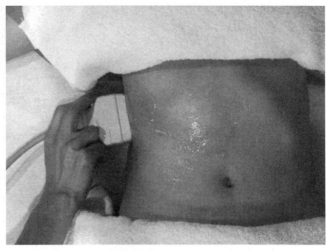

A

B

FIGURE 22. A: Intercostal scan in longitudinal plane of anterior branch (Ant) of right portal vein. PV5, branch to anteroinferior segment; PV8, branch to anterosuperior segment; GB, gallbladder. B: The probe position of intercostal scanning.

best seen on transverse scans whereas longitudinal scans will demonstrate cross-sections of the portal vessels.

In the hepatoduodenal ligament the main portal vein is located posterior to the bile duct and the hepatic artery. The normal mean diameter of the portal vein is 10 to 12 mm; its size is affected by various factors, including respiration, activity, position, and medications.

The portal vein enters the liver at the porta hepatis and divides into the main right and left portal vein (Fig. 20). The main right portal vein divides into anterior and posterior branches (Fig. 21). The anterior branch then provides anterosuperior portal veins (segment 8 branches) and the anteroinferior portal veins (segment 5 branches) (Fig. 22). More often the segment 8 branches consist of two branches: the ventral branch and the dorsal branch.

Frequently, the ventral branch comes off the trunk of the segment 5 branch or off one of the segment 5 branches. The segment 5 branches frequently consist of three or four branches. The posterior branch of the main right portal vein then provides the posterosuperior branch (segment 7 branch, usually only one branch) and the posteroinferior branches (segment 6 branches, often one or two branches) (Fig. 23). The main left portal vein starts with the initial transverse or horizontal portion, coursing anterior to the caudate lobe. The vein then abruptly turns anteriorly to form the ascending or umbilical portion of the left portal vein. At the beginning, this portion gives off the lateral superior branch (segment 2). At its end, the ascending portion gives off the lateral inferior branch

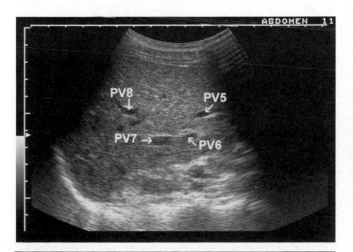

FIGURE 23. Segmental branches of right portal vein. PV5, anteroinferior; PV6, posteroinferior; PV7; posterosuperior, PV8; anterosuperior.

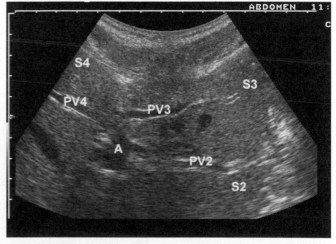

FIGURE 24. Segmental branches of left portal vein. A, ascending portion of the left portal vein; PV2, lateral superior branch; PV3, lateral inferior branch; PV4, medial branch; S2, S3, S4, parenchymal segments.

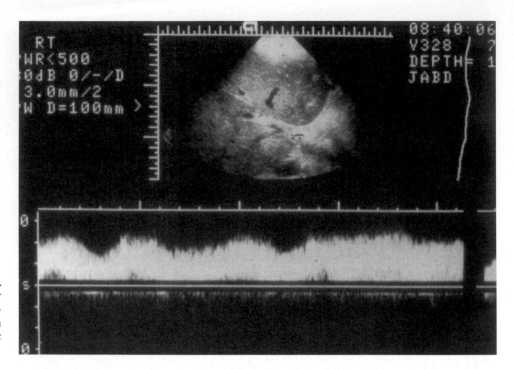

FIGURE 25. Duplex Doppler tracing of portal vein flow demonstrating higher velocity than normal in a patient with hepatic metastases.

(segment 3) laterally and the medial branch (segment 4) medially (Fig. 24). Because TAUS of the left lobe of the liver is usually performed subcostally, segment 3 and its portal branches are located superficially (closer to the transducer surface) and segment 2 and its portal branch are located more deeply on TAUS images. Similarly, segment 4a is superficial to segment 4b. Although both main right and left portal veins provide branches to the caudate lobe, the transverse portion of the left portal vein often gives off relatively large branches that can be delineated sonographically.

Variations of the portal venous system are relatively uncommon. One variation is the absence of the transverse portion of the left portal vein. Another is the ab-

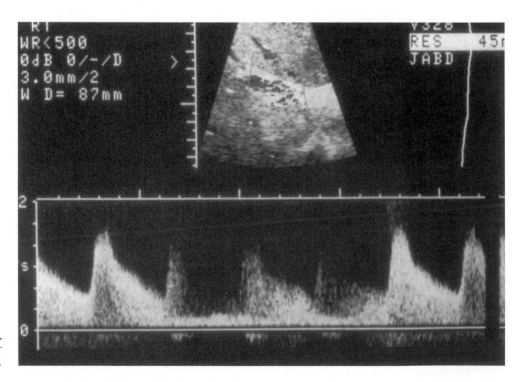

FIGURE 26. Duplex Doppler tracing of hepatic arterial flow.

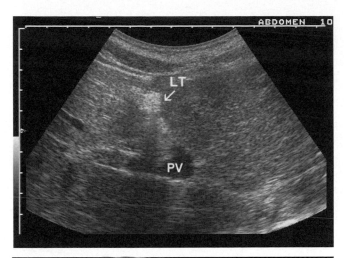

FIGURE 27. Transverse scan of ligamentum teres (LT). PV, ascending portion of the left portal vein.

Doppler ultrasound imaging may be helpful for identifying hepatic vascular structures and for detecting normal and abnormal flow patterns. Flow in the hepatic veins and IVC is usually bidirectional due to the cardiac cycle and respirations. The portal and splenic veins have a low-velocity, continuous flow toward the liver with minor undulations due to cardiac activity (Fig. 25). The hepatic arteries demonstrate characteristics of a low-resistance type of vessel with a biphasic spectral waveform that continues forward during diastole (Fig. 26). This is in contradistinction to the high-resistance waveform of muscular arteries, which demonstrate a triphasic pattern with flow reversal. The hepatic artery demonstrates more spectral banding than large vessels such as the aorta because in smaller arteries flow velocities in the lumen vary. Higher velocities are observed toward the center of the vessel and lower velocities near the wall. In larger vessels, intraluminal velocities are more equal.

sence of the main right portal vein in which case the portal vein at the porta hepatis divides into three branches (anterior right, posterior right and main left); this variation is referred to as trifurcation of the portal vein.

The proper hepatic artery is located anterior to the portal vein and medial to the bile duct and divides into the right and left hepatic arteries. Intrahepatic arterial branches accompany the portal vein branches. Hepatic artery branches are difficult to identify and to distinguish from the intrahepatic bile ducts with B-mode TAUS.

Ligaments and Diaphragm

The ligamentum teres and ligamentum venosum are embryologic remnants that can be visualized by TAUS (7). The ligamentum teres is the remnant of the umbilical vein running between the umbilicus and the left portal vein. It is located at the inferior border of the falciform ligament and enters the liver in the umbilical fissure. In the transverse plane it appears as a bright (hyperechoic) round structure about 1 cm in size located between the caudal portions of the medial and lateral segments of the

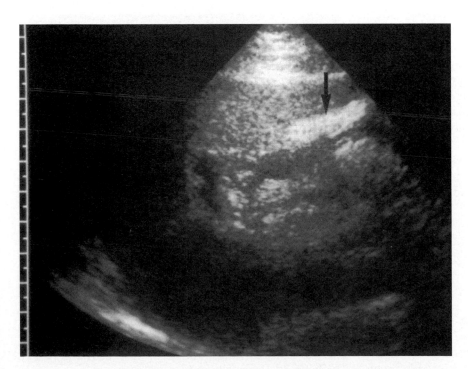

FIGURE 28. Longitudinal scan of ligamentum teres (*arrow*).

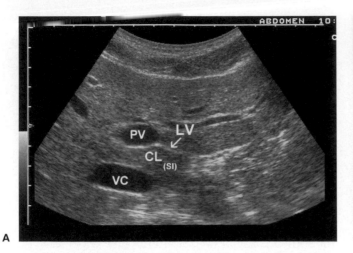
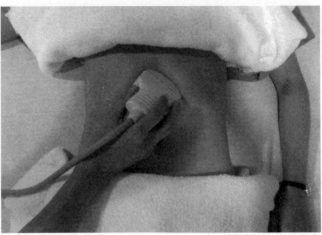

A   B

FIGURE 29. A: Ligamentum venosum (LV). PV, left portal vein; CL (S1), caudate lobe; VC, vena cava. B: The probe position to obtain this image.

left lobe (Fig. 27). In the longitudinal plane, the ligamentum teres appears as an echogenic band extending from the anterior surface of the liver to the porta hepatis (Fig. 28). A prominent ligamentum teres may mimic a hyperechoic mass and occasionally may demonstrate acoustic shadowing.

The ligamentum venosum is a remnant of the ductus venosum that connects the fetal left portal vein with the IVC. It separates the caudate lobe from the lateral segment of the left lobe. Sonographically, it appears as an echogenic line or band (Fig. 29). This hyperechoic ligament at times causes acoustic shadowing so that the caudate lobe appears hypoechoic relative to the rest of the liver. The caudate lobe should not be mistaken for a focal lesion in this situation.

The diaphragm is a prominent landmark during hepatic sonography. It is a highly echogenic curving line posterior to the liver (Fig. 30). Viewed sagittally it defines the pleural and subphrenic spaces. The diaphragm typically produces a mirror image artifact in which it appears that there is liver tissue both above and below the diaphragm (Fig. 31). Occasionally, slips of diaphragm or intercostal muscle may indent the lateral aspect of the liver and mimic mass lesions on cross-section. In such a circumstance, rotating the ultrasound transducer should allow proper interpretation.

Pathologic Ultrasound Anatomy of the Liver

Diffuse Abnormalities

Diffuse parenchymal abnormalities are generally represented as either an increase or decrease in normal liver echogenicity (11). Hyperechoic patterns are most commonly seen with fatty infiltration, cirrhosis, and chronic hepatitis (Fig. 32). The dense liver attenuates sound and could potentially obscure deeper focal lesions. When the liver is diffusely hyperechoic, low-frequency transducers (2.5 MHz) may be helpful to improve sound penetration and far-field visualization. The liver may be hypoechoic when edematous as with right-sided heart failure or severe acute viral hepatitis. In acute alcoholic hepatitis, the liver is more echogenic due to fat deposition. Infiltration with leukemia or lymphoma can also occasionally produce a hypoechoic scan. With a hypoechoic liver, the normally reflective portal vein walls may appear even brighter

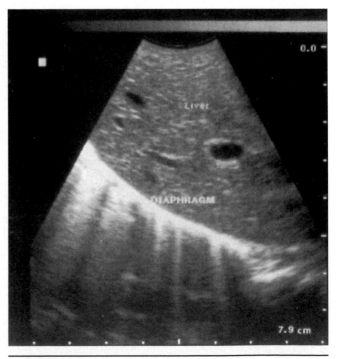

FIGURE 30. Diaphragm, longitudinal scan.

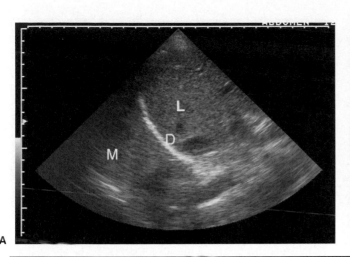

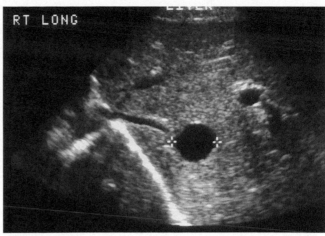

A   B

FIGURE 31. **A, B:** Both images show echogenic diaphragm (D) with liver (L) to right and mirror image artifact (M) to left of diaphragm.

than usual and the liver parenchyma may be less echogenic than the adjacent renal cortex. This has been referred to as a "starry-night liver" but is an uncommon finding.

Fatty Infiltration

Fatty infiltration is most commonly associated with alcohol in adults and malnutrition in children. It can also be seen with diabetes mellitus, hyperlipidemia, obesity, parenteral hyperalimentation, corticosteroid access, pregnancy, and Reye's syndrome (5,10,11). A more homogeneous dense pattern and liver enlargement favor a diagnosis of fatty infiltration over cirrhosis where the pattern is dense and more heterogeneous and the liver size may be reduced.

Fatty infiltration may be geographic rather than diffuse. Focal fat usually has defined borders, and entire lobes or segments can be affected (Fig. 33) (11,12). Areas of focal fat sparing are also common within a fatty infiltrated liver (Fig. 34). Focal sparing commonly occurs in segments 5 and 4 adjacent to the gallbladder; it has been suggested that the blood supply of the gallbladder influences the distribution of fat in the adjacent liver (13).

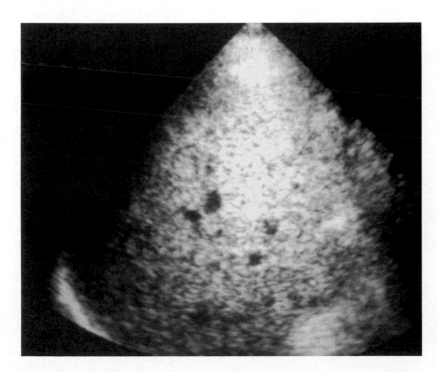

FIGURE 32. Hyperechoic liver due to fatty infiltration.

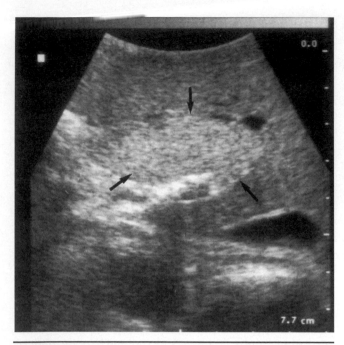

FIGURE 33. Focal fatty infiltration with well-defined margin (*arrows*).

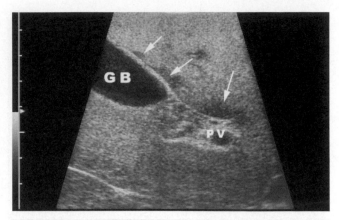

FIGURE 34. Areas of focal fat sparing (*arrows*). These hypo-echoic areas are located adjacent (anterior) to the gallbladder (GB) and the portal vein (PV).

Other common locations of fat sparing are the porta hepatis (anterior to the portal vein), adjacent to the falciform ligament, the dorsal left lobe, and the caudate lobe (11).

Both focal hepatic fat and focal fat sparing might simulate a neoplastic mass (12,14). Differentiation depends on recognition of the typical appearance and location of these processes. Focal fat and sparing tend to have a pyramidal shape with tapered margins (11). Unlike malignant masses, these do not displace adjacent vessels and a peripheral halo is absent.

Cirrhosis

The cirrhotic liver is hyperechoic and heterogeneous (Fig. 35). The overall size of the liver may be reduced but the caudate lobe or the lateral segment of the left lobe may be enlarged, whereas the right lobe is small (volume redistribution). Ratios of the size of the caudate lobe to the right lobe have been used to diagnose cirrhosis but are not always accurate (15). The liver edge may have a lobulated contour that can be better appreciated if there is ascites (11). Focal masses may represent regenerative

FIGURE 35. Cirrhotic liver. Note irregular, hyperechoic pattern. Lobulated contour is easily appreciated because of ascites (*black area anterior to the liver*).

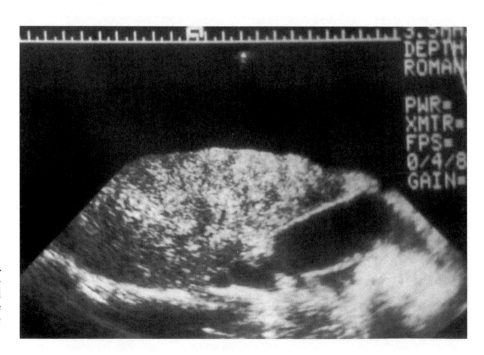

nodules or hepatocellular carcinoma. Sonographic findings of portal hypertension may be present including absent or diminished respiratory variation in portal vein size and flow, hepatofugal flow, portosystemic shunts, splenomegaly, and portal vein thrombosis.

Hepatic Cysts

The sonographic hallmarks of a simple hepatic cyst are a smooth, anechoic, round or oval structure with well-defined walls (Fig. 36). The posterior wall is typically sharp and there is posterior acoustic enhancement. Lateral or edge shadows are caused by refraction of the sound beam at the cyst margins. Internal echoes signify a complicated cyst with dense fluid, hemorrhage, infection, or a solid lesion. Occasionally a hypoechoic, homogeneous solid lesion simulates characteristics of a cyst. In this circumstance, the gain and time–gain compensation settings on the ultrasound console can be manipulated and low-level internal echoes may be detected in the solid lesion. In polycystic liver disease, multiple anechoic masses of varying size may be seen as well as associated renal cysts.

Liver Abscesses

The sonographic appearance of hepatic abscesses is variable depending on the age and cause of the lesion. Most pyogenic and amebic abscesses are primarily fluid filled, so they are hypoechoic with good sound transmission. They also contain debris and septation, so they are com-

plex with internal echoes (16). Pyogenic abscesses have a variable internal echo pattern that is often irregular and coarse (17). Amebic abscesses tend to contain more even, low-level echoes and are often found at the periphery of the liver (18). Fungal abscesses may appear as multiple, small, hypoechoic foci; they may have a target or "bull's-eye" appearance with a hyperechoic center and a hypoechoic peripheral ring (5). The presence of gas in an abscess produces a very hyperechoic reflection with acoustic shadowing or reverberation artifacts.

Echinococcal disease of the liver also produces cystic lesions with internal debris and echoes due to daughter cysts and septations (19). A double wall representing the endocyst and pericyst may be seen. Calcification in the wall of chronic hydatid cysts casts acoustic shadows.

Hematoma

The appearance of a hematoma in the liver varies by age (20). Initially, a well-defined hyperechoic mass is seen. Later it becomes hypoechoic and demonstrates characteristics of a complex cyst with septations and internal echoes. The subcapsular or intrahepatic location of a hematoma can be readily determined.

Cavernous Hemangioma

Cavernous hemangiomas are common benign lesions in the liver and often have a characteristic ultrasound appearance (21) (Fig. 37). Classically, these are small (most less than 3 cm), well-defined, rounded masses. They have

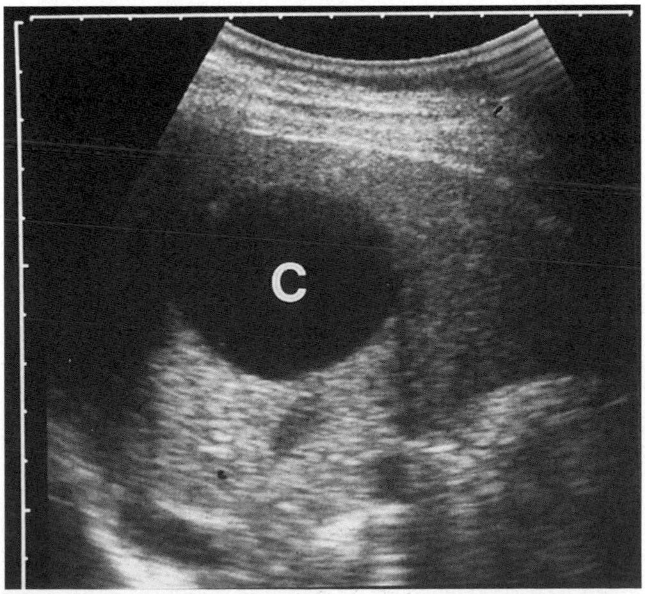

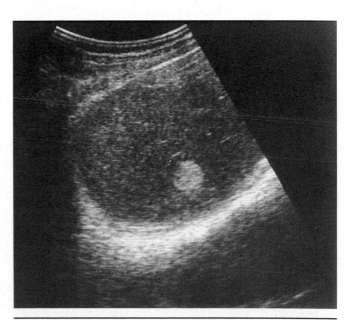

FIGURE 36. Simple hepatic cyst (C). Note smooth round margin, anechoic interior, posterior enhancement and edge shadows.

FIGURE 37. Hepatic hemangioma, showing a typical hyperechoic feature.

a homogeneous, dense echogenic pattern. Posterior enhancement may be seen. Some hemangiomas, particularly if they are larger, have an atypical appearance; they may be irregular and more heterogeneous in echogenicity and must be differentiated from other mass lesions, including malignancy.

Hepatic Adenoma and Focal Nodular Hyperplasia

Hepatic adenoma and focal nodular hyperplasia are two solid lesions that must be distinguished from cancers. The clinical features and imaging characteristics facilitate distinction of these two lesions (22–24). Unfortunately, sonographic findings are not diagnostic. Hepatic adenomas most commonly are solitary, well-defined echogenic masses. They may have irregular hypoechoic areas due to hemorrhage and necrosis, which occurs in a large proportion of the lesions. In patients with glycogen storage disease, adenomas may be multiple and may ap-

pear hypoechoic due to the increased echogenicity of the surrounding fatty liver (20). Focal nodular hyperplasia is variably echogenic and occasionally, although not commonly, will have a central scar visible as a nonshadowing hyperechoic focus (25).

Hepatocellular Cancer

Primary hepatocellular cancer can have variable sonographic findings. Smaller tumors (less than 3 cm) are usually hypoechoic and commonly demonstrate posterior enhancement (26–30). Typical characteristics of larger tumors are a mosaic internal echo pattern, posterior echo enhancement, lateral shadows, and a peripheral hypoechoic halo (27,29,30). Except for a peripheral halo, these features are uncommonly found in metastatic liver cancers (30). Daughter nodules may be detected (Fig. 38) as well as extension into major hepatic vessels.

Metastatic Tumors

Metastatic tumors are the most common hepatic malignancies. The sonographic appearance of tumors metastatic to the liver depends on multiple factors including size, histologic type, growth pattern, vascularity, and secondary changes such as necrosis, fibrosis, and hemorrhage. The

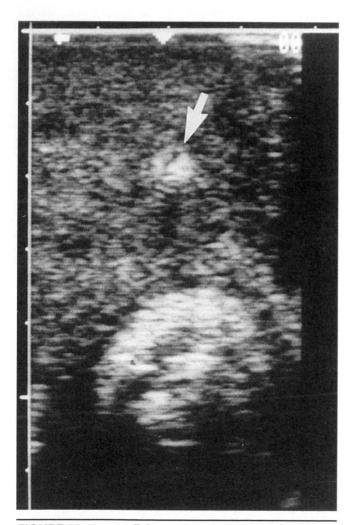

FIGURE 38. Hepatocellular carcinoma with hyperechoic mixed pattern, thin halo, and daughter nodule (*arrow*).

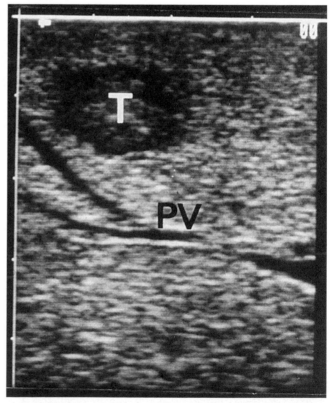

FIGURE 39. Hypoechoic metastatic liver tumor (T). PV, portal vein branch.

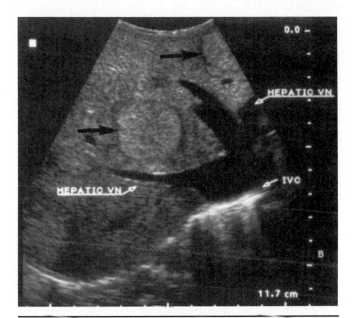

FIGURE 40. Multiple, slightly hyperechoic metastatic tumors (*black arrows*) with hypoechoic margins. Relationship to hepatic veins near inferior vena cava nicely demonstrated.

echogenic pattern may be hypoecloic, hyperechoic, isoechoic, or mixed. In general, smaller tumors are hypoechoic relative to the normal hepatic parenchyma (Fig. 39). Larger tumors tend to be more heterogeneous with hyperechoic and mixed areas (Fig. 40). A marginal hypoechoic zone or halo is characteristically seen around many metastatic liver tumors (Fig. 41). This may be referred to as a target or bull's-eye pattern. The presence of a halo nearly always suggests that the liver tumor is malignant. The shape and borders of metastatic tumors are often irregular. The retrotumoral echo pattern can be absent or demon-

strate irregular shadowing but is rarely enhanced. Some classic sonographic features of primary hepatocellular cancers are rarely observed in metastatic liver cancers; these include mosaic pattern, posterior echo enhancement, and bilateral edge shadows (30). (See also Chapter 15.)

Clinical Results of Liver Ultrasound

TAUS has proved highly accurate for the detection of liver tumors. Although the reported specificity of TAUS for identification typically exceeds 95%, sensitivity tends to be lower and more variable with figures ranging from 40% to 95% (31–34). TAUS is more accurate than carcinoembryonic antigen (CEA) levels as a screening test for hepatic metastases from colorectal cancer but it is less sensitive than CT or MRI, particularly in the detection of smaller lesions (32,33,35). Duplex and color Doppler sonography improve the accuracy of tumor detection. They also aid distinction between malignant and benign lesions and between primary hepatocellular cancer and metastatic cancers (36,37). TAUS is more accurate than CT to distinguish liver cysts from solid tumors, particularly when lesions are small and uncharacterizable by CT.

Because of its diagnostic accuracy, TAUS has become a valuable screening tool for primary hepatocellular carcinoma in patients with cirrhosis (31,38–41). It is more sensitive than serum α-fetoprotein and in some studies was superior to CT, MRI, angiography, or laparoscopy (39,41–43). Modern techniques of Doppler sonography, such as power Doppler or contrast-enhanced Doppler, have been useful for differentiating small hepatocellular cancers from benign regenerative nodules (44,45).

BILIARY TRACT

Indications

Some of the clinical indications for biliary ultrasound are shown in Table 4. The indication for TAUS that is most familiar to general surgeons is for the diagnosis of gallstone disease in patients who may have upper abdominal pain, abnormal liver or pancreatic chemistries, or other upper gastrointestinal symptoms. TAUS can also facilitate the diagnosis of acute cholecystitis by demonstrating typical sonographic findings in the appropriate clinical

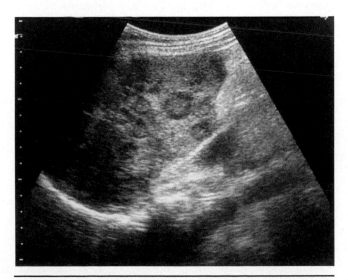

FIGURE 41. Typical hypoechoic halos of multiple metastatic tumors from a breast cancer.

▶ **TABLE 4 Clinical Indications for Transabdominal Ultrasound of the Biliary Tract**

- Detection of gallstones
- Evaluation of abnormal liver or pancreatic chemistries
- Evaluation of jaundice
- Assessment for postoperative complications
- Guidance for percutaneous interventions

situation. TAUS is not as reliable for the detection of stones in the common bile duct.

TAUS has been a standard initial imaging study for the evaluation of patients with abnormal liver enzymes to detect hepatic parenchymal or biliary tract abnormalities. For jaundiced patients, in particular, it is indicated to identify bile duct dilatation as evidence for possible mechanical obstruction. When obstructive jaundice is present, TAUS can help determine the level of obstruction and the potential cause.

If biliary tract tumors are suspected, TAUS can yield important information as to the extent of liver invasion, the presence of liver or lymph node metastases, and vascular involvement. Additional studies, such as contrast cholangiography, CT, or magnetic resonance cholangiopancreatography (MRCP), are usually necessary prior to planning resection.

TAUS can be valuable for the postoperative assessment of potential problems following cholecystectomy or other biliary operations. Specifically, it is indicated to detect subhepatic or subphrenic fluid collections that may be bilomas or abscesses. TAUS can demonstrate bile duct dilatation, which may indicate a retained common duct stone or bile duct injury.

Finally, TAUS is indicated to guide percutaneous biliary interventions, particularly tube placement for cholecystostomy, drainage of postoperative fluid collections, and transhepatic cholangiography and drainage.

Normal Ultrasound Anatomy of the Biliary Tract

Gallbladder

The normal gallbladder is a anechoic, roughly oval-shaped structure (Fig. 42). The dimensions of a normal fasted gallbladder are 8 to 10 cm in the longitudinal axis and less than 4 cm in the transverse axis. The gallbladder is fluid filled, so it has the sonographic characteristics of a cyst with good sound transmission and posterior acoustic enhancement. Low-level internal echoes may be seen due to mucus or thick bile. The gallbladder walls are sharply defined with a normal thickness of up to 3 mm. Gallbladder wall thickness is measured anteriorly on transverse scans adjacent to the liver; the posterior wall may not be well seen due to acoustic enhancement and neighboring bowel gas. Increased wall thickness is a nonspecific finding that can be seen in many conditions (46,47).

TAUS identification of the gallbladder may be difficult or may fail if the gallbladder is contracted or calcified or if there is proximal biliary obstruction or excessive bowel gas (46,48). Recognition of the gallbladder's anatomic position at the end of the main lobar fissure may be useful. If the echogenic fissure can be identified extending inferiorly from the right portal vein, it can be followed downward to the gallbladder neck (sulcus sign) (49).

Normal variations in gallbladder anatomy can occasionally confound sonographic interpretation. About 15% of individuals will have septations or folds in the gallbladder (50). A fold in the gallbladder near the fundus is known as a phrygian cap. The junctional fold is found at the junction of the gallbladder body and neck (51). These folds may appear as echogenic foci and may even shadow, thus mimicking stones. Unusual anomalies of the gallbladder include ectopic locations (intrahepatic, left sided, falciform ligament, suprahepatic), congenital hypoplasia or absence, and variations of gallbladder duplication (52).

Bile Duct

The segment of the bile duct regularly visualized by TAUS is in the region of the common hepatic duct and proximal common bile duct. The duct is a sonolucent tubular

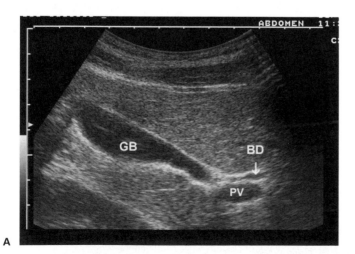

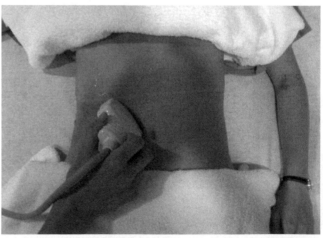

FIGURE 42. A: Long axis scan of gallbladder (GB) and common bile duct (BD) anterior to portal vein (PV). **B:** The probe position to obtain this image.

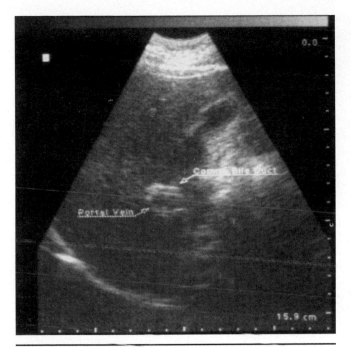

FIGURE 43. Normal bile duct (common hepatic duct) anterior to portal vein.

▶ TABLE 5 Ultrasound Criteria for Gallstones
1. Hyperechoic intraluminal focus
2. Posterior acoustic shadowing
3. Mobility

(53). The duct diameter may also increase up to 8 to 10 mm following cholecystectomy (54).

The distal common bile duct is more difficult to identify on TAUS and may be seen in fewer than half of patients (46). Interference from duodenal air and lack of a good acoustic window provided by the liver limits visualization. Unless dilated, the intrahepatic bile ducts are not normally well seen by TAUS. (See also Chapter 14).

Pathologic Ultrasound Anatomy of the Biliary Tract

Gallbladder

Cholelithiasis

Careful biplanar imaging of the entire gallbladder is required for the evaluation of cholelithiasis. There are three classic sonographic criteria for the diagnosis of gallstones (Table 5): (a) presence of a hyperechoic intraluminal focus, (b) posterior shadowing, (c) mobility: movement of the focus to a dependent position with changes in patient position (Fig. 44). If all three of these criteria are met, the diagnosis of gallstones is essentially assured (46). The diagnosis can be more difficult when all of these criteria are not satisfied. Small stones may not produce shadows (Fig. 45). Shadowing is best detected if the sound beam is focused at the level of the stone so that the beam is as narrow as possible at that site, ideally, narrower than the diameter of the stone.

structure anterior to the portal vein (Fig. 43). Because the cystic duct junction is not routinely identified, it is not possible to determine with certainty if the duct at this site is actually the common hepatic duct or the common bile duct. In transverse scans, the duct is a round structure lateral to the hepatic artery and anterior to the portal vein. An internal diameter of 6 mm is considered the upper normal size limit for the bile duct measured at this site (46,50). A duct diameter of more than 7 mm in an adult is considered dilated; a 6- to 7-mm-diameter duct is equivocal. Allowances are made for an increase in duct size with aging of about 1 mm per decade after 50 years

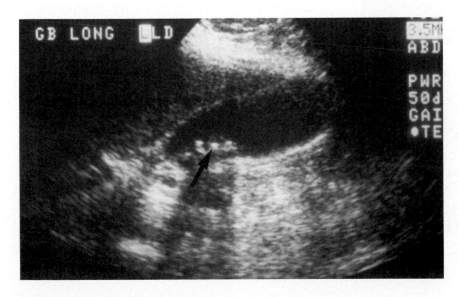

FIGURE 44. Typical sonographic features of gallstones (*arrow*) include hyperechoic foci with posterior acoustic shadowing.

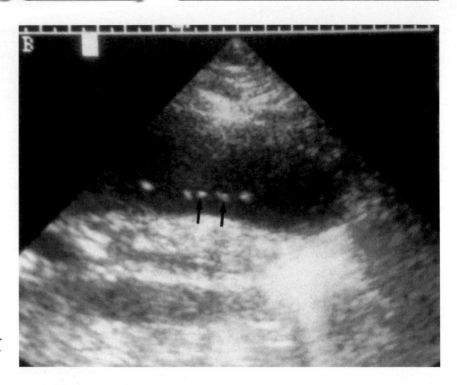

FIGURE 45. Small, floating gallstones (*arrows*) with minimal shadowing.

Lowering the gain may also facilitate detection of shadowing from small foci. A hyperechoic focus may shadow but not move. This could represent an impacted stone, but bowel gas, wall calcification, gallbladder folds or septations, or a cystic duct valve could cause similar findings. When the gallbladder is contracted, as in chronic cholecystitis, stones may be seen as hyperechoic, shadowing structures in the gallbladder fossa although the gallbladder lumen itself may not be seen. Gallbladder sludge, which is composed of calcium bilirubinate crystals and phospholipid, typically produces homogeneous low-level echoes in the dependent portion of the gallbladder (Fig. 46) (50). Sludge does not shadow, but it may move slowly with positional changes. Nonmobile sludge or a sludge ball may resemble a tumor.

Acute Cholecystitis

Sonographic features of acute calculous cholecystitis are listed in Table 6 and shown in Fig. 47 (46,50). Because the stone may be impacted in the neck or cystic duct, it may not move. Gallbladder wall thickening, pericholecystic fluid, and tenderness in the region of the gallbladder when examined with the ultrasound transducer are all nonspecific findings. Fewer than half of patients with acute cholecystitis may demonstrate wall thickening (55). Hypoechoic stripes or bands representing edema within the gallbladder wall may be seen. In emphysematous cholecystitis, air in the gallbladder wall produces dense echoes and irregular posterior shadows (56,57).

Hyperplastic Cholecystoses

The hyperplastic cholecystoses are benign proliferative conditions of the gallbladder that include choles-

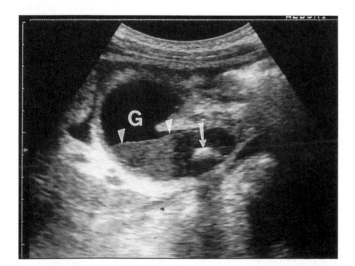

FIGURE 46. Gallstone (*arrow*) and a layering of sludge (*arrowheads*). G, gallbladder lumen.

▶ **TABLE 6 Ultrasound Features of Acute Calculous Cholecystitis**

1. Gallstones
2. Thick gallbladder wall (>3 mm)
3. Gallbladder distention
4. Pericholecystic fluid
5. Sonographic Murphy's sign

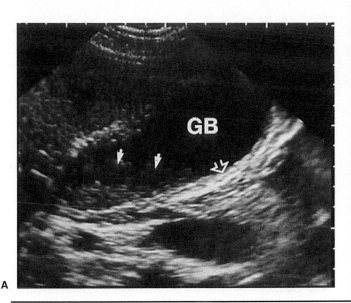
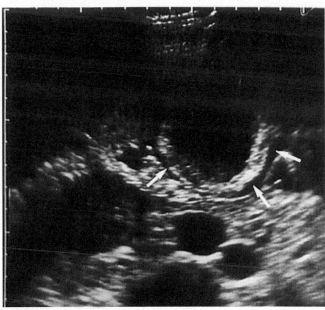

A

B

FIGURE 47. Acute cholecystitis. **A:** Gallbladder (GB) with sludge (*closed arrows*) and wall thickening (*open arrow*). **B:** Rim of pericholecystic fluid (*arrows*).

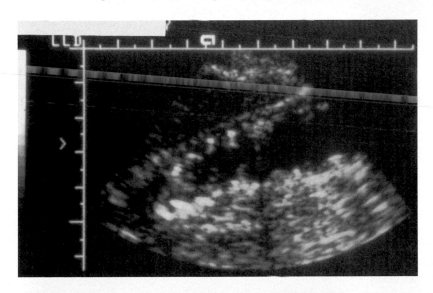

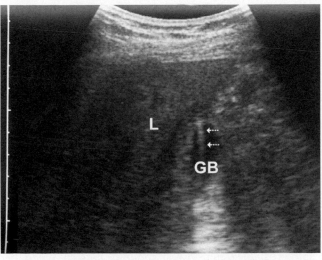
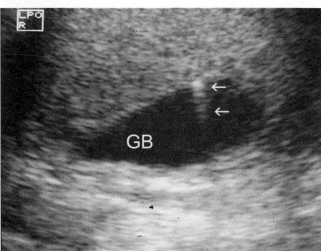

A

B

FIGURE 48. Cholesterolosis of gallbladder. Multiple, nonshadowing, nonmobile hyperechoic foci with "comet tail" reverberation artifacts.

FIGURE 49. **A, B:** Cholesterol polyp. Hyperechoic focus with comet tail artifact (*arrows*). GB, gallbladder, L, liver.

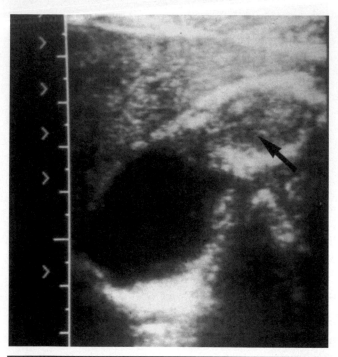

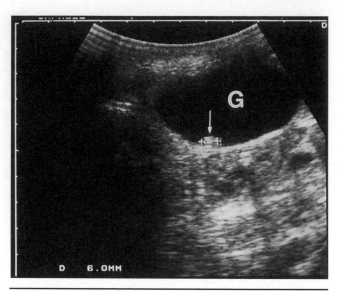

FIGURE 51. Gallbladder polyp (6 mm): nonshadowing, non-mobile echogenic focus (*arrow, cursors*). G, gallbladder lumen.

FIGURE 50. Fundal adenomyomatosis. Nonmobile, echogenic "pseudotumor" (*arrow*).

terolosis and adenomyomatosis (58). Cholesterolosis involves abnormal deposition of cholesterol precursors and lipids within macrophages in the gallbladder wall. The planar or diffuse form of cholesterolosis ("strawberry gallbladder") may yield a spotty appearance on ultrasound (Fig. 48). Hyperechoic intramural foci with "comet tail" artifacts may be seen In the polypoid form, cholesterol polyps develop attached to the gallbladder wall (Fig. 49) (59). These appear as nonmobile, nonshadowing echogenic masses within the gallbladder lumen and must be differentiated from neoplastic polyps. Some cholesterol polyps may cast weak shadows.

In adenomyomatosis, there is hyperplasia of the gallbladder mucosa and muscularis. Mucosal invaginations known as Rokitansky–Aschoff sinuses are found within the gallbladder wall and may be seen as hyperechoic foci. Segmental, diffuse, and focal forms of adenomyomatosis are recognized. Focal involvement of the fundus is most commonly seen (Fig. 50). Ultrasound imaging demonstrates wall thickening; focal forms are identified as echogenic masses that often mimic gallbladder neoplasms (60).

Neoplasms

Gallbladder polyps are echogenic intraluminal masses that typically do not shadow or move (Fig. 51). Neoplastic polyps may be adenomas or cancers; the likelihood of malignancy increases with polyps larger than 10 mm (61). Ultrasound characteristics, including size, echogenicity, and growth pattern, can be useful for differentiating

neoplastic polyps from cholesterol polyps, but these features are not perfect discriminants (62). Generally, neoplastic polyps are less echogenic than cholesterol polyps.

Gallbladder cancers may have several sonographic appearances (63–65). Fungating tumors demonstrate non-shadowing intraluminal echoes (Fig. 52). Localized infiltrating tumors present as hyperechoic or hypoechoic wall thickening with a transition zone to normal gallbladder wall. Tumors that are diffusely infiltrating show irregular wall thickening. TAUS is useful for detecting gallbladder cancer and for evaluating the local extent of disease such as liver infiltration. However, its accuracy for detecting metastases to lymph nodes or peritoneum is limited (66).

Bile Ducts

Bile Duct Obstruction

Dilatation of the intrahepatic or extrahepatic bile ducts is the sonographic hallmark of biliary obstruction (Fig. 53). As previously noted, the upper limit of extra-hepatic bile duct size by sonographic criteria is 6 to 7 mm. The smaller, intrahepatic branches of the bile duct are not normally seen on TAUS. Dilated intrahepatic ducts have an irregular appearance with multiple branches. The total number of ducts appears increased. The bile ducts are adjacent to the portal vein branches and are considered dilated if their caliber is equal to or larger than that of the adjacent portal vein (Fig. 54). On longitudinal scans, the dilated duct and portal vein branch have a "double channel" appearance; on transverse scans, the same structures may give a "shotgun" pattern. When there is marked intrahepatic duct dilatation, the bile ducts taper

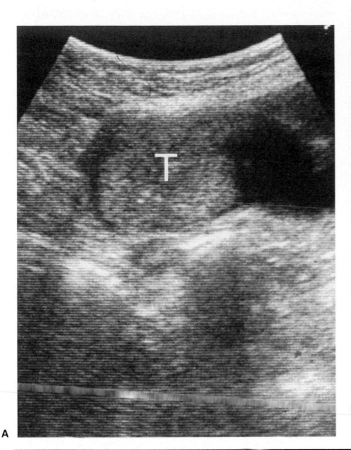
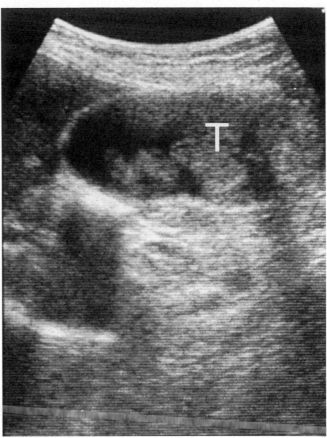

A   B

FIGURE 52. A, B: Gallbladder cancer: echogenic intraluminal mass (T).

less smoothly toward the periphery than the portal vein branches (67).

When bile duct dilatation is present, additional ultrasound information may indicate the cause of obstruction. Attempts should be made to identify the level of obstruction, the presence of stones or masses, and whether the

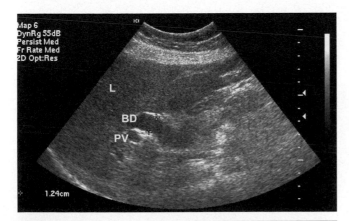

FIGURE 53. Dilated extrahepatic bile duct (BD), 12.4 mm. Note that duct is larger than portal vein (PV). L, liver. (Courtesy of Dr. Maurice Arregui.)

pattern of intrahepatic bile duct dilatation is diffuse or focal. If the obstruction is distal, the head of the pancreas should be carefully examined.

Choledocholithiasis

TAUS is not a sensitive method for visualizing stones in the distal bile duct. This is unfortunate because this is the site where they most commonly are found. The distal duct may be difficult to identify because of adjacent bowel gas, if the bile duct is not dilated or the bile duct stone does not shadow. When a bile duct stone is detected sonographically, however, it is a highly specific finding (Fig. 55). Common bile duct stones may be best detected during TAUS on sagittal scans with the patient in the 45-degree left posterior oblique position or by transverse scanning with the patient erect (4,68).

Pneumobilia

Air in the bile duct exhibits hyperechogenicity and shadowing, which must be differentiated from calculi. Air bubbles frequently produce reverberation or comet tail (ring down) artifacts (Fig. 56). This helps distinguish pneumobilia from biliary calculi because rever-

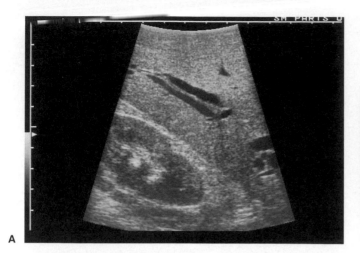
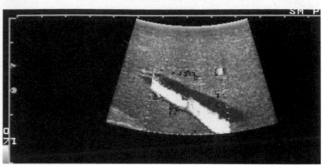

A   B

FIGURE 54. A: Dilated intrahepatic bile duct and portal vein branch appear as parallel channels. B: Color Doppler ultrasound demonstrates flow in portal vein. (See Color Plate 16.)

beration artifacts are not seen with the latter. (See also Chapter 14.)

Clinical Results of Biliary Tract Ultrasound

The clinical results of biliary TAUS are best described according to the clinical indication for which TAUS was obtained. The accuracy of TAUS for the detection of cholelithiasis exceeds 95% (69). One of the most common diagnostic errors occurs when stones impacted in the gallbladder neck or cystic duct are not recognized. Inac-

curacies can also result when stones are small or when imaging of the gallbladder is difficult due to contraction, bowel gas, or obesity.

TAUS is unreliable for diagnosing common bile duct stones. The sensitivity of TAUS based on actual sonographic visualization of duct stones is low, ranging from 10% to 45% (70,75). The sonographic finding of bile duct dilatation is also an unreliable indicator of choledocholithiasis. Among patients undergoing cholecystectomy, 30% to 40% with dilated ducts by TAUS do not have duct stones. Conversely, 20% to 33% of patients with choledocholithiasis do not have dilated ducts (70–,75). However,

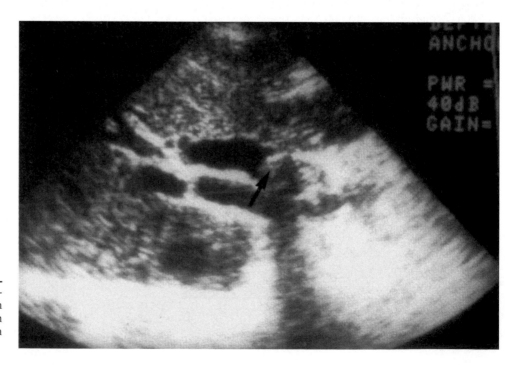

FIGURE 55. Choledocholithiasis. Shadowing stone (arrow) in distal common bile duct with proximal dilatation. Portal vein is seen posteriorly.

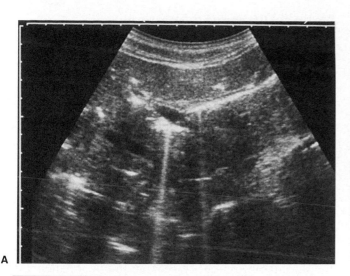
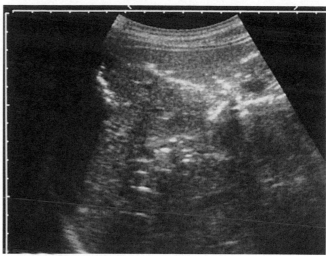

FIGURE 56. A, B: Pneumobilia in intrahepatic ducts with echogenicity and ring-down artifact.

on occasions when TAUS does visualize a common bile duct stone, it is a highly specific finding with a positive predictive value approaching 100%.

TAUS examination of the liver, biliary tract, and pancreas is frequently performed during the evaluation of patients with abnormal liver enzyme elevations. Significant abnormalities such as gallstones, hepatic parenchymal disease or malignancy have been diagnosed by ultrasound in over 60% of asymptomatic patients with abnormal biochemical liver tests (76). The sonographic demonstration of bile duct dilatation in nonjaundiced patients subsequently shown to have extrahepatic obstruction suggests that ultrasound is a more sensitive indicator of bile duct obstruction than serum bilirubin (77,78).

TAUS has long been used to evaluate jaundiced patients. Diffuse liver disease as a cause of jaundice can be diagnosed by ultrasound in a substantial percentage (60%) of patients (79). Yet the primary goal of ultrasound in jaundice is to identify or exclude bile duct dilatation; this presumes that dilated ducts indicate mechanical obstruction whereas nondilated ducts indicate nonobstructive or hepatic jaundice.

Prospective studies have compared the results of TAUS to those of endoscopic retrograde cholangiopancreatography (ERCP) for the diagnosis of mechanical obstruction (80–82). The specificity of TAUS is 92% to 95% but the sensitivity is lower (55% to 84%). The accuracy of TAUS for diagnosing duct dilatation has also been evaluated by comparing preoperative TAUS findings to intraoperative cholangiograms obtained during cholecystectomy (74,75). Lichtenbaum and colleagues reported ultrasound sensitivity of only 25% for detecting a common bile duct diameter greater than 8 mm on intraoperative cholangiography and concluded that preoperative ultrasound was neither sensitive nor specific for diagnos-

ing common bile duct dilatation (74). Different results were noted by Stott et al., who found that preoperative ultrasound accurately identified common bile duct dilatation (sensitivity 96%, specificity 95%) (75). These disparate findings might be explained by differences in the methods for determining duct size from intraoperative cholangiography, in the time intervals between studies, in controlling for injection pressure during cholangiography and by selection bias. Nonetheless, it is clear that mechanical obstruction of the common bile duct can exist without sonographic dilatation and that sonographic dilatation does not necessarily indicate obstruction.

Despite these limitations, TAUS has traditionally been the preferred initial imaging study for jaundiced patients because of its ease, availability, relative inexpensiveness, and high positive predictive value. Furthermore, TAUS has been valuable for determining the level and cause of blockage in patients with known obstructive jaundice. In a series of 102 patients, Okuda and Tsuchiya were able to detect the approximate level of obstruction in 101 patients and to identify the obstructing lesion itself in 69 (69).

MRI could supersede TAUS for screening patients with suspected biliary tract disease if it were more widely and readily available and less expensive. One study has shown that the sensitivity of MRI is higher than that of ultrasound or of ERCP for the diagnosis of jaundiced patients and patients with upper abdominal pain without jaundice (83).

PANCREAS

Indications

The primary indications for TAUS of the pancreas are for the evaluation of neoplastic disease and for the identifi-

▶ TABLE 7 Indications for Transabdominal
Ultrasound of the Pancreas

- Detection of neoplastic lesions
- Staging pancreatic malignancy, determination of resectability
- Acute pancreatitis
    - Gallstones
    - Fluid collections
    - Ascites
- Pancreatic pseudocysts
    - Detection
    - Serial follow-up
- Guidance for percutaneous interventions

cation and follow-up of complications of pancreatitis (Table 7). Although CT is more frequently used for evaluating pancreatic tumors, TAUS can be performed as an initial examination. For example, in patients with jaundice, TAUS may detect pancreatic head tumors. Resectability of pancreatic cancer may be determined by assessing vascular invasion or liver metastases. Islet cell tumors may be localized by TAUS preoperatively.

In acute pancreatitis, TAUS is performed to verify the presence or absence of gallstones as a potential etiologic factor. TAUS findings can also be used to diagnose and follow acute pancreatic fluid collections, pancreatic ascites, or associated pleural effusions.

TAUS is particularly useful for the diagnosis and follow-up of pseudocysts complicating chronic pancreatitis. One of the criteria for the interventional management of pseudocysts associated with chronic pancreatitis is pseudocyst enlargement. Pseudocyst size can be conveniently monitored with serial TAUS examinations.

Normal Ultrasound Anatomy of the Pancreas

The pancreas is located posterior to the stomach in the lesser sac and the head is surrounded by the duodenum. Posterior to the pancreas are several major blood vessels that are important landmarks for scanning the pancreas (Fig. 57). The shape and size of the pancreas vary with age and body habitus. The normal thickness (anterior to posterior diameter) of the pancreas is 2.5 to 3.5 cm for the head and 2.0 to 3.0 cm for the body (5,20,84).

Sonographically, the pancreas in adults is homogeneous and moderately echogenic. The echogenicity is greater than or equal to that of the liver. In the elderly, fatty replacement of the glandular tissue occurs and the echogenicity increases further, to become equal to that of the surrounding retroperitoneal fat. In this situation, the border of the pancreas is obscured and the gland blends into the background retroperitoneal tissue. In children, the pancreas may be less echogenic than the liver.

The main pancreatic duct is a tubular structure with echogenic walls. It appears as two parallel echoes separated by an anechoic lumen or as a single linear echo. The diameter of the normal duct measures about 3 mm in the head, 2 mm in the body, and 1.5 mm in the tail (20). A duct diameter larger than 2 mm in the midline is considered abnormal in individuals younger than 60 years (85).

The splenic vein courses posterior to the pancreatic body. The confluence of the splenic vein and the superior mesenteric vein is wrapped by the pancreatic head and the uncinate process; a part of the uncinate lies posterior to the vein. The border and the extent of the uncinate process are sometimes obscured, especially in the elderly.

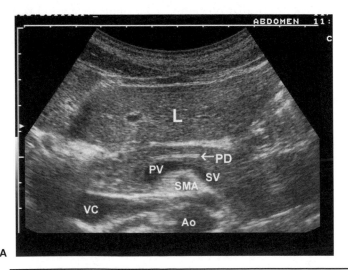

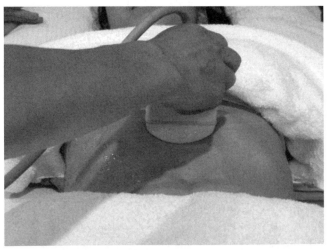

A   B

FIGURE 57. A: Transverse scan of pancreas. L, liver; PD, pancreatic duct; PV, portal vein; SV, splenic vein; SMA, superior mesenteric artery; VC, vena cava; Ao, aorta. Hypoechoic channel between aorta and SMA is left renal vein. **B:** The probe position.

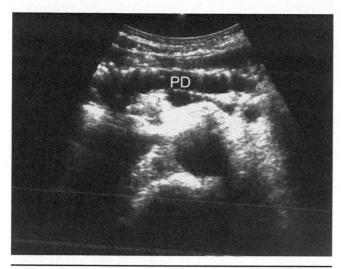

FIGURE 58. Chronic pancreatitis. Dilated pancreatic duct (PD) anterior to splenic and portal vein.

The proximal portion of the superior mesenteric artery courses posterior to the pancreatic body. Cephalad to the pancreatic body, the celiac axis and its branches are visualized. Caudad to the body, the left renal artery and vein are visualized. (See also Chapter 10).

Pathologic Ultrasound Anatomy of the Pancreas

Chronic Pancreatitis

The sonographic findings in chronic pancreatitis are varied and can be significant. These findings include increased echogenicity, focal or diffuse enlargement, focal dense echoes, pseudocyst formation, and common bile duct dilatation (5,20,84,86,87). Pancreatic parenchymal calcifications may interfere with sonographic imaging. The main pancreatic duct may be of normal size or may be dilated; pancreatic duct calculi may be detected as hyperechoic foci with or without acoustic shadowing (Fig. 58). At times, the duct may have combinations of strictures and dilated areas producing a "chain of lakes" appearance. Ectatic branches of the main pancreatic duct may appear as small cysts.

Pseudocysts

TAUS is particularly well suited to the identification and localization of pancreatic pseudocysts. Pseudocysts are anechoic or hypoechoic with posterior enhancement (Fig. 59). They may have internal echoes due to debris or blood (Fig. 60). Serial sonograms are valuable for assessing the evolution or resolution of pancreatic pseudocysts and peripancreatic fluid collections.

Acute Pancreatitis

The sonographic features of acute pancreatitis vary with severity and stage of the disease (5,20,84). In contrast to chronic pancreatitis, acute pancreatitis is characterized

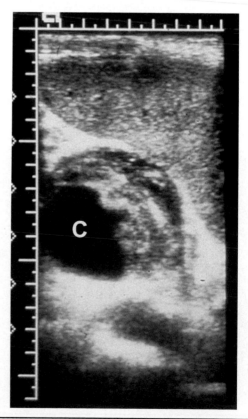

FIGURE 60. Pseudocyst (C) in tail of pancreas next to spleen. Note echogenic blood within pseudocyst.

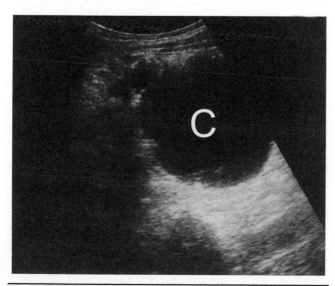

FIGURE 59. Pancreatic pseudocyst (C).

by relative hypoechogenicity of the parenchyma due to edema. In mild acute pancreatitis, there may be no changes detectable by TAUS. Hemorrhage and necrosis produce echogenic areas, and associated pancreatic or peripancreatic fluid collections may be seen. Pancreatic abscesses have cystic characteristics, but they contain debris and are not often well defined by TAUS. Evaluation of the biliary tract for gallstones or bile duct dilatation is an important component of the ultrasound examination for patients with acute pancreatitis.

Pancreatic Carcinoma

Pancreatic adenocarcinomas are usually relatively hypoechoic compared to the normal pancreatic tissue, although larger tumors have a mixed echogenic pattern (Figs. 61 and 62) (5,20). TAUS can identify tumors as small as 1 cm if the gland is adequately visualized (84). Dilatation of the common bile duct or main pancreatic duct caused by tumor obstruction can be recognized. Pancreatic cancer may be associated with enlargement of the gland or irregularity in contour. TAUS can provide useful staging information in some cases of pancreatic malignancy, such as demonstration of portal vein or superior mesenteric vein invasion or hepatic metastases. When vascular invasion is present, the echogenic wall of the vessel is distorted or destroyed (Fig. 63).

Cystic Neoplasms

Besides pancreatic pseudocysts, TAUS can delineate other cystic diseases of the pancreas and their relation to surrounding structures. However, the distinction be-

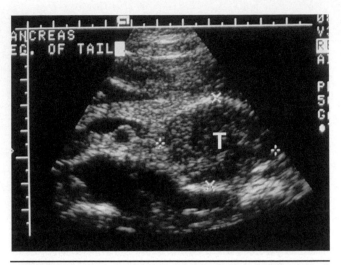

FIGURE 62. Hypoechoic tumor (T) in tail of pancreas.

tween mucinous (macrocystic) and serous (microcystic) cystadenoma and between cystadenoma and cystadenocarcinoma is difficult to make. Serous cystadenoma appears as multiple small cysts or even as an echogenic mass. Mucinous cystadenoma contains larger cysts, and papillary tumor growth may be seen within the cysts (Fig. 64). Involvement or distortion of adjacent blood vessels suggests cystadenocarcinoma.

Islet Cell Tumors

A pancreatic islet cell tumor (including insulinoma and gastrinoma) appears as a distinct, round, homogeneous, hypoechoic mass within the pancreas (Fig. 65). Less frequently, it may be isoechoic with the surrounding pancreas with a hypoechoic rim. TAUS may detect islet cell tumors of 5 to 10 mm. If a possible lesion is encountered, the probe should be rotated 90 degrees while the lesion is kept in view, then the lesion is scanned in the perpendicular plane to ensure that it is a true lesion (i.e., round in all directions). Once the tumor has been identified, its distance to the margin of the pancreas and its relationship to the pancreatic duct and adjacent structures can be ascertained. The entire pancreas should be screened to diagnosis or exclude multiple tumors. (see also Chapter 16).

Clinical Results of Pancreas Ultrasound

The accuracy of TAUS for detection of adenocarcinoma of the pancreas is 80% to 95%. The sensitivity for diagnosing liver metastases in patients with pancreatic malignancy exceeds 90% (84). Endoscopic ultrasonography is superior to TAUS and to CT scans for the diagnosis of periampullary tumors and also for tumor staging and for the detection of lymph node metastases or vascular invasion (88,89). However, TAUS is superior to endoscopic ul-

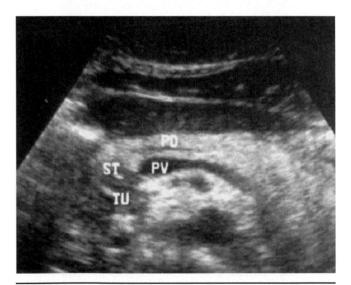

FIGURE 61. Transverse scan of cancer in pancreatic head without portal vein invasion. PD, pancreatic duct; PV, portal vein; ST, bile duct stent; TU, tumor.

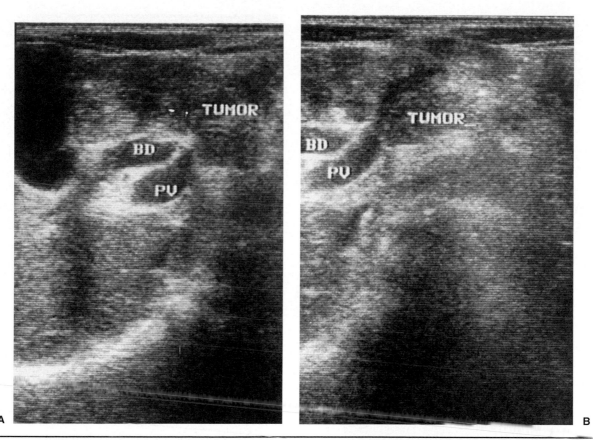

FIGURE 63. A, B: Longitudinal scans of pancreas cancer obstructing the bile duct (BD) and invading the portal vein (PV).

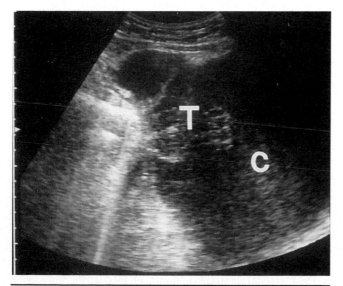

FIGURE 64. Pancreatic cystadenocarcinoma with tumorous (T) and cystic (C) components.

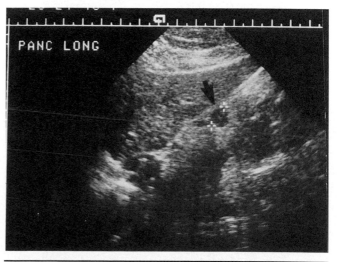

FIGURE 65. Hypoechoic insulinoma (*black arrow*) in body of pancreas. This is a sagittal scan through the left lobe of the liver.

ultrasound and comparable to CT scan for identifying distant metastases from periampullary tumors (89). TAUS is effective in the detection of about 60% of small (less than 2 cm) pancreatic islet cell tumors, which is comparable to CT (90). In the spectrum of islet cell tumors, it is least successful for visualizing insulinomas, since these β cell tumors are typically small and the patients are often obese (91). TAUS is useful for diagnosing pancreatic pseudocysts, but its accuracy is not as high as that of CT, largely due to technically inadequate studies (92).

INTERVENTIONAL TRANSABDOMINAL ULTRASOUND

Background

Ultrasound is a well-established imaging guide for the performance of a number of transabdominal procedures on the liver, biliary tract, and pancreas. TAUS-guided interventions entail placement of different types of needles and catheters for both diagnostic and therapeutic purposes. Ultrasound and CT are complementary image guidance techniques. TAUS guidance is preferred over CT

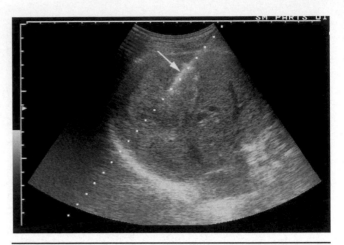

FIGURE 67. Transabdominal ultrasound guided liver biopsy. Needle (*arrow*) seen along puncture guide marks. Note tumor with halo.

guidance in certain circumstances, particularly when expediency and portability are at a premium. The direction of needle placement may also be more flexible with ultrasound guidance. For example, biopsy of a liver lesion located near the diaphragm using CT guidance may require traversing the lung, a route that might be avoided using an ultrasound-directed subcostal or intercostal approach. In other situations, the presence of impediments to sonographic visualization, such as air and bone, will give CT superior guidance capability.

The general principles that govern all ultrasound-guided interventions apply to hepatobiliary and pancreatic procedures as well (see Chapter 4). TAUS-guided interventions are usually performed under local anesthesia with or without conscious sedation. Percutaneous needle or catheter placement is done during direct real-time visualization of the target; typically a needle guidance system is used (Fig. 66). Since the 1970s, a variety of interventional hepatobiliary and pancreatic procedures have been performed using TAUS guidance including needle biopsy, drainage of liver abscesses, cyst aspiration, cholecystostomy, transhepatic cholangiography and biliary drainage, drainage of pancreatic pseudocysts or fluid collections, ablation of hepatic tumors, and even pancreatic duct puncture for aspiration or ductography and puncture of the portal vein branches for portography.

Ultrasound-Guided Needle Biopsy

TAUS-directed needle biopsies of the liver and pancreas are performed to obtain specimens for both cytologic and histologic examinations. For cytology, fine needle aspiration biopsy is performed with a 21- to 23-gauge needle without a stylet, a 10-cm-long 18-gauge needle to accommodate the fine needle, a 10-ml syringe, a needle guide, sterile acoustic coupling gel, and a sterile tray. The trans-

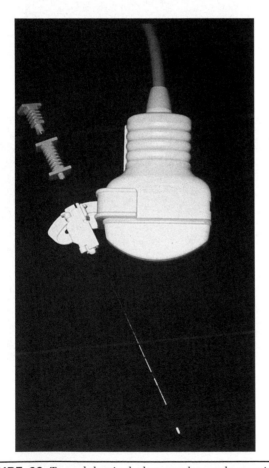

FIGURE 66. Transabdominal ultrasound transducer with attached needle guidance system.

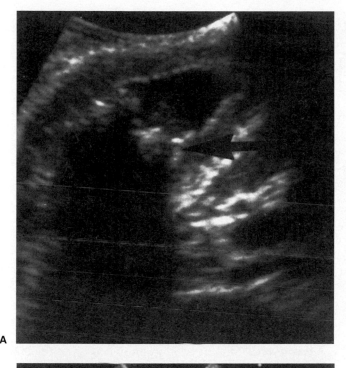

A

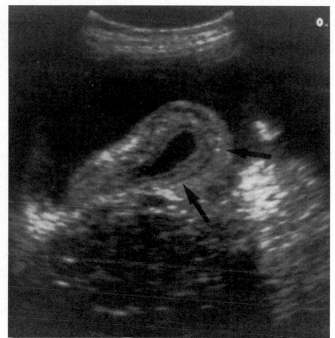

B

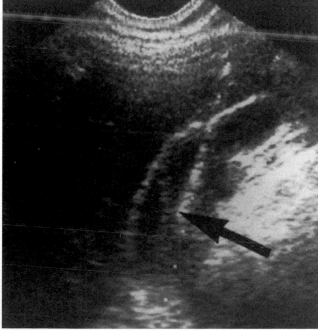

C

FIGURE 68. Acute cholecystitis. **A:** Gallbladder with gallstones (*arrow*). The walls of the gallbladder are inflamed. **B:** Splitting of layers in the gallbladder wall. Gallbladder (*arrow*) seen in pool of ascites. **C:** Ultrasound-guided puncture of the gallbladder. Note the needle-tip echo (*arrow*).

ducer is positioned with the electronic puncture guide on the scanner screen and traversing the target. The anticipated entry point of the needle is marked on the skin. The gel used for the initial scan is wiped off, the skin is cleaned and the area draped as for minor surgery, and local anesthetic is administered. The needle guidance system is mounted on the sterilized or draped transducer and sterile gel is applied. The transducer is again positioned so that the puncture line intersects the target and the 18-gauge guide needle is inserted through the needle

guidance system. The guide needle is only inserted 1 or 2 cm depending on the thickness of the abdominal wall. The fine needle attached to the 10-mL syringe is then inserted through the guide needle. It is seen moving along the puncture line as a bright spot indicating the position of the needle tip (Fig. 67). Not uncommonly, the needle deviates slightly and may have to be retracted and reinserted. Loss of the tip echo indicates deviation. The transducer may be tilted back and forth slightly until the needle echo is found. When the needle is inside the target,

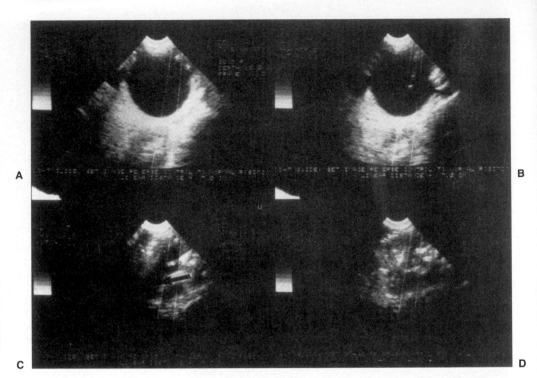

FIGURE 69. Ultrasound-guided puncture of a pancreatic pseudocyst. **A:** The cyst is seen traversed by the puncture line. **B:** The needle tip (*arrow*) is seen in the cyst. **C:** There has been substantial emptying of the cyst. The remaining fluid is marked with an arrow. **D:** The cyst is nearly empty.

full suction is applied with the syringe and the needle is moved in and out of the lesion several times. Then the needle is removed. Normally up to three needle passes are made sampling different areas of the target.

For histologic specimens, a core-cutting needle of 18 to 20 gauge is used. The needle is inserted in the same way as previously described and advanced with the stylet in place. A small skin incision is recommended to overcome resistance to needle passage. The biopsy is taken by advancing the cutting needle into the target (manually or automatically depending on needle design). The needle is removed and the tissue core is gently dislodged onto a small piece of paper. Typically, two or three needle passes are performed.

Currently, hepatic lesions are more frequently biopsied for histology using a core needle, particularly with an automated spring-loaded biopsy gun. Pancreatic lesions are commonly examined by fine needle aspiration cytology. The success rate for cytologic or histologic biopsy is high and complications, although possible, are uncommon (93–96).

Cholecystostomy

The gallbladder is readily accessible for needle aspiration and puncture catheterization for both diagnosis and treatment (97–100). Percutaneous cholecystostomy may obviate the need for cholecystectomy in certain high-risk patients. The transhepatic puncture route is preferred to avoid bile leaks (Fig. 68). Either the trocar or the

Seldinger technique may be used (see Chapter 4). Soft pig tail or balloon catheters are most frequently used because they secure the catheter in place. Other occasional indications for ultrasound-guided puncture of the gallbladder include diagnostic aspiration for chemical or bacterial examination, diagnostic cholecystocholangiography, and fine needle biopsy.

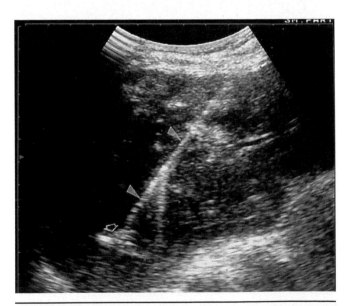

FIGURE 70. Ultrasound-guided percutaneous placement of cannula (*arrowheads*) for radiofrequency ablation of liver tumor (*open arrow*).

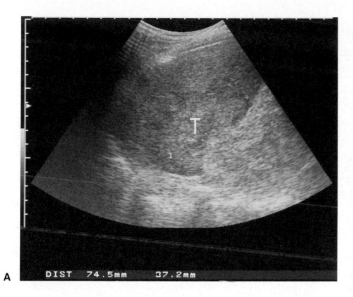

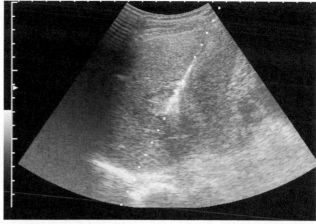

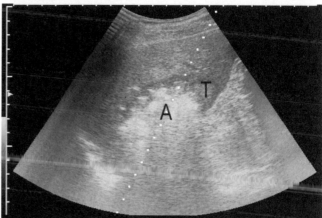

FIGURE 71. **A:** A 7.5-cm metastatic tumor (T) from sigmoid colon cancer in segment 6 extending to segment 7. **B:** An electrode cannula was inserted into the tumor under transabdominal ultrasound guidance. **C:** First the posterior areas of the tumor were ablated. The ablated areas (A) became hyperechoic. T indicates the anterior area of the tumor to be ablated subsequently.

Pancreatic Pseudocyst Puncture

Pancreatic pseudocysts or fluid collections can be punctured for either diagnostic or therapeutic purposes using TAUS guidance (Fig. 69) (101,102). For diagnostic aspiration, an 18- or 20-gauge needle is used. The aspirated fluid is checked for amylase, and culture and cytologic examination are carried out. Percutaneous catheter drainage of pseudocysts is performed using pigtail catheters varying in size from 6F to 10F or sometimes larger. The puncture route may be transperitoneal, retroperitoneal, or transgastric. The indications for percutaneous drainage of any pancreatic collection, as well as the most appropriate method of drainage (operative, percutaneous, endoscopic), should be made on an individual basis in consultation with an experienced pancreatic surgeon.

Hepatic Tumor Ablation

Percutaneous ablation of hepatic tumors can be accomplished under TAUS guidance (Fig. 70) (103,104). Treatment may involve injection of chemical agents or application of various energy sources for destruction of tumor cells by heating or freezing. Depending on tumor size and

location, TAUS allows percutaneous placement of energy delivering electrodes or probes into the lesion and monitoring the ablation process (Fig. 71). Tumors located beneath the diaphragm or on the inferior surface of the liver are not as well treated percutaneously because of poorer detection by TAUS or the risk of injury to adjacent organs, especially the gastrointestinal tract. The details of ultrasound-guided ablation of liver tumors are described in Chapters 4, 13, and 15.

ADVANTAGES AND DISADVANTAGES OF TAUS

TAUS has considerable advantages when compared with other methods of body imaging such as CT or MRI (Table 8). Modern ultrasound transducers and computer-enhanced machines provide images that are superbly detailed and accurate. TAUS can be performed rapidly, within minutes, which is a tremendous asset in the acute care setting and for the efficient elective evaluation of any patient. TAUS studies can be repeated as quickly and as often as necessary to verify results or to assess a

▶ TABLE 8 Advantages and Disadvantages
of Transabdominal Ultrasound

Advantages
- Accurate
- Rapid
- Easily repeatable
- Versatile
- Portable
- Available
- Safe

Disadvantages
- Interference from air, bone, fat
- Lower resolution than intraoperative ultrasound

changing clinical situation. Ultrasound is extremely versatile, with a wide range of probes suitable to examination of virtually any anatomic site. The portability of ultrasound machines cannot be matched by other body imaging modality. TAUS can be performed anywhere: in the office, in the emergency room, in the operating room, in the intensive care unit, or at the bedside. Critically ill or unstable patients need not be transported. Ultrasound imaging is cost effective, and capable ultrasound machines are widely available. Finally, ultrasound imaging is extremely safe. Patients are not exposed to ionizing radiation, and the biomechanical effects of diagnostic sound waves are negligible.

The primary limitations of TAUS result from anatomic or mechanical factors that interfere with image acquisition. Fat, air, and bone are confounding elements. Because the sound waves must penetrate the abdominal wall, TAUS requires the use of lower frequency transducers than does intraoperative or laparoscopic ultrasound. Therefore, the resulting images will have lower resolution. In general, the larger the abdominal wall, the poorer the image. In the upper abdomen, the ribs limit probe placement and produce shadows that eliminate segments of the image. Bowel gas is a common impediment to good TAUS imaging. Proper patient preparation and the use of various maneuvers can overcome these limitations to a degree, but not entirely.

CONCLUSIONS

Surgeons who are competent in TAUS have added value for the assessment of patients with suspected disease of the liver, biliary tract, or pancreas, both preoperatively and postoperatively. TAUS can provide focused and clinically relevant information that may directly influence the management of a patient's condition. For selected patients, TAUS can guide the surgeon in the performance of a number of diagnostic and therapeutic interventions.

REFERENCES

1. American Institute of Ultrasound in Medicine. *Standard presentation and labeling of ultrasound images*, 1999.
2. Tempkin BB. *Ultrasound scanning principles and protocols*, 2nd ed. Philadelphia: WB Saunders, 1998.
3. Okuda K, Tsuchiya Y. Ultrasonic anatomy of the biliary system. *Clin Gastroenterol* 1983;12:49–63.
4. Laing FC, Jeffrey RB, Wing WW. Improved visualization of choledocholithiasis by sonography. *AJR Am J Roentgenol* 1984;143:949–952.
5. Sauerbrei EE, Nguyen KT, Nolan RL. *Abdominal sonography*. New York: Raven Press, 1992.
6. Bismuth H. Surgical anatomy and anatomical surgery of the liver. *World J Surg* 1982;6:3–9.
7. Parulaker SG. Ligaments and fissures of the liver: sonographic anatomy. *Radiology* 1979;130:409–411.
8. Kane RA. Sonographic anatomy of the liver. *Semin Ultrasound* 1981;2:190–197.
9. Couinaud C. *Le foie. Etudes anatomiques et chirurgicales*. Paris: Masson, 1957.
10. Igidbashian VN, Jibin L, Goldberg BB. Hepatic ultrasound. *Semin Liver Dis* 1989;9:16–31.
11. Tchelepi H, Ralls PW, Radin R, et al. Sonography of diffuse liver disease. *J Ultrasound Med* 2002;21:1023–1032.
12. Quinn SF, Gosink BB. Characteristic sonographic signs of hepatic fatty infiltration. *AJR Am J Roentgenol* 1985;145:753–755.
13. Aubin B, Denys A, LaFortune M, et al. Focal sparing of liver parenchyma in steatosis: role of the gallbladder and its vessels. *J Ultrasound Med* 1995;13:77–80.
14. White EM, Simmeone JF, Mueller PR, et al. Focal periportal sparing in hepatic fatty infiltration: a cause of hepatic pseudomass on ultrasound. *Radiology* 1987;162:57–59.
15. Giorgio A, Ambroso P, Lettieri G, et al. Cirrhosis: value of caudate to right lobe ratio in diagnosis with ultrasound. *Radiology* 1986;161:443–445.
16. Subramanyam BR, Balthazor EJ, Raghavendra BN, et al. Ultrasound analysis of solid appearance abscesses. *Radiology* 1983;146:487–491.
17. Newlin N, Silver TM, Stuck J, et al. Ultrasonic features of pyogenic liver abscesses. *Radiology* 1981;139:155–159.
18. Ralls PW, Barnes PF, Radin DR, et al. Sonographic features of amebic and pyogenic liver abscesses: a blinded comparison. *AJR Am J Roentgenol* 1987;149:499–501.
19. Beggs I. The radiologic appearances of hydatid disease of the liver. *Clin Radiol* 1983;34:555–563.
20. Krebs C, Giyanani VL, Eisenberg RL. Ultrasound atlas of disease processes. Norwalk, CT: Appleton & Lange, 1993.
21. Mirk P, Rubaltelli L, Bazzocchi M, et al. Ultrasonographic patterns in hepatic hemangiomas. *J Clin Ultrasound* 1982;10:373–378.
22. Rogers JV, Mack LA, Freeny PC, et al. Hepatic focal nodular hyperplasia: angiography, CT, sonography and scintigraphy. *AJR Am J Roentgenol* 1981;137:983–990.
23. Sandler MA, Petrocelli RD, Marks DS, et al. Ultrasonic features and radionuclide correlation in liver cell adenoma and focal nodular hyperplasia. *Radiology* 1980;135:393–397.
24. Welch TJ, Sheedy PA, Johnson CM, et al. Focal nodular hyperplasia and hepatic adenoma: comparison of angiography, CT, US and scintigraphy. *Radiology* 1985;156:593–595.
25. Scatarige JC, Fishman EK, Sanders RC. The sonographic "scar sign" in focal nodular hyperplasia of the liver. *J Ultrasound Med* 1982;1:275–278.
26. Sheu JC, Chen DS, Sung JL, et al. Hepatocellular carcinoma: ultrasound evolution in the early stage. *Radiology* 1985;155:463–467.
27. Higashi T, Tobe K, Asano K, et al. Ultrasonographic characteristics of small hepatocellular carcinoma. *Acta Med Okayama* 1988;42:151–157.
28. Takayasu K, Moriyama N, Muramatsue Y, et al. The diagnosis of small hepatocellular carcinomas: efficacy of various

imaging procedures in 100 patients. *AJR Am J Roentgenol* 1990;155:49–54.

29. Choi BI, Kim CW, Han MC, et al. Sonographic characteristics of small hepatocellular carcinoma. *Gastrointest Radiol* 1989;14:255–261.

30. Yoshida T, Matsue H, Okazaki N, et al. Ultrasonographic differentiation of hepatocellular carcinoma from metastatic liver cancer. *J Clin Ultrasound* 1987;15:431–437.

31. Tanaka S, Kitamura K, Nakanishi K, et al. Recent advances in ultrasonographic diagnosis of hepatocellular carcinoma. *Cancer* 1989;63:1313–1317.

32. Glover C, Douse P, Kane P, et al. Accuracy of investigations for asymptomatic colorectal liver metastases. *Dis Colon Rectum* 2002;45:476–484.

33. Yoshida T, Matsue H, Suzuki M, et al. Preoperative ultrasonography screening for liver metastases of patients with colorectal cancer. *Jpn J Clin Oncol* 1989;19:112–115.

34. Scholmerich J, Volk BA, Gerok W. Value and limitations of abdominal ultrasound in tumor staging-liver metastasis and lymphoma. *Eur J Radiol* 1987;7:243–245.

35. Wernecke K, Rummeny E, Bongartz G, et al. Detection of hepatic masses in patients with carcinoma: comparative sensitivities of sonography, CT and MR imaging. *AJR Am J Roentgenol* 1991;157:731–739.

36. Reinhold C, Hammers L, Taylor CR, et al. Characterization of focal hepatic lesions with duplex sonography; findings in 198 patients. *AJR Am J Roentgenol* 1995;164:1131–1135.

37. Leen E, Angerson WT, Wotherspoon H, et al. Detection of colorectal liver metastases: comparison of laparotomy, CT, US and Doppler perfusion index and evaluation of postoperative follow-up results. *Radiology* 1995;195:113–116.

38. Tanaka S, Kitamura T, Ohshima A, et al. Diagnostic accuracy of ultrasonography for hepatocellular carcinoma. *Cancer* 1986;58:344–347.

39. Sheu JC, Sung JL, Chen DS, et al. Early detection of hepatocellular carcinoma by real-time ultrasonography: a prospective study. *Cancer* 1985;56:660–666.

40. Maringhini A, Cottone M, Sciarrino E, et al. Ultrasonography and alpha-fetoprotein in diagnosis of hepatocellular cancer in cirrhosis. *Dig Dis Sci* 1988; 33:47–51.

41. Larcos G, Sorokopud H, Berry G, et al. Sonographic screening for hepatocellular carcinoma in patients with chronic hepatitis or cirrhosis: an evaluation. *AJR Am J Roentgenol* 1998;171:433–435.

42. Gandolfi L, Muratori R, Solmi L, et al. Laparoscopy compared with ultrasonography in the diagnosis of hepatocellular carcinoma. *Gastrointest Endosc* 1989;35:508–511.

43. Ebara M, Ohto M, Kondo F. Strategy for early diagnosis of hepatocellular carcinoma. *Ann Acad Med Singapore* 1989; 18:83–89.

44. Francanzani AL, Burdick L, Borzio M, et al. Contrast-enhanced Doppler ultrasonography in the diagnosis of hepatocellular carcinoma and premalignant lesions in patients with cirrhosis. *Hepatology* 2001;34:1109–1112.

45. Koito K, Namieno T, Morita K. Differential diagnosis of small hepatocellular carcinoma and adenomatous hyperplasia with power Doppler sonography. *AJR Am J Roentgenol* 1998;170:157–161.

46. Cohen SM, Kurtz AB. Biliary sonography. *Radiol Clin North Am* 1991;29:1171–1198.

47. Ralls P, Quinn MF, Juttner HU, et al. Gallbladder wall thickening: patients without intrinsic gallbladder disease. *AJR Am J Roentgenol* 1981;137:65–68.

48. Hammond DI. Unusual causes of sonographic nonvisualization or nonrecognition of the gallbladder: a review. *J Clin Ultrasound* 1988;16:77–85.

49. Callen PW, Filly RA. Ultrasonographic localization of the gallbladder. *Radiology* 1979;133:687–691.

50. Krebs C, Giyanni VL, Eisenberg RL. Biliary system: In: *Ultrasound atlas of disease processes*. Norwalk, CT: Appleton & Lange,1993:51–83.

51. Sukov RJ, Sample WF, Sarti DA, et al. Cholecystography: the junctional fold. *Radiology* 1979;133:435–436.

52. Linder HH. Embryology and anatomy of the biliary tree. In: Way LW, Pellegrini CA, eds. *Surgery of the gallbladder and bile ducts*. Philadelphia: WB Saunders, 1987:3–22.

53. Wu CC, Ho YH, Chen CY. Effect of aging on common bile duct diameter; a real time ultrasonographic study. *J Clin Ultrasound* 1984;12:473–478.

54. Niederau C, Muller J, Sonnenberg A, et al. Extrahepatic bile duct in healthy subjects, in patients with cholelithiasis, and in post-cholecystectomy patients: a prospective ultrasound study. *J Clin Ultrasound* 1983;11:23–27.

55. Saunders RC. The significance of sonographic gallbladder wall thickening. *J Clin Ultrasound* 1980;8:143–146.

56. Hunter ND. Acute emphysematous cholecystitis: an ultrasonic diagnosis. *AJR Am J Roentgenol* 1980;134:592–593.

57. Parulekar SG. Sonographic findings in acute emphysematous cholecystitis. *Radiology* 1982;145:117–119.

58. Berk RN, Begt JH, Lichtenstein JE. The hyperplastic cholecystoses: cholesterolosis and adenomyomatosis. *Radiology* 1983;146:593–601.

59. Ruhe AH, Zachman JP, Mulder BD, et al. Cholesterol polyps of the gallbladder: ultrasound demonstration. *J Clin Ultrasound* 1979;7:386–388.

60. Rice J, Sauerbrei EE, Semogas P, et al. Sonographic appearance of adenomyomatosis of the gallbladder. *J Clin Ultrasound* 1981;9:336–337.

61. Koga A, Watanabe K, Fukuyama T, et al. Diagnosis and operative indications for polypoid lesions of the gallbladder. *Arch Surg* 1988;123:26–29.

62. Kubota K, Bandai Y, Noie T, et al. How should polypoid lesions of the gallbladder be treated in the era of laparoscopic cholecystectomy? *Surgery* 1995;117:481–487.

63. Yum HY, Fink AH. Sonographic findings in primary carcinoma of the gallbladder. *Radiology* 1980;134:693–696.

64. Ruiz R, Teynann H, Ferrandes N, et al. Ultrasonic diagnosis of primary carcinoma of the gallbladder, a review of 16 cases. *J Clin Ultrasound* 1980;8:489–495.

65. Tsuchiya Y. Early carcinoma of the gallbladder: macroscopic features and US findings. *Radiology* 1991;179:171–175.

66. Bach AM, Loring LA, Hann LE, et al. Gallbladder cancer: can ultrasonography evaluate extent of disease? *J Ultrasound Med* 1998;17:303–309.

67. Laing FC, London LA, Filly RA. Ultrasonographic identification of dilated intrahepatic bile ducts and their differentiation from portal venous structures. *J Clin Ultrasound* 1978;6:90–94.

68. Parulekar SG, McNamara MP Jr. Ultrasonography of choledocholithiasis. *J Ultrasound Med* 1983;2:395–400.

69. Okuda K, Tsuchiya Y. Ultrasonography of the biliary tract. *Prog Liver Dis* 1982;7:285–297.

70. Koo KP, Traverso LW. Do preoperative indicators predict presence of common bile duct stones during laparoscopic cholecystectomy? *Am J Surg* 1996; 171:495–499.

71. Cronan JJ, Mueller PR, Simeone JF, et al. Prospective diagnosis of choledocholithiasis. *Radiology* 1983;146:467–469.

72. Gross BH, Harter LP, Gore RM, et al. Ultrasonic evaluation of common bile duct stones: prospective comparison with endoscopic retrograde cholangiography. *Radiology* 1985; 146:471–474.

73. O'Connor HJ, Hamilton I, Ellis WR, et al. Ultrasound detection of choledocholithiasis: prospective comparison with ERCP in the post cholecystectomy patient. *Gastrointest Radiol* 1986;11:161–164.

74. Lichtenbaum RA, McMullen HF, Newman RM. Preoperative abdominal ultrasound may be misleading in risk stratification for presence of common bile duct abnormalities. *Surg Endosc* 2000;14:254–257.

75. Stott MA, Farrands PA, Guyer PB, et al. Ultrasound of the common bile duct in patients undergoing cholecystectomy. *J Clin Ultrasound* 1991;19:73–76.

76. Ekberg O, Aspelin P. Ultrasonography in asymptomatic patients with abnormal biochemical liver tests. *Scand J Gastroenterol* 1986;21:573–576.

77. Weinstein BJ, Weinstein DP. Biliary tract dilatation in the nonjaundiced patient. *AJR Am J Roentgenol* 1980;134:899–906.
78. Gilbert FJ, Calder JF, Bayliss AP. Biliary tract dilatation without jaundice demonstrated by ultrasound. *Clin Radiol* 1985;36:197–198.
79. Taylor KJW, Rosenfield AT, Spiro HM. Diagnostic accuracy of gray scale ultrasonography for the jaundiced patient: a report of 275 cases. *Arch Intern Med* 1979;139:60–63.
80. Borsch G, Wegener M, Wedmann B, et al. Clinical evaluation ultrasound, cholescintigraphy and endoscopic retrograde cholangiography in cholestasis: a prospective comparative clinical study. *J Clin Gastroenterol* 1988;10: 185–190.
81. O'Connor KW, Snodgrass PJ, Swonder JE, et al. A blinded prospective study comparing four current noninvasive approaches in the differential diagnosis of medical versus surgical jaundice. *Gastroenterology* 1983;84:1498–1504.
82. Lindsell DR. Ultrasound imaging of pancreas and biliary tract. *Lancet* 1990;335:390–393.
83. Hakansson K, Ekberg O, Hakansson HO, et al. MR and ultrasound in screening patients with suspected biliary tract disease. *Acta Radiol* 2002;43:80–86.
84. Lees WR. Pancreatic ultrasonography. *Clin Gastroenterol* 1984;13:763–789.
85. Bryan PJ. Appearance of the normal pancreatic duct: a study using real time ultrasound. *J Clin Ultrasound* 1982; 10:63–66.
86. Alpern MB, Sandler MA, Kellman GM, et al. Chronic pancreatitis: ultrasonic features. *Radiology* 1985;155:215–219.
87. Huntington DK, Hill MC, Steinberg W. Biliary tract dilatation in chronic pancreatitis: CT and sonographic findings. *Radiology* 1989;172:47–50.
88. Chen CH, Tseng LJ, Yang CC, et al. The accuracy of endoscopic ultrasound, endoscopic retrograde cholangiopancreatography, computed tomography and transabdominal ultrasound in the detection and staging of primary ampullary tumors. *Hepatogastroenterology* 2001;48:1750–1753.
89. Chen CH, Tseng LJ, Yang CC, et al. Preoperative evaluation of preampullary tumors by endoscopic sonography, transabdominal sonography, and computed tomography. *J Clin Ultrasound* 2001;29:313–321.
90. Gunther RW, Klose KJ, Ruckert K, et al. Islet-cell tumors: detection of small lesions with computed tomography and ultrasound. *Radiology* 1983;148:485–488.

91. Shawker TH, Doppman JL, Dunnick NR, et al. Ultrasonic investigation of pancreatic islet cell tumors. *J Ultrasound Med* 1982;1:193–200.
92. Williford ME, Foster WL Jr, Halvorsen RA, et al. Pancreatic pseudocyst: comparative evaluation by sonography and computed tomography. *AJR Am J Roentgenol* 1983;140: 53–57.
93. Smith EH. Complications of percutaneous abdominal fine needle biopsy. *Radiology* 1991;178:253–258.
94. Fornari F, Civardi G, Cavanna L, et al. Complications of ultrasonically guided fine-needle abdominal biopsy: results of a multicenter Italian study and review of the literature. *Scand J Gastroenterol* 1989;24:949–955.
95. Nolsoe C, Nielsen L, Torp-Pedersen S, et al. Major complications and deaths due to interventional ultrasonography: a review of 8000 cases. *J Clin Ultrasound* 1990;18:179–184.
96. Livraghi T, Damascelli B, Lombardi C, et al. Risk in fine needle abdominal biopsy. *J Clin Ultrasound* 1983;11:77–81.
97. McGahan JP, Lindfors KK. Percutaneous cholecystectomy: an alternative to surgical cholecystostomy for acute cholecystitis? *Radiology* 1989;173:481–485.
98. Lohela P, Soiva M, Suramo I, et al. Ultrasound guidance for percutaneous puncture and drainage in acute cholecystitis. *Acta Radiol* 1986;27:543–546.
99. VanSonnenberg E, Wittich RG, Casola G, et al. Diagnostic and therapeutic percutaneous gallbladder procedures. *Radiology* 1986;160:23–26.
100. Vogelzang LR, Nemcek AA Jr. Percutaneous cholecystostomy. Diagnosis and therapeutic efficacy. *Radiology* 1988;168:29–34.
101. VanSonnenberg W, Wittich RG, Casola G, et al. Percutaneous drainage of infected and noninfected pancreatic pseudocysts: experience in 101 cases. *Radiology* 1989;170: 757–761.
102. Torres EW, Even BM, Baumgartner RB, et al. Percutaneous aspiration and drainage of pancreatic pseudocysts. *AJR Am J Roentgenol* 1986;147:1007–1009.
103. Rhim H, Dodd GD III. Radiofrequency ablation of liver tumors. *J Clin Ultrasound* 1999;5:221–229.
104. Curley SA, Izzo F, Delrio P, et al. Radiofrequency ablation of unresectable primary and metastatic hepatic malignancies: results in 123 patients. *Ann Surg* 1999;230:9–11.

Chapter 12

Other Transabdominal Ultrasound

José M. Velasco and Tina J. Hieken

Evaluation of the abdomen using real-time ultrasound has both diagnostic and therapeutic usefulness in the management of abdominal pathologic processes. Surgeons are particularly well suited to use ultrasound because of their knowledge of anatomy, their technical aptitude, and the opportunity to compare ultrasound images with intraoperative findings. Increasingly, sophisticated ultrasound equipment with multifrequency transducers, color Doppler imaging capabilities, and reusable biopsy guide attachments allow for simultaneous diagnostic and therapeutic interventions at the patient's bedside, as well as in the ambulatory setting and in the operating room.

Interventional ultrasound is used not only as an adjunct to guide biopsies (e.g., retroperitoneal masses) but also to guide therapeutic intervention (e.g., abscess drainage). Particularly relevant, given the escalation of health care costs, is the fact that ultrasound is less expensive than other imaging modalities. It is also safe and accessible. In this chapter, the indications for abdominal ultrasound, instrumentation, technique, clinical applications, advantages, and limitations will be reviewed as they apply to the surgeon. This chapter describes ultrasound of abdominal and retroperitoneal organs other than the liver, biliary tract, and pancreas, which are covered in Chapter 11.

INDICATIONS

Indications for abdominal ultrasound are continuously expanding. The patient with an acute abdomen frequently challenges the surgeon, particularly in the areas of diagnosis and operative decision making. Over the past several years, a plethora of innovative approaches have been introduced to enhance the treatment of these patients. These include patient care algorithms, evidence-based pathways, and imaging modalities such as helical computed tomography (CT), magnetic resonance imaging (MRI), isotope scanning, and minimally invasive techniques. Due to their cost, restricted availability, and

time-consuming nature, none of these approaches has gained widespread acceptance (1).

In the atraumatic acute abdomen, ultrasound can be an initial diagnostic test because it complements clinical findings, helps in selecting other diagnostic studies, provides a safe means of specimen procurement, and aids in establishing operative indications. Some patients benefit from ultrasound more than others do, including those with equivocal clinical findings, women with suspected appendicitis, patients with diverticulitis, inflammatory bowel disease, bowel obstruction, and even those with suspected perforated viscus or ischemic bowel.

Ultrasound of the abdominal wall, including the inguinal region, can aid in the differential diagnosis of hernias, postoperative seromas, and abdominal wall tumors. Moreover, ultrasound accurately defines the presence of abdominal wall adhesions (2).

Ultrasound is a powerful tool in diagnosing and managing postoperative complications, such as abscess, hemorrhage, acute cholecystitis, perforated viscus, and mechanical bowel obstruction. Other indications include the surveillance of solid organ injuries, evaluation of transplant grafts, and assessment of patency of portosystemic shunts. Ultrasound is being used also for biopsy of abdominal wall masses and retroperitoneal adenopathy, and for diagnosis and drainage of abdominal wall and intraabdominal lesions and fluid collections. Most importantly, interventional procedures can be performed with a high degree of accuracy and safety (Table 1) (3).

INSTRUMENTATION AND SCANNING TECHNIQUE

In general, ultrasound examination of the abdomen requires an ultrasound device equipped with a multifrequency sector (phased array), curvilinear array (convex), or linear array transducer (2.5 to 5 MHz). A higher frequency transducer (7.5 to 12 MHz) provides higher resolution, but at the cost of lower penetration; these probes are more suitable for examination of the abdominal wall

> **TABLE 1** Indications for Abdominal Ultrasound

1. Initial Diagnostic Test
   - Complements clinical findings
   - Guides diagnostic and therapeutic procedures
   - Aids in operative planning
2. Preoperative
   - Equivocal clinical findings
   - Women with suspected appendicitis
   - Inflammatory bowel disease, diverticulitis
   - Bowel obstruction
3. Postoperative
   - Abdominal wall: hernia, seroma
   - Intraabdominal fluid collections: drainage
   - Bleeding
   - Surveillance of solid organs

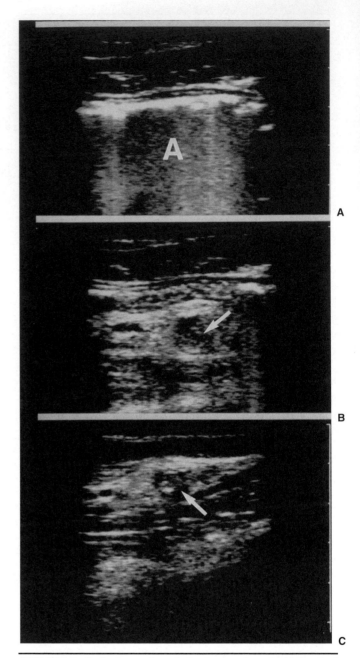

FIGURE 1. Technique of graded compression. **A:** Abdominal wall musculature and anterior wall of the terminal ileum are visible. Air trapped in the ileum results in reflection artifacts. **B:** Continuous pressure applied with the ultrasound probe displaces gas of the terminal ileum and a target lesion (*arrow*) located underneath the ileum, is identified. **C:** Further compression results in displacement of the ileum, allowing the identification of an 8-mm noncompressible target of acute appendicitis (*arrow*).

or for abdominal scanning in children. Color Doppler imaging capabilities optimize identification and definition of vascular structures; this knowledge is invaluable, particularly when interventional procedures are contemplated. In addition, a video printer and digital image storage system permit documentation for inclusion in the medical record, and for quality assurance and credentialing purposes.

The initial ultrasound examination of the abdomen starts with the patient in a supine position by systematically scanning the entire abdomen, not just the area of concern, for evidence of additional pathology (4). Examination of abdominal organs, including detection of fluid in dependent areas, can be performed first by placing the transducer in the subxiphoid area and by tilting it cephalad toward the pericardium. Next, the probe is moved toward the right midaxillary line, and scanning is continued subcostally and intercostally to visualize the liver, right kidney, right diaphragm, subhepatic space, and Morison's pouch. Placing the patient in the lateral decubitus position may facilitate detection of free fluid and pneumoperitoneum. Subsequently, the transducer is moved to the left anterior, middle, and posterior axillary lines to evaluate the left kidney, spleen, and left diaphragm intercostally. Next, the pancreas, upper gastrointestinal tract, retroperitoneum, and major upper abdominal vessels are scanned. Finally, it is important to move the probe to the midline, just superior to the symphysis pubis, because as little as 50 mL of fluid can be detected in the pouch of Douglas. An ultrasound-guided peritoneal tap and lavage, using a 21- or 22-gauge needle, may be performed in a safe and accurate manner (5). After the entire abdomen has been assessed, a more careful, detailed scan of suspicious areas must be performed. The abdominal wall, particularly the rectus sheath and inguinal region, should be scanned.

The technique of graded compression, as described by Puylaert (6), reduces the distance between the transducer and the bowel, and displaces gas, feces, intestine, or mesentery, thereby reducing or eliminating artifacts and interfaces. Gentle compression is gradually applied with the probe at the points of maximal tenderness in case of, for example, suspected acute appendicitis; continuous

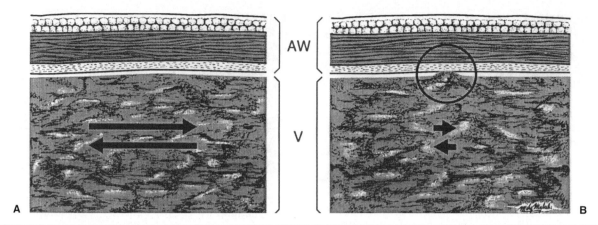

FIGURE 2. Schematic drawing of viscera slide (AW, abdominal wall; V, viscera). **A:** Normal viscera slide showing a wide excursion (*long arrows*) of viscera. **B:** Restricted viscera slide caused by an adhesion to the abdominal wall (*within circle*) that is characterized by a shorter excursion of viscera (*short arrows*). (From Sigel B, Golub RM, Loiacono LA, et al. Technique of ultrasonic detection and mapping of abdominal wall adhesions. *Surg Endosc* 1991;5:161–165, with permission.)

application of pressure improves the image (Fig. 1). As long as pressure is applied slowly and gently, the patient will tolerate it amazingly well.

Another useful technique involves the detection of restricted motion of viscera in reference to the abdominal wall for diagnosis of abdominal adhesions. Access to the abdominal cavity during laparotomy or laparoscopy may be problematic in the presence of adhesions since tedious dissection is required and organ injury may ensue. Intraabdominal adhesions restrict the normal motion of intraabdominal organs, including the bowel, liver, omentum, and stomach, with respect to each other and to the abdominal wall. Visceral slide occurs either spontaneously as a result of respiratory movements or can be induced by compression of the abdomen. A real-time linear array or curvilinear transducer with a wide footprint is desirable to provide the longest field of view. Restricted viscera slide is defined as an ultrasonically detected movement of viscera of less than 1 cm in relation to the abdominal wall (Fig. 2). Both spontaneous and induced viscera slide are noted. When a normal spontaneous slide exists, it is not mandatory to perform an induced slide (Figs. 3 and 4). Should restricted spontaneous viscera slide be present during respiration and/or exaggerated

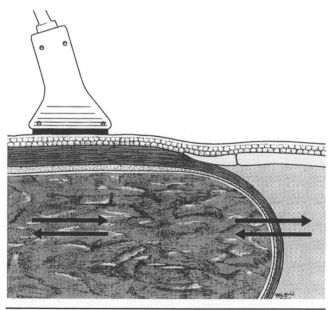

FIGURE 3. Schematic drawing of spontaneous viscera slide. Respiratory movement of the diaphragm (*right arrows*) produces a viscera slide (*left arrows*) beneath the transducer on the abdominal wall. (From Sigel B, Golub RM, Loiacono LA, et al. Technique of ultrasonic detection and mapping of abdominal wall adhesions. *Surg Endosc* 1991;5:161–165, with permission.)

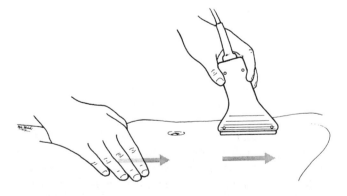

FIGURE 4. Manual compression (*left arrow*) of the abdominal wall produces induced viscera slide (*right arrow*) beneath the transducer. The direction of compressive force lies along the scan path of the transducer (linear axis of the transducer). (From Sigel B, Golub RM, Loiacono LA, et al. Technique of ultrasonic detection and mapping of abdominal wall adhesions. *Surg Endosc* 1991;5:161–165, with permission.)

breathing, it should be confirmed by longitudinal and transverse induced slide methods. The extent of restriction at a particular site must be compared with that at other sites to define whether the restriction is a localized or a generalized phenomenon (2,7).

INTERVENTIONAL ULTRASOUND TECHNIQUE

Interventional ultrasound has been used as a diagnostic adjunct to guide biopsies as well as a therapeutic procedure to guide drainage of intraabdominal fluid collections (8,9). The basics of interventional ultrasound are detailed in Chapter 4. For interventional abdominal ultrasound, a needle guidance system (needle guide) is frequently used. The needle guide should have a puncture canal of sufficient length (3 to 4 cm) and it should allow release of the needle easily since catheter placement may follow the initial puncture. In addition, needle guides of different calibers from 14 to 23 gauge must be available to accommodate different needles; alternatively, an adjustable needle-steering device is available (12 to 20 gauge). It is advisable to use the thinnest needle possible so as to avoid complications. An electronically generated puncture-line and echogenic needles aid greatly, especially during one's initial experience. The appropriate needle size for aspiration of fluid collections, cysts, and abscesses is 18 to 20 gauge, whereas 22- to 23-gauge needles are used for cytology. Either a Menghini or a True-Cut needle of 14 to 21 gauge can be used to obtain tissue core biopsies. A spring-loaded automated biopsy needle device facilitates both aspiration and tissue biopsy.

Two basic methods of percutaneous drainage exist: puncture drainage of a collection with subsequent lavage through an 18-gauge needle or insertion of a drainage catheter. The usual drainage catheter is a multihole, pigtail type measuring from 6F to 10F, inserted either by a guidewire exchange (Seldinger) technique or a one-step trocar technique. It is imperative that the tip of the catheter, and preferably the entire catheter, constantly be kept under direct visualization. The drainage can be accomplished in most cases with local anesthesia, although in some cases conscious sedation may be required.

Interventional abdominal ultrasound is an invasive procedure; therefore, the patient's history determines any preprocedural testing. In addition, equipment should be sterilized and the patient's abdomen should be prepared. Though the published mortality and morbidity falls below 0.05% (10), an informed consent from the patient is mandatory (11). While fine needle aspiration of a midabdominal fluid collection can be performed safely, even in the presence of intervening bowel loops, the passage of a large-gauge drainage catheter into that same collection could result in a catastrophic intestinal injury (12).

▶ **TABLE 2 Ultrasound for Acute Abdomen**

- Acute appendicitis
- Cholecystitis and biliary obstruction
- Intestinal obstruction
- Hernia
- Intestinal perforation
- Acute colonic diverticulitis

Disadvantages of ultrasound do exist. Because ultrasound does not penetrate bone or air well, its efficacy may be limited in the midabdomen due to intestinal gas. Mechanisms for sterilization are cumbersome, frequently mandating the use of sterile covers. Finally, the relatively steep learning curve may dampen the neophyte surgeon's enthusiasm. Therefore, it is often the case that initially the assistance of an experienced ultrasonographer is invaluable.

ULTRASOUND OF ABDOMINAL DISEASES

In general, ultrasound of the abdomen can provide direct visualization of a diseased viscus and can identify indirect signs such as inflammatory wall thickening or periintestinal fluid collections. A western European database of abdominal conditions requiring urgent operative intervention identified six diagnoses amenable to ultrasound characterization (Table 2) (13). In addition, ultrasound can be used in the imaging of abdominal wall and retroperitoneal pathologic processes as well as splenic and abdominal vascular diseases (14).

Abdominal Wall

Ultrasound of the abdominal wall provides the surgeon with important information (Table 3) about palpable masses, particularly in the difficult-to-examine obese or comatose patient. Ultrasound can accurately discern whether the mass is solid or cystic, whether it originates from the abdominal cavity, and its location in relation to the abdominal wall structures. When a mass is palpable in an incision made from a previous cancer operation, an ultrasound-guided needle biopsy can be performed

▶ **TABLE 3 Ultrasound of Abdominal Wall**

- Incisional, ventral and groin hernias
- Fluid collections: abscess, seroma
- Rectus sheath hematoma
- Tumors: diagnosis, biopsy
- Intestinal adhesions
- Operative planning: laparoscopic trocar insertion

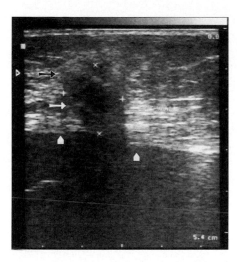

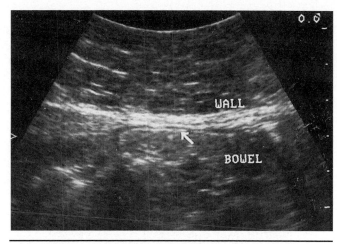

FIGURE 7. Small bowel immediately posterior to the abdominal wall (*arrow*).

FIGURE 5. Subcutaneous metastatic sarcoma (*solid arrows, cursors*) with intact fascia posteriorly (base pad).

quickly and safely to diagnose or rule out an abdominal wall metastasis (Fig. 5). Rectus sheath hematoma most commonly occurs spontaneously, particularly in patients on anticoagulation therapy. The ultrasound appearance of a rectus sheath hematoma depends both on its location and on the age of the hematoma. Above the arcuate line, the characteristic appearance is of a lens-shaped mass (Fig. 6). Below the arcuate line, the hematoma can spread across the midline and to the pelvis, even indenting the bladder.

Preoperatively, ultrasound of the abdominal wall can precisely define the presence of adherent bowel by using the technique of viscera slide, as described previously, helping the surgeon to avoid intestinal injury (2,7,15,16) (Fig. 7). Incisional hernias may present with pain and gastrointestinal symptoms alone, in the absence of a palpable mass. Both the fascial defect and, frequently, the hernia contents can be identified with ultrasound (Figs. 8 and 9). Tenderness directly over the ventral hernia may indicate compromised bowel. Spigelian hernias occur at the junction of the linea semilunaris and arcuate line and are often undiagnosed preoperatively when based on

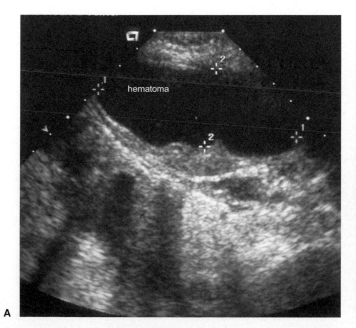

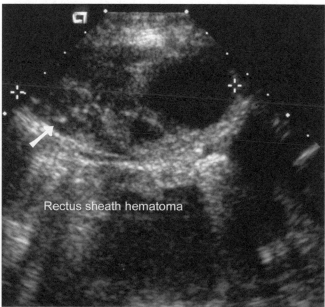

FIGURE 6. Hypoechoic rectus sheath hematoma sagittal (**A**) and transverse (**B**) views (*cursors, arrow*).

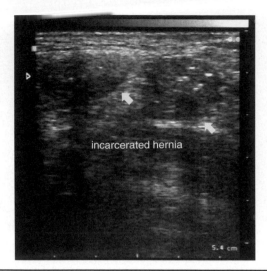

FIGURE 8. Incarcerated small bowel (*arrows*) in a groin hernia.

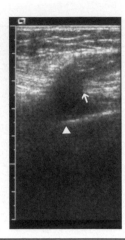

FIGURE 10. Spigelian hernia with an *arrow* indicating hernia sac. Note interruption of hyperechoic fascia (*arrowheads*).

clinical signs and symptoms alone (17,18). The diagnostic findings on ultrasound consist of the demonstration of a defect at any point on the linea semilunaris independent of the presence of herniated bowel (Fig. 10).

The groin region can be divided into two sonographically distinct areas: the inguinal region and the femoral triangle. Groin hernias, whether direct, indirect, or femoral, are occasionally difficult to confirm based on clinical findings alone, especially in the morbidly obese patient (19). Ultrasound is useful in depicting cysts, undescended and retractile testis, as well as intestinal peristalsis associated with groin hernias (20). Unfortunately, while ultrasound can confirm the presence of a mass, unless that mass is demonstrated to be a hydrocele, a varicocele, or a femoral artery aneurysm, or shown to contain bowel, an exact diagnosis may remain nebulous, particularly in cases of inguinal adenopathy as opposed to ab-

scess (21,22). Fluid-filled bowel, omentum, and lymph nodes can all have similar echo patterns, making differentiation difficult.

Sonographic features of a suspicious or metastatic lymph node include a spherical (rather than ellipsoid) shape, a thickness-to-length ratio greater than 2:3, a diameter greater than 5 mm, and the presence of low-level internal echoes (23) (Fig. 11). Ultrasound with high-frequency transducers has been used for both the initial evaluation and follow-up of high-risk melanoma patients as a highly sensitive technique to assess at-risk lymphatic draining areas and nodal basins (24,25). In cases of inguinal adenopathy and deeper soft-tissue metastases

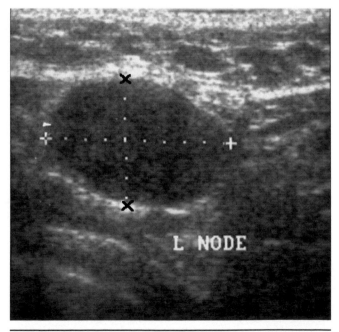

FIGURE 11. Inguinal lymph node (*cursors*) containing metastatic melanoma.

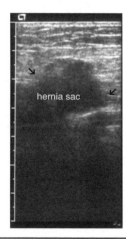

FIGURE 9. Ventral hernia with *arrowheads* indicating fascial defect.

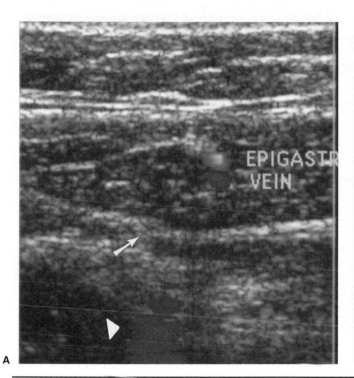

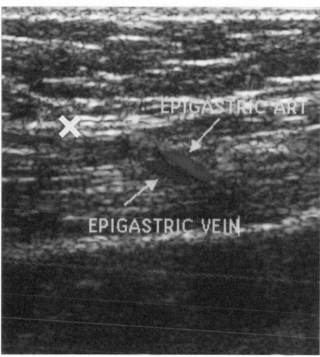

A

B

FIGURE 12. Transverse **(A)** (See Color Plate 17) and longitudinal **(B)** (See Color Plate 18) views of inguinal region using color Doppler imaging. Note epigastric vessels, iliac vessels (*triangle*), transversalis fascia (*arrow*), and aponeurosis (X).

(which may be small and near major vascular structures), ultrasound-guided needle aspiration or core biopsy is safe and efficacious.

Most recently, color and power Doppler ultrasound has been used in an attempt to define different types of hernias (e.g., direct or indirect) and to establish intestinal viability in cases of incarcerated hernias (26,27) (Fig. 12). This technique is extremely useful in the assessment of femoral masses (28). In addition, color Doppler ultrasound permits identification of false aneurysms following femoral artery access. Thrombin-mediated obliteration of false aneurysms under ultrasound guidance has become the treatment of choice for these vascular complications (29). Acute scrotal pain may pose a diagnostic dilemma in the preoperative and postoperative settings. A 5- to 7.5-MHz linear array transducer with color Doppler imaging capabilities reliably diagnoses the cause of such a condition with a sensitivity of 95% and a specificity of 94% (30). Furthermore, in this era of laparoscopic preperitoneal hernia repair, patients often present with troublesome inguinal swelling or masses in the early postoperative period; ultrasound can help to differentiate recurrent hernias from seromas and spermatic cord hematomas (Fig. 13).

Peritoneal Cavity

Ultrasound with a 3.5- to 5-MHz curvilinear array transducer is an excellent tool for visualizing pathologic in-

traabdominal collections and pneumoperitoneum. A recent study found ultrasound to be more sensitive and accurate than plain radiographs in detecting free intraperitoneal air (31) (Fig. 14).

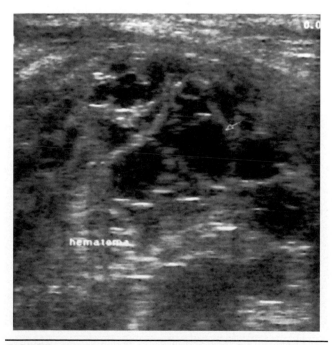

FIGURE 13. Spermatic cord hematoma after laparoscopic preperitoneal hernia repair.

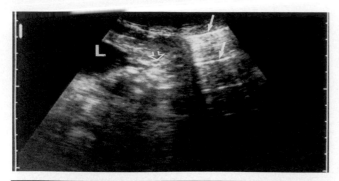

FIGURE 14. Pneumoperitoneum. Free intraabdominal air in a patient with perforated gastric ulcer: the gas artifacts appear as reverberation artifacts (*arrows*) posterior to the abdominal wall. The stomach is hardly visible (*open arrow*) medially to the liver (L).

Ultrasound guidance facilitates paracentesis in patients, especially those with multiple prior operations and loculated fluid collections. Ultrasound also can be used to perform percutaneous peritoneal catheter placement to palliate patients with large-volume malignant ascites who would otherwise require frequent paracentesis (32).

Gastrointestinal Tract

Ultrasound images can give great detail of the bowel wall and major vascular structures of the gastrointestinal tract. The ultrasound appearance of normal intestine is that of a target with an echogenic central area and a hypoechoic rim on cross-section. The wall has an average thickness of 5 mm on ultrasound (33). In real time, using the graded compression technique, bowel loops are often shown to be compressible. Most recent, and of increasing interest to the surgeon, is the use of ultrasound as an adjunct to the clinical evaluation of appendicitis and diverticulitis.

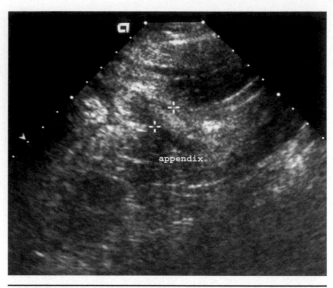

FIGURE 16. Sonographic appearance of distended appendix (*cursors*) in acute appendicitis. The luminal diameter is 12 mm.

Appendicitis

In 1986, Puylaert initially described the use of ultrasound as an aid in the diagnosis of acute appendicitis (6). Other investigators have duplicated and refined this initial work (34). It is helpful to have the patient point to the region of maximal pain or discomfort. Examination of the area of interest routinely should include both longitudinal and transverse images. While Puylaert initially reported that the diagnosis of acute appendicitis mandated the appearance of a blind-ended and aperistaltic tube arising from the cecum, others have found that a normal appendix can be visualized with ultrasound (35). In the proper clinical setting, visualization of an appendix

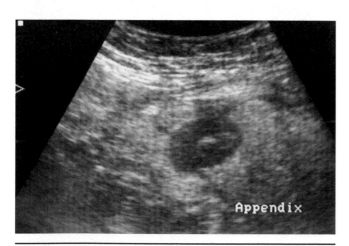

FIGURE 15. "Target sign" indicative of acute appendicitis.

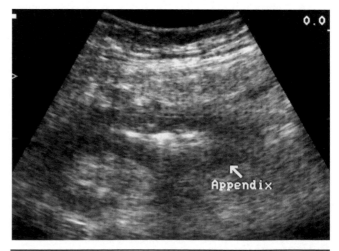

FIGURE 17. Noncompressible dilated appendix (*arrow*) indicative of acute appendicitis.

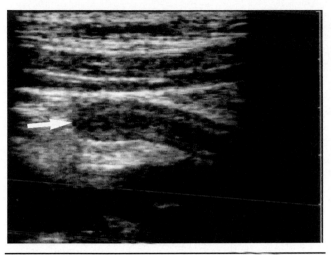

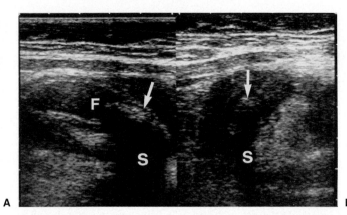

FIGURE 18. Nonperforated appendicitis in longitudinal view: a longitudinal tubular structure 10 mm in diameter is seen with a blind-ending tip (*arrow*). The submucosal interface (bright innermost layer) and the muscularis (hypoechogenic outer layer) are visualized.

FIGURE 19. Confined perforation in acute appendicitis: an obstructing fecalith (*arrows*) with posterior acoustic shadowing (S) causing acute appendicitis. The longitudinal section (**A**) depicts intraluminal fluid (F) retention and dilatation. The appendix is surrounded by fluid similar in sonolucency to the intraluminal fluid, suggesting a suppurative fluid collection. The axial section (**B**) demonstrates complete obstruction of the base of the appendix by fecalith.

should always be regarded as ultrasound evidence of appendicitis. The features of acute appendicitis include the target sign (Fig. 15), a 6- to 12-mm diameter (Fig. 16), noncompressibility (Fig. 17), lack of peristalsis, and presence of a blind-ending tip (Fig. 18, Table 4). Perforated appendicitis may be difficult to diagnose with ultrasound because of regional ileus, abdominal wall rigidity, or even disintegration of the appendix. However, perforated appendicitis can be suspected by mesenteric edema, fluid collections, and associated loops of adynamic ileus, which are found relatively easily by ultrasound (Figs. 19 and 20).

The impact of ultrasound, its relative value in comparison with computed tomography (CT) scanning and its overall applicability, continue to be a matter of controversy (36–38). Its value depends on its availability, the operator experience and its inclusion as an added tool to the patient's clinical evaluation. In this context, an accuracy rate over 90% (sensitivity about 80% to 90%, specificity higher than 95%) and a reduction in negative laparotomies to below 10% have been reported (1,39). Although CT scan has been purported to be the imaging study of choice in patients presenting with a presumed diagnoses of appendicitis (37,38), critical analysis of its application has failed to provide a clear and absolute advantage over ultrasound as the preferred initial test in the acute setting (36).

▶ **TABLE 4** **Ultrasound Criteria for the Diagnosis of Acute Appendicitis**

1. Direct
   - Blind-ended tip, aperistaltic tube
   - Target sign
   - 6- to 12-mm diameter
   - Noncompressibility
2. Indirect
   - Mesenteric edema
   - Regional ileus
   - Fluid collection

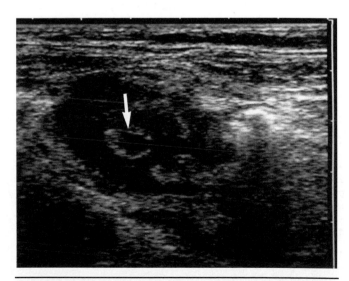

FIGURE 20. Perforated appendicitis in transverse view: appendiceal phlegmon due to perforated appendicitis. The appendix is hardly visible, and only a "remnant" target pattern (*arrow*) is seen. Note the irregular shape of the inflammatory pseudotumor secondary to periappendiceal spread of inflammation.

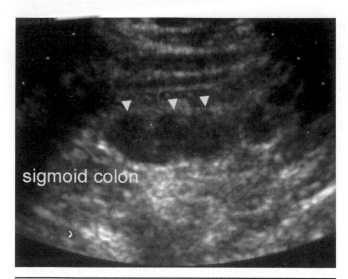

FIGURE 21. Sigmoid diverticulitis. *Arrowheads* indicating inflamed diverticula.

Diverticulitis

The ultrasound features of acute diverticulitis consist of a thickened intestinal wall, lack of compressibility, and diminished peristalsis. Once the long axis of the thickened intestinal loop is identified, rotating the transducer 90 degrees may help identify inflamed diverticula as grape-like, hypoechogenic structures beyond the thickened intestinal wall (Fig. 21). Inflammatory changes in the mesenteric fat may be visualized as poorly defined hypoechoic areas (40). Associated abscess formation can also be detected by ultrasound (Fig. 22). While ultrasound may be useful in evaluating diverticulitis, especially in the presence of associated abscess formation, its main drawback is the failure to differentiate diverticulitis from other inflammatory or neoplastic conditions. For

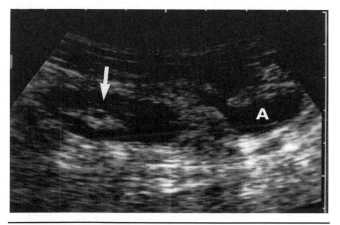

FIGURE 22. Confined perforation of a diverticulum in colonic diverticulitis: hypoechogenic target (*arrow*) displaying asymmetric thickening of the wall and a small, well-confined abscess (A) lateral to the sigmoid colon.

example, inflammatory bowel disease, particularly Crohn's disease but also ulcerative colitis, may be demonstrated by ultrasound. A uniformly thickened bowel wall with impaired peristalsis and minimal compressibility may be identified in these bowel diseases (Fig. 23) (14).

Bowel Obstruction

Intraluminal fluid and distention present in bowel obstruction can be accurately identified by ultrasound. In one study, ultrasound was found to be more accurate in diagnosing ileus and mechanical obstruction than radiographic obstructive series (41). A systematic longitudinal and transverse scan of the abdominal cavity is performed using a 3.5- to 5-MHz transducer. In the longitudinal view, the bowel wall is thickened to 3 to 5 mm, and appears as a compressible, multilayered sandwich structure (Fig. 24). The small intestine is collapsed and easily compressed. The transverse view shows the characteristic target appearance (Fig. 25); this target (diameter of the bowel) measures 10 to 20 mm for the small bowel and 30 mm for the colon. Adynamic bowel is identified by the presence of distended, fluid-filled bowel loops without peristalsis. On the other hand, concomitant collapsed and distended loops of bowel with variable degrees of peristalsis may aid in the diagnosis of mechanical obstruction (1) (Table 5).

Bowel obstruction may occur in the immediate postoperative period and is often caused by adhesions. Generally, these are incomplete obstructions and can be managed expectantly. Conversely, closed-loop obstruction is a complete mechanical blockade that often rapidly progresses to strangulation. Early in the presentation, abdominal films may show gas distal to the obstruction, giving the surgeon a false sense of security. Additional imaging studies, such as ultrasound or CT scan, may provide critical evidence of an isolated fluid-filled bowel loop with a thickened wall and thereby facilitate earlier intervention.

Although ultrasound is very sensitive in showing the presence of distended bowel, it is not so specific, except in cases of intestinal intussusception (1). Intussusception is one of the few conditions in bowel obstruction where ultrasound is diagnostic. Plain abdominal radiographs are usually nondiagnostic. Sonographic evidence of a mass with two lumens (bull's-eye sign) confirms the diagnosis of intussusception (Fig. 26). Ultrasound has been used to predict and monitor the efficacy of hydrostatic reduction of intussuscepted bowel in children (42).

Retroperitoneum

Routine scanning is performed with a 3.5- or 5-MHz transducer in longitudinal and transverse planes. Even though ultrasound does not consistently identify masses or lymph nodes of less than 1 cm, a 98% accuracy rate has

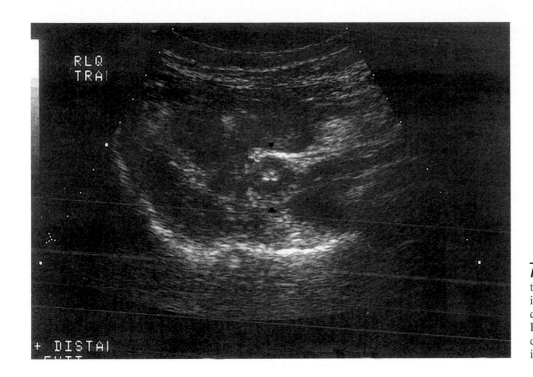

FIGURE 23. Right colon with thickened minimally compressible bowel wall. Target lesion demonstrated by solid arrows. Laparoscopy revealed Crohn's disease involving the terminal ileum.

been reported for retroperitoneal lymph nodes larger than 2 cm in lymphoma patients (43) (Fig. 27). Doppler ultrasound aids in identifying nodes and their relationship to neighboring vessels. The differential diagnosis of adenopathy includes soft-tissue masses, abscesses, hematomas, and inflammatory masses. Lymph nodes usually present as hypoechoic structures of variable size and shape. Larger nodal masses may displace adjacent structures. There are no definitive features that reliably distinguish benign from malignant nodes, although benign nodes tend to be more elongated and rarely have central necrosis. The hilar fat sign is often difficult to demonstrate, but it is a sign of benignancy (43). Other pathologic lesions, such as tumors, abscesses, and retroperitoneal infections, may be amenable to ultrasound examination; however, generally other imaging modalities, especially CT, are more suitable for their diagnosis.

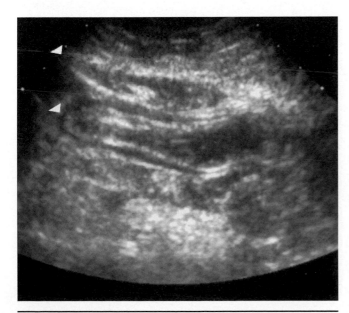

FIGURE 24. Stacked loops of obstructed small bowel (*arrowheads*).

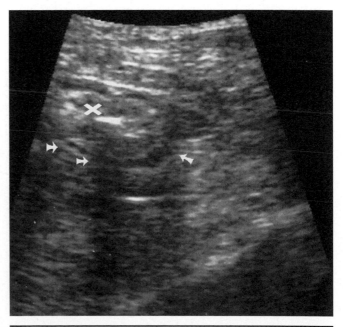

FIGURE 25. Transverse view of obstructed small intestine. Note wall thickness (*arrows*) and hyperechoic center (X).

TABLE 5 **Ultrasound for Bowel Obstruction**

1. Technique
   - 3.5- to 5-MHz transducer
   - Gentle compression
   - Visceral slide technique
2. Criteria
   - The normal intestine is collapsed and compressible
   - Bowel diameter greater than 10–20 mm
   - Aperistaltic fluid-filled bowel (ileus)
   - Concomitant collapsed and distended bowel with peristalsis (mechanical obstruction)
   - Bull's eye sign (intussusception)
3. Indications
   - Postoperative ileus versus obstruction
   - Intussusception
   - Incarcerated hernia
   - Pseudointestinal obstruction

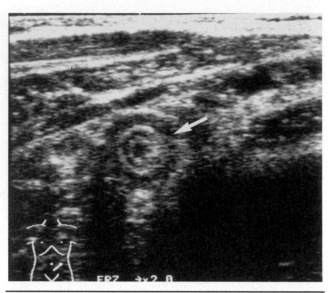

FIGURE 26. Ileoileal intussusception in a child, showing typical sign of the multiple concentric rings (*arrow*) or bull's-eye sign in transverse section.

Kidney

Ultrasound is an excellent modality for renal examination (Table 6); its sensitivity for hydronephrosis approaches 100% by showing dilatation of the collecting system (Fig. 28). In addition, it is an excellent screening modality for renal tumors in conjunction with CT.

Ultrasound can be used for radiofrequency ablation (RFA) of renal tumors by guiding the placement and deployment of multielectrode probes (44). While the volume of treated tissue is difficult to monitor sonographi-

cally during RFA, characteristic hyperechoic changes due to outgassing are seen and provide a rough estimation of the treatment sphere (Fig. 29). This technique is finding increasing applicability in the treatment of cancer patients with significant comorbid illnesses, unresectable tumors, or a solitary kidney. It can be a renal-sparing technique for patients with multiple bilateral tumors

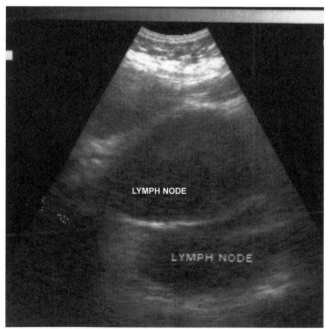

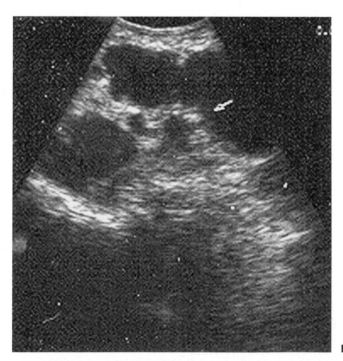

A

B

FIGURE 27. Retroperitoneal adenopathy in a patient with lymphoma. Note hypoechoic, heterogeneous lymph nodes (A). Note the aorta (*arrow*) surrounded by lymph nodes (B).

▶ **TABLE 6** **Ultrasound for Renal Disease**

1. Hydronephrosis
2. Renal calculi
3. Renal tumors
4. Guidance for ablation of renal tumors
5. Evaluation of the transplanted kidney
   a. Lymphocele
   b. Hematoma
   c. Urinoma
   d. Arterial Doppler flow studies
   e. Guidance for needle aspiration and/or biopsy

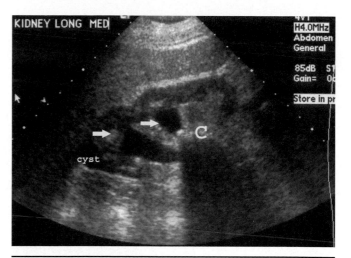

FIGURE 28. Sonographic view of the kidney with a cyst, hydronephrosis (*arrows*) and a renal calculus (C). Note acoustic shadowing of a calculus.

such as those with von Hippel–Lindau syndrome. Ultrasound-guided RFA also has been described for ablating selected adrenal and splenic tumors (44,45).

Early diagnosis and treatment of technical problems associated with transplanted organs, such as the kidney, is crucial to their long-term viability (see Chapter 18). Ultrasound provides valuable information regarding vascular integrity, as well as parenchymal features that aid the transplant surgeon in management of graft dysfunction. Ultrasound allows for relatively easy evaluation of a transplanted kidney graft because the transplanted kidney is usually located in the lower abdomen (46). Lymphoceles, hematomas, and urinomas may be easily recognized and sampled using ultrasound-guided needle aspiration. Increased dimensions of the renal pelvis and ureter may signal distal obstruction. Doppler flow studies may provide useful information regarding the patency of the renal artery and vein. A significant deterioration in the Doppler appearance is to be expected in the first 24 to 48 hours postoperatively (47). If the Doppler appearance fails to improve, or if it deteriorates further, rejection should be strongly suspected. Other signs of acute rejection are a rapid increase in graft size and increased density of the parenchymal echo pattern. Chronic rejection is usually demonstrated by decreasing parenchymal size. Finally, ultrasound-guided biopsy of renal transplant grafts increases the safety and accuracy of the procedure.

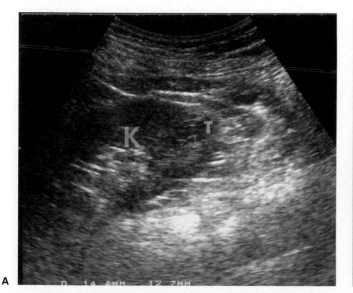

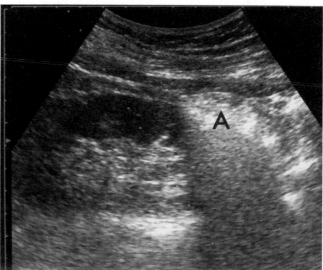

FIGURE 29. Ultrasound-guided radiofrequency ablation of a renal tumor. **A:** 14-mm tumor (T) was detected at the lower pole of right kidney (K). **B:** Percutaneous ablation was performed under ultrasound guidance and monitoring. Note a hyperechoic ablated lesion (A).

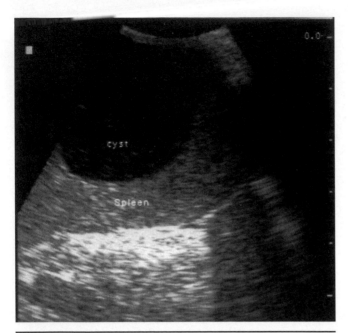

FIGURE 30. Simple cyst of the spleen. Note posterior enhancement.

Spleen

A transducer frequency of 3.5 to 5.0 MHz is suited for splenic examination. The sonographic architecture of the spleen is similar, albeit slightly hyperechoic as compared with the liver. The use of ultrasound in trauma has been firmly established and it is discussed in Chapter 9. In the nontrauma patient, ultrasound can readily identify cystic lesions of the spleen as anechoic simple or complex cysts (Fig. 30). Most true cysts are parasitic in areas of endemic

▶ **TABLE 7** **Ultrasound for Splenic Disease**

1. Cyst
   a. Simple cyst
   b. Complex cyst
   c. Pseudocyst
2. Abscess
3. Infarct
4. Lymphoma

hydatid diseases. CT scan further characterizes true cysts. On the other hand, most pseudocysts are traumatic in origin, and up to half of such cysts contain calcifications. Pancreatic pseudocysts located in the pancreatic tail should be considered in the differential diagnosis (14).

Splenic abscesses are similar to those found in other solid organs (i.e., hypoechoic areas with echogenic foci of debris and gas) (Fig. 31). Their clinical presentation is often insidious, especially in the critically ill patient. Treatment depends on whether the cyst is unilocular, in which case percutaneous drainage is successful in excess of 90% of patients, or multilocular, which mandates splenectomy. Although CT scan generally makes the diagnosis of splenic abscesses more accurately, such diagnosis also may be made by ultrasound. Ultrasound may become most useful in the drainage of splenic abscesses associated with sickle cell anemia or following embolization of the splenic vessels. Splenic infarcts can initially resemble splenic abscesses sonographically, and clinical correlation is necessary to differentiate them. With time, splenic infarcts will become increasingly echogenic. Lym-

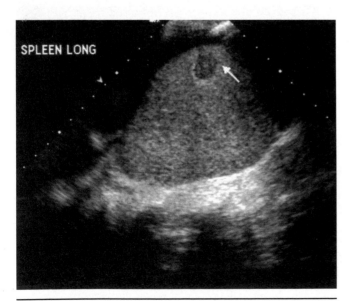

FIGURE 31. Unilocular splenic abscess (*arrow*).

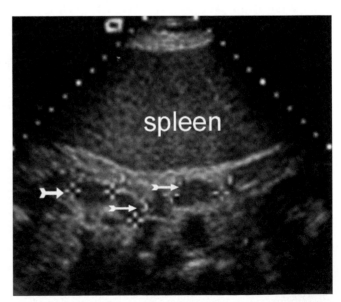

FIGURE 32. Multiple lymphadenopathy (*arrows*) at the splenic hilum.

phomatous involvement of the spleen may be determined by the presence of multiple hypoechoic, rounded parenchymal lesions and by the presence of lymph nodes at the splenic hilum that can be safely biopsied under ultrasound guidance (Table 7, Fig. 32) (14,43).

POSTOPERATIVE EVALUATIONS

Ultrasound is extremely useful in the postoperative period. A critically ill patient may be spared a potentially dangerous trip out of the intensive care unit to the radiology suite by having the diagnosis of an intraabdominal abscess made by ultrasound at the bedside. Interventional procedures such as ultrasound-guided paracentesis can be performed with a high degree of accuracy and safety.

Fluid tends to collect in the most dependent points of the abdomen and frequently shifts with body positioning. When only a small amount of fluid is present, ultrasound examination can detect it most reliably in the right perihepatic space (43). With massive ascites, ultrasound may demonstrate central displacement of the intestine. Intraabdominal bleeding should be clinically suspected in the postoperative patient who remains unstable despite fluid resuscitation. Ultrasound can be useful in identifying intraabdominal blood collections as a cause in these situations, thereby sparing the patient the morbidity of an unnecessary laparotomy.

Abscess

On ultrasound, an abscess has a variable appearance. Most often it appears as an irregular fluid collection, containing septations and fluid debris; occasionally, gas bubbles may be identified. It may have air-fluid levels, it may resemble a completely cystic mass (Fig. 33), or it may resemble an echogenic solid mass (Fig. 34). Location and associated clinical signs and symptoms help to narrow the diagnosis. The diagnosis of intraabdominal abscess should be entertained in any patient who has undergone a recent intraabdominal procedure and who, after several days, manifests fever, leukocytosis, or persistent ileus. If physical examination does not reveal evidence of wound infection, pneumonic process, or other evident cause, an ultrasound or CT scan should be performed. While CT scan is generally viewed as being a more accurate imaging technique in these cases, ultrasound offers the advantage of being quick, portable, and relatively inexpensive. An experienced operator can perform this test with a high degree of accuracy and may be able to offer the patient immediate intervention with ultrasound-guided drain placement if clinically appropriate (14). Certain types of intraabdominal abscesses (e.g.,

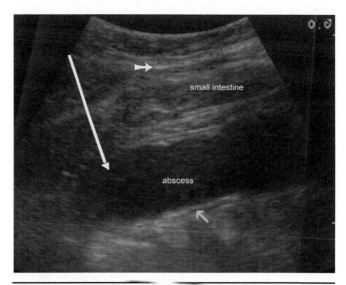

FIGURE 33. Intraabdominal abscess (*deep arrow*). Note small intestine interposed between abscess and abdominal wall (*superficial rrow*). Percutaneous drainage of the abscess was accomplished avoiding the intestine (*long solid line*).

subphrenic and perihepatic) are common, easily recognized, and generally amenable to ultrasound-guided drainage (Fig. 35). Lower abdominal and midabdominal fluid collections or abscesses may be more difficult to detect because of bulky dressings, open wounds, or interference with bowel gas (Table 8).

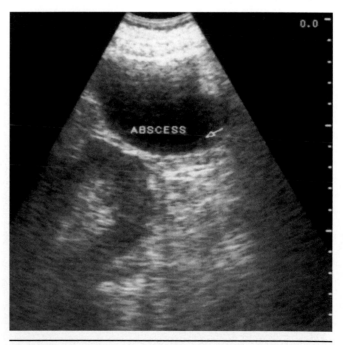

FIGURE 34. Echogenic debris floating on top of fluid within an abscess (*arrow*).

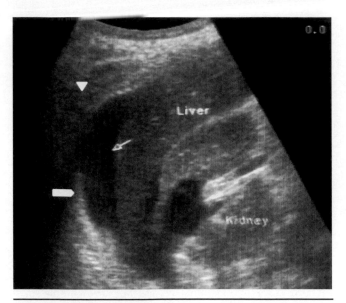

FIGURE 35. Right subphrenic abscess (*arrow*). Note pleural effusion (*triangle*) and hyperechoic diaphragm (*solid bar*).

The decision to aspirate or drain is based on considerations of the patient and abscess and on the surgeon's experience. Using standard aseptic technique, an ultrasound-guided guidewire exchange (Seldinger) technique is used most commonly for the placement of drainage catheters. Follow-up by ultrasound can be performed as indicated based on the patient's clinical course.

Diaphragm

The diaphragm is easily visualized by ultrasound due to its proximity to solid organs. The diaphragm-lung inter-

▶ **TABLE 8 Ultrasound for Abdominal Abscess**

1. Criteria
   - Cystic
   - Septations and debris, gas
   - May resemble a solid mass
2. Use for diagnosis and management
   - Quick bedside use, particularly postoperative use
   - Certain abscesses (subphrenic, perihepatic) easy to diagnose
   - Lower or mid-abdominal abscesses difficult to image
   - CT scan is generally more accurate
   - Ultrasound-guided aspiration or drainage: easier and quicker than CT-guidance

face appears as a thick echogenic line; reverberation artifacts from air in the lung may be seen as well as mirror image of the liver–diaphragm interface (Fig. 36). A transverse scan over the xyphoid allows simultaneous views of both hemidiaphragms.

Diaphragmatic paralysis may result from injury to the phrenic nerve following cardiac or hepatic surgery. In such instances, assessment of diaphragmatic motion can be performed with the use of real-time ultrasound (48). Paralysis is demonstrated by paradoxical motion of the affected diaphragm and exaggerated excursion of the normal side. Finally, diaphragmatic hernias can be detected even in the prenatal stage; posterior Bochdalek hernias are most common and are easier to image than the anterior (Morgagni) hernias. Preoperative detection of traumatic diaphragmatic hernias by ultrasound is more difficult due to the frequency of associated injuries that obscure the field and due to poor patient cooperation.

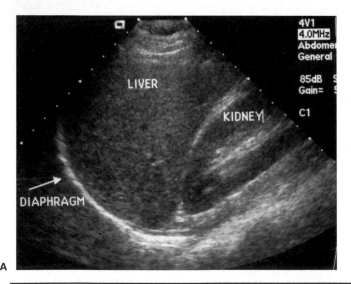

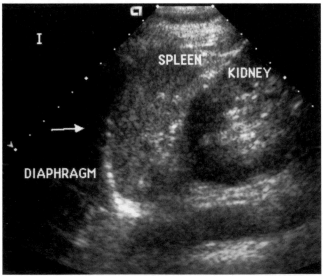

FIGURE 36. Sonographic view of normal right (**A**) and left (**B**) hyperechoic hemidiaphragms (*arrows*). Note mirror image of the liver on the other side of the diaphragm (A).

CONCLUSIONS

Real-time ultrasound of the abdomen by surgeons has many applications and advantages. As we have described in this chapter, ultrasound can be used to evaluate intraabdominal and retroperitoneal organs and structures and various disease states as well as hepatobiliary and pancreatic diseases. Transabdominal ultrasound is a safe, quick, and cost-effective method for guiding interventional procedures such as biopsy, drainage, and ablation.

ACKNOWLEDGMENTS

I thank Elsa Abraham and Kathy Martin for their contributions in the preparation of this manuscript.

REFERENCES

1. Zielke A. Ultrasound of the acute abdomen. In: Machi, J, Sigel B, eds. *Ultrasound for surgeons*. New York: Igaku-Shoin Medical Publishers, 1997:42–71.
2. Sigel B, Golub RM, Loiacono LA, et al. Technique of ultrasonic detection and mapping of abdominal wall adhesions. *Surg Endosc* 1991;5:161–165.
3. Torp-Pedersen S, Skjoldbye B. Interventional abdominal ultrasound. In: Staren ED, ed. *Ultrasound for the surgeon*. Philadelphia: Lippincott–Raven Publishers, 1997:161–179.
4. Röthlin M, Bouillon B, Klotter HJ. *Checkliste sonographie für chirurgen*. New York: Thieme Medical Publishers, 1991.
5. Goletti O, Ghiselli G, Lippolis PV, et al. The role of ultrasonography in blunt abdominal trauma: results in 250 consecutive cases. *J Trauma* 1994;36:178–181.
6. Puylaert JB. Acute appendicitis: ultrasound evaluation using graded compression. *Radiology* 1986;158:355–360.
7. Machi J, Sigel B, Kokecki R. Ultrasound detection of abdominal wall adhesions prior to surgery. In: Machi, J, Sigel B, eds. *Ultrasound for surgeons*. New York: Igaku-Shoin Medical Publishers, 1997:93–103.
8. Berlyne GM. Ultrasonics in renal biopsy: an aid to determination of kidney position. *Lancet* 1961;2:750–751.
9. Hanke S, Holm HH, Koch F. Ultrasonically guided percutaneous fine needle biopsy of the pancreas. *Surg Gynecol Obstet* 1975;140:361–364.
10. Nolsoe C, Nielsen L, Torp-Pedersen S, et al. Major complications and deaths due to interventional ultrasonography: a review of 8000 cases. *J Clin Ultrasound* 1990;18:179–184.
11. Staren ED, Torp-Pedersen S. General interventional ultrasound. In: Staren ED, ed. *Ultrasound for the surgeon*. Philadelphia: Lippincott–Raven Publishers, 1997:137–160.
12. Charboneau JW, Reading CC. Ultrasound-guided biopsy of the abdomen and pelvis. In: Rumack CM, Wilson SSR, Charboneau JW, eds. *Diagnostic ultrasound*. St. Louis: Mosby-Year Book, 1991:429–442.
13. de Dombal FT. Objective medical decision making: acute abdominal pain. In: Beneken JEW, Thevenin V, eds. *Advances in biomedical engineering*. Amsterdam: IOS Press, 1993:65–87.
14. Velasco JM, Vallina VL, Kummerer RG. General abdominal ultrasound. In: Staren ED, ed. *Ultrasound for the surgeon*. Philadelphia: Lippincott–Raven Publishers, 1997:17–33.
15. Caprini JA, Arcelus JA, Swanson J, et al. The ultrasonic localization of abdominal wall adhesions. *Surg Endosc* 1995; 9:283–285.
16. Kodama I, Loiacono LA, Sigel B, et al. Ultrasonic detection of viscera slide as an indicator of abdominal wall adhesions. *J Clin Ultrasound* 1992;20:375–380.
17. Weiss Y, Lernau OZ, Nissan S. Spigelian hernia. *Ann Surg* 1974;180:836–839.
18. Deitch EA, Engel JM. Spigelian hernia: an ultrasonic diagnosis. *Arch Surg* 1980; 115:93.
19. Deva AK, Quinn MJ, Nettle WJ. The difficult problem of a groin lump in a morbidly obese patient. *Aust N Z J Surg* 1993;63:664–665.
20. Shadbolt CL, Heinze SB, Dietrich RB. Imaging of groin masses: inguinal anatomy and pathologic conditions revisited. *Radiographics* 2001; 21:S261–S271.
21. Lineaweaver W, Vlasak M, Muyshondt E. Ultrasonic examination of abdominal wall and groin masses. *South Med J* 1983;76:590–592.
22. Horn TW, Harris JA, Martindale R, et al. When a hernia is not a hernia: the evaluation of inguinal hernias in the cirrhotic patient. *Am Surg* 2001;67:1093–1095.
23. Uren RF, Howman-Giles R, Thompson JF, et al. High-resolution ultrasound to diagnose melanoma metastases in patients with clinically palpable lymph nodes. *Australas Radiol* 1999;43:148–152.
24. Voit C, Schoengen A, Schwurzer-Voit M, et al. The role of ultrasound in detection and management of regional disease in melanoma patients. *Semin Oncol* 2002;29:353–360.
25. Hoffman U, Szedlak M, Rittgen W, et al. Primary staging and follow-up in melanoma patients: monocenter evaluation of methods, costs and patient survival. *Br J Cancer* 2002;87: 151–157.
26. Zhang GQ, Sugiyama M, Hagi H, et al. Groin hernias in adults: value of color Doppler sonography in their classification. *J Clin Ultrasound* 2001;29:429–434.
27. Babkova VV, Bozhko VV. Ultrasound assessment in diagnosis of uncomplicated inguinal hernia. *Khirurgiia* 1999;2: 46–50.
28. Loftus WK, Hewitt PM, Metrewcli C, et al. Case report: femoral hernia causing small bowel obstruction-ultrasound diagnosis. *Clin Radiol* 1998;53:618–619.
29. Norman DR, Mahute M, Kristenson W, et al. Successful thrombin injection treatment of a large post-catheterization pseudoaneurysm arising from a synthetic aortofemoral graft. *J Vasc Technol* 2000;24:125–127.
30. Blaivas M, Sierzenski P, Lambert M. Emergency evaluation of patients presenting with acute scrotum using bedside ultrasonography. *Acad Emerg Med* 2001;8:90–93.
31. Chen SC, Yen ZS, Wang HP, et al. Ultrasonography is superior to plain radiography in the diagnosis of pneumoperitoneum. *Br J Surg* 2002; 89:351–354.
32. O'Neill MJ, Weissleder R, Gervais DA, et al. Tunneled peritoneal catheter placement under sonographic and fluoroscopic guidance in the palliative treatment of malignant ascites. *AJR Am J Roentgenol* 2001;177:615–618.
33. Fleischer AC, Muhletaler CA, James AE. Sonographic assessment of the bowel wall. *AJR Am J Roentgenol* 1981;136:887–891.
34. Jeffrey RB, Laing FC, Townsend RR. Acute appendicitis: monographic criteria based on 250 cases. *Radiology* 1988; 167:327–329.
35. Abu-Yousef MM, Bleicher JJ, Maher JW, et al. High-resolution sonography of acute appendicitis. *AJR Am J Roentgenol* 1987;149:53–58.
36. Morris KT, Kavanagh M, Hansen P, et al. The rational use of computed tomography scans in the diagnosis of appendicitis. *Am J Surg* 2002;183:547–550.
37. Walker S, Haun W, Clark J, et al. The value of limited computed tomography with rectal contrast in the diagnosis of acute appendicitis. *Am J Surg* 2000;180:450–455.
38. Horton MD, Counter SF, Florence MG. A prospective trail of computed tomography and ultrasonography for diagnosing appendicitis in the atypical patient. *Am J Surg* 2000;179: 379–381.
39. Schwerk WB, Wiehtrup B, Rüschoff J, et al. Acute and perforated appendicitis: current experience with ultrasound-aided diagnosis. *World J Surg* 1990;14:271–276.
40. Parulekar SG. Sonography of colonic diverticulitis. J Ultrasound Med 1985;4:659–666.

41 Meisel G. Gastrointestinale Ultrasschalldiagnostik: Chirurgische Bedeutung fassbarer Befunde. *Ultraschall Klin Prax* 1987;2:137–145.

42. Babcock DS. Sonography of the acute abdomen in the pediatric patient. *J Ultrasound Med* 2002;21:887–899.

43. Sauerbrei EE, Nguyen KT, Nolan RL. *Abdominal sonography*. New York: Raven Press, 1992.

44. Pavlovich CP, Walther MM, Choyke PL, et al. Percutaneous radio frequency ablation of small renal tumors: initial results. *J Urol* 2002;167:10–15.

45. Wood BJ, Ramkaransingh JF, Fojo T, et al. Percutaneous tumor ablation with radiofrequency. *Cancer* 2002;94:443–451.

46. Silver TM, Campbell D, Wicks JD, et al. Peritransplant fluid collections. *Radiology* 1981;138:145–151.

47. Stevens PE, Gwyther SJ, Hanson ME, et al. Interpretation of duplex Doppler ultrasound in renal transplants in the early postoperative period. *Nephrol Dial Transplant* 1993;8:255–258.

48. Diament MJ, Boechat MI, Kangarloo H. Real time sector ultrasound in the evaluation of suspected abnormalities of diaphragmatic motion. *J Clin Ultrasound* 1985;13:539–543.

Chapter 13

Overview of Intraoperative and Laparoscopic Ultrasound

Junji Machi, Andrew J. Oishi, Nancy L. Furumoto, and Robert H. Oishi

An accurate diagnosis is essential for surgical decision making; however, even with the improvement of preoperative imaging studies, accurate diagnostic information cannot always be obtained before surgery. Often surgeons still have to make intraoperative decisions based on findings noted during the operation. Meticulous exploration by inspection and palpation is essential. However, even during open surgery, exploration may not always be accurate or possible; this is particularly true in evaluation of solid organs or deep structures. Intraoperative imaging methods can provide useful and, at times, critical information. Intraoperative ultrasound (IOUS) is a valuable and widely applicable modality because it provides high-resolution images of the operative field in real time, which cannot be obtained by other intraoperative studies.

Over the last several years, the application of laparoscopic surgery has expanded to include various and more complex types of abdominal problems. While a laparoscopic approach has a number of advantages, including minimal invasiveness, patient comfort, less pain, and quicker recovery, it has certain disadvantages and limitations as well. In particular, the lack of sufficient tactile feedback from the tissues and little or no capability of palpation limits the possibility of intraoperative assessment of organs or lesions during laparoscopy. Laparoscopic ultrasound (LUS) is a form of IOUS that allows surgeons to visualize and evaluate the interior of organs and deep structures. This imaging capability of LUS can compensate remarkably for the inherent limitation of laparoscopic examination.

We have been using IOUS during various open surgical operations since 1980, and LUS during laparoscopic operations since 1990. Based on our experience with IOUS and LUS in more than 4,000 operations and a review of the literature, this chapter presents an overview of IOUS and LUS (1–7). First, the history of IOUS and LUS is briefly reviewed. Instrumentation and basic techniques of IOUS and LUS are described. The normal ultrasound anatomy and the ultrasound appearances of typical pathologic lesions that are frequently encountered during abdominal surgery are presented. General indications and specific organ indication are summarized. Following this is a review of the advantages and limitations of IOUS and LUS. Finally, intraoperative color Doppler imaging and IOUS- or LUS-guided procedures are described. Although IOUS has been applied to a wide variety of surgical fields, including hepatobiliary, pancreatic, endocrine, neurologic, urologic, gynecologic, and cardiovascular surgery, the overview of IOUS in this chapter is focused mainly on abdominal surgery. This chapter also is an introduction to the following chapters, which describe organ- or disease-specific applications of IOUS or LUS.

HISTORY

Although intraoperative radiographic modalities such as intraoperative cholangiography were used as early as the 1930s or 1940s, the development of IOUS/LUS did not start until the 1960s. There are three remarkable periods in the history of IOUS/LUS: the first period in the 1960s was the beginning of IOUS/LUS utilizing A-mode or static B-mode ultrasound; the second period in the late 1970s and the 1980s was due to the expansion of IOUS with real-time B-mode ultrasound; and the third period occurred in the 1990s with the application of intraoperative color Doppler imaging and the expansion of LUS (8).

French and Wild first attempted IOUS in the 1950s for detection of brain tumors using A-mode ultrasound (9). In the 1960s, Schlegel employed A-mode IOUS to locate renal calculi; Hayashi, Knight, and Eiseman applied IOUS to detection of biliary calculi; and Tanaka used IOUS for localization of brain tumors (10–14). Interestingly, the first attempt of LUS occurred at the same time around the 1960s. Yamakawa used a prototype 5-mm-diameter, 30-cm-long probe laparoscopically to visualize gallstones and gastric cancer (15). Although the need for appropriate Intraoperative imaging methods in the operating room was recognized almost 40 years ago, A-mode or primitive B-mode ultrasound used at that time was not easily performed or interpreted, making intraoperative application difficult, and did not lead to widespread use of IOUS or LUS.

In the 1970s, the advances in ultrasound technology and the refinement of instruments led to the development of real-time B-mode imaging. The introduction of high-frequency, high-resolution or so-called small-parts ultrasound led to particular interest in IOUS in the late 1970s. Early applications of real-time B-mode IOUS were reported by Cook for localizing renal calculi in 1977 (16), by Makuuchi for detecting hepatic tumors in 1977 (17), and by Lane and Sigel for diagnosing biliary calculi in 1979 (18,19). In the United States, cylindrical sector probes were employed during operation at that time, whereas flat linear array probes were developed in Japan by Makuuchi in 1977, mainly for IOUS scanning of the liver (17,20). In the early 1980s, B-mode IOUS was introduced to various surgical fields: by Rubin, Dohrmann, and Shkolnik during neurosurgery in 1980 and 1981 (21,22), by Sigel and Lane during endocrine surgery (i.e., parathyroid, islet cell tumors) in 1981 and 1982 (23,24), and by Sahn during cardiac surgery in 1982 (25). Sigel and Machi reported on IOUS during pancreatic and vascular surgery at that time (26,27). During the 1980s, IOUS was applied in a wide variety of surgical fields, especially hepatobiliary, pancreatic, endocrine, neurologic, and cardiovascular surgery. In the 1980s, several books on IOUS, describing its value during open surgery, were published (28–30).

In the 1990s, two new ultrasound modalities were incorporated into IOUS: color or power Doppler imaging, which enhanced the value of IOUS; and LUS, which extended the usefulness of IOUS (8,31). Intraoperative color Doppler imaging was found to be useful particularly in cardiovascular surgery (32,33). It also facilitated image interpretation of IOUS by delineating blood vessels in color during general surgical procedures and transplantation (34).

Although prototype B-mode LUS instruments were attempted in the 1980s, rigid and flexible probes specifically made for LUS that were inserted through the current 10-mm trocars became available in the early to mid-1990s (35–39). LUS rapidly became popular among laparoscopic surgeons because LUS could compensate for the principal limitations of laparoscopy (i.e., paucity of tactile feedback from tissues and impossibility of examining deep structures). Shortly after the performance of video laparoscopic cholecystectomy become routine, LUS was first introduced for evaluation of the biliary system. Subsequently, LUS was performed and proved useful as an adjunct during exploratory laparoscopy for ab-dominal malignant tumors. The same instruments were also used as thoracoscopic ultrasound during thoracoscopic surgery.

Despite this progress in IOUS and LUS, the main obstacle to the wider use of IOUS/LUS among surgeons has been the difficulty in obtaining sufficient training and achieving technical proficiency. Training and credentialing in ultrasound for surgeons has emerged as an important issue. During the last several years, the educational and training issue of ultrasound including IOUS/LUS has been addressed by many surgical residency programs and surgical organizations, such as the American College of Surgeons.

INSTRUMENTATION

The standard ultrasound instrument for current use consists of a hand-held probe incorporating transducer crystals (elements), a pulse processing scanner, a monitor screen, and a recorder. The ultrasound system provides B-mode ultrasound, duplex ultrasound, or color/power Doppler imaging. The equipment of choice for IOUS and LUS is a "small parts scanner," which is a high-frequency, high-resolution, real-time ultrasound system, using transducers with frequencies of 5 MHz or higher (1–8,28–30, 38,39). While ultrasound at higher frequency does not penetrate deeply, it provides greater resolution of images; this is an ideal trade-off for IOUS/LUS because penetrating the body wall is not an issue. To meet special requirements of intraoperative and laparoscopic applications, several manufacturers have developed high-frequency probes specifically designed for use within the operative field.

Transducer: Probe

For IOUS and LUS, transducer frequencies ranging from 5 to 10 MHz have generally been employed. A 7.5-MHz or 7- to 8-MHz transducer provides a depth of sound penetration of 6 to 10 cm, and is used most commonly. Since IOUS/LUS scanning is carried out directly on the areas of interest and the sound does not need to penetrate the body wall, a sound penetration of 6 to 10 cm is usually sufficient. With the greater resolution of IOUS/LUS, small lesions such as 1-mm calculi and 3- to 5-mm tumors can be detected.

There are two principal types of probes: linear array and sector probes (Fig. 1) (also see Chapters 2 and 3). Linear array probes are composed of a series of small transducer crystals aligned in a row and usually electronically pulse and receive sound sequentially. They produce

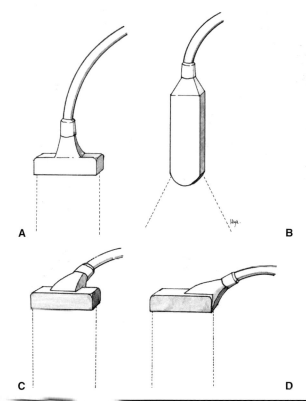

FIGURE 1. Principal types of intraoperative ultrasound probes (linear array and sector). **A:** Linear array, T-shaped, end-viewing. **B:** Sector or convex, cylindrical, end-viewing. **C:** Linear array, flat T-shaped, side-viewing. **D:** Linear array, flat I-shaped, side-viewing.

manipulation in the restricted operative field. Two basic shapes of IOUS probes are flat and cylindrical (Figs. 1 and 2). Flat probes are linear array or convex, and are configured into a "T" or "I" shape. T-shaped probes have either side or end (front) viewing. Cylindrical probes are convex or phased array. They are pencil-like, often with flattened sides to achieve greater slimness, and usually have an end viewing. The use of a particular probe is dictated by the special requirements of IOUS, which are related to accessibility and footprint. Flat probes have longer footprints of 4 to 6 cm, which provide wide images in the near field. These probes are suitable for examination of relatively large organs such as liver, pancreas, kidney, and gastrointestinal tract. Flat side-viewing probes are especially important for the optimal scanning of the liver because the probe must be often placed in the limited space between the anterior or superior surface of the liver and the diaphragm (see Figure 10 in Chapter 15). On the other hand, cylindrical probes have shorter footprints, usually 3 cm or less, but provide wider sector images in the far field. Such slim probes are useful for examination of small target organs such as the extrahepatic biliary duct, spinal cord and peripheral vessels (see Figures 33 and 35 in Chapter 14), especially when areas of interest are situated deep in the operative field where manipulation of the probe is limited. It is ideal to possess various flat and cylindrical probes. However, if only one IOUS probe were available to perform intraabdominal IOUS, we would recommend a T-shaped side-viewing flat probe (linear array or convex) (e.g., Fig. 2G, J, or L) because this is the most versatile and with it abdominal organs can almost always be scanned.

LUS probes consist of transducer crystals mounted on or near the tip of a slender shaft (6,7,38,39). The shaft is usually 10 mm (some up to 12 mm) in diameter and approximately 30 to 70 cm in length and is introduced into the peritoneal cavity by way of a 10- to 12-mm trocar. Several types of LUS probes are presently available (Figs. 2 and 3), utilizing linear array, convex, or sector systems. A probe can be either end viewing (scanning plane parallel to the probe shaft) or side viewing (scanning plane at a right angle to the probe shaft). An end-viewing sector probe is suitable for scanning of the extrahepatic bile duct or the pancreas, whereas a side-viewing linear array or convex probe is more frequently used currently, can be applicable to almost all organs of the abdomen, and is essential for scanning of the liver. Manufacturers originally made a rigid-shaft probe; at present, a flexible probe is also available for side viewing. This has a flexible tip that is mobile in two or four directions (bi- or quadridirectional). A flexible tip facilitates scanning of areas that are difficult to delineate with a rigid probe (e.g., behind the dome of the liver), reduces the number of trocar insertion sites, and decreases the scanning time. Disadvantages of

rectangular images. The span of tissue in contact with linear array probes for IOUS/LUS is usually 3 to 6 cm and is displayed on the monitor screen as the "footprint" that corresponds to the length of linear array. When electronic transducer crystals are aligned in a curved fashion, they are curvilinear array, and are often called convex probes. Sector probes are mechanical or electronic phased array. A mechanical sector scanner with a single transducer crystal is rarely used currently. Sector probes produce pie- or fan-shaped images, and the footprint is shorter (usually 1 to 3 cm). Convex probes also produce pie-shaped or truncated images, but their field of image is not as wide as a sector image. Currently, many manufacturers are making mostly electronic linear array or convex systems rather than sector systems for the use of IOUS and LUS.

Transducer crystals are housed within probes that should meet certain requirements for intraoperative use during open and laparoscopic surgery. The essential features of IOUS probes during open surgery (i.e., laparotomy) are their size and shape (1–7,28–30). A probe of relatively small size with a long flexible cable is required for

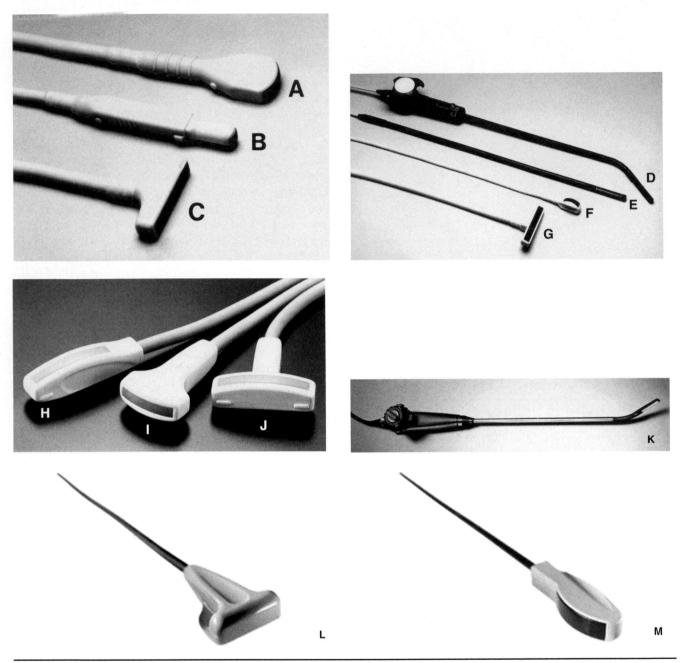

FIGURE 2. Intraoperative ultrasound probes and laparoscopic ultrasound (LUS) probes. Transducer frequencies are 5 to 10 MHz. **A:** Convex, cylindrical, end-viewing. **B:** Sector, cylindrical, end-viewing (for burr hole of neurosurgery). **C:** Linear array, T-shaped, end-viewing. **D:** Flexible LUS probe, linear array, side-viewing. **E:** Rigid LUS probe, linear array, side-viewing. **F:** Convex, flat I-shaped, side viewing. **G:** Linear array, flat T-shaped, side-viewing. **H:** Convex, flat I-shaped, side-viewing. **I:** Convex, T-shaped, end-viewing. **J:** Convex, flat T-shaped, side-viewing. **K:** Flexible LUS probe, linear array, sideviewing. **L:** Convex, flat T-shaped, side-viewing. **M:** Convex, flat I-shaped, side viewing. (A to G courtesy of Aloka, H to K courtesy of Toshiba Medical, L and M courtesy of B&K Medical.)

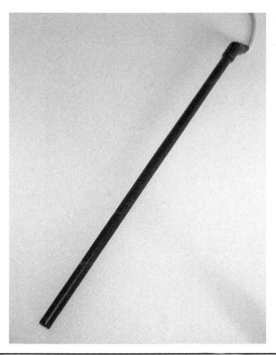

FIGURE 3. End-viewing sector rigid laparoscopic ultrasound (LUS) probe. This is a newer LUS probe with needle guidance capability (see Fig. 41). (Courtesy of Aloka.)

a flexible probe are inability to apply adequate pressure to tissues by the tip and more working parts with requirement for more demanding skills. Also, LUS-guided needle placement may be slightly more difficult with a flexible probe.

During laparoscopic exploration, a probe with biplane transducers, which is utilized for endorectal ultrasound examination, can be inserted in the peritoneal cavity through a small incision. This probe provides both longitudinal and transverse images without changing the position, and may be useful for evaluation of abdominal organs such as the liver and pancreas.

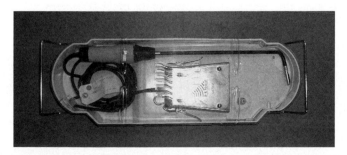

FIGURE 4. A flexible laparoscopic ultrasound probe in the Steris sterilization system. (Courtesy of B&K Medical.)

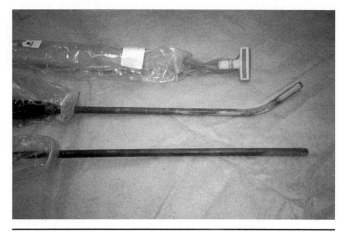

FIGURE 5. Intraoperative and laparoscopic ultrasound probes placed in sterile covers.

Probe Sterilization

IOUS or LUS probe sterility for intraoperative use is achieved by cold gas sterilization or utility of a plastic sterile cover. Ethylene oxide gas is usually used for cold gas sterilization. Because aeration is also required to remove the gas after sterilization, the sterilized probe generally can be used only once a day. Chemical solutions such as alcohol or glutaraldehyde may be used. Soaking of the probe for a short period results only in disinfection and thus is not appropriate for intraoperative use. Sterilization requires a longer soaking of approximately 10 hours. A newer sterilization method such as a low-temperature chemical sterilization (e.g., Steris using liquid peracetic acid, Sterrad using hydrogen peroxide gas plasma), which can sterilize instruments in 30 to 60 minutes, is available, and some probes are amenable to this method (Fig. 4). A disposable sterile probe cover has been commonly used. Various long plastic (polyethylene) and/or latex sleeves (covers) that cover the probe and the cable are commercially available (Fig. 5). To obtain acoustic coupling between the transducer surface and the plastic cover, acoustic coupling gel is introduced into the closed end of the sleeve (Fig. 6). Only a thin layer of gel is needed at the contact between the probe and the cover. It is important to eliminate air bubbles which may be trapped on the transducer surface and obscures images. The use of a plastic cover is cumbersome; however, with this method one probe can be used repeatedly during different operations as many times as desired per day. Even when a probe cover is used, a short soaking (10 to 20 minutes) in chemical solution is recommended because of the possible occurrence of a tear in the cover during IOUS/LUS procedures.

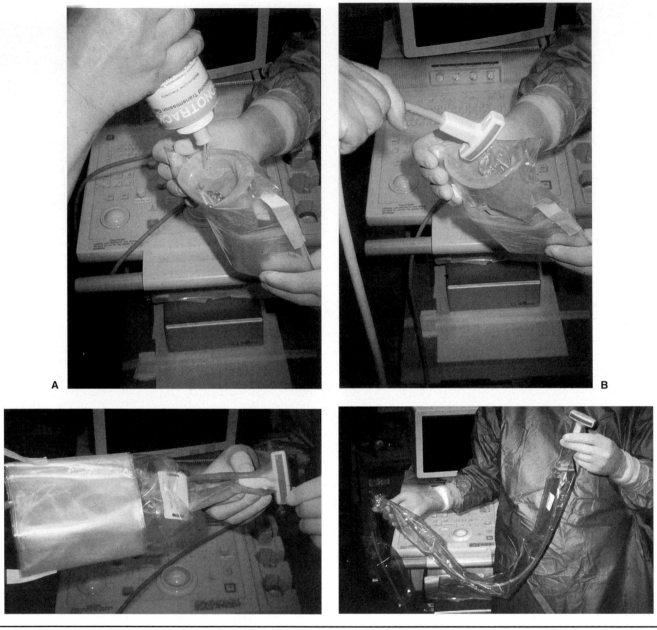

FIGURE 6. The process of sterile cover placement for intraoperative ultrasound probe. **A:** A gel is placed inside the cover. **B:** Ultrasound probe is placed inside the cover. **C, D:** The cable of the probe is covered by a sterile sheath. It is important to get rid of all air from the transducer surface.

BASIC TECHNIQUES

Deployment of Instruments

It is recommended to set up IOUS or LUS instruments and have the sterile probe in the operative field before the actual scanning to minimize the use of operating time for these preparations. The control settings of the scanner should be adjusted and the recording system checked. Generally, a person performing the scanning should be in the surgeon's position. The ultrasound system is best placed on the opposite side of the patient from where the surgeon stands (Fig. 7 and 8), although this setting requires an assistant to manipulate the controls and adjust the ultrasound images. The monitor is placed to permit easy viewing of both the screen and the operative field with minimal change-of-gaze movement. For LUS, in which the surgeon needs to look at both ultrasound images and laparoscopic images, ultrasound images can be displayed on the same video monitor as a "picture-in-picture" (Fig. 9). A picture-in-picture feature may be helpful to quickly develop appropriate hand–eye coordi-

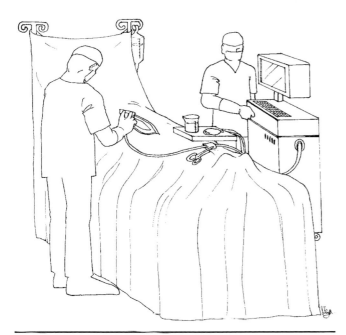

FIGURE 7. Deployment of ultrasound instruments and systems in the operating room. The sterile probe cable is fixed on the operative table. The examiner usually stands at the same position as the operating surgeon. The ultrasound system is on the opposite side of the patient from where the examiner stands. An assistant who is familiar with the ultrasound system should be available to control images.

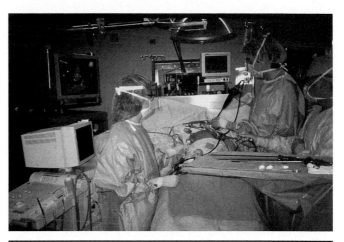

FIGURE 8. Operating room setting for laparoscopic ultrasound. The monitor for laparoscopy and the ultrasound monitor screen should be placed close to each other on the same side, if picture-in-picture images are not used.

nation in LUS scanning techniques. Alternatively, a surgeon can scan with one hand and control images with the other hand by himself or herself. In this situation, the ultrasound system is placed on the same side where the surgeon stands, and the control panel is covered by a sterile transparent cover or sheet (Fig. 10)

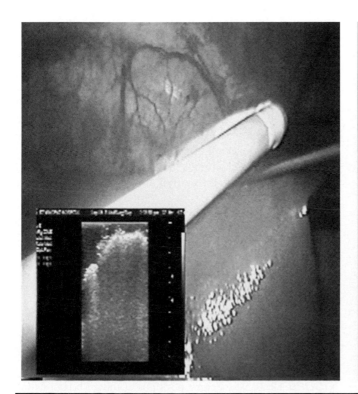

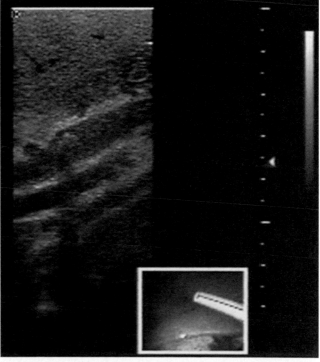

FIGURE 9. "Picture-in-picture" images used for laparoscopic ultrasound. The anatomic location of laparoscopic ultrasound probe (laparoscopic image) and its actual ultrasound images can be visualized simultaneously in one screen. (Courtesy of Dr. Maurice Arregui.)

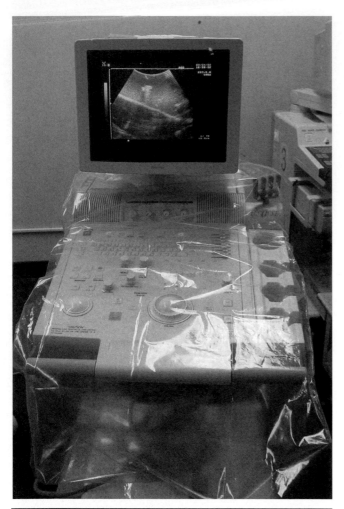

FIGURE 10. The control panel of ultrasound machine is covered by a sterile sheet so that the examiner can touch it in a sterile manner.

Probe Placement

Ultrasound scanning is a two-step process: probe placement and probe movement (7,29,30). Knowing the exact position of the probe in the operative field is essential; therefore, we often insert the probe in a "dry" field for optimal visual placement and subsequently add saline as needed for acoustic coupling (Fig. 11). Since saline used for probe immersion may become blood tinged and obscure anatomic landmarks, whenever the position of the probe becomes unclear, the saline solution should be aspirated and the probe-to-target position reset in a dry field.

Two basic probe placement techniques of IOUS and LUS are contact scanning and probe-standoff scanning (Fig. 12). In contact scanning, the probe is placed directly on the tissue or organ surface, whereas in probe-standoff scanning it is positioned 0.5 to 2.0 cm from the surface of

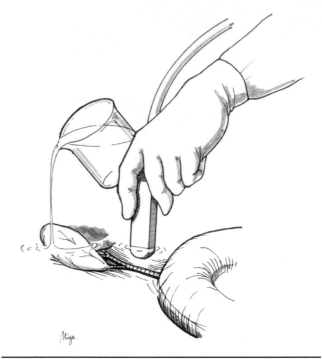

FIGURE 11. After the probe is placed in a "dry" field, saline solution is introduced to obtain acoustic coupling between the probe and the tissue. This shows probe-standoff scanning using a cylindrical probe to image the longitudinal section of the extrahepatic bile duct.

structure. The region of interest is best examined at the focal distance or in the focal zone of transducer and should not be positioned in the "near field" (between the transducer and the focal distance) where the ultrasound resolution is low. Therefore, the distance from the probe to the area of interest in the organ as well as the size of the target organ determines which scanning technique should be employed. Contact scanning is usually used to examine the interior of organs such as the liver, pancreas, and brain. During contact scanning, only a small amount of saline is introduced to make the organ surface wet

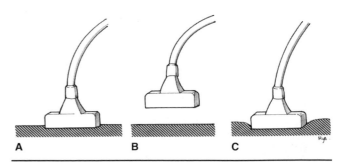

A   **B**   **C**

FIGURE 12. Basic scanning positions of the probe in relation to the tissue or organ. **A:** Contact scanning. **B:** Probe-standoff scanning. **C:** Compression scanning.

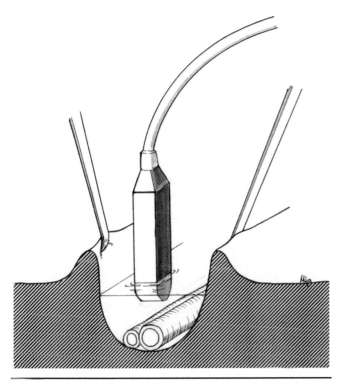

FIGURE 13. Retraction of the wound edges to perform probe-standoff scanning. The skin edges are retracted upward to permit the introduction of enough saline solution into the operative field.

▶ **TABLE 1** Advantages of Probe-Standoff Scanning

1. Ability of placement of region of interest at the appropriate focal zone
2. Clear visualization of surface or superficial areas
3. No compression of tissue by probe
4. Allowance for more scanning maneuvers
5. Not affected by irregular surface of organ or tissue

enough to achieve an adequate acoustic coupling. Coupling gel that is commonly utilized in body scanning is not necessary.

On the other hand, probe-standoff scanning is done when an image of the surface or a superficial area of organs is needed. For examination of relatively small structures such as the extrahepatic bile ducts and the peripheral blood vessels, this technique is of particular importance. During probe-standoff scanning, a larger amount of saline is introduced for acoustic coupling until the transducer surface is immersed beneath the solution (Fig. 11). During laparotomy, it is easy to keep saline in the abdominal cavity. However, when the target structures are not easily submerged, such as at the time of peripheral vascular surgery, it is helpful to retract the edges of the wound upward so that a sufficient "saline pool" is maintained (Fig. 13). To minimize the production of air bubbles that interfere with ultrasound imaging, the best way to introduce saline is by decanting it from a container or a basin. Saline instillation using a bulb syringe should be avoided because it produces more air bubbles.

In contrast to contact scanning, probe-standoff scanning is a unique IOUS and LUS technique that is not commonly performed in percutaneous body scanning. Although saline immersion is always required, the probe-

standoff technique has several advantages that are summarized in Table 1. With probe-standoff scanning, the distance from the probe to the target area of interest can be adjusted, thus allowing for placement of the target or region of interest at the optimal focal point. As already described, it is critical to perform probe-standoff scanning to clearly visualize the organ surface or other superficial areas. In addition, excessive tissue or organ compression by the probe which may distort the anatomy is avoidable by the use of this technique. Because the probe can be moved freely in the saline bath (because there is no need for persistent contact with tissue), a greater variety of scanning maneuvers can be applied (see the next section on probe movement). For example, the angulation technique (rocking or tilting) of the probe is more readily and effectively carried out with probe-standoff scanning than with contact scanning. At times, the irregular surface of an organ or tissue (e.g., the surface of a cirrhotic liver) does not allow good probe contact, causing the development of artifacts due to air between the transducer surface and tissue. This can be avoided by saline immersion with probe-standoff scanning. For IOUS and LUS, the appropriate use of both contact and probe-standoff scanning is important. At times, both methods

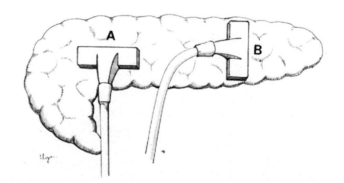

FIGURE 14. An example of scanning planes of the pancreas during intraoperative ultrasound. **A:** A longitudinal scanning for the pancreas because it is along the long axis of the pancreas and this image shows the main pancreatic duct in its longitudinal section. **B:** A transverse scanning plane for the pancreas because it is perpendicular to the long axis of the pancreas and this image exhibits the main pancreatic duct in its transverse or cross-section.

may be employed together by placing a part of the transducer surface in contact with tissue and the remainder not in tissue contact.

An additional technique that is useful is compression scanning, in which the tissue is gently compressed intentionally by the probe (Fig. 12). This method helps to eliminate air between the transducer surface and tissue or between tissues or structures. Air in the gastrointestinal tract lumen that overlies a region of interest can also be displaced by compression. This is particularly useful when gas in the duodenum obscures the distal common bile duct (see Figure 14 in Chapter 14). Compression scanning can also be employed to distinguish veins from arteries. The compressibility of veins is readily recognized on real-time IOUS/LUS, whereas arteries are not as easily compressed.

Scanning Planes and Views

There are two basic scanning planes of ultrasound; longitudinal and transverse. For transabdominal ultrasound (TAUS), the scanning planes are referred to the long axis of the body (see Figure 4 in Chapter 11). Longitudinal scanning with TAUS includes the sagittal plane (which transects the body from anterior to posterior) and the coronal plane (which transects the body from right to left). Transverse scanning with TAUS follows the short axis of the body and cuts through the body perpendicular to the long axis. The transverse plane shows cross-sectional anatomy similar to that demonstrated with computed tomography.

Describing or presenting images of longitudinal and transverse scanning for TAUS and IOUS/LUS can be confusing. Occasionally, particularly in IOUS/LUS, the scanning planes are described in reference to the long axis of the organ rather than the axis of the body. For example, sagittal (longitudinal) scanning of the pancreas in TAUS shows the transverse cross-section of the pancreas. Conversely, in IOUS/LUS, longitudinal scanning of the pancreas usually means imaging along the long axis of pancreas, and thus shows the main pancreatic duct in its longitudinal section (Fig. 14).

During IOUS/LUS, a target or suspected lesion should be scanned from various positions and directions. An organ should be scanned in a systematic fashion for a thorough IOUS/LUS examination. Although the scanning method varies depending on the organ examined, it is usually important to obtain longitudinal, transverse, and, sometimes, oblique views of a lesion or organ. A longitudinal view is the ultrasound image parallel to the long axis of the structure or organ being examined, whereas a transverse view is the image at the right angle to the long axis. Oblique views are intermediate in position between longitudinal and transverse views (Fig. 15). For large organs such as the liver, a combination of longitudinal, transverse, and oblique view scanning is used to systematically examine the entire organ. For smaller tubular structures, such as the extrahepatic bile duct and blood vessels, longitudinal scanning is initially performed, and then transverse scanning is performed. Whenever suspected lesions are identified, it is important to obtain multiple images from longitudinal to transverse views in real time, which provide three-dimensional information about the lesions. This is particularly important in distinguishing an oval or circular lesion from a blood vessel or a duct in cross-section.

Probe Movement in IOUS

The second step in ultrasound scanning is probe movement. There are four basic IOUS scanning maneuvers for probe movement (as with TAUS): sliding, rotating, rocking, and tilting (Table 2). In sliding, the probe is slid across the surface of a tissue or organ while the probe-to-surface geometry is maintained (Fig. 16). For example, the probe is slid in contact with the surface of the liver or pancreas during imaging of these organs (see Figure 14 in Chapter 3 and Figure 6 in Chapter 16). Sliding is usually the commonest probe manipulation during systematic scanning of an entire organ. In rotating, the probe is turned along the direction of the sound beam, either clockwise or counterclockwise, while the region of interest is maintained in the image during the entire time of scanning (Fig. 17; see also Figure 11 in Chapter 15). With this technique, lesions or structures are delineated continually from longitudinal to oblique to transverse views, or vice versa, and thus three-dimensional information on lesions can be acquired. In rocking and tilting, the probe's head (transducer surface side) remains in relatively stationary position while the shaft of the probe is moved or swung to different angles. Such angulation technique is called rocking when the direction of angulation is parallel to the scanning plane, and tilting when the direction of angulation is perpendicular to the scanning plane (Fig. 18; see also Figures 12 and 13 in Chapter 15). This technique is especially useful in a deep and restricted operative field where sliding the probe is limited or impossible. These basic maneuvers can be combined simultaneously, and combination maneuvers are commonly performed during IOUS.

Basic Scanning Techniques in LUS

The basic scanning techniques of LUS are similar to those of IOUS. In general, IOUS scanning during open surgery is easier because the probe can be manipulated freely in the operative field. LUS is technically more demanding because of restricted freedom of probe movement.

Probe placement and probe movement during LUS are essentially the same as for IOUS. In addition to con-

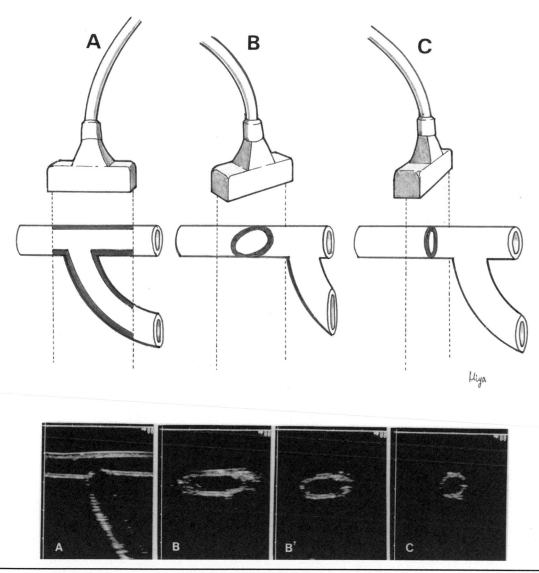

FIGURE 15. Longitudinal (**A**), oblique (**B**), and transverse (**C**) views of the target structures such as blood vessels or ductal systems. The sonograms shown are obtained by scanning a rubber tube (T tube) in a water bath in longitudinal (A), oblique (B and B'), and transverse (C) views.

tact scanning, probe-standoff scanning with saline immersion is frequently used during LUS (e.g., during LUS scanning of the bile ducts). When saline solution is introduced in the abdominal cavity, the patient's position often must be changed so that the transducer surface and the tissue are appropriately immersed. Freedom of probe movement during LUS is limited compared with IOUS. Sliding and rotating (or tilting in case of a side-viewing LUS probe) movements are two major maneuvers of the LUS probe (Fig. 19; see also Figures 2 and 3 in Chapter 14). Rocking of the probe shaft is difficult with a rigid probe, whereas rocking (upward and downward flexion) can be performed quite readily with a flexible tip probe.

IOUS is technically much easier to master and greatly facilitates the performance of LUS. Therefore, surgeons who intend to perform LUS should learn IOUS before or while learning LUS. Surgeons who intend to use LUS

▶ **TABLE 2 Probe Movement**

1. Sliding: along longitudinal or transverse scan paths
2. Rotating: clockwise or counterclockwise
3. Rocking: change of direction (angulation) parallel to the scanning plane
4. Tilting: change of direction (angulation) perpendicular to the scanning plane

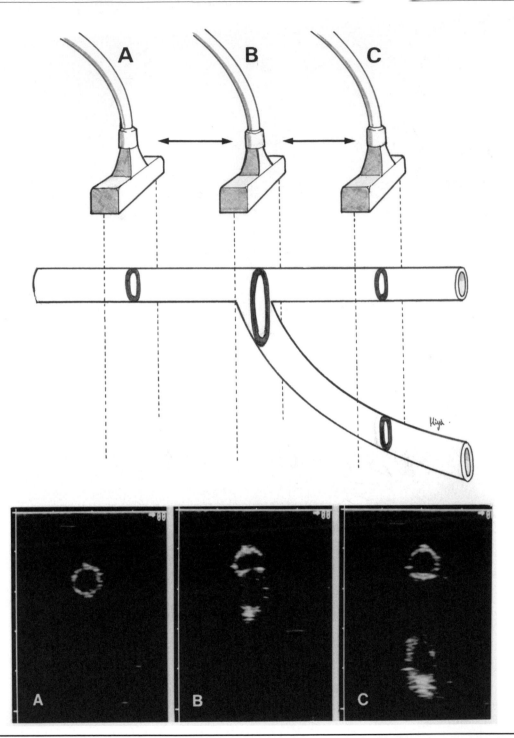

FIGURE 16. Sliding the probe along the longitudinal scan path of the target structure while the transverse views of the structure are maintained. **A:** One transverse view of the tubular structure is seen. **B:** The bifurcation of the structure is displayed. **C:** Two transverse sections are seen. The sonograms are the corresponding images obtained in a water bath.

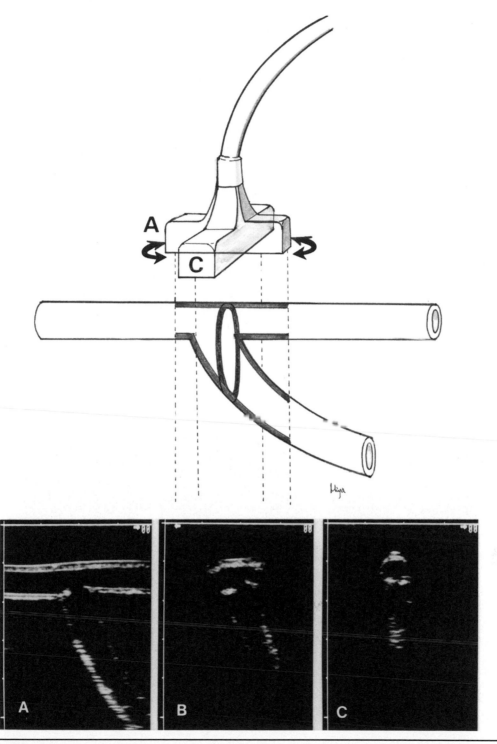

FIGURE 17. Rotating the probe at the same location. The target structure is imaged in longitudinal (**A**), oblique (**B**), and transverse (**C**) views by this rotating maneuver. The sonograms are corresponding images obtained in a water bath.

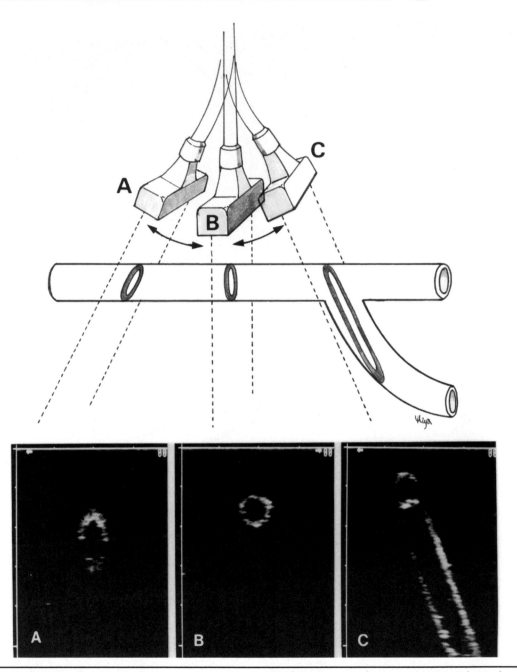

FIGURE 18. Tilting the probe to examine various areas of the structure from one position. The probe is angulated (tilted), perpendicular to the scanning plane, to different directions along the longitudinal scan path of the structure. The sonograms (**A–C**) obtained in a water bath are the images corresponding to the probe positions (A–C) illustrated.

should be able to perform open IOUS, just as surgeons who perform laparoscopic cholecystectomy should know how to perform open cholecystectomy.

Image Interpretation

Several points should be kept in mind for interpretation of IOUS/LUS images. The images of IOUS/LUS are usu-

ally more magnified than those of percutaneous body ultrasound. Most ultrasound systems provide image magnification and zooming; for example, the images can be magnified on the monitor as large as three or four times their actual size. Attention to electronic calipers marking distance, usually displayed at the top or the left side of the monitor, is important for proper interpretation of image size. Before scanning is begun, it is a good routine

A

B

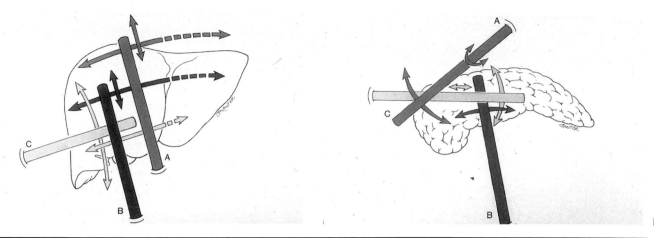

FIGURE 19. **A:** Laparoscopic ultrasound (LUS) scanning of the liver using a rigid LUS probe. Scanning is performed via the subxiphoid (A), umbilical (B), and right subcostal (C) ports. The sliding and rotating techniques are appropriately used to scan and screen the entire liver. **B:** LUS scanning of the pancreas using a rigid LUS probe. Scanning is performed via the subxiphoid (A), umbilical (B), and right subcostal (C) ports. The scanning of the pancreatic head (A) is essentially the same as the scanning of the distal bile duct using sliding and rotating techniques. The entire pancreas should be visualized.

to understand the orientation (right or left) of the image on the screen in relation to each side of the probe. One can determine which portion of the probe window is associated with the right or left side of the image by gently touching either side of the transducer surface and observing the monitor screen at the near-field area of image. During scanning, particularly when the probe position is changed or rotated, the right–left relation of images may be altered. As a rule, the left side of the image on the monitor screen should be maintained toward the patient's right side or toward the patient's head. This is accomplished by utilizing the right–left orientation control of the ultrasound system and changing the direction of image whenever necessary.

Ultrasound images are best read at the focal zone of the transducer. With a high-frequency transducer such as 7.5 MHz, the image resolution within 0.5 to 1.0 cm from the transducer surface (near field) is poor (Fig. 20). Thus,

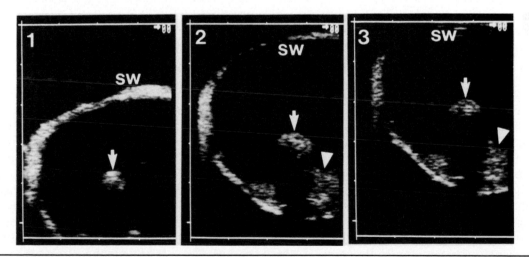

FIGURE 20. Reading images in the focal zone of the transducer. These sonograms are obtained by scanning an excised gallbladder containing a gallstone (*arrow*) and sludge (*arrowhead*) in a water bath. **1:** The superficial wall (SW) of the gallbladder is well visualized in the focal zone by probe-stand-off scanning. **2:** The superficial wall (SW) is not well demonstrated because of its location in the near field of the transducer, although a gallstone is clearly delineated in the focal zone. **3:** In this contact scanning with the gallbladder, the superficial wall is hardly seen.

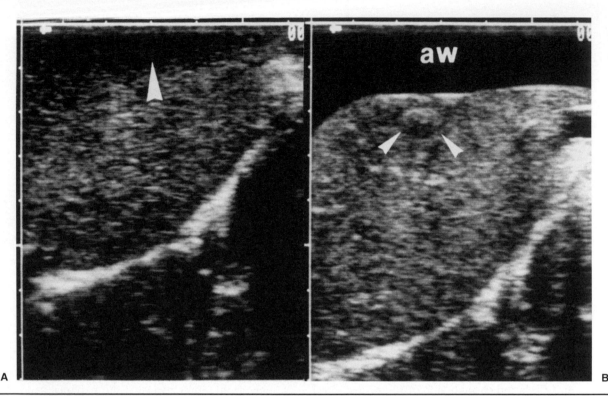

FIGURE 21. Placement of the target lesion or area in the focal zone using the probe-standoff technique. The lesion was a metastatic tumor (*arrowheads*) in the superficial area of the left lateral segment of the liver. **A:** In the contact scanning, the lesion was in the near field and was not well delineated. **B:** In the probe-standoff scanning, in which an acoustic window (aw) was achieved with saline immersion, the lesion was clearly demonstrated.

interpretation of images at this near field should be avoided. If an abnormal lesion is situated in the near field during contact scanning, it is less likely to be detected (Fig. 21). In such an instance, probe-standoff scanning should be appropriately used to place the lesion at the focal distance. Similarly, images in the far field beyond the focal zone or images beyond adequate sound penetration cannot be read appropriately (Fig. 22). Although sound penetration depends on the character of tissue to be scanned, its depth is inversely related to the frequency of ultrasound. The approximate depth of sound penetration within soft tissue in reference to the ultrasound frequency is summarized in Table 3.

Finally, images from innumerable directions are delineated in real time during IOUS/LUS examination. At times, unfamiliar images that are never seen by TAUS are obtained. Understanding the orientation of scanning planes in relation to the anatomy of the target or the organ is critical to interpretation of IOUS/LUS images. Whenever the probe is moved using various scanning maneuvers, the location and orientation of the transducer window should be understood and should be confirmed, if necessary, by directly observing the operative

field where the probe is placed. Hand–eye–image coordination is a key process that must be developed in the learning of IOUS/LUS.

Time of Scanning

IOUS or LUS can be conducted at any time during the operation, depending on the purpose or indication for examination (see the next section on indications). Early in the course of operation, IOUS/LUS is performed to obtain new information that is not evident during preoperative studies or during initial surgical exploration before tissue dissection. Such information may help determine the approach and type of procedure to be performed. For example, immediately after laparotomy or laparoscopy for intraabdominal malignancy, IOUS/LUS is used to evaluate the liver and lymph nodes as well as the primary lesion. IOUS/LUS can also be employed during the main surgical procedure. Under IOUS/LUS guidance, various surgical manipulations, such as needle placement or tissue dissection, can be carried out. Following surgical procedures but prior to closure, IOUS/LUS can be used

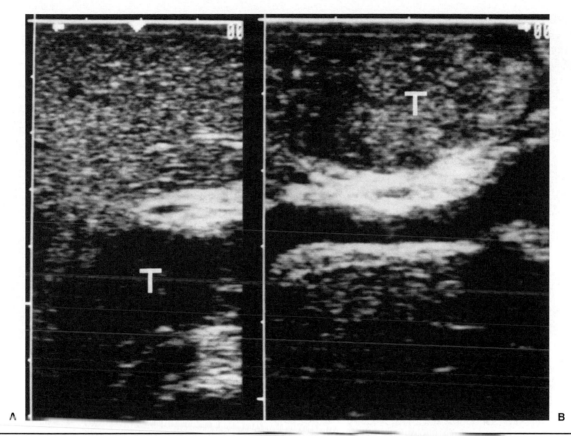

FIGURE 22. A metastatic tumor in the caudate lobe of the liver that was imaged from different positions. **A:** The tumor (T) was scanned from the anterior (ventral) surface of the liver. It was not well seen or was falsely delineated as a hypoechoic tumor because it was located beyond the focal zone and behind the portal vein. **B:** The same tumor (T) was scanned from the inferior surface of the liver. It was clearly delineated, and its echogenicity and echo pattern were appropriately determined.

as a completion examination to confirm the result of procedures and to look for problems that still may be corrected. For example, extraction of calculi or resection of tumors can be verified. IOUS and LUS can be repeated as often as necessary during operation. Therefore, it is advised to keep the probe sterile and the equipment available until completion.

▶ **TABLE 3** Frequency and Penetration of Ultrasound

Ultrasound Frequency (MHz)	Sound Penetration (cm)
3.5	About 15 or more
5	About 10–15
7.5	About 6–10
10	About 5–7

NORMAL ULTRASOUND ANATOMY

Normal ultrasound anatomy of abdominal organs is described in detail in Chapter 11, in which TAUS images are shown. Ultrasound images during IOUS and LUS are demonstrated here; also see subsequent chapters for normal IOUS and LUS anatomy images. Figure 23 shows IOUS or LUS images of the normal liver. Figure 24 shows IOUS or LUS images of the normal pancreas and surrounding vascular structures. Figure 25 shows IOUS or LUS image of the normal biliary system.

TYPICAL IMAGE OF PATHOLOGY

Typical ultrasound image findings of lesions that are frequently encountered during IOUS and LUS examination are briefly presented.

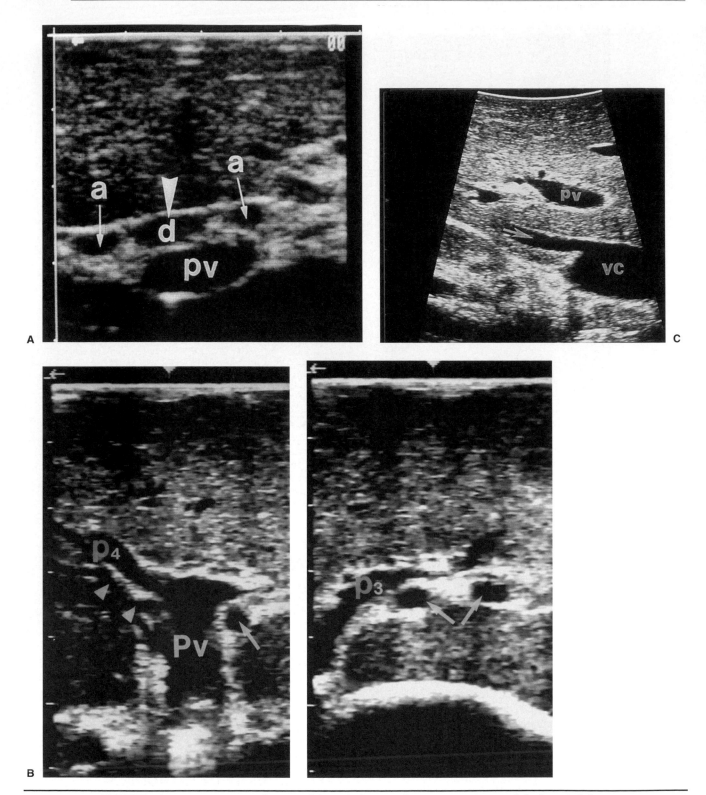

FIGURE 23. A: Intraoperative ultrasound (IOUS) showing the transverse image of the hepatic hilum. The hepatic artery (a, *arrow*) and the bile duct (d, *arrowhead*) are located anterior to the portal vein (pv). **B:** Laparoscopic ultrasound (LUS) of the left lobe of the liver, in transverse views. **Left:** The ascending portion of the left portal vein (Pv) and its medial branch, segment 4 branch (P4). The bile duct (*arrow*) and the hepatic artery (*arrowheads*) are also seen. **Right:** Segment 3 portal vein branch (P3). The bile duct (*arrows*) is located posterior to the portal vein in this location. **C:** IOUS of the main right portal vein (pv) in a transverse view of the liver. There is a large hepatic vein (*arrow*) draining into the vena cava (vc). This is the inferior right hepatic vein. This is the draining vein of segment 6 area of the liver. It is present in approximately 10% to 15% of the population.

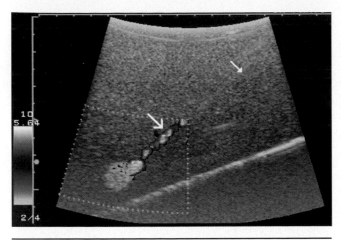

COLOR PLATE 1. Color motion marking for better visualization of the location of the needle using color Doppler imaging. Under color or power Doppler imaging, a needle or a stylet is moved back and forth. This movement produces color motion marking (*large arrow*). This needle is not well visualized in the area of B-mode ultrasound imaging (*small arrow*). (See Figure 44 in Chapter 4.)

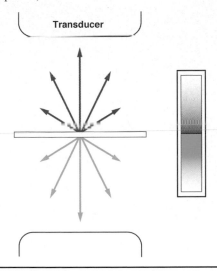

COLOR PLATE 2. Color representation is usually set up with all vectors toward the transducer red and away from the transducer blue (except with venous imaging). (See Figure 2 in Chapter 8.)

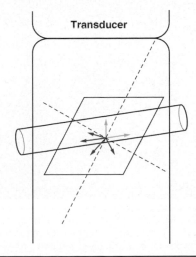

COLOR PLATE 3. With the usual color representation vectors toward the head (conventionally set up to the left of the image if this was a carotid artery) are red. (See Figure 3A in Chapter 8.)

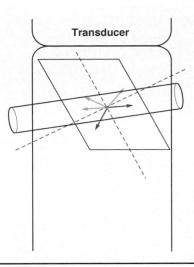

COLOR PLATE 4. With steering of the color box to the right most vectors toward the head would now be blue. (See Figure 3B in Chapter 8.)

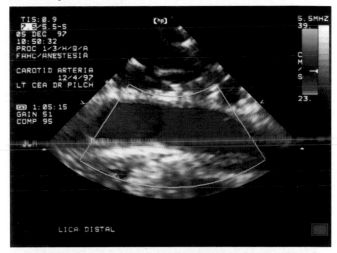

COLOR PLATE 5. Blood cells are traveling from right to left, but they have different color representations because their color vectors are different. This is not reversal of flow nor aliasing. (See Figure 4A in Chapter 8.)

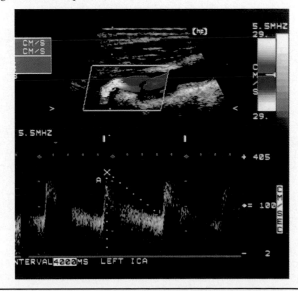

COLOR PLATE 6. Blood is traveling left to right, but color aliasing is evident when red changes to blue with intervening white or yellow (high velocities). (See Figure 4B in Chapter 8.)

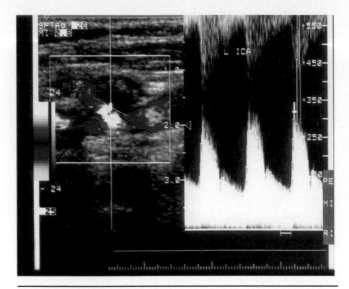

COLOR PLATE 7. Internal carotid artery stenosis is defined by the peak systolic velocity (310 cm/sec here) and the end-diastolic velocity (113 cm/sec here) placing this stenosis in the 80% to 99% range. (See Figure 6 in Chapter 8.)

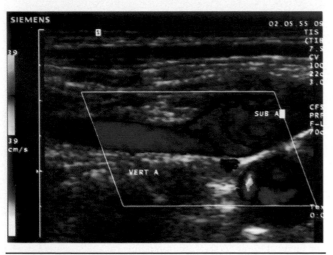

COLOR PLATE 8. The right vertebral origin from the subclavian can frequently be visualized. In this patient a 7.5-MHz linear probe is used. (See Figure 7A in Chapter 8.)

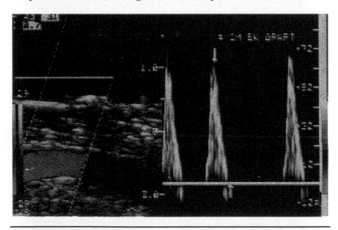

COLOR PLATE 9. Intraoperative graft velocity spectra before papaverine injection. (From Johnson BL, Bandyk DF, Back MR, et al. Intraoperative duplex monitoring of infrainguinal vein bypass procedures. *J Vasc Surg* 2000;31:678–690, with permission). (See Figure 13A in Chapter 8.)

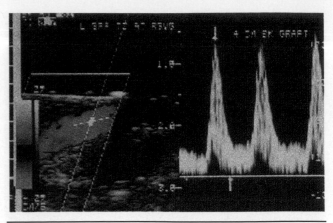

COLOR PLATE 10. Intraoperative graft velocity spectra after papaverine injection. (From Johnson BL, Bandyk DF, Back MR, et al. Intraoperative duplex monitoring of infrainguinal vein bypass procedures. *J Vasc Surg* 2000;31:678–690, with permission). (See Figure 13B in Chapter 8.)

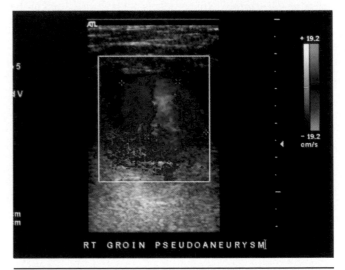

COLOR PLATE 11. Pseudoaneurysm of the common femoral artery shows back-and-forth color distinctive from arterial flow seen beneath the pseudoaneurysm. (See Figure 20 in Chapter 8.)

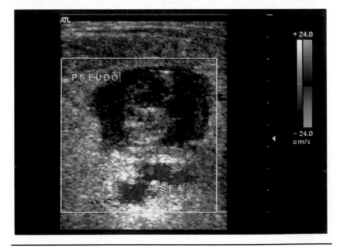

COLOR PLATE 12. After thrombin injection, there is no flow in the pseudoaneurysm cavity on color Doppler imaging. An echogenic thrombus is seen. (See Figure 22 in Chapter 8.)

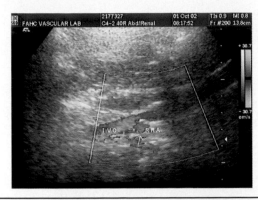

COLOR PLATE 13. The right renal artery (RRA) passing beneath the inferior vena cava (IVC) serves as a landmark for inferior vena cava filter placement. (See Figure 26 in Chapter 8.)

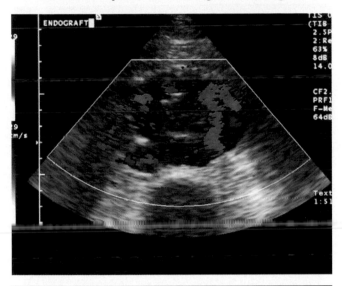

COLOR PLATE 14. Type I endoleak after aortic endograft has back-and-forth pattern similar to that in femoral catheterization–related pseudoaneurysms. (See Figure 27 in Chapter 8.)

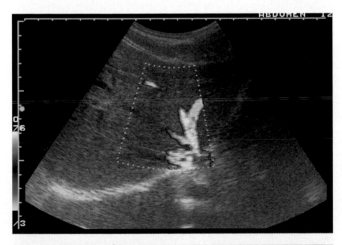

COLOR PLATE 15. The same hepatic veins with color Doppler flow. (See Figure 19B in Chapter 11.)

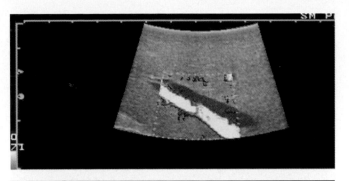

COLOR PLATE 16. Color Doppler ultrasound demonstrates flow in portal vein. (See Figure 54B in Chapter 11.)

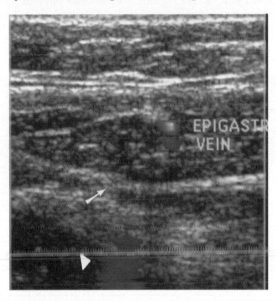

COLOR PLATE 17. Transverse views of inguinal region using color Doppler imaging. Note epigastric vessels, iliac vessels (*triangle*), transversalis fascia (*arrow*), and aponeurosis (X). (See Figure 12A in Chapter 12.)

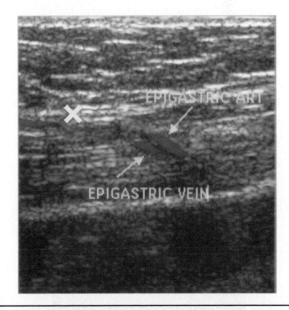

COLOR PLATE 18. Longitudinal views of inguinal region using color Doppler imaging. Note epigastric vessels, iliac vessels (*triangle*), transversalis fascia (*arrow*), and aponeurosis (X). (See Figure 12B in Chapter 12.)

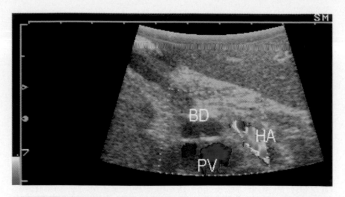

COLOR PLATE 19. B-mode and color Doppler intraoperative ultrasound of the bile duct and vascular structures. Color Doppler imaging of the same structures. The bile duct (BD) without blood flow, hepatic artery (HA), and portal vein (PV) with blood flow in color are readily identified. (See Figure 25B in Chapter 13.)

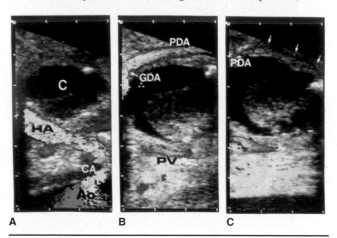

COLOR PLATE 20. Intraoperative color Doppler imaging of the vascular structures around the pancreatic head during an operation for a pseudocyst (C). The course of branches of the celiac artery (CA) was clearly demonstrated. **A:** Ao, aorta; HA, common hepatic artery. **B:** GDA, gastroduodenal artery; PDA, pancreatico-duodenal artery; PV, portal vein, which was partially compressed. **C:** The distal branch (*arrows*) of the PDA was visualized. The pseudocyst contained debris. (See Figure 33 in Chapter 13.)

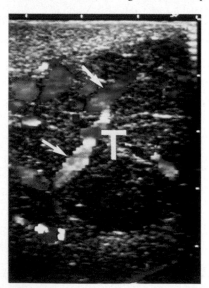

COLOR PLATE 21. Intraoperative color Doppler imaging of a hepatocellular carcinoma. The tumor (T) had multiple large intratumoral vessels (*arrows*), which were difficult to identify with B-mode imaging alone. (See Figure 34 in Chapter 13.)

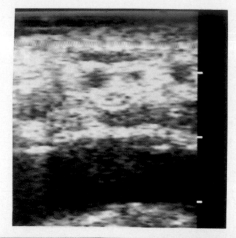

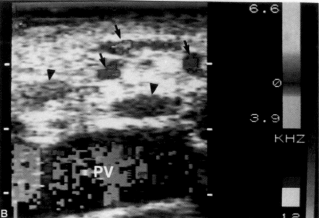

COLOR PLATE 22. Distinction of hypoechoic areas by intraoperative color Doppler imaging. **A:** During an operation for chronic pancreatitis with severe inflammation, B-mode imaging showed multiple hypoechoic areas. **B:** Intraoperative color Doppler imaging demonstrated blood flow in the blood vessels (*arrows*) in color, thus quickly distinguishing them for other tissue spaces (*arrowheads*). PV, portal vein. (See Figure 35 in Chapter 13.)

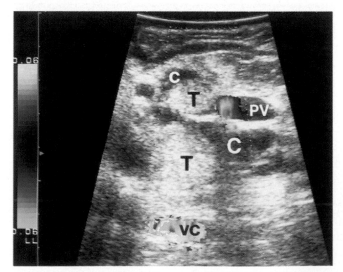

COLOR PLATE 23. Intraoperative color Doppler imaging demonstrating the portal vein (PV) and the vena cava (VC) in color, which were readily distinguished from other hypoechoic areas. This shows cystadenoma containing cystic (C) and tumorous (T) components. The tumor was partly encasing the portal vein; however, the wall and the lumen of the vein were well maintained, indicating the benign character of the tumor. (See Figure 36 in Chapter 13.)

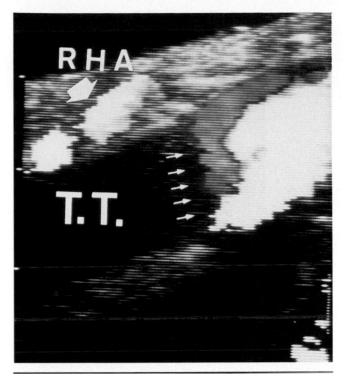

COLOR PLATE 24. Tumor thrombus of a hepatocellular carcinoma. The presence and the extent (*arrows*) of a tumor thrombus (TT) in the right portal vein were quickly determined by the use of intraoperative color Doppler imaging. It was especially helpful when the thrombus was very hypoechoic, as shown here. RHA, right hepatic artery. (See Figure 37 in Chapter 13.)

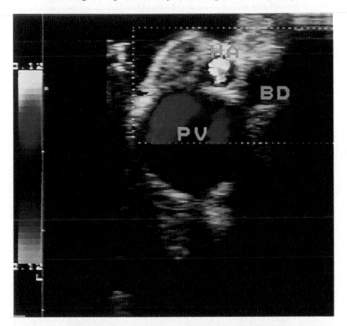

PLATE 25. On color Doppler imaging, the bile duct (BD) without color flow and the hepatic artery (HA) with color flow can be immediately identified. In this image, the artery is the right hepatic artery (not proper hepatic artery), located on the patient's right. PV, portal vein. (See Figure 7A in Chapter 14.)

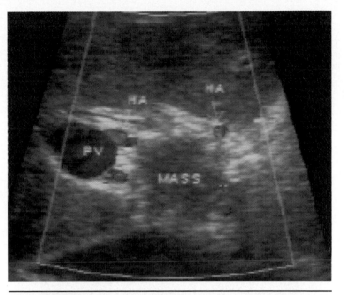

COLOR PLATE 26. A resectable cholangiocarcinoma ("mass"), which does not invade any vascular structures, is shown here. HA, hepatic artery; PV, portal vein. (Courtesy of Dr. Steven Strasberg). (See Figure 31 in Chapter 14.)

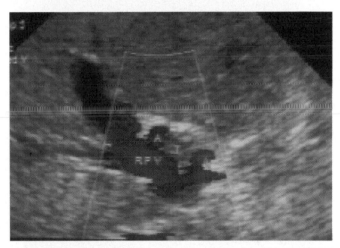

COLOR PLATE 27. Staging laparoscopy with use of laparoscopic ultrasound shows that the cholangiocarcinoma (T) intimately abuts the right portal vein (RPV) and right hepatic artery (A). (Courtesy of Dr. Steven Strasberg). (See Figure 32 in Chapter 14.)

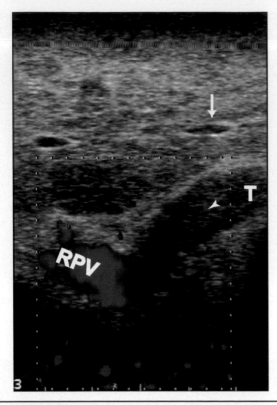

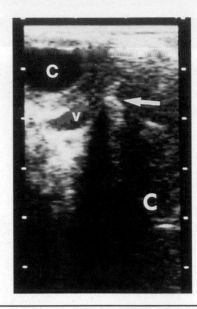

COLOR PLATE 28. Tumor invasion with thrombosis of the main left portal vein. The arrowhead denotes the edge of the tumor thrombus (T) in the left portal vein. The arrow notes a small vein with echogenic tumor thrombus within it. The right portal vein (RPV) has flow indicated by color Doppler imaging. (See Figure 59 in Chapter 15.)

COLOR PLATE 30. A vein detected by intraoperative color Doppler imaging between pseudocysts during an operation for chronic pancreatitis. After cystotomy of the large cyst, a metal probe (*arrow*) was introduced into the large cyst to examine the relation of the two cysts to the intervening vein (v). (See Figure 25B in Chapter 16.)

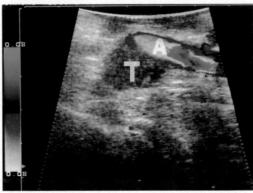

COLOR PLATE 31. Pelvic recurrent cancer in a patient with previous surgery and radiation for a rectal cancer. During laparotomy, surgical exploration was difficult to identify this recurrent cancer. Tumor was located adjacent to the right iliac artery (A), demonstrated by color Doppler imaging. (See Figure 60B in Chapter 16.)

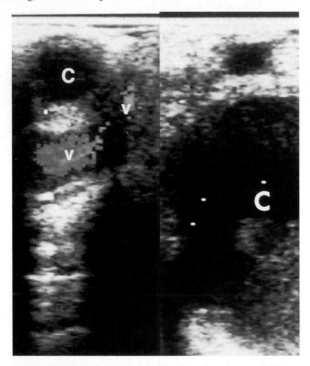

COLOR PLATE 29. A vein detected by intraoperative color Doppler imaging between pseudocysts during an operation for chronic pancreatitis. Color Doppler imaging demonstrated a venous branch (v) between a preoperatively known large pseudocyst (C) and an intraoperative ultrasound–detected small pseudocyst (C). (See Color Plate 29). (See Figure 25A in Chapter 16.)

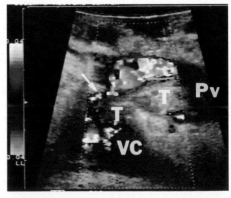

COLOR PLATE 32. Anastomotic stricture and thrombus formation of a portacaval shunt. Intraoperative ultrasound demonstrated a stricture (*arrow*) at the anastomosis between the portal vein (Pv) and vena cava (VC). Intraoperative color Doppler imaging was valuable to recognize the significance of stricture and the extent of thrombus formation (T). (See Figure 62 in Chapter 16.)

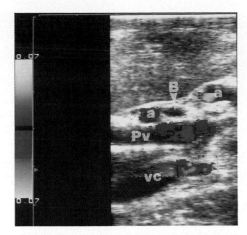

COLOR PLATE 33. Laparoscopic ultrasound image of the hepatic hilum in the transverse view. Color Doppler imaging showing blood flow in the portal vein (Pv), hepatic artery (a), and vena cava (vc). The bile duct (B, *arrowhead*) can be readily distinguished from the artery because of the absence of blood flow. (See Figure 2B in Chapter 17.)

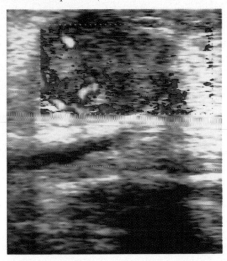

COLOR PLATE 34. Acinar cell adenoma. Power Doppler imaging demonstrated intratumoral blood vessels. Laparoscopic distal pancreatectomy was performed. (See Figure 28B in Chapter 17.)

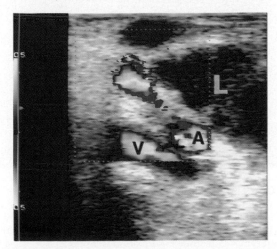

COLOR PLATE 35. Retroperitoneal lymphoma. Laparoscopic ultrasound (LUS) (color Doppler imaging) quickly localized multiple enlarged lymph nodes (L) in the retroperitoneum and demonstrated their relation to vascular structures such as the splenic artery (A) and vein (V). (See Figure 36A in Chapter 17.)

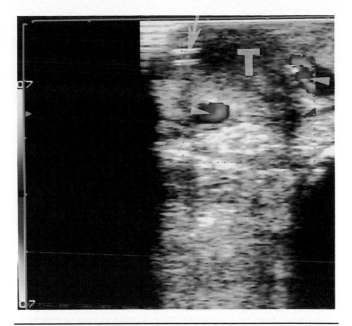

COLOR PLATE 36. Recurrent pelvic lymphoma. A large tumor (T) surrounding the left ureter was localized by laparoscopic ultrasound (LUS) (color Doppler imaging) in the left side of the pelvis. An arrow indicates a stent in the ureter. Arrowheads indicate ileac vessel branches. (See Figure 37A in Chapter 17.)

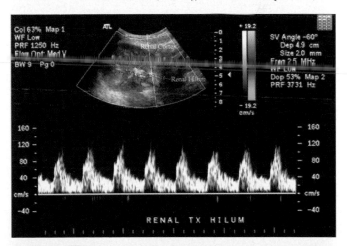

COLOR PLATE 37. Ultrasound with Doppler spectrum of the transplant kidney demonstrating excellent flow in the renal artery and renal vein. (See Figure 1 in Chapter 18.)

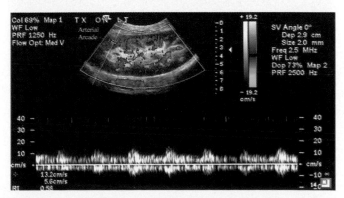

COLOR PLATE 38. Vascular resistive index (RI) is obtained from the arcuate arterials within the cortex of the kidney. In this sonogram, the RI is 0.58. (See Figure 4 in Chapter 18.)

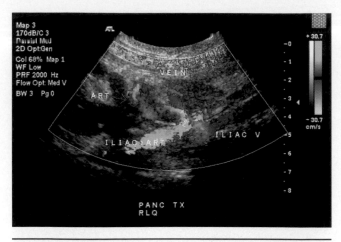

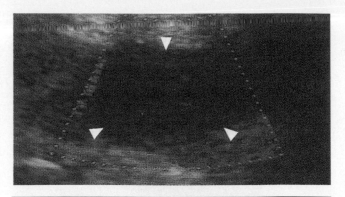

COLOR PLATE 42. Contrast-enhanced color Doppler image obtained after percutaneous ethanol injection showing the disappearance of color flow signals in the treated hepatocellular carcinoma (*arrowheads*). (See Figure 5B in Chapter 21.)

COLOR PLATE 39. Ultrasonic depiction of the portal vein flow into the iliac vein and adjacent arterial flow via the reconstructed arterial conduit of the pancreas graft. (See Figure 7 in Chapter 18.)

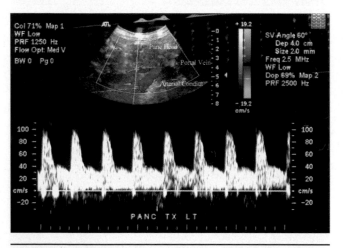

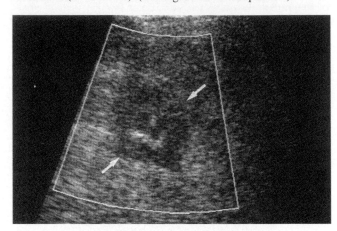

COLOR PLATE 40. Ultrasound with Doppler spectrum depicting the arterial reconstruction and arterial inflow to the transplant pancreas. (See Figure 8 in Chapter 18.)

COLOR PLATE 43. Ultrasound images from a patient with hepatocellular carcinoma following radiofrequency ablation. Unenhanced power Doppler ultrasound image performed after radiofrequency ablation that shows an area of low echogenicity (*arrows*) without intratumoral flow indicative of ablation. (See Figure 6A in Chapter 21.)

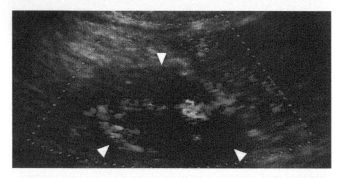

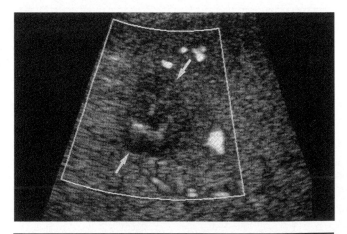

COLOR PLATE 41. Contrast-enhanced color Doppler image with Levovist obtained prior to percutaneous ethanol injection of a hepatocellular carcinoma. Note the intratumoral flow signals (*arrowheads*). (See Figure 5A in Chapter 21.)

COLOR PLATE 44. Ultrasound images from a patient with hepatocellular carcinoma following radiofrequency ablation. Contrast-enhanced power Doppler ultrasound showing no flow signal within the ablated area (*arrows*) but with obvious flow in surrounding tissue. (See Figure 6B in Chapter 21.)

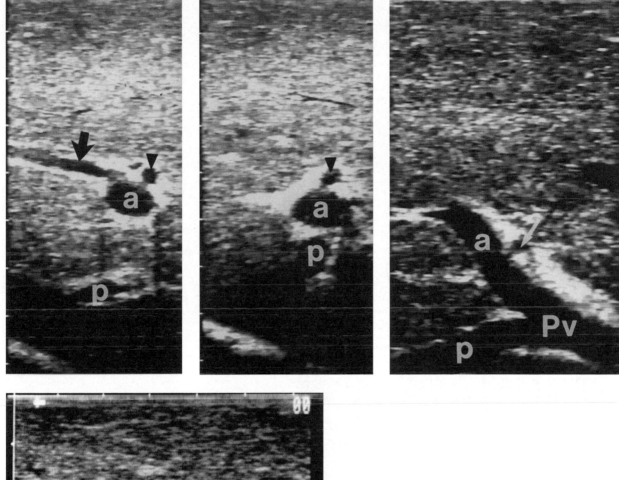

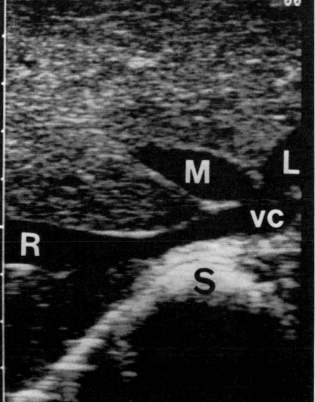

FIGURE 23. *Continued* **D:** LUS of the right portal vein branches. **Right:** The bifurcation of the right portal vein (Pv) into the anterior branch (a) and the posterior branch (p). *White arrow* represents the bile duct. **Middle:** The segment 5 branch (*black arrowhead*) is seen coming from the anterior branch (a). **Left:** The segment 8 branch (*black arrow*) is coming from the anterior branch. In order to follow these segmental or subsegmental branches of the portal vein, the examiner needs to manipulate the probe using sliding and rotating techniques. **E:** IOUS of three hepatic veins. In order to see the hepatic veins in IOUS, the probe must be slid upward toward the dome of the liver or tilted superiorly. Here the right (R), middle (M), and left (L) hepatic veins are coming into the vena cava (VC). S, spine.

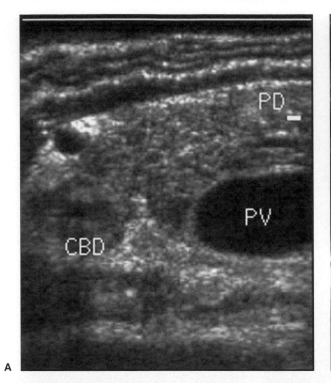

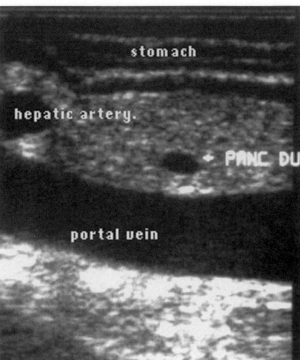

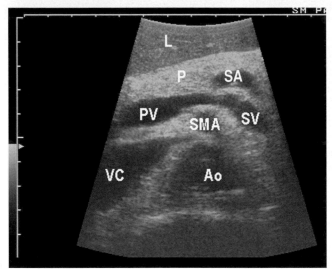

FIGURE 24. **A:** Transgastric laparoscopic ultrasound showing the pancreatic head to the neck. **Left:** The longitudinal (longitudinal to the long axis of the pancreas) view of the head of the pancreas. The common bile duct (CBD) and the pancreatic duct (PD) are seen. PV, portal vein. **Right:** The transverse (perpendicular to the long axis of the pancreas, cross-section of the pancreas) view of the neck of the pancreas. The pancreatic neck is located anterior to the portal vein. Again, the pancreatic duct (Panc Du) is visualized. (Courtesy of Dr. Maurice Arregui.) **B:** Intraoperative ultrasound showing the pancreas neck to body (P) and surrounding vascular structures. The scanning was performed through the left lobe of the liver (L). The portal vein (PV) and splenic vein (SV) are located posterior to the pancreas. SA, splenic artery; SMA, superior mesenteric artery; VC, inferior vena cava; Ao, aorta.

Tumors

The ultrasound features of tumors vary significantly with the tissue type and are affected by multiple factors, such as histologic type, tumor size, growth pattern, vascularity, and secondary changes including degeneration or necrosis. Differentiation between benign and malignant tumors is often difficult even with high-resolution IOUS or LUS, although attention to image characteristics such as shape and border of tumor, echogenicity, echo pattern, and changes in posterior echo may be helpful. Echo-genicity and echo pattern refer to prevailing gray scale appearance: iso-, hyper-, or hypoechoic in reference to surrounding tissue. If more than one pattern is present, the echo pattern is mixed or heterogeneous. In general, tumors can be described as hypoechoic, isoechoic, hyperechoic, mixed, and target patterns. Malignant tumors, when small, are most frequently hypoechoic relative to surrounding normal tissue (Fig. 26). With growth, tumors tend to exhibit a mixed pattern of hypoechoic and hyperechoic areas. A target or so-called "bull's eye" pattern (Fig. 27) is often seen in solid organ tumors, in par-

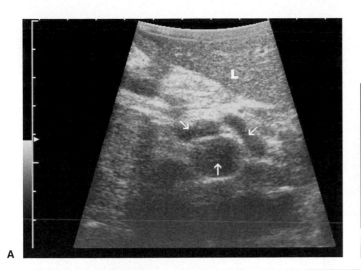
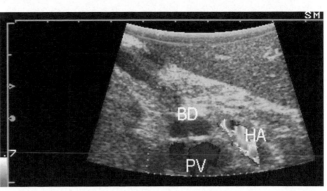

FIGURE 25. B-mode and color Doppler intraoperative ultrasound of the bile duct and vascular structures. **A:** A transverse view of the hepatoduodenal ligament showing three tubular structures of the portal triad (*arrows*). L, left lobe of the liver. **B:** Color Doppler imaging of the same structures. The bile duct (BD) without blood flow, hepatic artery (HA), and portal vein (PV) with blood flow in color are readily identified. (See Color Plate 19.)

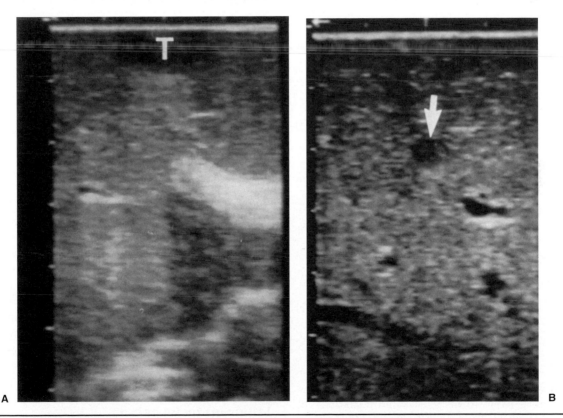

FIGURE 26. Hypoechoic liver metastases from a colon cancer. **A:** A hypoechoic 10 × 17 mm tumor (T) in the medial segment (segment 4) of the left lobe. This tumor was visible and palpable. **B:** A hypoechoic 4 × 5 mm tumor (*arrow*) in the anterior inferior segment (segment 5) of the right lobe. This tumor was unknown preoperatively and was not palpable during surgery.

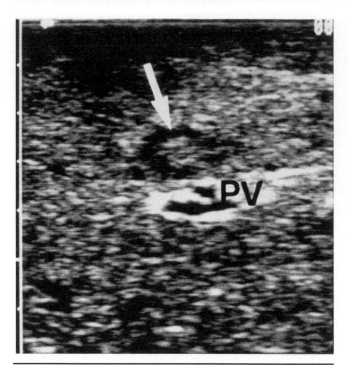

FIGURE 27. An occult liver metastasis with a "bull's eye" appearance. The tumor was not previously recognized. During surgery for a rectal cancer, intraoperative ultrasound was used and detected this tumor (*arrow*) adjacent to the branch of the right portal vein (PV) in the anterior superior segment (segment 8) of the right lobe. The tumor measured 10 × 15 mm, was 2.2 cm in depth from the liver surface, was nonpalpable, and exhibited a "bulls eye" sign.

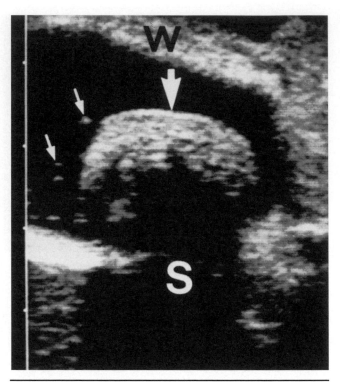

FIGURE 28. A calculus (*arrow*) detected in the gallbladder. It was hyperechoic and was associated with an acoustic shadow (S). Small arrows indicate sludge without shadowing. W, thickened gallbladder wall.

ticular liver tumors, and almost always suggests malignancy. Additional IOUS/LUS images of tumors are found in Chapters 15 and 17 for liver tumors, Chapter 14 for biliary tumors, Chapters 16 and 17 for pancreatic tumors, and Chapters 16 and 17 for endocrine tumors.

Calculi and Air (Gas)

Calculi are hyperechoic (Fig. 28). Focal hyperechogenicity is usually associated with a posterior acoustic shadow, although rarely there are calculi without a shadow. Biliary calculi are usually movable, which can be confirmed by externally manipulating the gallbladder or bile duct. On the other hand, pancreatic duct calculi and kidney calculi are more likely to be fixed. Air or gas may be sometimes difficult to distinguish from calculi; however, air or gas is frequently accompanied by reverberation artifacts, which are unusual with calculi. For example, pneumobilia is associated with reverberation such as ring down artifact as well as shadowing (Fig. 29). Additional IOUS/LUS sonograms are found in Chapter 14 for

biliary calculi and pneumobilia, and in Chapter 16 for pancreatic calculi.

Cystic Lesions

IOUS and LUS are very accurate in the diagnosis of cysts. Typical cysts are anechoic and are associated with posterior enhancement (Fig. 30), although some cysts have debris. Once cysts are complicated by infection or hemorrhage, more internal echoes are visualized. Because of these echoes, at times abscesses may not be easily distinguished from tumors (Fig. 31). In such instances, ultrasound-guided aspiration is recommended. More IOUS/LUS sonograms are seen in Chapter 15 for liver cysts and Chapter 16 for pancreatic cysts.

Inflammatory Lesions

An acute inflammatory process such as acute pancreatitis shows either a hypoechoic or mixed echo pattern, depending on the degree of tissue edema and the presence of necrosis or hemorrhage. On the other hand, chronic inflammatory lesions such as chronic pancreatitis usu-

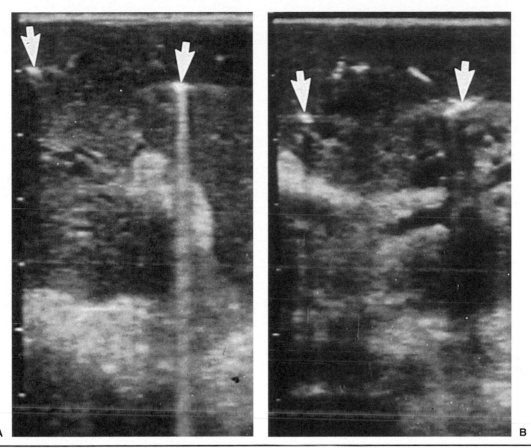

FIGURE 29. Pneumobilia (*arrows*) detected in intrahepatic bile ducts by intraoperative ultrasound. Air exhibits shadowing (**B**) or ring-down reverberation artifacts (**A**) as shown here.

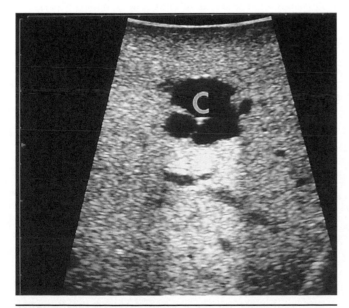

FIGURE 30. A liver cyst (C) detected by intraoperative ultrasound. The cyst was anechoic and was associated with posterior enhancement.

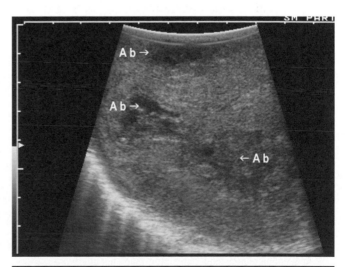

FIGURE 31. Ultrasound diagnosis of an abscess is more difficult than that of a cyst. This is because of the presence of internal echoes, irregular borders, and often the lack of posterior enhancement. This shows multiple abscesses (Ab, *arrows*) which were detected by intraoperative ultrasound.

ally display relative hyperechogenicity in comparison with normal tissue. See Chapter 16 for IOUS/LUS sonograms of pancreatitis.

GENERAL INDICATIONS

The four general indications for IOUS and LUS are listed in Table 4 (3–7,29). Acquisition of new or more accurate information that is not possible with preoperative imaging studies or intraoperative surgical exploration includes new diagnosis of unrecognized disease, localization or exclusion of previously identified lesions, and provision of other anatomic information. IOUS/LUS can be invaluable in assessing the extent of malignant disease (cancer staging). For example, liver metastasis and vascular invasion of hepatobiliary and pancreatic cancers can be diagnosed more accurately than by preoperative tests. During hepatic surgery for liver tumors, IOUS findings have changed previously planned surgical procedures in 30% to 50% of operations (40–44). When employed as a screening procedure, IOUS detects occult liver metastasis in 5% to 10% of operations (40,45,46). LUS can also provide more staging information of abdominal malignancy than laparoscopy alone, and laparoscopy with LUS has established unresectability in 20% to 50% of patients who preoperatively had been considered to have potentially resectable tumors (47,48). Prelaparotomy laparoscopy with LUS can significantly reduce unnecessary or nontherapeutic laparotomy for patients with unresectable cancers not diagnosed with preoperative imaging. Precise localization of nonpalpable lesions such as liver tumors, cysts and abscesses, intrahepatic calculi, pancreatic tumors, cysts and dilated ducts, and other intraabdominal lesions is possible. IOUS appears to be one of the best methods to localize islet cell tumors and parathyroid tumors. Preoperatively or intraoperatively suspected pathologic processes may be excluded by the use of IOUS/LUS. In addition to diagnosing focal lesions, important anatomic structures, including vascular anatomy, can be delineated prior to surgical dissection. By providing new imaging information, IOUS/LUS helps to select the best approach to lesions or choice of the most appropriate surgical operations.

▶ **TABLE 4 Indications for Intraoperative
                and Laparoscopic Ultrasound**

1. Acquisition of new diagnostic information not otherwise available
2. Complement to or replacement for intraoperative radiology
3. Guidance of surgical procedures
4. Confirmation of completion of operation

IOUS/LUS is indicated as a complement to or replacement for conventional intraoperative radiographic studies. During both open and laparoscopic cholecystectomy, IOUS/LUS has shown equal or superior accuracy to intraoperative cholangiography in the diagnosis of bile duct calculi (40,49–53). Therefore, IOUS/LUS can replace cholangiography when used as a routine screening examination, with cholangiography being reserved for selective application. Because IOUS/LUS and cholangiography have advantages and disadvantages, both tests should be used in complementary fashion. During vascular surgery, in comparison with intraoperative arteriography, IOUS has demonstrated equal accuracy in detecting vascular defects such as intimal flaps, strictures, and thrombi (3–5,27,54).

Guidance of various operative procedures can be performed with IOUS/LUS. IOUS/LUS-guided procedures are often indispensable and directly affect surgical outcome (see the following section on IOUS- and LUS-guided procedures).

Confirmation of completion of operation includes assessment of tissue excision and discovery of technical problems. IOUS or LUS is used to confirm adequate resection of tumors in solid organs such as the liver, complete removal of biliary or pancreas calculi, and extraction of foreign bodies. Discovery of technical problems after reconstructive operations such as cardiovascular surgery is possible, so that the problems can be corrected immediately. Operative complications, such as hematoma formation in organs, can be recognized intraoperatively. Intraoperative color Doppler imaging can provide blood flow information to organs immediately after operations such as organ transplantation.

There may be multiple indications of IOUS/LUS during a single operation. For example, during hepatic surgery, IOUS or LUS can be used first to obtain new information, then guide biopsy and resection, and finally confirm complete resection of lesions (see Fig. 44).

SPECIFIC ORGAN INDICATIONS

Indications for IOUS/LUS performed upon the following organs are considered in chapters dealing with these areas of IOUS/LUS.

Liver (see Chapters 15 and 17)
Biliary Tract (see Chapter 14)
Pancreas (see Chapters 16 and 17)
Other abdominal organs (see Chapters 16 and 17)
Endocrine system (see Chapters 6, 16, and 17)

Additional indications that are not discussed in other chapters are briefly reviewed below. These include IOUS indications for extraabdominal organs.

Cardiovascular System

During vascular surgery, IOUS can be used for pre-reconstruction evaluation of vascular abnormalities as needed when preoperative imaging information is not sufficient. However, the main indication of IOUS is post-reconstruction detection of peripheral vascular defects as a completion examination. After vascular reconstruction including bypass operation and endarterectomy, vascular defects such as intimal flaps, strictures, and thrombi that may cause postoperative complications should be detected and corrected. Intraoperative arteriography has been utilized for this purpose. In our studies on 519 vascular operations, vascular defects were detected by IOUS in 155 operations (29.9%). Of these, vascular defects in 48 operations (9.3%) were judged to be significant to endanger patency of reconstructed vessels and thus were repaired (3–5,27). In comparison to intraoperative arteriography, IOUS was equally accurate with a sensitivity of 93.1% and a specificity of 97.8% for diagnosing vascular defects. In addition, IOUS has several advantages over arteriography as described in the next section on advantages. Therefore, IOUS can be a first-choice screening test to examine vascular reconstructive sites. In particular, during carotid endarterectomy, IOUS is the only safe imaging method because of the risk associated with intraoperative carotid arteriography. By using IOUS, intraoperative arteriography can be used more selectively when IOUS results are not conclusive or when the distal arterial bed must be evaluated. Intraoperative color Doppler imaging provides additional blood flow information that may enhance the efficacy of IOUS. During endovascular procedures such as intravascular stent placement, intravascular IOUS often provides valuable information.

During cardiac surgery, IOUS can be used directly on the heart (epicardially); however, intraoperative transesophageal echocardiography with color Doppler imaging has become especially useful. Using these IOUS methods after the completion of cardiac procedures, the adequacy of the repair can be assessed during open heart surgery for valvular or congenital heart disease (32,55). In addition to anatomic information, dynamic blood flow and cardiac functional information can be obtained with color Doppler imaging. Epicardial IOUS may be used during coronary artery bypass operation to select the optimal site for distal anastomosis before reconstruction and to evaluate anastomotic sites after reconstruction. Thoracic aortic dissection can also be assessed before and after the repair (32).

Brain and Spinal Cord

Indications for IOUS during brain and spinal cord operations include localization and assessment of lesions, guidance of neurosurgical procedures, and confirmation of operative procedures (56,57). Lesions for which IOUS has been used during neurosurgery are brain and spinal cord tumors, cysts, abscesses, hematomas, syringomyelias, vascular abnormalities (aneurysms and arteriovenous malformations), hydrocephalus, disk hernias, and foreign bodies. IOUS localization and needle guidance (Fig. 32) are frequently used, and this method is much simpler than stereotactic computed tomography.

Kidney

In the management of urinary tract calculi, introduction of nonsurgical techniques such as extracorporeal shock wave lithotripsy have remarkably reduced open surgical nephrolithotomy. However, when open surgery is needed, IOUS is often indicated to localize intrarenal calculi, guide extraction, and confirm complete calculus removal (30,58). IOUS is quicker, easier to perform, and more accurate in detecting renal calculi than intraoperative radiography. During surgery for renal tumors, IOUS can be performed for localization of nonpalpable tumors or for evaluation of tumor extension in the renal vein or vena cava (29,59). Tumor thrombi extending to the heart are

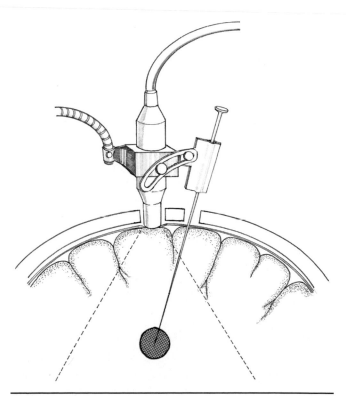

FIGURE 32. Intraoperative ultrasound–guided needle placement in a brain lesion using an end-viewing sector probe. A needle is advanced toward the target lesion along the guide line on the monitor screen. This technique can be used for aspiration, biopsy, or catheterization.

also visualized with intraoperative transesophageal echocardiography. With increased use of laparoscopic nephrectomy, LUS may be used more frequently intraoperatively for evaluation of renal lesions.

Lung and Mediastinum

IOUS can be used during operations for malignant tumors of the lung and mediastinum to evaluate cardiovascular invasion and lymph node involvement during thoracotomy. Cardiovascular invasion of lung cancer has been more accurately diagnosed by IOUS than by preoperative imaging studies (29,60). The liver can also be scanned intraoperatively from the thoracic cavity through the diaphragm. Thoracoscopic ultrasound has recently been performed using laparoscopic ultrasound probes. Thoracoscopic ultrasound can be used to detect and localize lung nodules that are not identifiable by thoracoscopy alone.

Breast

With more frequent use of ultrasound by surgeons, IOUS of the breast has been lately recognized as a valuable tool, particularly for localization and guidance of excision of nonpalpable breast lesions or cancers (61,62). See Chapter 5 for breast ultrasound in detail.

Foreign Bodies

Although radiologic studies are important initial tests in the diagnosis of foreign bodies, during surgery to remove them, nonpalpable foreign bodies are often difficult to locate even with intraoperative radiography or fluoroscopy. In such instances, IOUS is indicated for precise localization. IOUS can eliminate blind or radiographic exploration, and can guide removal of foreign bodies more quickly and safely (3,5,29). Assistance of IOUS is especially valuable for foreign bodies in critical organs such as the heart or brain.

ADVANTAGES, LIMITATIONS, AND COMPLICATIONS

Advantages and Limitations of IOUS

In comparison to intraoperative radiography such as cholangiography, IOUS has multiple advantages as listed in Table 5 (1–7,28–30). IOUS is inherently safer than contrast radiography because cannulation, contrast injection, and irradiation are not required. Because of its safety, IOUS can be used for a prolonged period or repeated as necessary during the course of an operation.

▶ **TABLE 5   Advantages and Disadvantages of Intraoperative Ultrasound**

Advantages
1. Safety: no contrast, no radiation
2. Repeatability
3. Speed
4. High accuracy
5. More imaging information: real time, multiplanar
6. Wider applicability
7. Capability to guide procedures

Disadvantages
1. Limitations in certain imaging abilities
2. Slow learning curve, examiner dependency
3. Requirement of specific instruments

Once learned, the scanning itself is relatively simple and image interpretation is done immediately during surgery using real-time images. The scanning time depends on the purpose of IOUS: usually IOUS is completed in a short time. For example, screening of lesions such as liver metastasis or bile duct calculi can be completed in approximately 5 minutes. Detailed examination of cancer spread or guidance of surgical procedures may require 10 to 20 minutes. However, information provided by IOUS actually reduces overall operating time because unnecessary tissue dissection time is reduced. IOUS-guided procedures are usually much faster and safer than "blind" procedures without IOUS (1–7).

IOUS is generally more accurate than preoperative imaging studies such as computed tomography and TAUS or to conventional surgical exploration by inspection and palpation. IOUS demonstrates equal or superior accuracy to intraoperative contrast radiography such as cholangiography and arteriography. IOUS provides multiplanar images from various locations and angles; therefore, more imaging views can be obtained than are obtained by radiologic means. By displaying two-dimensional images in real time, three-dimensional information about lesions, organs, and vascular structures can be acquired. IOUS has been applied to a variety of surgical procedures including hepatobiliary, pancreatic, endocrine, cardiovascular, neurosurgical, gastrointestinal, urologic, gynecologic, thoracic, and other operations. The unique capability of IOUS in guiding various procedures cannot be replaced by intraoperative radiography.

IOUS also has disadvantages and limitations (Table 5). Limitations in imaging capabilities relate to detectability of small lesions and delineation of ductal or tubular structures. For example, tumors less than 3 to 5 mm are usually undetectable even with high-resolution ultrasound. Furthermore, even larger tumors, if isoechoic, may not be detected. Generally, IOUS displays smaller fields of views than radiography. An entire ductal system such as biliary tracts and pancreatic ducts or vascular trees cannot be displayed in a single image. Small fistulas (e.g., biliary or pancreatic fistulas) that are identifiable by contrast radiography are difficult to delineate with IOUS.

The result of IOUS examination is dependent upon the operator's experience, diligence and ability. This operator dependency is also related to the learning curve. The learning curve for developing competency in various examinations or procedures differs, depending on the target organ or lesion, the purpose of IOUS and the complexity of the images. To master IOUS, for example, approximately 20 to 30 examinations are needed for screening of the liver or the bile duct. For guidance of hepatic or pancreatic operations, probably 30 to 40 examinations (or even more) are required. However, surgeons who are familiar with performance and interpretation of percutaneous or other general ultrasound can learn IOUS faster. Specific instruments for IOUS including probes that are small and easily maneuverable in the operating field are required. Currently, each high-frequency IOUS probe costs in the range of $6,000 to $10,000.

Advantages and Limitations of LUS

LUS combined with laparoscopic exploration compensates for the major disadvantages of laparoscopy, particularly the loss of tactile sensation and the inability to examine deeply located structures or lesions (6, 7, 38, 39). The advantages of LUS over preoperative imaging studies and intraoperative radiography are overall the same as those of IOUS. The disadvantages or limitations are also similar (Table 6).

Because the same high-frequency instruments are employed during LUS as during IOUS, the resolution of LUS and IOUS imaging should be essentially the same. However, LUS scanning techniques are generally more demanding than IOUS scanning performed during laparotomy. For example, complete examination of the entire liver is more difficult using LUS than IOUS. Therefore, diagnostic accuracy of LUS should be close to, but may not be as high as, that of open IOUS (6,63). The time needed to scan the same organ or lesion is longer with

LUS than IOUS. The learning curve for LUS is also longer. In addition, because LUS probes are relatively new, their availability is still limited, and they are still costly. LUS equipment should be more refined, particularly in the development of an appropriate needle guidance system, which currently is not widely available.

Possible Complications Related to the Use of IOUS and LUS

There are no confirmed biologic effects on patients or examiners caused by present ultrasound equipment, including that used for IOUS and LUS. Although potential complications include organ injuries due to probe manipulation and contamination due to disruption of a sterile cover, such complications are very rare during diagnostic IOUS or LUS.

There are possible complications associated with therapeutic or interventional IOUS/LUS (IOUS/LUS-guided procedures). For example, IOUS/LUS-guided needle placement for biopsy may cause bleeding, infection, or bile or pancreatic leakage. However, because a needle is advanced under ultrasound imaging, IOUS/LUS-guided needle placement is safer than blind needle placement with inspection and palpation alone. Complications associated with more advanced IOUS/LUS-guided procedures such as tumor ablation and resection are caused by the procedures themselves, not by IOUS/LUS.

INTRAOPERATIVE COLOR DOPPLER IMAGING

Color or power Doppler imaging displays blood flow in color within real-time B-mode gray scale images. This ultrasound modality has been introduced in cardiovascular surgery and general surgery, and provides blood flow information in addition to anatomic information (32–34, 55). During general surgery, several benefits can be realized with the use of intraoperative color or power Doppler imaging as compared with B-mode imaging alone: (a) detection and localization of small blood vessels (including intratumoral vessels) that are difficult or impossible to identify by surgical exploration or B-mode IOUS (Figs. 33 and 34); (b) rapid and definitive distinction of blood vessels from other hypoechoic areas such as tissue spaces, ducts or cystic lesions (Figs. 35 and 36); (c) determination of the relation of tumors to vascular structures such as vascular invasion of cancer or detection of tumor thrombi (Figs. 36 and 37); (d) confirmation of blood flow to organs after surgical operations such as major organ resection or transplantation (see Figures 1, 4, 7, 8, and 16 in Chapter 18); and (e) clearer needle localization for guidance of needle placement by color motion marking

▌ **TABLE 6 Advantages and Limitations of Laparoscopic Ultrasound**

1. Compensation for limitations of laparoscopic exploration
2. Overall advantages and disadvantages: similar to those of open intraoperative ultrasound
3. Technically more demanding than open intraoperative ultrasound
4. Diagnostic accuracy: close to, but maybe not as accurate as, open intraoperative ultrasound

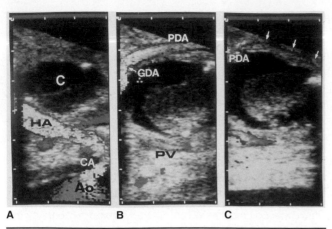

A   B   C

FIGURE 33. Intraoperative color Doppler imaging of the vascular structures around the pancreatic head during an operation for a pseudocyst (C). The course of branches of the celiac artery (CA) was clearly demonstrated. **A:** Ao, aorta; HA, common hepatic artery. **B:** GDA, gastroduodenal artery; PDA, pancreaticoduodenal artery; PV, portal vein, which was partially compressed. **C:** The distal branch (*arrows*) of the PDA was visualized. The pseudocyst contained debris. (See Color Plate 20.)

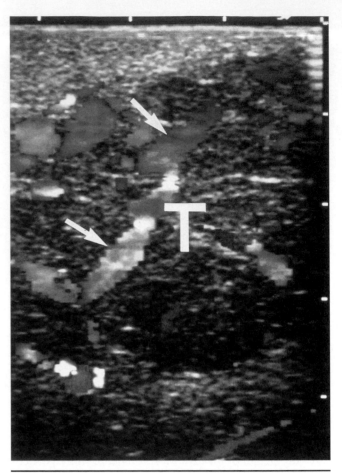

FIGURE 34. Intraoperative color Doppler imaging of a hepatocellular carcinoma. The tumor (T) had multiple large intratumoral vessels (*arrows*), which were difficult to identify with B-mode imaging alone. (See Color Plate 21.)

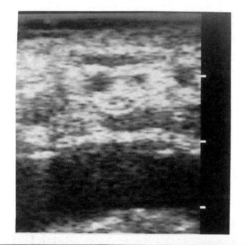

A

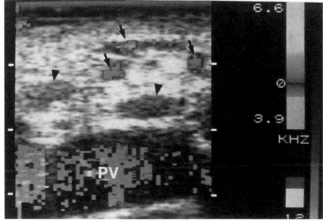

B

FIGURE 35. Distinction of hypoechoic areas by intraoperative color Doppler imaging. **A:** During an operation for chronic pancreatitis with severe inflammation, B-mode imaging showed multiple hypoechoic areas. **B:** Intraoperative color Doppler imaging demonstrated blood flow in the blood vessels (*arrows*) in color, thus quickly distinguishing them for other tissue spaces (*arrowheads*). PV, portal vein. (See Color Plate 22.)

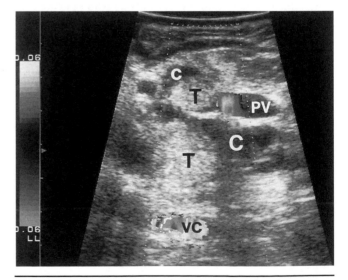

FIGURE 36. Intraoperative color Doppler imaging demonstrating the portal vein (PV) and the vena cava (VC) in color, which were readily distinguished from other hypoechoic areas. This shows cystadenoma containing cystic (C) and tumorous (T) components. The tumor was partly encasing the portal vein; however, the wall and the lumen of the vein were well maintained, indicating the benign character of the tumor. (See Color Plate 23.)

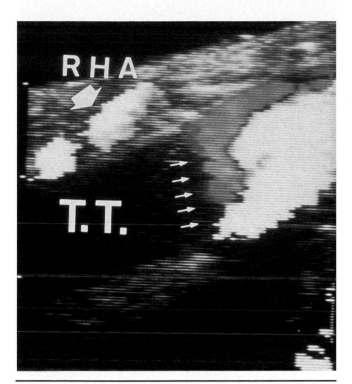

FIGURE 37. Tumor thrombus of a hepatocellular carcinoma. The presence and the extent (*arrows*) of a tumor thrombus (TT) in the right portal vein were quickly determined by the use of intraoperative color Doppler imaging. It was especially helpful when the thrombus was very hypoechoic, as shown here. RHA, right hepatic artery. (See Color Plate 24.)

(see Figure 42 in Chapter 4). During the majority of IOUS/LUS examinations, B-mode ultrasound alone is generally sufficient. However, color or power Doppler imaging is helpful, particularly to quickly identify blood vessels and distinguish them from other tubular or ductal structures (e.g., distinction between the bile duct and the hepatic artery during LUS).

IOUS- AND LUS-GUIDED PROCEDURES

Various operative procedures can be guided by IOUS/LUS. This indication for IOUS/LUS is unique because the assistance it provides is more than simply supplying diagnostic information and because the use of ultrasound in this context may directly affect the therapeutic outcome of surgery. Surgical procedures or manipulations guided by IOUS/LUS are classified in two categories: intraoperative needle, cannula, or ablation probe placement; and surgical tissue dissection (1–7,29,40) (see Tables 1 and 2 in Chapter 4).

IOUS/LUS-Guided Techniques

For IOUS-guided needle, cannula or ablation probe placement, the freehand technique or the technique using a needle guidance system (see Chapter 4 in detail; see also Figures 12 to 26 in Chapter 4) are selected, based on the size, location and depth of the target lesion and the condition of the operative field (accessibility of the lesion), after weighing the advantages and disadvantages of each method. In general, needle or cannula placement in superficially situated, larger lesions can be performed by the freehand technique, whereas deeply situated, smaller lesions require use of a needle guidance system (Figs. 38 and 39). With more experience, the surgeon can use the freehand technique more often. The optimal needle guidance system for side-viewing LUS probes is not widely available, except for one LUS probe with biopsy guidance system provided by B&K Medical (Fig. 40). Therefore, the freehand method is usually used for laparoscopic operations. LUS-guided needle placement is technically more demanding because of the lack of this guidance system, greater distance to the target lesion (owing to peritoneal insufflation), and limited access for LUS probe placement. At times, it is difficult to visualize the entire needle shaft and tip during needle insertion under LUS guidance. Recently, an end-viewing LUS probe with a needle guidance system has become available (Fig. 41). This type of probe will become useful for LUS guidance procedures. When a cryoablation probe or thermal ablation cannula is placed under IOUS/LUS guidance, the ablation process is also monitored by IOUS/LUS imaging (ice ball formation for cryoablation and hyperechoic changes for thermal ablation).

The parenchyma of organs (most frequently the liver) or tissue can be dissected for incision or resection under IOUS/LUS guidance. Unlike needle placement, the dissection itself is not visualized in real-time. Rather, IOUS/LUS is performed repeatedly, and the dissection plane is intermittently visualized in relation to surrounding structures. The dissection or transection plane, which contains air bubbles, is delineated as a hyperechoic glittering line on IOUS/LUS (Fig. 42). The plane can be recognized also by inserting a surgeon's finger into it (Fig. 43). The tissue dissection can be also assisted by the needle localization technique. In this technique, a needle is inserted into the planned plane of dissection under IOUS/LUS guidance, and the tissue is incised along the needle. Examples of IOUS-guided tissue dissection procedures are briefly described.

IOUS-Guided Hepatectomy

Using IOUS imaging, the resection areas are marked on the surface of the liver by electrocautery (Fig. 44). The

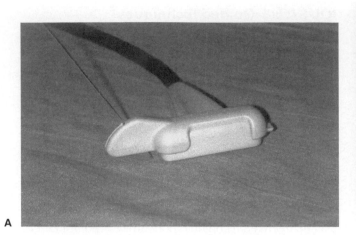

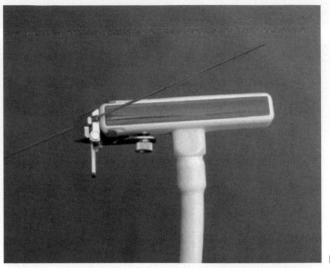

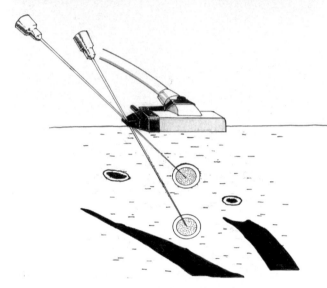

FIGURE 38. A: T-shaped intraoperative ultrasound (IOUS) probe with needle guidance system. (Courtesy of B&K Medical.) B: T-shaped IOUS probe with needle guidance system. (Courtesy of Aloka.) C: IOUS-guided needle placement to the target lesions within the liver parenchyma. In many instances, needle placement is accomplished by the freehand method. However, for deeply located lesions or small lesions, the needle guidance system, as shown here, is helpful.

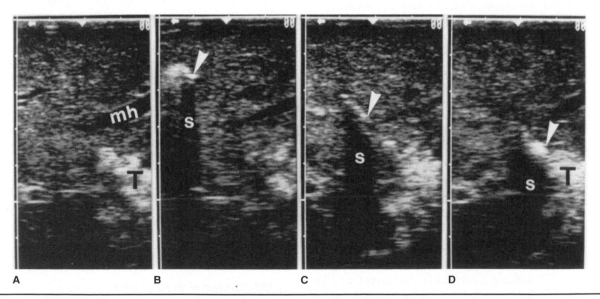

FIGURE 39. Intraoperative ultrasound guidance of needle placement for biopsy. A: A tumor (T) was detected in the posterior inferior segment (segment 6) of the right lobe. mh, middle hepatic vein. **B–D:** A biopsy needle (*arrowhead*), which was associated with an acoustic shadow (s), was introduced into the liver and advanced to the tumor. An injury to the vein was avoided. The tumor was a metastasis from a rectal cancer.

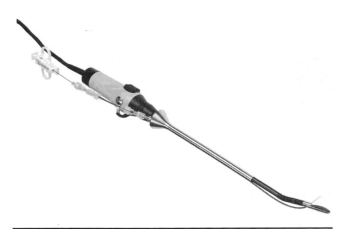

FIGURE 40. Biopsy needle guidance system specifically made for a laparoscopic ultrasound (LUS) probe by one company. So far, this is the only needle guidance system available for a flexible LUS probe. This is a special biopsy needle that can only be used in this particular probe. (Courtesy of B&K Medical.)

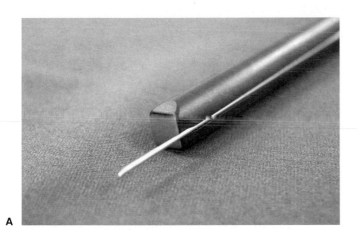

A

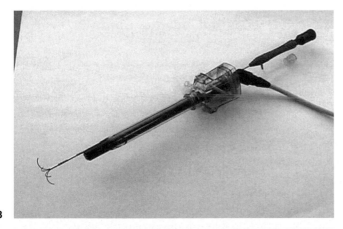

B

FIGURE 41. End-viewing rigid laparoscopic ultrasound probe that has a needle guidance capability. (Courtesy of Aloka.) **A:** Biopsy needle. **B:** Radiofrequency ablation electrode-cannula. (Courtesy of RITA Medical.)

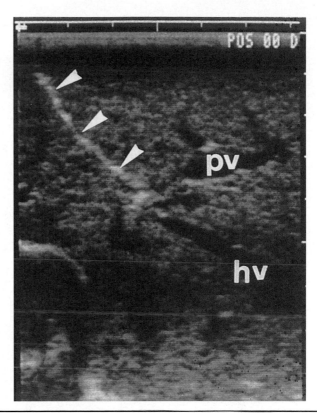

FIGURE 42. Sonogram showing hepatic tissue dissection guided by intraoperative ultrasound. The dissection plane (*arrowheads*) is visualized well in relation to intrahepatic vascular structures such as the portal vein (pv) branch and the hepatic vein (hv) branch.

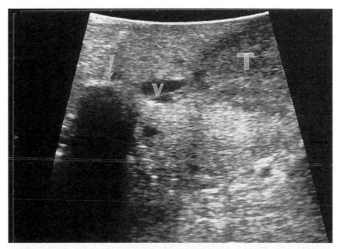

FIGURE 43. Intraoperative ultrasound (IOUS) guidance of hepatic resection. This sonogram was obtained during a resection of a metastatic liver tumor (T). The tumor was located in the medial segment of the left lobe (segment 4). A branch of the left hepatic vein (v) was seen. When the resection was halfway finished, IOUS was repeated to clarify the resection line in its relation to the tumor and the branch of the hepatic vein. An arrow indicates a finger of the surgeon placed in the resection plane. From this image, it was understood that the resection line was close to this branch of the hepatic vein but away from the tumor. With continuation of this resection line, good surgical margin would be obtained. As shown in this sonogram, repeat IOUS is helpful in order to guide surgical resection of a liver tumor.

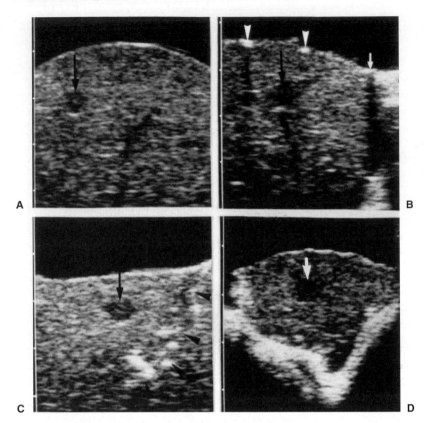

FIGURE 44. Intraoperative ultrasound (IOUS)–guided hepatectomy for a small nonpalpable tumor. **A:** A 5-mm nonpalpable hepatocellular carcinoma (*black arrow*) in a cirrhotic liver was localized by IOUS in the anterior inferior segment (segment 5) of the right lobe. Because of poor liver function, a anatomic hepatic resection such as lobectomy or segmentectomy could not be performed; therefore, a limited nonanatomic hepatectomy was planned. **B:** Liver surface markings were made with an electrocautery. Two white arrowheads indicate the location of the tumor, and a white arrow indicates the starting point of hepatic resection. **C:** The hepatic resection was underway. The hepatic transectioning plane was visualized as a hyperechoic line (*black arrowheads*), and the relation of the resection line to the tumor was clearly demonstrated. **D:** A resected specimen containing the tumor (*white arrow*) was scanned in the water bath to confirm the adequacy of resection.

direction of the plane of transection is determined. Once parenchymal dissection is begun, IOUS is used repeatedly. The transection plane is delineated, and its relationship to the target lesion and major vascular structures (mainly the portal veins and hepatic veins) is recognized. By repeated IOUS, the direction and extent of the dissection planes are confirmed and corrected if needed. When a landmark for dissecting the liver parenchyma is desired, a blue dye can be injected into the parenchyma (tattooing technique) after IOUS-guided needle placement. For IOUS-guided anatomic subsegmentectomy, each subsegment is identified by a staining technique, in which the subsegmental portal vein branch is punctured and a dye is injected (see Chapter 15 in detail).

IOUS-Guided Pancreatotomy

For opening the pancreatic duct during Puestow's operation (pancreaticojejunostomy), the duct is imaged longitudinally, and a needle is inserted into the center of the duct under IOUS guidance (Fig. 45). The pancreatic parenchyma is then incised along the needle, and the duct is opened. The same technique can be used for opening a pancreatic cyst. For enucleation of islet cell tumors, IOUS is first used to select the most direct route to the tumors through the least amount of surrounding pancreatic tissue. Once the site of parenchymal incision is deter-

mined and dissection is begun, IOUS is repeated to assist or direct the tissue dissection. Alternatively, IOUS-guided needle localization of the tumor can be performed first, with the tissue dissection carried out along the needle.

IOUS/LUS-Guided Needle, Cannula, or Ablation Probe Placement

IOUS/LUS can be used to guide placement of a needle, cannula, or ablation probe. IOUS/LUS-guided needle placement aids biopsy of tumors (especially nonpalpable tumors), fluid aspiration of cystic lesions, injection of contrast or other agents, and catheter introduction into the ducts or lesions. Following needle placement under IOUS/LUS guidance, biopsy is performed for hepatobiliary and pancreatic tumors. Needle biopsy of suspicious lymph nodes can be performed. IOUS/LUS-guided needle biopsy is particularly indispensable for deeply located, invisible, nonpalpable tumors or lymph nodes (Fig. 39). IOUS/LUS-guided fluid aspiration is mainly performed for cystic lesions, such as liver and pancreatic cysts, and abdominal abscesses. Aspiration is also used to confirm the location of the bile duct and to decompress the biliary system. IOUS/LUS-guided agent injection is performed during operations on the liver, biliary tract, and pancreas. Various agents can be injected: alcohol is injected directly into malignant tumors or for celiac nerve block,

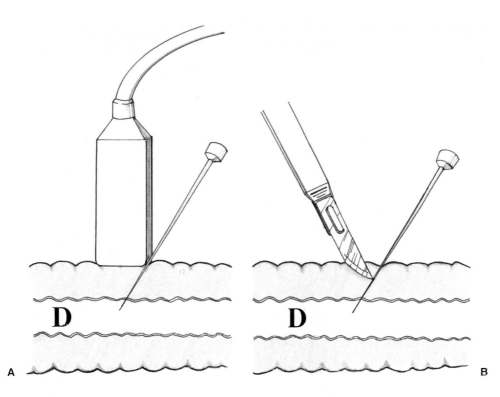

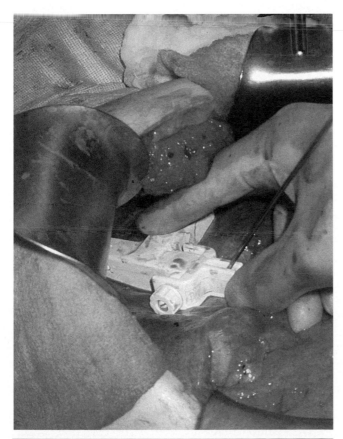

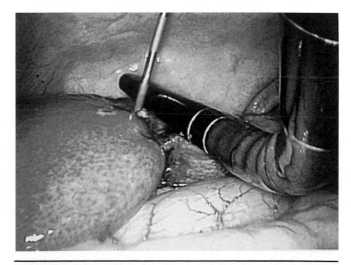

FIGURE 45. Intraoperative ultrasound (IOUS)–guided pancreatotomy for opening the pancreatic duct. **A:** The probe is positioned over the center of the pancreatic duct (D). An exploratory needle is inserted under IOUS guidance. **B:** A pancreatic incision is made along the needle.

and contrast materials are injected for intraoperative radiographic examination (such as intraoperative cholangiography or pancreatic cystography). Under IOUS/LUS guidance, catheters can be introduced and placed for drainage of the intrahepatic biliary ducts for bile, into cysts for fluid, and into abdominal abscesses for pus.

With IOUS/LUS guidance, ablation cannula or probe placement is performed for nonresectional tumor treat-

FIGURE 46. Intraoperative ultrasound (IOUS)–guided radiofrequency thermal ablation by open surgical approach. Using IOUS with a needle guidance system, an electrode-cannula was inserted into a tumor for thermal ablation.

FIGURE 47. Laparoscopic ultrasound (LUS)–guided radiofrequency thermal ablation by laparoscopic approach. An electrode-cannula was inserted from subxiphoid region into the peritoneal cavity and advanced into a tumor in the left lateral segment (segment 3) under LUS guidance by a freehand method.

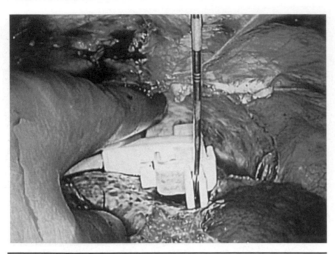

FIGURE 48. Hand-assisted laparoscopic radiofrequency thermal ablation. An electrode-cannula can be guided by a conventional intraoperative ultrasound probe with a needle guidance system during hand-assisted laparoscopic surgery.

ments such as cryoablation or thermal ablation (radiofrequency or microwave) (see Table 5 in Chapter 4; see also Figs. 45 to 47 in Chapter 4). Recently, radiofrequency thermal ablation has found increasing use because of excellent local control of tumors and fewer associated complications (64,65). Depending on the tumor and the patient condition, radiofrequency thermal ablation can be performed percutaneously, laparoscopically, open surgically, or hand-assisted laparoscopically (65,66). These ablation therapies are currently performed mainly for unresectable malignant liver tumors; however, their indications may expand to include tumors of other abdominal and extraabdominal organs. The ablation process can be precisely planned and monitored with IOUS/LUS (Figs. 46 to 51).

IOUS/LUS-Guided Tissue Dissection

IOUS-guided tissue dissection can assist incision or resection of solid organs such as the liver, pancreas, or other intraperitoneal-retroperitoneal tissues. During operations for chronic pancreatitis, dilated pancreatic ducts and small pancreatic pseudocysts often are not palpable. In such instances, incision of the pancreatic parenchyma (pancreatotomy) or incision of the cyst wall is guided by IOUS for internal drainage (e.g., Puestow's operation or cystogastrostomy). For enucleation of islet cell tumors of the pancreas, especially those that are nonpalpable, IOUS-guided pancreatotomy is carried out until the tumor is visualized. The abdominal abscess cavity wall is incised under IOUS guidance to achieve wide surgical drainage. Foreign bodies in various organs or tissues can be extracted using IOUS-guided needle localization and tissue incision.

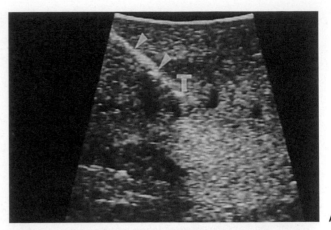

A

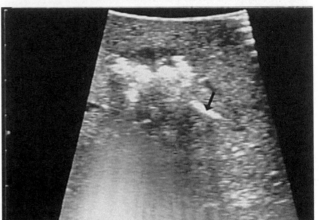

B

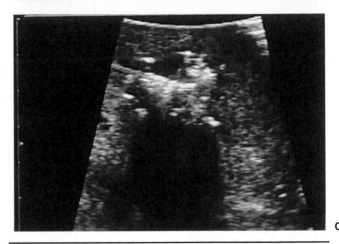

C

FIGURE 49. The process of intraoperative ultrasound–guided radiofrequency thermal ablation. **A:** A cannula (*arrowheads*) was inserted into a tumor (T). **B:** During thermal ablation, the ablated area became hyperechoic due to outgassing. This hyperechoic ablated area caused shadowing artifact. **C:** The ablation lesion a few minutes after the completion of thermal ablation.

IOUS-guided tissue dissection for resection is performed in various organs; however, it is used most frequently during hepatic resection. Resection procedures of the liver that are guided by IOUS include lobectomy, segmentectomy, subsegmentectomy, and other nonana-

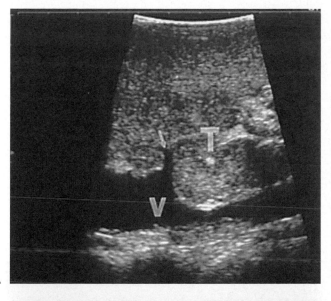

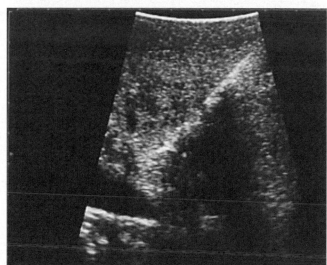

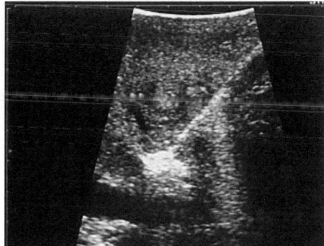

FIGURE 50. Intraoperative ultrasound (IOUS)-guided radiofrequency thermal ablation of an unresectable metastatic liver tumor from sigmoid colon cancer. **A:** Sagittal view of the tumor (T) in segments 4 to 1 (caudate lobe), 6 cm in size, which was invading the left hepatic vein (*arrow*) and the vena cava (V). This tumor required multiple overlapping radiofrequency thermal ablation sessions. **B:** First, an electrode-cannula was inserted under IOUS guidance into the most superior and posterior (deep) area of this tumor. Accurate placement of the cannula was possible under guidance of IOUS. **C:** Echogenic changes of the ablated area.

tomic resections (see Chapter 15 for details). These operations are performed in most instances for the management of primary and metastatic malignant tumors, and in fewer instances for the management of benign tumors, intrahepatic calculi, or other benign diseases. During hepatectomy, the transecting plane of the liver is clearly delineated on IOUS images, and thus, IOUS can direct appropriate hepatic resection. Tumors of the pancreas or biliary system can be also resected with the assistance of IOUS guidance. Furthermore, new surgical operative techniques, such as IOUS-guided systematic subsegmentectomy of the liver, have been developed as a result of the introduction of IOUS (28,67). When laparoscopic surgery is performed for these operations (e.g., cystogastrostomy, hepatectomy), LUS guidance can be used in a manner similar to open IOUS guidance for incision or resection.

Advantages of IOUS/LUS-Guided Procedures

IOUS/LUS guidance is directly relevant to various surgical procedures and can therefore benefit surgical management. In comparison to operations performed using surgical inspection and palpation alone, certain surgical procedures can be performed more safely under IOUS/LUS guidance. "Blind" procedures, such as blind biopsy or blind resection, are avoided, and thus bleeding, bile or pancreatic leakage or fistula, and other surgical complications associated with blind procedures can be reduced. Repeated needle placement or unnecessary surgical tissue dissection is avoided or minimized with the use of IOUS/LUS guidance. Consequently, overall operating time can be shortened. IOUS/LUS guidance may enable surgeons to perform procedures that are otherwise im-

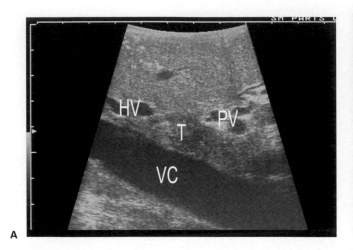

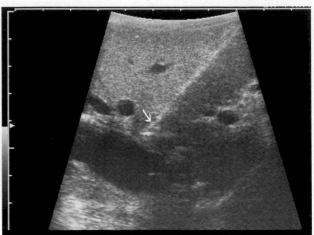

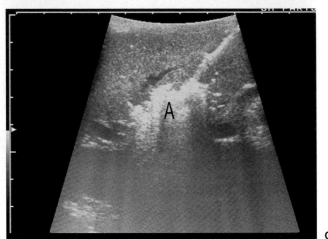

FIGURE 51. Intraoperative ultrasound (IOUS)–guided radiofrequency thermal ablation of metastatic gastrinoma to the liver. During laparotomy, IOUS detected a total of six tumors. **A:** One of the tumors (T) in segment 1 (caudate lobe) just anterior to the vena cava (VC). It was located close to the left portal vein (PV) and left and middle hepatic veins (HV). **B:** Under IOUS guidance, an electrode-cannula was introduced into the tumor accurately (*arrow*). **C:** Hyperechoic ablated lesion (A) during thermal ablation treatment. The tumor (like this) close to the major vessels can be ablated safely under IOUS guidance and monitoring.

possible to conduct. For example, needle placement into nonpalpable and invisible lesions, such as deep-seated hepatic tumors, can be achieved only with the assistance of IOUS/LUS guidance. Cryoablation or thermal ablation is currently performed mostly under IOUS/LUS guidance. These various IOUS/LUS guidance methods cannot be substituted by other intraoperative radiographic techniques. Finally, IOUS guidance has opened the way for the design of new surgical operations.

CONCLUSIONS

Based on our own experience with IOUS and LUS and this review of the literature, an overview of IOUS/LUS is presented. The equipment of choice, high-resolution B-mode ultrasound systems and basic techniques of IOUS/LUS are described in detail. General indications for IOUS/LUS are acquisition of new diagnostic information, complement to or replacement for intraoperative radiography, guidance of surgical procedures, and confirmation of completion of operation. Intraoperative needle placement and surgical tissue dissection are enhanced by IOUS/LUS guidance and at times impossible without it.

IOUS/LUS possesses many advantages, including safety, speed, high accuracy, extensive imaging information, and wide array of applications. IOUS/LUS is particularly useful during operations to localize nonpalpable lesions, detect occult lesions, determine cancer resectability, and guide procedures. The disadvantages include limitations in certain imaging capability, a slow learning curve, and specific equipment requirements. We believe that the advantages of IOUS/LUS outweigh the disadvantages. The problem related to learning and equipment can be solved when there is sufficient commitment of time and resources to the application of IOUS/LUS. Intraoperative color Doppler imaging will enhance the benefits of IOUS/LUS. The appropriate use of IOUS and LUS can have a remarkable impact on surgical management, including improvement of intraoperative decision making, reduction in surgical tissue manipulation and dissection, reduction in the need of intraoperative radiography, reduction in operation time, potential reduction in operative complication or disease recurrence, and development of new surgical procedures. New ultrasound technologies, such as ultrasound contrast enhancement, three-dimensional ultrasound, and high-intensity focused ultrasound, will be utilized more during future IOUS and

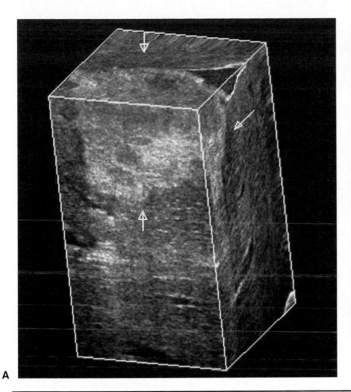

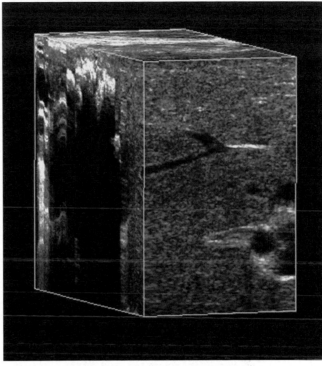

A   B

FIGURE 52. A: Three-dimensional intraoperative ultrasound (IOUS) image of a solid liver tumor (*arrows*). **B:** Three-dimensional IOUS image of a calcified liver lesion. The relationship of these lesions with intrahepatic vascular structures is much easier to understand in three-dimensional images. (Courtesy of B&K Medical.)

LUS, and will likely improve surgical outcome (31) (Fig. 52).

For general surgeons, particularly hepatobiliary, pancreatic, and endocrine surgeons and laparoscopic surgeons, it will become critically important to master IOUS and LUS. The American College of Surgeons is offering the postgraduate course "Abdominal Ultrasound: Transabdominal/Intraoperative/Laparoscopic." Taking such courses is helpful for surgeons, especially for the ultrasound neophyte, who are interested in getting started in IOUS and LUS.

REFERENCES

 1. Machi J, Sigel B. Overview of benefits of operative ultrasonography during a ten year period. *J Ultrasound Med* 1989; 8:647–652.
 2. Machi J, Sigel B, Kurohiji T, et al. Operative ultrasound guidance for various surgical procedures. *Ultrasound Med Biol* 1990;16:37–42.
 3. Machi J, Sigel B. Intraoperative ultrasonography. *Radiol Clin North Am* 1992;30:1085–1103.
 4. Machi J, Sigel B. Operative ultrasound in general surgery. *Am J Surg* 1996;172:15–20.
 5. Machi J, Sigel B. Intraoperative ultrasound. *Probl Gen Surg* 1997;14:94–106.
 6. Machi J. Intraoperative and laparoscopic ultrasound. *Surg Oncol Clin North Am* 1999;8:205–226.
 7. Machi J, Sigel B. Intraoperative and laparoscopic ultrasound: a surgical tool of great versatility. In: Baker RJ, Fischer JE, eds. *Mastery of surgery,* 4th ed. Philadelphia: Lippincott Williams & Wilkins, 2001:226–237.
 8. Makuuchi M, Torzilli G, Machi J. History of intraoperative ultrasound. *Ultrasound Med Biol* 1998;24:1229–1242.
 9. French LA, Wild JJ, Neal D. The experimental application of ultrasonics to the localization of brain tumors. Preliminary report. *J Neurosurg* 1951;8:198–203.
10. Schlegel JU, Diggdon P, Cuellar J. The use of ultrasound for localizing renal calculi. *J Urol* 1961;86:367–369.
11. Hayashi S, Wagai T, Miyazawa R, et al. Ultrasonic diagnosis of breast tumor and cholelithiasis. *West J Surg* 1962;70:34–40.
12. Knight RP, Newell JA. Operative use of ultrasonics in cholelithiasis. *Lancet* 1963;1:1023–1025.
13. Eiseman B, Greenlaw RH, Gallagher JQ. Localization of common duct stones by ultrasound. *Arch Surg* 1965;91:195–199.
14. Tanaka K, Ito K, Wagai T. The localization of brain tumors by ultrasonic techniques. A clinical review of 111 cases. *J Neurosurg* 1965;23:135–147.
15. Yamakawa K, Naito S, Azuma K, et al. Laparoscopic diagnosis of intraabdominal organs. *Jpn J Gastroenterol* 1958;55: 741.
16. Cook JH, Lytton B. Intraoperative localization of renal calculi during nephrolithotomy by ultrasound scanning. *J Urol* 1977;117:543–546.
17. Makuuchi M, Hasegawa H, Yamazaki S. Newly devised intraoperative probe. *Image Technol Info Display Med* 1979;11: 1167–1169.
18. Lane RJ, Crocker EF. Operative ultrasonic bile duct scanning. *Aust N Z J Surg* 1979;49:454–458.
19. Sigel B, Spigos DG, Donahue PE, et al. Intraoperative ultrasonic visualization of biliary calculi. *Curr Surg* 1979;36:158–159.
20. Mukuuchi M, Hasegawa H, Yamazaki S. Intraoperative ultrasonic examination for hepatectomy. *Jpn J Clin Oncol* 1981;11:367–390.

21. Rubin JM, Mirfakhraee M, Duda EE, et al. Intraoperative ultrasound examination of the brain. *Radiology* 1980;137:831–832.

22. Shkolnik A, McLane DG. Intraoperative real-time ultrasonic guidance of ventricular shunt placement in infant. *Radiology* 1981;141:515–517.

23. Sigel B, Kraft AR, Nyhus LM, et al. Identification of a parathyroid adenoma by operative ultrasonography. *Arch Surg* 1981;116:234–235.

24. Lane RJ, Coupland GA. Operative ultrasonic features of insulinomas. *Am J Surg* 1982;144:585–587.

25. Sahn DJ, Barratt-Boyes BG, Graham K, et al. Ultrasonic imaging of the coronary arteries in open-chest humans: evaluation of coronary atherosclerotic lesions during cardiac surgery. *Circulation* 1982;66:1034–1044.

26. Sigel B, Coelho JC, Nyhus LM, et al. Detection of pancreatic tumors by ultrasound during surgery. *Arch Surg* 1982;117:1058–1061.

27. Sigel B, Machi J, Anderson KW, et al. Operative ultrasonic imaging of vascular defects. *Semin Ultrasound CT MR* 1985;6:85–92.

28. Makuuchi M. *Abdominal intraoperative ultrasonography.* Tokyo: Igaku-Shoin Medical Publishers, 1987.

29. Machi J. *Operative ultrasonography: fundamentals and clinical applications (in Japanese).* Tokyo: Life Science, 1987.

30. Sigel B. *Operative ultrasonography,* 2nd ed. Philadelphia: Raven Press, 1988.

31. Makuuchi M, Machi J, Torzilli G. The future of biomedical ultrasound. Clinical foresight (Part II: Clinical application): intraoperative procedures (Intraoperative ultrasound). *Ultrasound Med Biol* 2000;26(Suppl 1):S140–S143.

32. Takamoto S, Kyo S, Adachi H, et al. Intraoperative color flow mapping by real-time two-dimensional Doppler echocardiography for evaluation of valvular and congenital heart disease and vascular disease. *J Thorac Cardiovasc Surg* 1985;90:802–812.

33. Machi J, Sigel B, Roberts AB, et al. Operative color Doppler imaging for vascular surgery. *J Ultrasound Med* 1992;11:65–71.

34. Machi J, Sigel B, Kurohiji T, et al. Operative color Doppler imaging for general surgery. *J Ultrasound Med* 1993;12:455–461.

35. Jakimowicz JJ. Review: intraoperative ultrasonography during minimal access surgery. *J R Coll Surg Edinb* 1993;38:231–238.

36. Stiegmann GV, McIntyre RC Jr. Principles of endoscopic and laparoscopic ultrasound. *Surg Endosc* 1993;7:360–361.

37. Windsor JA, Garden OJ. Laparoscopic ultrasonography. *Aust N Z J Surg* 1993;63:1–2.

38. Garden OJ. *Intraoperative/laparoscopic ultrasound.* Cambridge: Blackwell Science, 1995.

39. Kane RA. *Intraoperative, laparoscopic and endoluminal ultrasound.* New York: Churchill Livingstone, 1999.

40. Machi J, Sigel B, Zaren HA, et al. Operative ultrasonography during hepatobiliary and pancreatic surgery. *World J Surg* 1993;17:640–646.

41. Castaing G, Emond J, Bismuth H, et al. Utility of operative ultrasound in surgical management of liver tumors. *Ann Surg* 1986;204:600–605.

42. Makuuchi M, Hasegawa H, Yamazaki S, et al. The use of operative ultrasound as an aid to liver resection in patients with hepatocellular carcinoma. *World J Surg* 1987;11:615–621.

43. Rifkin MD, Rosato FE, Branch HM, et al. Intraoperative ultrasound of the liver. An important adjunctive tool for decision making in the operating room. *Ann Surg* 1987,205:466–472.

44. Parker GA, Lawrence W, Horsley JS, et al. Intraoperative ultrasound of the liver affects operative decision making. *Ann Surg* 1989;209:569–577.

45. Machi J, Isomoto H, Yamashita Y, et al. Intraoperative ultrasonography in screening for liver metastases from colorectal cancer: comparative accuracy with traditional procedures. *Surgery* 1987;101:678–684.

46. Olsen AK. Intraoperative ultrasonography and the detection of liver metastases in patients with colorectal cancer. *Br J Surg* 1990;77:998–999.

47. John T, Greig J, Crosbie JL, et al. Superior staging of liver tumors with laparoscopy and laparoscopic ultrasound. *Ann Surg* 1994;220:711–719.

48. Barbot DJ, Marks JH, Feld RI, et al. Improved staging of liver tumors using laparoscopic intraoperative ultrasound. *J Surg Oncol* 1997;64:63–67.

49. Sigel B, Machi J, Beitler JC, et al. Comparative accuracy of operative ultrasound and cholangiography in detecting common bile duct calculi. *Surgery* 1983;94:715–720.

50. Jakimowicz JJ, Rutten H, Jurgens PJ, et al. Comparison of operative ultrasonography and radiography in screening of common bile duct for calculi. *World J Surg* 1987;11:628–634.

51. Birth M, Ehlers KU, Delinikolas K, et al. Prospective randomized comparison of laparoscopic ultrasonography using a flexible-tip ultrasound probe and intraoperative dynamic cholangiography during laparoscopic cholecystectomy. *Surg Endosc* 1998;12:30–36.

52. Thompson DM, Arregui ME, Tetik C, et al. A comparison of laparoscopic ultrasound with digital fluorocholangiography for detecting choledocholithiasis during laparoscopic cholecystectomy. *Surg Endosc* 1998;12:929–932.

53. Machi J, Tateishi T, Oishi AJ, et al. Laparoscopic ultrasonography versus operative cholangiography during laparoscopic cholecystectomy: review of the literature and a comparison with open intraoperative ultrasonography. *J Am Coll Surg* 1999;188:360–367.

54. Lane RJ, Ackroyd N, Appleberg M, et al. The application of operative ultrasound immediately following carotid endarterectomy. *World J Surg* 1987;11:593–597.

55. Ungerleider RM, Greely WJ, Sheikh KH, et al. The use of intraoperative echo with Doppler color flow imaging to predict outcome after repair of congenital cardiac defects. *Ann Surg* 1989;210:526–534.

56. Chandler WF, Rubin JM. The application of ultrasound during brain surgery. *World J Surg* 1987;11:558–569.

57. Rubin JM, Chandler WF. The use of ultrasound during spinal cord surgery. *World J Surg* 1987;11:570–578.

58. Alken P, Thuroff JW, Hammer C. The use of operative ultrasonography for the localization of renal calculi. *World J Surg* 1987;11:586–592.

59. Marshall FF, Holdford SS, Hamper UM. Intraoperative sonography of renal tumors. *J Urol* 1992;148:1393–1396.

60. Machi J, Hayashida R, Kurohiji T, et al. Operative ultrasonography for lung cancer surgery. *J Thorac Cardiovasc Surg* 1989;98:540–545.

61. Snider HC Jr, Morrison DG. Intraoperative ultrasound localization of nonpalpable breast lesions. *Ann Surg Oncol* 1999;6:308–314.

62. Harlow SP, Krag DN, Ames SE, et al. Intraoperative ultrasound localization to guide surgical excision of nonpalpable breast carcinoma. *J Am Coll Surg* 1999;189:241–246.

63. Tandan VR, Asch M, Margolis M, et al. Laparoscopic versus open intraoperative ultrasound of the liver: a controlled study. *J Gastrointest Surg* 1997,1:146–151.

64. Siperstein AE, Rogers SJ, Hansen PD, et al. Laparoscopic thermal ablation of hepatic neuroendocrine tumor metastases. *Surgery* 1997;122:1147–1155.

65. Machi J, Uchida S, Sumida K, et al. Ultrasound-guided radiofrequency thermal ablation of liver tumors: percutaneous, laparoscopic and open surgical approaches. *J Gastrointest Surg* 2001;5:477–489.

66. Machi J, Oishi AJ, Mossing A, et al. Hand-assisted laparoscopic ultrasound-guided radiofrequency thermal ablation of liver tumors: a technical report. *Surg Laparosc Endosc* 2002;12:160–164.

67. Makuuchi M, Hasegawa H, Yamazaki S. Ultrasonically guided subsegmentectomy. *Surg Gynecol Obstet* 1985;161:345–350.

Chapter 14

Intraoperative and Laparoscopic Ultrasound of the Biliary Tract

Emily R. Winslow and Nathaniel J. Soper

Intraoperative imaging of the biliary tract with ultrasound is certainly not new; it was attempted as early as the 1960s (1,2). When real-time B-mode ultrasound became available in the late 1970s, it became more practical for the surgeon to use this technology in the operating room (3,4). By the middle of the 1980s, several large studies were conducted in which the use of intraoperative ultrasound (IOUS) to detect common bile duct stones during open cholecystectomy was directly compared to the use of intraoperative cholangiography (IOC) (5,6). In both of these studies, IOUS was at least equivalent to and in some respects was superior to traditional IOC. Despite this evidence, the use of IOUS during open cholecystectomy did not gain widespread popularity. For the most part, surgeons continued to rely on IOC for bile duct screening, likely because there was no obvious incentive to switch to an unfamiliar new technology without marked superiority.

The advent of laparoscopic cholecystectomy brought another opportunity to determine the optimal imaging method for screening of the common bile duct. Because there were initially some technical and logistical barriers to IOC during laparoscopy, ultrasound became an obvious alternative. Over the last decade, many groups have reported their experience with intraoperative laparoscopic ultrasound (LUS) during laparoscopic cholecystectomy. Importantly, the majority of these reports have found this method of screening the common bile duct to be comparable to IOC in terms of the sensitivity and specificity of detecting stones. In addition, many groups have shown that LUS is faster, less expensive, and more convenient to perform than IOC. For these reasons, it has been referred to by some as the "stethoscope of the surgeon" (7). Thus, in contrast to the experience with open cholecystectomy, LUS during laparoscopic cholecystectomy has been embraced by a variety of biliary surgeons, and it is becoming an essential element in the training of all future surgeons.

In this chapter, we will focus primarily on the technique and outcomes of LUS during laparoscopic chole- cystectomy because this is the most commonly performed procedure. In addition, we will discuss other indications for the use of IOUS of the biliary tree, including its use in the difficult open cholecystectomy, and in the resection of cholangiocarcinomas and gallbladder carcinomas.

INSTRUMENTATION

When surgeons began to study the use of ultrasound during laparoscopic cholecystectomy, the instrumentation was primitive. One group (8) adapted a probe developed for endoluminal sonography of the bladder to use for imaging of the hepatoduodenal ligament. Others (9) used early rigid devices that made scanning more difficult. Several major advances in the instrumentation significantly improved the quality of LUS imaging and made its use more practical.

One of these advances was the development of LUS probes with flexible tips. Because any instrument placed through a trocar is fixed in space at the level of the body wall, there are significant limitations to the use of the rigid probes, as they cannot always adequately contact the tissue. The flexible tips have the advantage of moving in two or more directions, so that the tissue can be optimally contacted and can be more easily scanned both longitudinally and transversely. Another important technology that was incorporated is the capability to use color flow and pulsed Doppler sonography. This is particularly useful when a given tubular structure is difficult to identify. Because such Doppler scanning clearly differentiates the biliary system from its neighboring arteries and veins, it is possible to identify an accessory or aberrant biliary duct and safely distinguish it from an anomalous artery.

Most probes used today for LUS of the biliary tree use side-viewing linear or curvilinear array (convex) technology and have frequencies that vary between 5 and 10 MHz, with 7.5 MHz being the most common (see Chapter 13). The length of the probes varies between approximately 30 and 70 cm, and they fit through a 10-mm trocar. The probe that we are using has a flexible tip that articulates in two planes with a curvilinear array probe design at its tip (B&K Medical Systems, North Billerica, MA). Some manufacturers have produced front-viewing sector LUS probes, which are also useful for biliary LUS scanning (see Chapter 13).

Because the probes are covered with a plastic sheath that can be damaged by the trocar valves, our preference is to place the probes directly through the abdominal wall to avoid the somewhat costly repair of the sheaths. There are several methods for sterilization of LUS or IOUS probes, as described in Chapter 13. Some of the current designs allow sterilization in Steris or Sterad systems.

A video mixer is also an extremely helpful addition to the performance of LUS because it allows both the view from the laparoscope and the view from the ultrasound probe to be displayed simultaneously on the same video monitor. This set up is commonly referred to as "a picture within a picture," and it helps the surgeon to correlate the sonographic anatomy with the laparoscopic view more easily.

When a laparoscopic procedure is converted to an open procedure, LUS can still be used in the open operative field. However, during open biliary surgery small IOUS probes are obviously much easier to manipulate. See Chapter 13 regarding instrumentation of open IOUS probes.

SCANNING TECHNIQUES

Bile Duct Imaging During Laparoscopic Cholecystectomy

The procedure is begun in the usual fashion with the placement of trocars and establishment of pneumoperitoneum. While some surgeons advocate LUS imaging of the bile duct before any dissection has been done (9–11), we generally prefer to first proceed as usual with the initial dissection of Calot's triangle. Once the cystic duct is identified and the "critical view of safety" achieved, a single clip is placed across the junction of the gallbladder neck with the cystic duct to preclude stone passage during subsequent manipulation. At this point, LUS images of the bile duct are obtained. If the cystic duct cannot be readily identified or the anatomy is otherwise unclear, the LUS probe can be inserted earlier to help define the relevant anatomy. It is important to emphasize that although LUS images can help to delineate some dissection-pertinent anatomy, the safest way to avoid biliary injury is through careful dissection.

Using the "American technique" of laparoscopic cholecystectomy, one 10-mm port is usually placed at the umbilicus and a second in the epigastrium. The LUS probe can be inserted through either of these access ports. If placed through the epigastric port (Fig. 1), the probe will be oriented so that the portal structures are running perpendicular to the axis of the transducer and the images including the bile duct will be obtained in transverse section (Fig. 2). If placed through the umbilical port, the probe will be parallel to the portal structures and the images obtained will be in longitudinal section (Fig. 3). During laparoscopic cholecystectomy, the laparoscope is generally placed through the umbilical port; thus, it is most convenient to place the LUS probe through the epigastric port, obtaining images in transverse section. If the probe is placed through the umbilical port, the laparoscope must be repositioned to the epigastric port, which gives some difficulty with mirror image viewing of the ultrasound probe. We routinely obtain only transverse views through the epigastric trocar. One group (12) has demonstrated that some small stones are visible from only one position. They and others (13) have therefore advocated obtaining both transverse and longitudinal views of the bile duct. The technique from both positions is described below.

Epigastric Scanning Position

The grasping forceps are placed on the fundus of the gallbladder and are used to elevate the gallbladder and roll the liver superiorly, exposing the porta hepatis. The transducer is first placed on the gallbladder wall itself and is moved slowly from fundus to infundibulum. During this maneuver, the image can be fine tuned (adjusting the gain, time-gain compensation, depth, and so forth) to allow for optimal visualization. In addition to simply documenting stones within the gallbladder lumen (Fig. 4), the surgeon should also look carefully for unsuspected gallbladder polyps or masses (Fig. 5). The probe should then be placed as superiorly as possible in gentle contact with the portal structures. It is important that only gentle pressure is applied as the most superficial structures may be occluded and therefore not recognized when excessive pressure is applied. The portal structures are usually readily apparent, with the portal vein being the largest and most posterior structure. The bile duct lies anteriorly and to the patient's right, whereas the hepatic artery lies anteriorly and to the patient's left. The appearance of the portal triad in transverse section has been aptly described as a "Mickey Mouse" (head and ears) appearance (Fig. 6).

In most cases, the portal structures are easily visualized without additional maneuvers. However, in patients with very little intraabdominal fat it may be difficult to visualize the bile duct. This is not only because contact

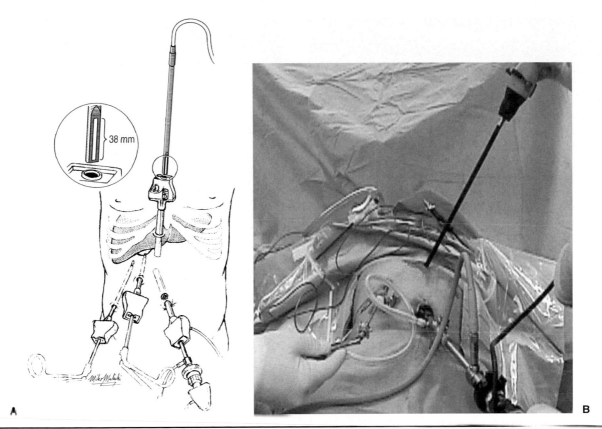

FIGURE 1. A, B: The laparoscopic ultrasound probe is placed through the epigastric port with the laparoscopic camera placed through the periumbilical trocar. Note in the figure **(B)** that the probe is placed directly through the skin incision with the trocar removed.

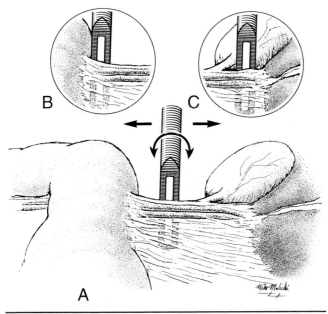

FIGURE 2. In order to obtain transverse images, the laparoscopic ultrasound probe is placed on the lateral edge of the hepatoduodenal ligament **(A)**. The ligament can be scanned superiorly **(C)** to the hilum of the liver and inferiorly **(B)** to the antimesenteric wall of the duodenum.

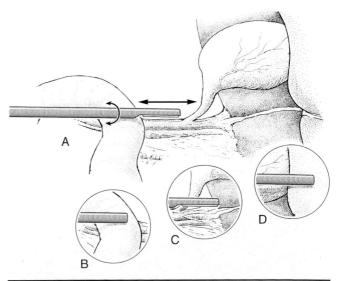

FIGURE 3. In order to obtain longitudinal images, the laparoscopic ultrasound probe is placed through the umbilical port and the portal structures are scanned along their long axis as shown **(A)**. To image the intrapancreatic bile duct, transduodenal scanning is necessary **(B)**. The probe should be advanced superiorly to the hepatic hilum **(C)** after which it can then be placed on the anterior surface of the liver to allow imaging of intrahepatic ducts **(D)**.

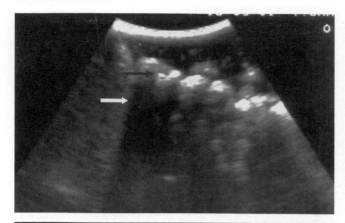

FIGURE 4. With the probe placed directly on the gallbladder wall, multiple stones (*black arrow*) can be shown in the dependent portion of the gallbladder lumen. As depicted, gallbladder stones produce characteristic acoustic shadowing (*white arrow*).

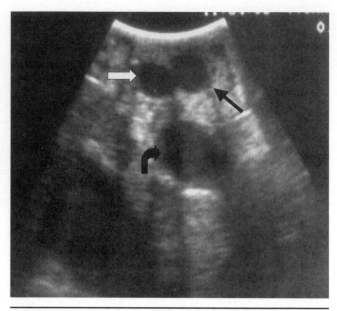

FIGURE 6. The portal triad in cross-section with the common bile duct superficially on the patient's right (*white arrow*), the hepatic artery superficially on the patient's left (*straight black arrow*), and the portal vein posteriorly (*curved black arrow*). This shows the "Mickey Mouse" appearance.

scanning may cause compression to the bile duct but also because the duct is placed in the near field of the transducer (out of the focal zone) where ultrasound images are suboptimal. In this case, probe-standoff scanning should be performed by instillation of sterile irrigant (sa-

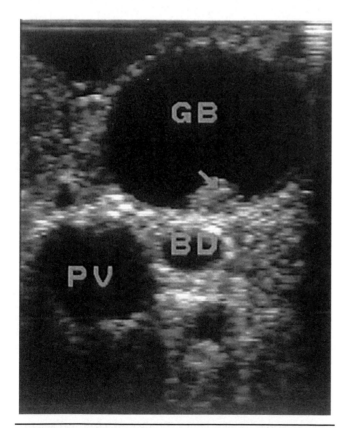

FIGURE 5. Gallbladder pathology other than gallstones can be detected by laparoscopic ultrasound. This shows a polyp (*arrow*) of the gallbladder (GB). PV, portal vein; BD, bile duct.

line solution) in the operative field as an acoustic coupler and acoustic window (see Chapter 13 regarding contact scanning versus probe-standoff scanning with saline immersion). Some surgeons recommend the routine use of the saline immersion technique during LUS scanning of the biliary tract (13). It may also be difficult to visualize the portal structures in patients with extensive inflammatory tissue changes and those with excess intraabdominal fat. In difficult cases it is helpful to use the Doppler capability to confirm correct identification of the bile duct. Both the hepatic artery and portal vein will display flow signals, whereas the bile duct will not exhibit flow (Fig.7).

Once a view of the portal structures is adequately obtained, the transducer should be moved (slid) slowly and gently, inferiorly along the edge of the hepatoduodenal ligament (Fig. 8). Depending on its size, the cystic duct will then come into view. Initially, it appears as a small structure separate from the common hepatic duct, usually to the far right within the porta (Fig. 9). As the probe is moved inferiorly, the junction of the cystic duct and the hepatic duct can be demonstrated (Fig. 10). As the operator continues to slide the probe inferiorly, the orientation of the scan becomes such that the common bile duct is imaged slightly obliquely (Fig. 8).

After imaging the suprapancreatic bile duct, attention should be turned toward evaluation of the intrapancreatic bile duct. This section of the duct is the most difficult to examine; however, its clear visualization is essential because stones are commonly located in this portion of

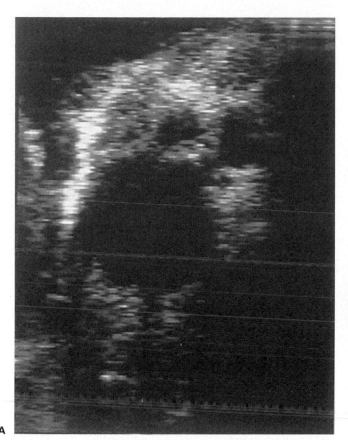

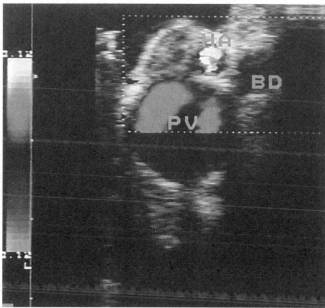

FIGURE 7. A: B-mode laparoscopic ultrasound showing the transverse section of the portal vein, bile duct and hepatic artery. The duct and the artery cannot be readily distinguished because of their similar size. **B:** On color Doppler imaging, the bile duct (BD) without color flow and the hepatic artery (HA) with color flow can be immediately identified. In this image, the artery is the right hepatic artery (not proper hepatic artery), located on the patient's right. PV, portal vein. (See Color Plate 25.)

the duct. In order to best image the distal bile duct from the epigastric position the transducer must be slowly rotated in a clockwise direction after abutting the transducer tip to the antimesenteric wall of the duodenum. The goal is to image the duct through the pancreatic head just posterior and medial to the duodenum (Fig. 11). In this way, the junction of the common bile duct and pancreatic duct are usually well visualized. It is also possible to visualize the entry of the duct into the medial wall of the duodenum (Fig. 12), as well as the ampullary muscle complex itself (Fig. 13). The latter appears as a well-defined hypoechoic ring at the edge of the pancreatic substance.

If the distal duct cannot be completely visualized, several scanning techniques can be employed (Table 1). The probe can be repositioned and placed directly on the antimesenteric (lateral or anterolateral) surface of the duodenum. At this location, the air in the duodenum may obscure the LUS image. With gentle pressure, the duodenum is slowly compressed so as to redistribute the air, which otherwise causes bright reverberation or shadow-

ing artifacts. In most instances, the distal most bile duct and its entry into the duodenum are seen reliably with this "probe-compression" technique (Fig. 14) (also see Chapter 13). If this is still inadequate, two additional maneuvers can be attempted to improve the imaging qualities. First, fluid can be instilled into the patient's stomach through a nasogastric tube with the hope that it will fill the duodenum and eliminate the interfering gas. A second possibility employed in the early experience of one group (14) was to place a cholangiocatheter into the cystic duct and to irrigate the duct with saline in an attempt to distend it. Obviously, this requires the same steps as a cholangiogram, and the logical argument is that if a catheter has to be placed, it would be most appropriate to obtain a cholangiogram.

After the surgeon is satisfied that the distal duct has been well visualized and is free of abnormality, the probe should be replaced on the inferior edge of the hepatoduodenal ligament and is slid superiorly up toward the liver, reexamining the common duct in reverse. Although the cystic duct–common hepatic duct junction can usually be

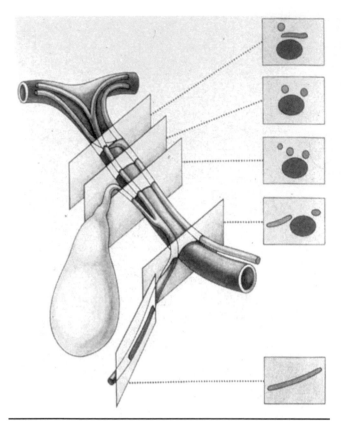

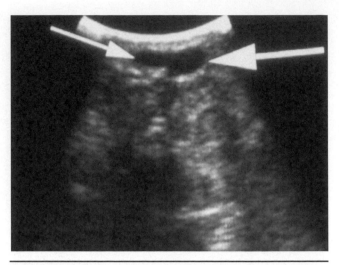

FIGURE 10. The cystic duct (*thin white arrow*) and the hepatic duct (*thick white arrow*) join here to form the common bile duct.

FIGURE 8. The structures of the portal triad and their cross-sectional relationship to one another along the length of the hepatoduodenal ligament are depicted here. (From Rothlin M, Largiader F. The anatomy of the hepatoduodenal ligament in laparoscopic sonography. *Surg Endosc* 1994;8:173–180, with permission.)

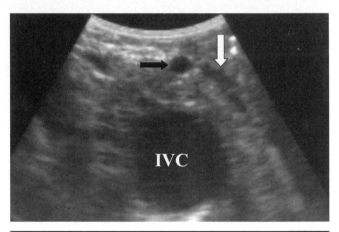

FIGURE 11. Imaging just posterior and medial to the duodenum. The common bile duct (*black arrow*) and the pancreatic duct (*white arrow*) can be seen within the pancreatic substance. IVC, inferior vena cava.

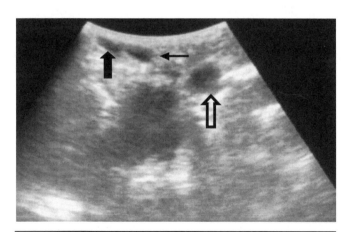

FIGURE 9. The cystic duct (*thick black arrow*) is shown just superior to its junction with the hepatic duct (*thin black arrow*). The hepatic artery (*arrow outline*) is situated on the patient's left.

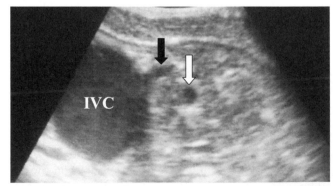

FIGURE 12. The common bile duct (*black arrow*) empties into the medial wall of the duodenum. The probe's surface is in contact with the anterolateral duodenal wall. *White arrow*, pancreatic duct; IVC, inferior vena cava.

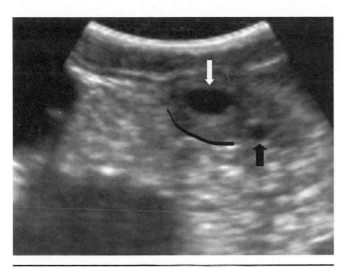

FIGURE 13. The ampullary complex is shown. The common bile duct (*white arrow*) and pancreatic duct (*black arrow*) are within the substance of the muscular complex (as outlined by a black line).

> **TABLE 1 Maneuvers to Assist in Visualization of the Intrapancreatic Bile Duct**

1. Place the probe directly on the duodenum and compress to eliminate the air.
2. Move the probe from the epigastric to the umbilical position or vice versa.
3. Instill fluid via a nasogastric tube to fill the duodenum.
4. Place a catheter transcystically and flush with saline to distend duct.
5. Mobilize the duodenum by the Kocher maneuver to image from the posterior aspect of pancreas.

ing the safety of the surgical dissection around this area. At this location, the LUS probe can also be rotated in a counterclockwise direction to follow the common hepatic duct further proximally toward the liver. The right and left hepatic ducts and their junction may be visualized (Fig. 15).

Umbilical Scanning Position

When the LUS probe is placed through the umbilical trocar, the laparoscope is placed through the epigastric trocar. The gallbladder can first be imaged transhepatically by placing the transducer on the anterior surface of the

reliably imaged, the more proximal cystic duct is often difficult to visualize due to its small size, lack of investing tissue, and superficial position. The location of the cystic duct–common hepatic duct junction by LUS is compared to the area of dissection in the laparoscopic view, ensur-

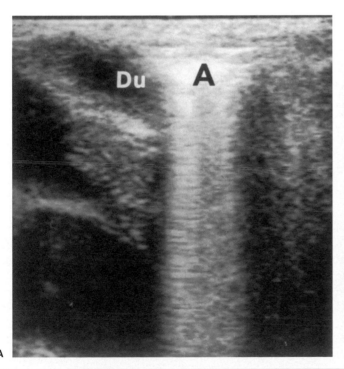

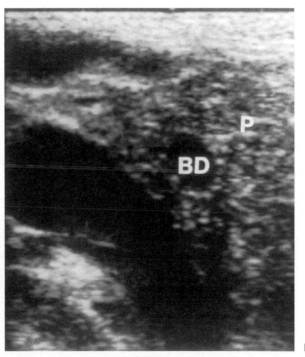

FIGURE 14. Transduodenal scanning of the intrapancreatic bile duct with the compression technique. **A:** Air (A) in the duodenum (Du) causing reverberation artifacts obscures the image. **B:** Mild compression of the duodenum eliminates the air, enabling visualization of the bile duct (BD) in the head of the pancreas (P). (From Machi J, Sigel B, Zaren HA, et al. Technique of ultrasound examination during laparoscopic cholecystectomy. *Surg Endosc* 1993;7:544–549, with permission.)

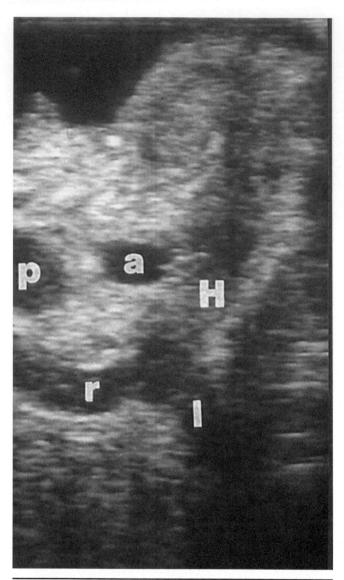

FIGURE 15. By rotating the laparoscopic ultrasound probe near the hepatic hilum, the hepatic duct (H) may be followed to the level of right (r) and left (l) hepatic duct junction. P, portal vein; a, hepatic artery.

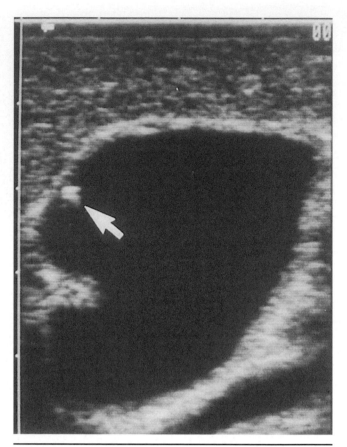

FIGURE 16. By positioning the transducer on the surface of the liver, the liver parenchyma is delineated. Transhepatic scanning of the gallbladder can be performed at this location. In this image, a small polyp (*arrow*) is detected.

liver (Fig. 16) so that the image quality can be optimized before proceeding. The axis of the probe should be parallel to the axis of the portal structures, giving longitudinal views. The probe is first placed as superiorly as possible on the porta hepatis. Again, the "lay of the land" should first be established, if necessary with the assistance of color flow Doppler. In longitudinal section, the bile duct and the portal vein (and often the inferior vena cava) are visualized, while generally the proper hepatic artery and the bile duct cannot be delineated simultaneously. However, the cross-section of the right hepatic artery is often seen between the bile duct (hepatic duct) and the portal vein (Figs. 8 and 17). Once the longitudinal view of the bile duct, hepatic artery, and portal vein is obtained, the

probe is slowly withdrawn so that the scanning continues inferiorly toward the pancreas. It is essential to keep the bile duct in view at all times during this maneuver. In order to accomplish this, the operator will likely need to rotate the probe slightly to the right or left, as the bile duct curves. The junction of the cystic duct and the common hepatic duct can be well visualized with this technique (Fig. 18).

In order to visualize the intrapancreatic portion of the duct, the probe can be placed directly on top of the first portion of the duodenum. With gentle compression of the duodenum to eliminate the artifact associated with air, the probe is changed from a vertical position to a position slightly to the patient's right. This allows the intrapancreatic bile duct to be visualized in cross or oblique section as it traverses the pancreas (Fig. 19). If the distal duct cannot be visualized in this fashion, the probe can be placed on the gastrocolic ligament just to the left of the pancreatic head. In this position, transduodenal imaging is avoided altogether.

If visualization of the proximal biliary ducts is necessary, it is easier to introduce the LUS probe through the

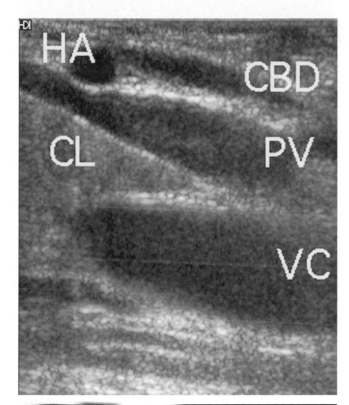

FIGURE 17. The longitudinal view of the proximal portal structures as obtained with the laparoscopic ultrasound probe placed via the umbilical port. The cross-section of the right hepatic artery (HA) is visualized between the common hepatic duct (CBD) and the portal vein (PV). VC, inferior vena cava; CL, caudate lobe. (Courtesy of Dr. Maurice Arregui.)

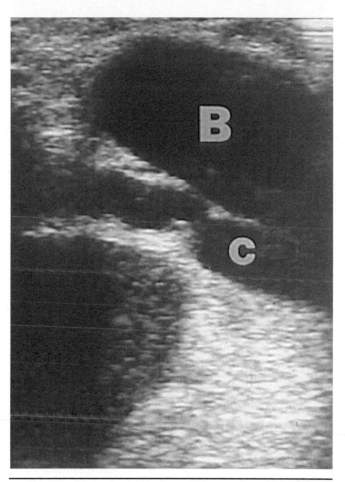

FIGURE 18. The junction of the cystic duct (c) and the common hepatic duct (B) is depicted in longitudinal section.

umbilical port. The gallbladder should be released and the liver allowed to assume its natural position. The probe can be placed directly on top of segment IV of the liver (transhepatic scanning). Using the hepatic parenchyma as an acoustic window facilitates views of the intrahepatic ducts and proximal common hepatic duct (Fig. 20).

Generally, longitudinal scanning of the bile duct and transhepatic scanning are more readily performed by the probe from the umbilical position. However, such scanning can also be performed from the epigastric position with the flexible-tip probe although it is technically more demanding and at times difficult. The probe tip is flexed upward, and the probe is placed parallel to the bile duct (Fig. 21).

Interpreting Abnormal Ultrasound Images

While scanning the bile duct, the surgeon must be alert for any abnormal findings. When the gallbladder itself is imaged, one should look carefully for masses or polyps, in addition to gallstones and sludge. Polyps or tumors can be differentiated from stones because they cause no

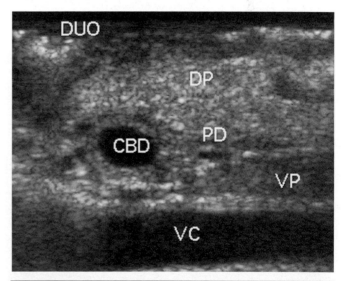

FIGURE 19. Transduodenal imaging of the intrapancreatic bile duct (CBD) with the laparoscopic ultrasound probe placed via the periumbilical port. DUO, duodenum; DP, pancreatic substance; PD, pancreatic duct; VP, portal vein; VC, inferior vena cava. (Courtesy of Dr. Maurice Arregui.)

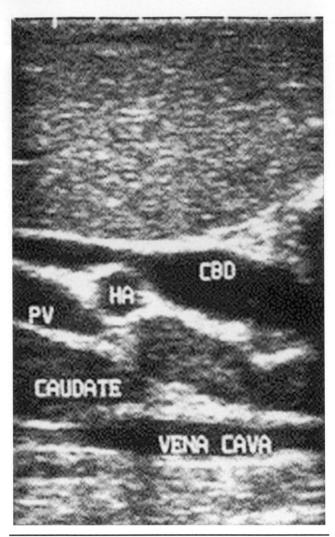

FIGURE 20. Transhepatic images of the proximal hepatic duct (CBD) in longitudinal section. The cross-section of the right hepatic artery (HA) is visualized between the duct and the portal vein (PV). (Courtesy of Dr. Maurice Arregui.)

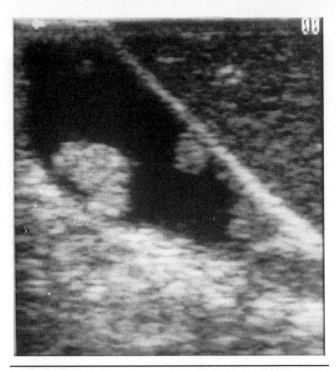

FIGURE 22. Polyps of the gallbladder can be differentiated from gallstones by the absence of acoustic shadows and other features.

acoustic shadow, are not dependent, and are not mobile with a change in body position (Fig. 22). As scanning continues along the biliary tree, the surgeon should be able to identify stones and/or sludge in the duct. Figure 23 depicts sludge in the suprapancreatic duct. After glucagon is given intravenously, a catheter is placed transcystically and the common duct can be flushed (Fig. 24). The duct can then be scanned again to document clearance of the sludge (Fig. 25). Figure 26 depicts a combination of sludge and small stones in the common bile duct on a longitudinal view. Because the pancreatic substance

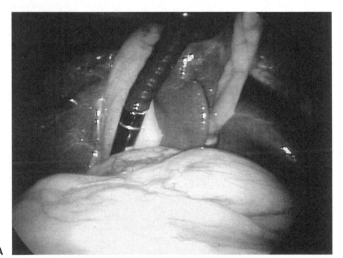

A

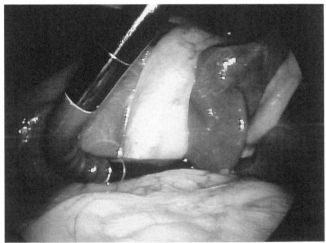

B

FIGURE 21. Laparoscopic views of laparoscopic ultrasound bile duct scanning using a flexible-tip probe from the epigastric position. **A:** Transverse scanning of the bile duct. **B:** Longitudinal scanning of the bile duct by flexing the probe tip upward.

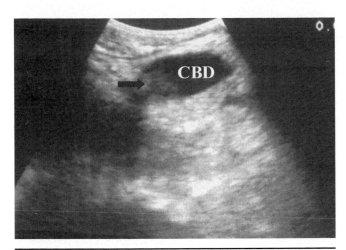

FIGURE 23. In transverse section, amorphous sludge (*black arrow*) is seen within the suprapancreatic common bile duct (CBD), which is mildly dilated.

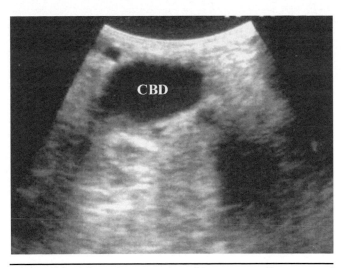

FIGURE 25. After administration of intravenous glucagon and saline irrigation through the catheter, the sludge is no longer detectable in the common bile duct (CBD).

is relatively hyperechoic (particularly in elderly patients), the search for stones should be methodical, and any suggestion of an echogenic structure with shadowing should prompt closer evaluation. Figure 27 depicts a small stone in the intrapancreatic duct in the transverse plane, and Figure 28 shows a larger stone in longitudinal section, Figure 29 shows a stone in the intrahepatic bile duct. Air in the bile duct (pneumobilia) also exhibits hyperechogenicity associated with shadowing, similar to a stone. Air is usually floating at the superficial area of the duct and is frequently accompanied by reverberation or comet tail (or ring down) artifacts, thus making distinction from a stone possible (Fig. 30). During IOC air may be introduced into the bile duct; therefore, generally LUS or

IOUS of the bile duct should be performed before IOC (if both methods are performed).

Other Applications of Laparoscopic Biliary Ultrasound

Another application of ultrasound evaluation of the biliary tree laparoscopically is in the setting of a staging laparoscopy for patients with biliary tumors, including extrahepatic biliary cancer and gallbladder cancer. Patients

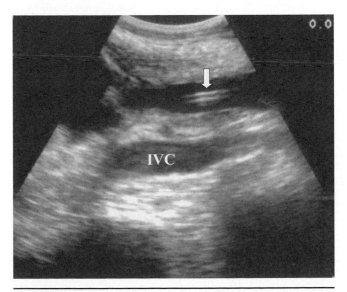

FIGURE 24. A transcystically placed catheter (*white arrow*) is seen within the lumen of the common bile duct. IVC, inferior vena cava.

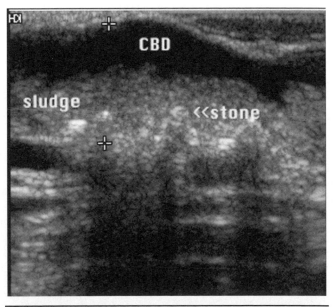

FIGURE 26. At times, small stones can be seen within the biliary sludge. Here the dilated common bile duct (CBD), between two markers, is seen in longitudinal section with a dependent mixture of sludge and stones. Note acoustic shadows associated with small stones. (Courtesy of Dr. Maurice Arregui.)

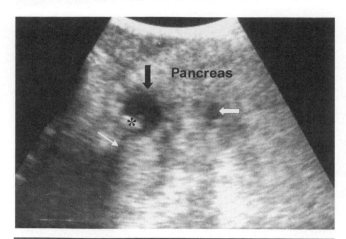

FIGURE 27. A small stone (*) with acoustic shadowing (*thin white arrow*) is seen in the intrapancreatic bile duct (*black arrow*). The pancreatic duct is depicted by a thick white arrow.

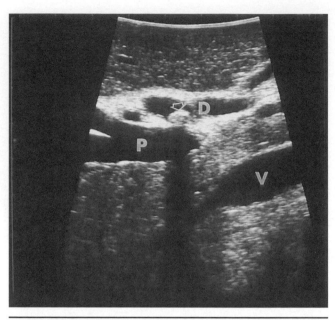

FIGURE 29. A stone (*open arrow*) with shadowing is detected in the right hepatic duct (D) by transhepatic scanning. P, right portal vein; V, vena cava.

with biliary tumors that appear potentially resectable may first undergo laparoscopic exploration with LUS, not only to rule out unsuspected metastasis but also to precisely define the extent of tumor within the porta and liver (15,16). The same type of flexible LUS probe is used, and the position of the probe depends on the location of the tumor. The use of color flow Doppler is at times critical in this setting, so that vascular invasion can be confidently ruled in or out (Figs. 31 and 32). In addition, LUS-guided lymph node or liver biopsy may be useful in determining the resectability and staging of tumor in these patients.

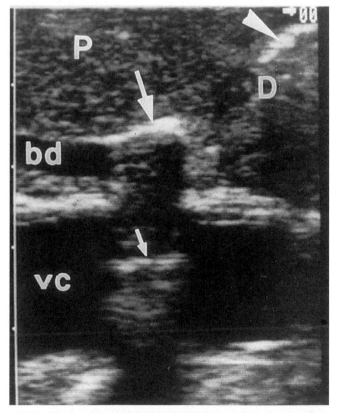

FIGURE 30. Air (pneumobilia) in the intrapancreatic distal bile duct (bd). A large arrow indicates the air, whereas a small arrow indicates a reverberation artifact. An arrowhead indicates air in the duodenum (D). P, pancreas; vc, vena cava.

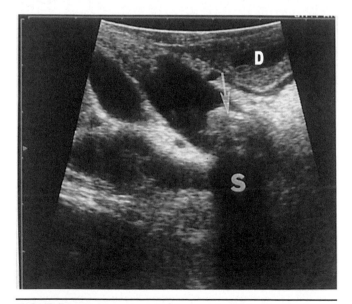

FIGURE 28. A 1 cm stone (*white arrow*) within the distal common bile duct is seen here in longitudinal section with acoustic shadowing (S). D, duodenum.

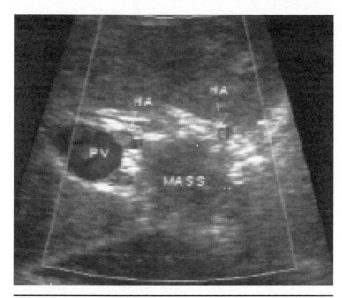

FIGURE 31. A resectable cholangiocarcinoma ("mass"), which does not invade any vascular structures, is shown here. HA, hepatic artery; PV, portal vein. (Courtesy of Dr. Steven Strasberg.) (See Color Plate 26.)

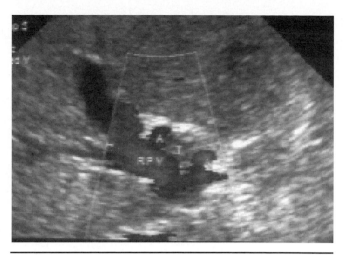

FIGURE 32. Staging laparoscopy with use of laparoscopic ultrasound shows that the cholangiocarcinoma (T) intimately abuts the right portal vein (RPV) and right hepatic artery (A). (Courtesy of Dr. Steven Strasberg.) (See Color Plate 27.)

Applications of Intraoperative Ultrasound During Open Biliary Procedures

The principles of scanning techniques for IOUS during open biliary surgery are similar to those of LUS. Actually, open IOUS scanning is technically less demanding be-cause of a wide operative wound where there is more freedom of manipulation of an IOUS probe. IOUS scanning techniques are illustrated in the following figures: selection of an IOUS probe (Fig. 33), IOUS scanning of the gallbladder (Fig. 34), IOUS probe-standoff scanning of the bile duct (Fig. 35), longitudinal and transverse scanning of the bile duct (Fig. 36), and transduodenal scanning (Fig. 37). (See also Chapter 13 for details re-

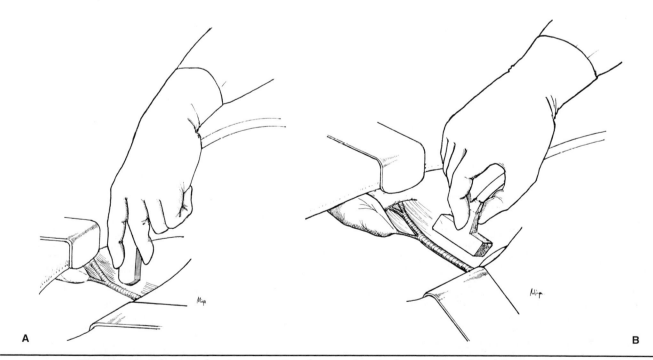

A

B

FIGURE 33. Selection of an intraoperative ultrasound probe for scanning of the bile duct. **A:** When the operative field at the hepatoduodenal ligament is limited, a cylindrical, end-viewing sector or convex probe is ideal. **B:** When the operative field is wide enough, a flat, end-viewing or side-viewing probe can be used.

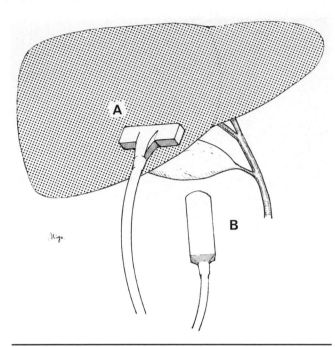

FIGURE 34. Intraoperative ultrasound scanning of the gallbladder. **A:** Transhepatic scanning of the gallbladder using a flat, T-shaped probe. **B:** Direct scanning of the gallbladder using a cylindrical probe. A flat probe is also usable. Probe-standoff scanning with saline immersion must be performed to image the superficial wall of the gallbladder.

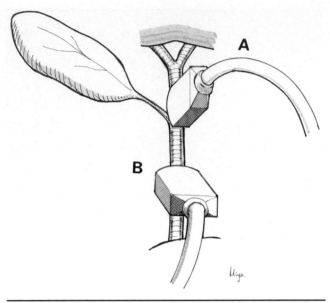

FIGURE 36. Longitudinal scanning **(A)** and transverse scanning **(B)** of the bile duct during laparotomy.

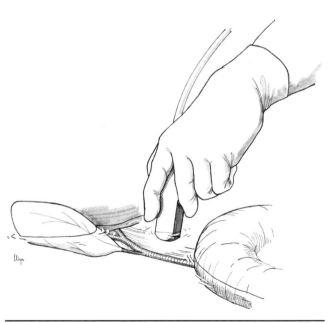

FIGURE 35. Probe-standoff scanning of the bile duct during intraoperative ultrasound. The probe is placed at least 1 cm away from the duct, and the saline immersion technique is used. Here the supraduodenal (suprapancreatic) portion of the duct is being scanned.

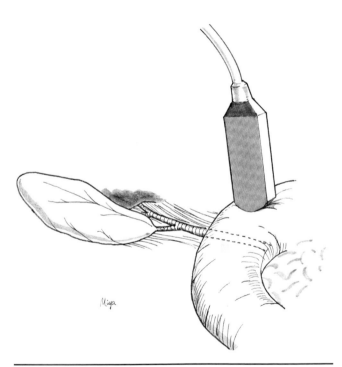

FIGURE 37. Transduodenal scanning of the intrapancreatic common bile duct. At times, a compression scanning technique is used as needed.

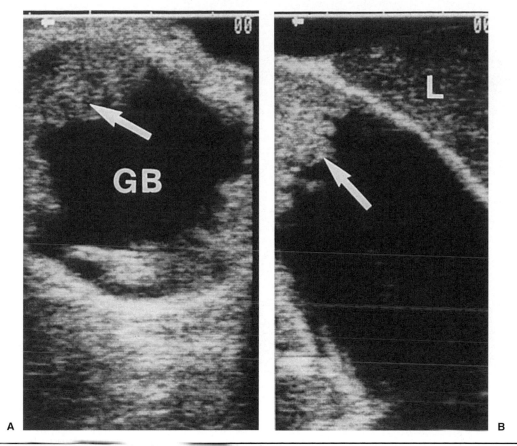

FIGURE 38. Transverse section **(A)** and longitudinal section **(B)** of the gallbladder (GD) showing a gallbladder cancer (*white arrow*). There is no invasion of the tumor into the liver parenchyma (L).

garding basic IOUS scanning techniques.) Currently, open IOUS is used more commonly during more complex biliary surgery than LUS. Therefore, image interpretation may be more difficult, although scanning technique is easier with IOUS than LUS.

Open IOUS is frequently used during surgery for biliary malignant tumors. Scanning of a tumor is performed not only for evaluation of local cancer extension (e.g., vascular invasion, liver parenchymal invasion) but also for assessment of the liver and lymph nodes for metasta-

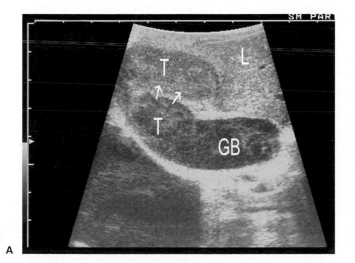
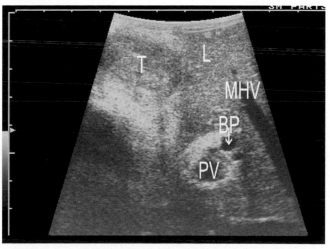

FIGURE 39. A gallbladder cancer with invasion into the liver. **A:** A tumor (T) of the gallbladder (GB) is invading (*arrows*) into the liver parenchyma (T). L, segment 4 of the liver. **B:** To evaluate the resectability, the relation of the invading tumor (T) to intrahepatic vessels is examined. The right portal vein (PV), intrahepatic bile duct (BD, arrow) and middle hepatic vein (MHV) are away from the tumor; it is therefore technically resectable.

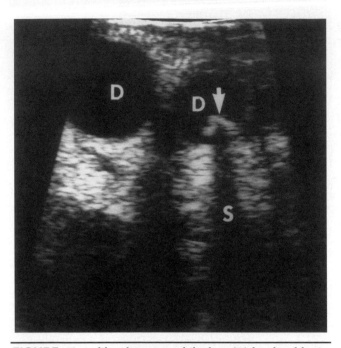

FIGURE 40. A dilated, tortuous bile duct (D) localized by intraoperative ultrasound during reoperation for recurrent bile duct stones. Initial surgical dissection and exploration failed to locate the duct. A bile duct stone (*arrow*) was also demonstrated. S, acoustic shadow.

ses. The use of IOUS during the resection of gallbladder cancers has been investigated (17). The most obvious application is in the determination of the depth of penetration, specifically if there is transmural extension into the hepatic parenchyma (Figs. 38 and 39). One group (18) has evaluated the use of color flow Doppler signals within the tumor prior to resection to attempt to differentiate the precise extent of wall penetration and thus to determine the stage of the tumor. It is important to visualize the tumor in many different planes; the IOUS probe must be moved and simultaneously rotated over the entire gallbladder surface.

A final application of IOUS of the biliary tree occurs in difficult biliary cases, such as open cholecystectomy for acute cholecystitis or reoperation. Because there is always significant inflammation or adhesions in these cases, the use of IOUS is often helpful in defining the location of the bile duct before proceeding with a "blind" dissection (5). If the location of the duct is well known by IOUS prior to significant dissection, it is presumed that duct injury may be more easily avoided. In addition, many of these patients should undergo screening of the bile duct to rule in or out choledocholithiasis (Fig. 40). However because of the scarring and inflammation, the surgeon may feel that cannulating the cystic duct is potentially hazardous or even impossible. In this situation, the duct can be safely evaluated with IOUS without the need for instrumentation of any part of the ductal system.

INDICATIONS

The major indications for LUS and IOUS of the biliary tree are outlined in Table 2. The most common application is to screen the bile duct for the presence of stones. This can be done either routinely or selectively during laparoscopic cholecystectomy. As described in the following section, LUS and IOC are complementary as intraoperative imaging studies. Because LUS has various advantages over IOC, LUS can be used as the first-choice screening procedure for bile duct stones. Furthermore, if IOC is attempted and cannulation is unsuccessful or considered dangerous due to extensive surrounding inflammation or the presence of cystic duct stones, LUS can be used in the place of IOC. In addition, in patients with a stone demonstrated in the bile duct, LUS can be repeated after management of the stone to document its clearance.

A second application of biliary LUS and IOUS is to assist in defining biliary anatomy when it is either unclear or an aberrant duct or vessel is suspected. In the case of routine laparoscopic cholecystectomy, the anatomy that is most helpful to demonstrate is the junction of the cystic duct and the bile duct. By using picture-in-picture technology, the surgeon can identify by LUS where the common hepatic and bile ducts lie in relation to the planned location of clip placement. It is by using this type of information that many proponents of ultrasound have asserted that the routine use of LUS should decrease biliary injuries during laparoscopic cholecystectomy. It can also be helpful during the dissection to be aware of aberrant arterial anatomy, especially a replaced right hepatic artery (Fig. 41). Using color Doppler imaging, the arterial anatomy can be studied and the course of an anomalous anatomy defined. Generally, IOC is more accurate in distinctly defining biliary anatomy and in diagnosing anomalies or variations of the biliary tract. However, with careful scanning LUS can detect or raise suspicion of such anomalies. Figure 42 demonstrates a separately inserting right posterior hepatic duct, which was indicated by LUS and confirmed by IOC. For the converted or planned open cholecystectomy, IOUS can be

▶ **TABLE 2 Indications for Laparoscopic and Open Intraoperative Biliary Ultrasound**

1. Screening the bile duct for stones
2. Helping to define obscured biliary anatomy during cholecystectomy or difficult biliary surgery
3. Determining the stage and resectability of biliary tumors (cholangiocarcinoma, gallbladder cancer): local invasion, liver and lymph node metastases
4. Screening the gallbladder for stones in nonbiliary operations

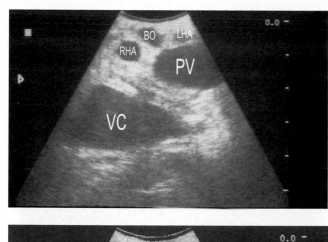

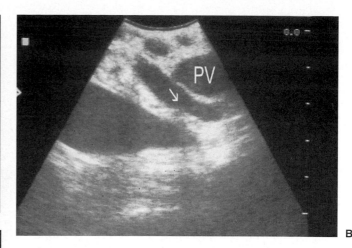

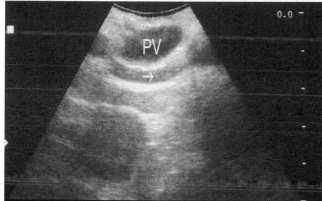

FIGURE 41. Replaced right hepatic artery identified by laparoscopic ultrasound (LUS). **A:** LUS transverse view of the portal triad shows the replaced right hepatic artery (RHA) in addition to the bile duct (BD) and the left hepatic artery (LHA) anterior to the portal vein (PV). VC, vena cava. **B, C:** This right hepatic artery is being followed (*arrows*) proximally; it courses posterior to the portal vein (PV) and the pancreatic head and is originated from the superior mesenteric artery. (Courtesy of Dr. Daniel J. Deziel.)

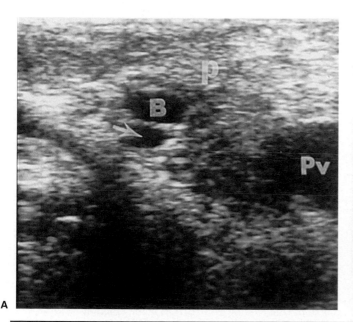

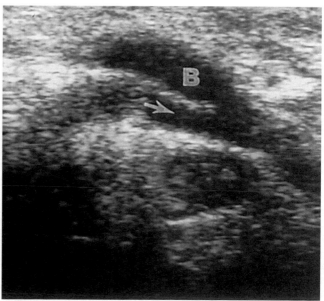

FIGURE 42. Separately inserting right posterior hepatic duct (so-called aberrant hepatic duct) suspected by laparoscopic ultrasound (LUS). **A:** LUS transverse view of the intrapancreatic common bile duct (B) showing another tabular structure (*arrow*) running posterior to the common bile duct. P, pancreas; PV, portal vein. **B:** Longitudinal view showing this structure (*arrow*) joining the common bile duct (B) distally in the pancreas. Based on this LUS finding, a separately inserting right posterior hepatic duct was suspected and was confirmed by intraoperative cholangiography.

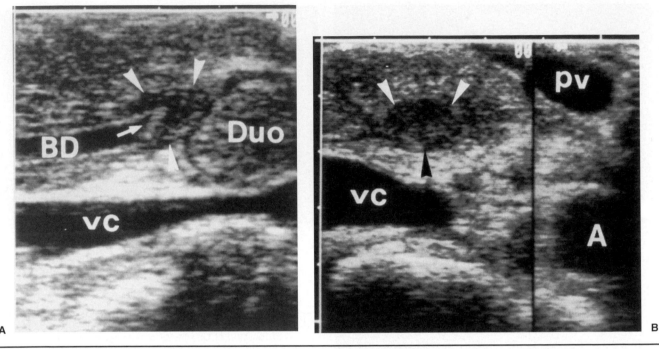

FIGURE 43. A small, resectable tumor at the terminal portion of the common bile duct. Despite the signs of biliary obstruction, preoperative ultrasound and computed tomography did not delineate any tumor. Intraoperative ultrasound immediately after laparotomy demonstrated this hypoechoic, 8 × 12 mm tumor, which was resected by pancreatoduodenectomy and was histologically confirmed to be a terminal common bile duct cholangiocarcinoma. **A:** Longitudinal view of the bile duct showing the tumor (*arrowheads*) causing the obstruction (*arrow*) of the bile duct (BD). vc, vena cava; Duo, duodenum. **B:** Transverse section of the tumor (*arrowheads*) showing its relation to the portal vein (Pv) and the vena cava (vc). A, aorta.

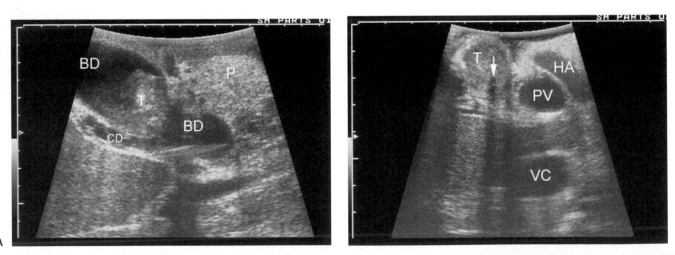

FIGURE 44. A resectable cholangiocarcinoma at the midportion of extrahepatic bile duct. **A:** Intraoperative ultrasound longitudinal view showing a tumor in the dilated bile duct (BD) near the junction with the cystic duct (CD). P, pancreatic head. **B:** Transverse view showing the tumor (T) without invasion to the portal vein (PV) or the hepatic artery (HA), thereby determining its resectability. An arrow indicates a biliary stent with acoustic shadowing. VC, vena cava.

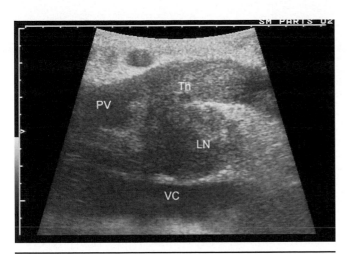

FIGURE 45. Metastatic lymph nodes with portal vein tumor thrombus detected by intraoperative ultrasound (IOUS) in a patient with a gallbladder cancer. IOUS scanning of the hepatoduodenal ligament demonstrated multiple hypoechoic enlarged lymph nodes (LN); intraoperative biopsy confirmed those to be metastatic. IOUS also detected echogenic thrombus (tumor thrombus, Th) in the portal vein (PV). These findings indicated unresectability of this gallbladder cancer. VC, vena cava.

helpful in defining the location of the ducts within an inflamed portal bed. In such circumstances, if IOC is still required, IOUS can be used to guide a needle directly into the bile duct for injection of contrast. Knowing the precise location of the duct can aid the surgeon in directing surgical dissection.

LUS or IOUS may be able to detect a small, preoperatively unknown periampullary cancer, including cholangiocarcinoma, in a patient with obstructive jaundice (Fig. 43). The major indications for LUS and IOUS for biliary malignant tumors are the staging and determination of the resectability. For cholangiocarcinomas, LUS and IOUS can be used to detect the superior and inferior extent of spread along the bile duct, as well as to detect infiltration of the vascular structures (Fig. 44). This type of information can be gathered during a staging laparoscopy, but it can also be useful immediately prior to resection. LUS and IOUS can also be used in evaluating potential gallbladder cancers. In this case, the extent of invasion into the liver can be defined prior to an attempted resection. For both cholangiocarcinoma and gallbladder cancer, liver and lymph node metastases can be assessed by LUS or IOUS (Fig. 45).

A final potential application that is rarely necessary is the screening of the gallbladder itself for stones. Because some stones are very small and beyond the resolution of transabdominal ultrasound, the surgeon may be able to diagnose previously undiscovered small stones by using LUS or IOUS. In patients undergoing operation for other reasons, LUS or IOUS can be used to document stones in the gallbladder if cholecystectomy would be considered. This is especially true when performing laparoscopic procedures, such as gastric bypass surgery, where direct palpation is not possible. Although most gallstones can be palpated during laparotomy, IOUS may be helpful in documenting smaller stones and in eliminating the need for dissection in patients with significant adhesions in the right upper quadrant that obviate easy palpation.

It is important to emphasize specifically that LUS or IOUS should not be used as a means by which the surgeon can rule out biliary injury. If injury is suspected, a traditional IOC should be obtained. Only with an IOC can the entire biliary tree be visualized and biliary injury definitively confirmed or ruled out.

ADVANTAGES AND LIMITATIONS

Advantages

As with any new technology, the relative advantages and disadvantages of LUS and open IOUS should be thoughtfully evaluated (Tables 3 and 4). One obvious advantage of LUS and IOUS is that the surgeon performs the ultrasound scanning and image interpretation, so that no additional personnel are needed. With IOC, a radiology technician is usually needed, which may be the limiting factor in terms of time while adding significant cost. When a surgeon performs LUS or IOUS, only the usual operating room personnel are needed. In addition, ultrasound does not require moving special equipment into the operative field (i.e., the fluoroscopic C-arm); only the probe is required, and it can be kept on the back table with the other instruments. Performance of ultrasound does not require the use of iodinated contrast material or ionizing radiation. A patient's allergy to contrast material is a contraindication to IOC. Although the lack of ionizing radiation is beneficial to the patient and allows a study to be performed safely even in a pregnant patient, the true benefit of lack of radiation probably pertains to

▌ **TABLE 3 Advantages of Laparoscopic Ultrasound and Open Intraoperative Ultrasound in Comparison with Intraoperative Cholangiography**

1. No additional personnel required (technician or radiologist)
2. No iodinated contrast material or ionizing radiation
3. Less costly to perform; no disposable equipment
4. Significantly faster
5. Feasible in virtually all patients; does not require cannulation of cystic duct
6. Easily repeatable throughout the operation
7. Structures can be visualized in more than one plane
8. Higher positive predictive value and specificity than cholangiography

> **TABLE 4** Limitations of Laparoscopic and Open Intraoperative Biliary Ultrasound

1. Lengthy learning curve for the novice
2. Operator dependent technology
3. Difficult to visualize the intrapancreatic duct in a small fraction
4. Less accurate than intraoperative cholangiography in certain biliary imaging capabilities (e.g., detailed biliary anatomy, bile duct injury)

the operating room personnel. Eliminating the use of heavy lead aprons and thyroid collars places less strain on the surgeon during the course of the operation. In addition, operating room personnel are often concerned about the potential effects of frequent (sometimes daily) exposure to radiation, and this worry can be eliminated with the use of LUS or IOUS rather than IOC.

Another important advantage of LUS and IOUS is that they are significantly less expensive to perform than IOC (19,20). Because IOC requires a disposable catheter, contrast material, fluoroscopic time, and a radiology fee, it costs more on a case-by-case basis. The ultrasound machine and probe are certainly expensive capital costs (as is the fluoroscopic equipment), but the machine can be used across a range of surgical specialties and the cost shared. In addition, it has been shown in almost every study that LUS and IOUS take significantly less time to perform than IOC. Because operative time is billed by the minute, this translates into significant savings. In addition, it means the patients' operative and anesthetic times are shorter, which may confer other benefits.

Because IOC requires cannulation of the cystic duct, it cannot be performed safely in a certain proportion of patients who have either a prohibitively small cystic duct or an obstructing stone that prohibits passage of the catheter. During the passage of the cholangiocatheter through the cystic duct, the duct can be inadvertently punctured or avulsed. Because neither LUS nor IOUS requires cystic duct cannulation, such problems are avoided. Because LUS and IOUS are technically possible in virtually all patients, they carry a higher rate of success in terms of visualizing the bile duct. In addition, they do not carry a risk of injury to any ductal structure. Furthermore, images of the duct can be obtained multiple times during the operation without any increase in risk to the patient or inconvenience to the operating room team.

Another potential advantage of LUS and IOUS over IOC is that they are more specific (14,21,22) for the identification of bile duct stones. This is important because it minimizes the number of negative common bile duct explorations that are undertaken in response to false-positive tests. These data will be discussed further in the following section.

Limitations

There are no absolute contraindications to the use of LUS or IOUS. Probe contact scanning may be difficult in patients who are extremely thin; in such instances, instillation of saline is usually required to perform probe-standoff scanning. Perhaps the biggest disadvantage of ultrasound, especially LUS, is that there is a substantial learning curve before the scanning can be efficiently performed and the images accurately interpreted (19,23). Ultrasound is a highly operator-dependent technology. Most experts suggest that practicing surgeons who wish to start acquiring LUS or IOUS skills perform both ultrasound and IOC on the first subset of patients until the sensitivity and specificity become similar to that reported in the literature.

Imaging the intrapancreatic portion of the bile duct has been described as the Achilles heel of LUS (24,25). In comparison to the suprapancreatic duct, the intrapancreatic duct is relatively well hidden in the substance of the pancreas and is often obscured by air in the overlying duodenum. However, it has been shown by many authors that use of a variety of the methods described above allows complete visualization of intrapancreatic duct in the vast majority of patients. Compared with IOC, LUS and IOUS have a few distinct disadvantages with regard to biliary imaging: they do not give as detailed of a "road map" of the anatomy; they do not demonstrate the functional emptying characteristics of the biliary tree; and they are not accurate in evaluating bile duct injury, biliary leakage or biliary fistula.

Perhaps the biggest hurdle to overcome in the use of LUS or IOUS is the transition from a familiar procedure with which the surgeon is comfortable to one that is distinctly unfamiliar. This type of change can be difficult and uncomfortable for the practicing surgeon. However, there are an increasing number of courses available to teach surgeons the basic principles of ultrasound and how to apply them in specific situations, such as screening the bile duct by LUS. In addition, as the new generation of surgical trainees becomes more skilled with the use of ultrasound through experience with it in various settings, such as trauma (i.e., the focused abdominal sonography for trauma, or FAST, examination) and in staging laparoscopy, the technology will become more familiar and the learning curve less daunting.

CLINICAL RESULTS

Since the mid-1990s, many authors have reported their experience using LUS during laparoscopic cholecystectomy. Most of these reports pertained to studies comparing LUS to IOC within a single institution. There are several problems inherent to this type of data. First, the majority of studies have compared the results of LUS to the results of IOC performed in sequence on the same patient. Obviously, the results of the test performed first are known to the surgeon and are likely to influence the results of the second study. One group attempted to control for this by randomizing the order in which the tests were performed (24). The results of this trial were not significantly different from those of other trials reported in terms of the accuracy of the two methods. Another group employed different operators blinded to clinical details to perform the two tests (26). The results of this study indicated that LUS was both more sensitive and more specific for the detection of bile duct stones than IOC.

To date, there has not been a trial in which patients were randomized to either LUS or IOC and the outcomes compared. The difficulty of carrying out this type of study comparing two surgical techniques is exemplified by the group who had planned a three-part study, with phase III being a randomized controlled trial comparing LUS with IOC (21). However, because the initial phases confirmed the reliability and accuracy of LUS, the surgeons did not feel that the randomized study was necessary and elected to proceed directly to routine LUS for all patients.

Another problem exists with the clinical studies of LUS. It is difficult to know for sure how the two techniques compare if there is not a separate test that serves as the gold standard. When IOC is considered to be, in effect, the gold standard, calculating its sensitivity and specificity is difficult. In addition, showing that a new test is more sensitive than the gold standard is not possible. For example, a stone seen by LUS but not confirmed by IOC may be considered a false-positive result for LUS when in fact it is a false-negative result for IOC.

Theoretically, the ideal way to solve this problem is for all patients to undergo bile duct exploration as the gold standard against which both techniques are compared. This is obviously impractical and would cause harm to the patient; therefore, surgeons have had to use surrogate markers to determine as best as possible the sensitivity and specificity of these tests. Most have chosen to explore the common duct of any patient with a positive result by either imaging method and to assume that the remainder of the ducts were free of stones unless the patient presents postoperatively with symptoms due to a retained stone. Because it is well known that small stones can pass spontaneously from the bile duct without causing symptoms, this assumption is not completely accurate; however, it allows the clinician to draw clinically relevant conclusions. Given the caveats just discussed, we compare the outcomes from the more recent clinical studies and discuss their implications.

Feasibility

The value of an imaging modality depends not only on its accuracy but also on the ability to successfully obtain the images. Because IOC requires cannulation of the cystic duct and free passage of contrast into the bile duct, it is not always technically possible to obtain an IOC. The data in Table 5 taken together indicate that surgeons obtained an intraoperative cholangiogram in 93.7% of the patients in whom IOC was attempted, compared to 97.8% of patients imaged by LUS. In our experience (27), we were able to obtain a cholangiogram in 97% of patients in whom IOC was attempted. The reasons for failure included a duct too small to cannulate, an avulsed cystic duct, and technical difficulty with the fluoroscopic equipment. In contrast, we were able to obtain LUS images in 99% of patients, with the failures only being due to technical issues relating to the equipment.

The more critical issue for LUS imaging is the ability to completely image the duct, especially the intrapancreatic

▶ **TABLE 5** **Summary of Feasibility and Time Required for Intraoperative Cholangiography and Laparoscopic Ultrasound in Clinical Series**

Study	*Number*	*Time (min)* *IOC*	*Time (min)* *LUS*	*Success* *IOC*	*Success* *LUS*
Rothlin (14)	100	13.5	4.5	90	100
Thompson (21)	360	10.9	6.6	NS	NS
Catheline (22)	150	17.6	11.6	96	83
Birth (24)	518	16	7	92.1	99.6
Wu (20)	607	15.1	5.3	97	100
Machi (28)	100	15.9	8.2	92	95
Kimura (29)	184	NS	NS	95.6	94.6
Siperstein (30)	300	NS	4	94	100
Tranter (26)	135	NS	NS	83	98

IOC, intraoperative cholangiography; LUS, laparoscopic ultrasound.

▶ **TABLE 6** Comparison of Sensitivity and Specificity of Intraoperative Cholangiography and Laparoscopic Ultrasound in Clinical Series

Study	Number	IOC Sensitivity	IOC Specificity	LUS Sensitivity	LUS Specificity
Rothlin (14)	100	64	100	91	100
Thompson (21)	360	98.1	98.1	90	100
Catheline (22)	150	78	97	80	99
Birth (24)	518	100	99	83.3	100
Machi (28)	100	87.5	97.6	88.9	100
Kimura (29)	184	93.3	98.2	82.4	100
Siperstein (30)	300	96.2	100	96.2	100
Menack (23)	360	98.1	98.1	90	100
Tranter (26)	135	90	99	98	100

IOC, intraoperative cholangiography; LUS, laparoscopic ultrasound.

portion of the distal bile duct. One group (22) has shown that while visualization of the proximal bile duct is possible in 100% of patients by LUS and 95% of patients by IOC, the distal one third of the duct was well visualized in only 83% of patients by LUS compared to 96% by IOC. A second group (24) reported similar numbers, with the intraligamental suprapancreatic segment of the duct well visualized in 99% of patients by both methods, but the periampullary duct well visualized in only 85% of patients by LUS, compared with 92% by IOC. However, it is clear that the ability to visualize the distal duct significantly improves with the number of cases performed and the surgeon's level of experience. In another series, visualization on the intrapancreatic bile duct was documented in only 7 of the first 20 cases, but increased to 16 of 20 after the first 40 procedures were performed (9). In our experience with 377 patients in whom LUS was completed (27), there were 18 patients (5%) in whom the middle portion of the common duct could not be visualized in continuity and 21 patients (6%) in whom the distal portion of the duct could not be visualized in continuity. Thus, a total of 36 patients (10%) had suboptimal imaging of some part of the common bile duct (in three patients neither segment was visualized in continuity).

Detection of Bile Duct Stones

The potential for each test to reveal bile duct stones when they are present and rule them out when they are absent is essential to its clinical utility. Because of the methodologic difficulties with the available data (discussed above) and the varying patient populations, each study yields slightly different values for sensitivity and specificity of LUS and IOC (Table 6). Assessing the data as a group, several features that distinguish the imaging modalities become clear.

First and foremost, false-positive results are extremely rare when LUS is used to screen the bile duct. The few false positives that have been reported have been due to two instances of a calculus lodged in the distal cystic duct that was mistaken for the common bile duct (9,22) and one instance of a juxtapapillary diverticulum (14). In two cases classified as false positives, a stone was seen by LUS but not confirmed by IOC (8). Although it is possible that the stones were cleared from the bile duct as the IOC was obtained, it is also possible that this was due to the learning curve (this was one of the first 20 cases for the operator involved). It is remarkable that in the more than 2,500 cases reported in these series, only a handful of false positives occurred with LUS. This is clinically essential because it indicates a much higher positive predictive value and means that the decision to explore the bile duct based on the LUS findings can be made confidently (28). Because the positive predictive value and specificity of IOC is slightly lower than for LUS, one could expect more negative bile duct explorations to result from reliance on IOC than on LUS. Some authors have even used LUS to rule out the presence of stones suggested by IOC (29).

A second difference in these screening methods is that a higher percentage of patients are found to have bile duct stones when LUS is employed as the screening modality. The reason for this is that it is often difficult to detect small stones on IOC, either because they are flushed out of the bile duct upon injection or because they are so small that they are easily obscured. LUS can detect not only small stones but also biliary sludge in the bile duct, which is impossible by any other technique. The precise clinical consequence of this difference is presently unclear. Much of the sludge and many of the small stones are likely to pass spontaneously and will not result in clinical consequence. On the other hand, it has been shown that both small stones and biliary sludge are associated with the occurrence of biliary pancreatitis. We currently employ a selective approach to patients with biliary sludge detected by LUS, treating some with glucagon infusion and flushing of the duct and others with conservative therapy.

Finally, it is clear that there are some false-negative LUS results. Because these patients can usually be treated by postoperative endoscopic retrograde cholangiopancreatography (ERCP), the consequences of this rare occurrence are small. Several strategies can be employed to minimize the number of false-negative results encountered. The first is to ensure adequate visualization of the entire common bile duct in continuity. If the entire duct cannot be visualized in continuity by LUS and stones are clinically suspected, we obtain an IOC. In addition, the duct should be scanned in both directions during LUS, superior to inferior and inferior to superior. Some have suggested that scanning the duct in multiple planes can reduce the chance of a false-negative result. This often requires moving the transducer from the epigastric port to the umbilical port, so that both longitudinal and transverse images can be obtained. Finally, if an abnormality is suspected but cannot be clearly demonstrated by LUS, particularly if the imaging is suboptimal, an IOC should be obtained.

Effect on Biliary Injury

The primary use of LUS imaging during laparoscopic cholecystectomy is to document the presence or absence of stones in the bile duct. However, as its use has expanded and surgeons have become quite adept at both the acquisition and interpretation of the LUS images, additional avenues for its use are being explored. A retrospective study including 842 patients was conducted at an institution in which two surgeons used LUS routinely and three surgeons adhered to a policy of selective cholangiography (10). Ultrasound was performed through the epigastric port both before dissection was begun and after dissection was complete, and if stones were suspected by LUS, an IOC was obtained. When the incidence of postoperative bile duct complications was examined with respect to each patient group, it was found that the patients who underwent routine LUS had significantly fewer complications than those who underwent selective IOC. Specifically, there were 5 (0.8%) bile duct injuries, 4 (0.7%) retained bile duct stones, and 6 (1%) postoperative bile leaks in the IOC group; there were no biliary complications in the LUS group. This finding was statistically significant and occurred despite the fact that the surgeons who used LUS performed fewer cholecystectomies per year and were more junior members of the faculty.

This group concluded that laparoscopic cholecystectomy with LUS is associated with fewer bile duct complications than laparoscopic cholecystectomy without adjunctive imaging. Although these data certainly suggest what others have conjectured, namely, that LUS may help to protect against iatrogenic biliary injury, they are certainly not conclusive. Because the imaging strategy was routine in one group and selective in the other, and two different groups of surgeons were compared, the differences between groups may be due only to the routine nature of the imaging strategy rather than the method by which the duct is imaged. Despite its weaknesses, this study makes one wonder if the complete absence of bile duct complications is indeed due to the advantages of LUS. Additional clinical studies are warranted to define the value of LUS in preventing biliary complications during laparoscopic cholecystectomy.

Time of Performance

One of the consistent findings across almost every study comparing LUS to IOC is that LUS takes significantly less time to perform than IOC. When the data in Table 5 are combined and the weighted average is computed, the mean time for completion of IOC is 14.7 minutes, compared with 6.7 minutes for LUS. The precise amount of time will vary with conditions within a given institution. In an early multicenter trial, the time for LUS was significantly shorter in some centers than others, but the range varied only from a mean of 5.5 minutes to 8.0 minutes (11).

The Learning Curve

There is clearly a learning curve involved in the adequate performance of LUS. Surgeons must not only acquire the technical skills to perform a clear and complete study, but also must learn how to interpret the LUS images. When the novice ultrasonographer was compared with the experienced ultrasonographer in one study (19), the perceived difficulty of LUS was found to be "easy" for 71% of the experienced group compared with only 24% of the novice group. Importantly, whereas 12% of the novice group found LUS to be "impossible," 0% of the experienced group did. This same group was also able to show a more than threefold increase in the percentage of experienced surgeons who were able to image the distal common bile duct compared with the novice. A similar effect of experience on LUS performance was shown by another surgeon who demonstrated that during his first 140 cases, he had four false-negative ultrasound examination results, compared with only one in his next 220 exams (23). A final group (14) was able to show that as the number of cases performed increased, so did the number of biliary and vascular variations that were detected by LUS.

Although it is clear that there is a learning curve for LUS, what remains unknown is how many procedures must be done before the curve flattens. No clear data exist to help define this. Some groups have left their first 20 cases out of their series for analysis, suggesting that these cases were certainly on the steep part of the learning curve. Another group reported that it took 10 to 20 cases for them to feel comfortable with the LUS technique (25). From experience, it is our impression that the learning curve for LUS is initially quite steep and that proficiency can probably be obtained after 10 to 20 cases. However, the learning curve no doubt continues well past this point and perhaps does not level off until more than 50 such procedures have been performed.

Cost

It has been shown in two separate studies that the cost of performing LUS is significantly less than that of performing IOC. In one study (20), the cost was calculated to be $198 for IOC and $53 for LUS. These figures do not include the radiologist's fee or the cost of the equipment. In a similar analysis (19), the cost of a LUS exam was $362 compared with $665 for an IOC.

CONCLUSIONS

The addition of ultrasound to a laparoscopic procedure gives back to the surgeon the ability to "see beyond" the visible surface. In the case of laparoscopic cholecystectomy, the use of LUS for documenting bile duct stones has been shown to be equivalent or even superior to IOC. LUS is faster to perform, less cumbersome, and less costly. It has a high sensitivity and a nearly perfect specificity. Despite these advantages, LUS is not likely to completely replace IOC because of certain limitations and disadvantages of LUS in comparison with IOC. Instead, the two techniques are complementary and should both be thought of as part of the surgeon's complete armamentarium. During the learning period for surgeons who are interested in LUS, it is recommended that both LUS and IOC be performed. Once mastered, LUS can be used as a first-choice screening method for bile duct stones during laparoscopic cholecystectomy. IOC is then used selectively, as indicated.

In our practice, we prefer to use LUS routinely and IOC selectively. If the entire bile duct can be demonstrated in continuity by LUS and is free of abnormalities, we complete the cholecystectomy without IOC. If the bile duct cannot be imaged completely by LUS and bile duct stones are not suspected clinically, we proceed with cholecystectomy without IOC. When bile duct stones are clinically suspected and the LUS imaging is suboptimal, we proceed to IOC. If stones or sludge are demonstrated

in the bile duct by LUS, we initially give a dose of intravenous glucagon and proceed with transcystic irrigation. The LUS is then repeated to document clearance of the abnormality. If the abnormality persists and is suspected to be clinically relevant, we either proceed with laparoscopic bile duct exploration or plan to obtain a postoperative ERCP, depending on the characteristics of the bile duct, the stone, and the patient. IOC should also be performed when the biliary anatomy is unclear by LUS and must be clarified or when bile duct injury is suspected. Although LUS cannot replace IOC completely, the routine use of LUS will result in a significant reduction in the need for IOC during laparoscopic cholecystectomy.

IOUS during open biliary surgery plays a valuable role, particularly because open surgery is currently performed for more complicated or difficult biliary diseases or conditions, including biliary malignancy. A variety of information can be obtained intraoperatively by using biliary IOUS, which helps both to determine the final diagnosis or pathologic staging and to select the most appropriate operation. Biliary surgeons who are interested in ultrasound are urged to master LUS and IOUS simultaneously.

REFERENCES

1. Knight R, Newell J. Operative use of ultrasonics in cholelithiasis. *Lancet* 1963;1:1023–1025.
2. Hayashi S, Wagai T, Miyazawa R. Ultrasonic diagnosis of breast tumor and cholelithiasis. *West J Surg* 1962;70:34–40.
3. Lane RJ, Coupland GA. Ultrasonic indications to explore the common bile duct. *Surgery* 1982;91:268–274.
4. Sigel B, Coelho JC, Nyhus LM, et al. Comparison of cholangiography and ultrasonography in the operative screening of the common bile duct. *World J Surg* 1982;6:440–444.
5. Machi J, Sigel B, Zaren H, et al. Operative ultrasonography during hepatobiliary and pancreatic surgery. *World J Surg* 1993;17:640–646.
6. Jackimowitcz J, Rutten H, Jurgens P, et al. Comparison of operative ultrasonography and radiography in screening of common bile duct for calculi. *World J Surg* 1987;11:628–634.
7. Holthausen U, Troidl H, Paul A. Ultrasonography: the stethoscope of the surgeon in the era of endoscopic surgery. *Surg Endosc* 1994;8:1163–1164.
8. Rothlin M, Largiader F. The anatomy of the hepatoduodenal ligament in laparoscopic sonography. *Surg Endosc* 1994;8: 173–180.
9. John TG, Banting SW, Pye S, et al. Preliminary experience with intracorporeal laparoscopic ultrasonography using a sector scanning probe. A prospective comparison with intraoperative cholangiography in the detection of choledocholithiasis. *Surg Endosc* 1994;8:1176–1180;discussion 1180–1181.
10. Biffl WL, Moore EE, Offner PJ, et al. Routine intraoperative laparoscopic ultrasonography with selective cholangiography reduces bile duct complications during laparoscopic cholecystectomy. *J Am Coll Surg* 2001;193:272–280.
11. Stiegmann GV, Soper NJ, Filipi CJ, et al. Laparoscopic ultrasonography as compared with static or dynamic cholangiography at laparoscopic cholecystectomy. A prospective multicenter trial. *Surg Endosc* 1995;9:1269–1273.
12. Santambrogio R, Bianchi P, Opocher E, et al. Prevalence and laparoscopic ultrasound patterns of choledocholithiasis and

biliary sludge during cholecystectomy. *Surg Laparosc Endosc Percutan Tech* 1999;9:129–134.

13. Machi J, Sigel B, Zaren HA, et al. Technique of ultrasound examination during laparoscopic cholecystectomy. *Surg Endosc* 1993;7:544–549.

14. Rothlin MA, Schob O, Schlumpf R, et al. Laparoscopic ultrasonography during cholecystectomy. *Br J Surg* 1996;83:1512–1516.

15. Tilleman EH, de Castro SM, Busch OR, et al. Diagnostic laparoscopy and laparoscopic ultrasound for staging of patients with malignant proximal bile duct obstruction. *J Gastrointest Surg* 2002;6:426–430;discussion 430–431.

16. Weber SM, DeMatteo RP, Fong Y, et al. Staging laparoscopy in patients with extrahepatic biliary carcinoma. Analysis of 100 patients. *Ann Surg* 2002;235:392–399.

17. Azuma T, Yoshikawa T, Araida T, et al. Intraoperative evaluation of the depth of invasion of gallbladder cancer. *Am J Surg* 1999;178:381–384.

18. Sato M, Ishida H, Konno K, et al. Localized gallbladder carcinoma: sonographic findings. *Abdom Imaging* 2001;26:619–622.

19. Falcone RA Jr, Fegelman EJ, Nussbaum MS, et al. A prospective comparison of laparoscopic ultrasound vs intraoperative cholangiogram during laparoscopic cholecystectomy. *Surg Endosc* 1999;13:784–788.

20. Wu JS, Dunnegan DL, Soper NJ. The utility of intracorporeal ultrasonography for screening of the bile duct during laparoscopic cholecystectomy. *J Gastrointest Surg* 1998;2:50–60.

21. Thompson DM, Arregui ME, Tetik C, et al. A comparison of laparoscopic ultrasound with digital fluorocholangiography for detecting choledocholithiasis during laparoscopic cholecystectomy. *Surg Endosc* 1998;12:929–932.

22. Catheline JM, Turner R, Rizk N, et al. Evaluation of the biliary tree during laparoscopic cholecystectomy: laparoscopic ultrasound versus intraoperative cholangiography: a prospective study of 150 cases. *Surg Laparosc Endosc Percutan Tech* 1998;8:85–91.

23. Menack MJ, Arregui ME. Laparoscopic sonography of the biliary tree and pancreas. *Surg Clin North Am* 2000;80:1151–1170.

24. Birth M, Ehlers KU, Delinikolas K, et al. Prospective randomized comparison of laparoscopic ultrasonography using a flexible-tip ultrasound probe and intraoperative dynamic cholangiography during laparoscopic cholecystectomy. *Surg Endosc* 1998;12:30–36.

25. Stiegmann GV, McIntyre RC, Pearlman NW. Laparoscopic intracorporeal ultrasound. An alternative to cholangiography? *Surg Endosc* 1994;8:167–171;discussion 171–172.

26. Tranter S, Thompson M. Laparoscopic ultrasound is capable of replacing operative cholangiography. *Br J Surg* 2002;89:63.

27. Halpin VJ, Dunnegan D, Soper NJ. Laparoscopic intracorporeal ultrasound versus fluoroscopic intraoperative cholangiography: after the learning curve. *Surg Endosc* 2002;16:336–341.

28. Machi J, Tateishi T, Oishi AJ, et al. Laparoscopic ultrasonography versus operative cholangiography during laparoscopic cholecystectomy: review of the literature and a comparison with open intraoperative ultrasonography. *J Am Coll Surg* 1999;188:360–367.

29. Kimura T, Umehara Y, Yoshida M, et al. Laparoscopic ultrasonography and operative cholangiography prevent residual common bile duct stones in laparoscopic cholecystectomy. *Surg Laparosc Endosc Percutan Tech* 1999;9:124–128.

30. Siperstein A, Pearl J, Macho J, et al. Comparison of laparoscopic ultrasonography and fluorocholangiography in 300 patients undergoing laparoscopic cholecystectomy. *Surg Endosc* 1999;13:113–117.

Intraoperative Ultrasound of the Liver

Reid B. Adams

Intraoperative ultrasound (IOUS) has an essential role in the evaluation and management of liver diseases amenable to surgical therapy (Table 1). Its successful use requires a fundamental understanding of ultrasound principles and normal three-dimensional hepatic anatomy. Together, this knowledge allows the surgeon great flexibility in managing hepatic neoplasms and other liver diseases. IOUS of the liver is the only real-time, intraoperative imaging technique for liver imaging available to the surgeon in the operating room. It has the advantage of allowing direct contact scanning with the organ of interest, which increases its sensitivity for the detection of small lesions and provides superb anatomic detail. IOUS allows the surgeon not only to do diagnostic studies but also to perform therapeutic procedures.

Prior to the introduction of IOUS, intrahepatic anatomic relationships and the location of nonpalpable hepatic tumors could only be inferred based on preoperative imaging studies. In the late 1970s, Makuuchi reported the initial use of IOUS during hepatic procedures (1). Since then, the use of IOUS has increased steadily. Currently, despite the fact that liver imaging modalities have improved dramatically, IOUS has become a critical tool for the safe and accurate conduct of liver surgery. It provides unparalleled information by confirming a diagnosis previously made on the basis of preoperative imaging. It detects occult lesions missed preoperatively or during intraoperative inspection and palpation. In addition, intrahepatic structures can be clearly defined at the time of the operation, and the relationship of hepatic tumors to these structures can be precisely determined. IOUS aids in the differential diagnosis of these tumors and allows targeted biopsy if necessary. IOUS facilitates intraoperative decision making and has allowed the development of a number of novel hepatectomy techniques. Lately, nonresectional management of tumors, such as that by radiofrequency thermal ablation, has been advanced with IOUS guidance.

This chapter describes the general uses of IOUS during hepatic surgery. Instrumentation and scanning techniques for examining the liver are reviewed in detail.

Normal hepatic anatomy as viewed during IOUS and the IOUS features of hepatic pathology are presented. The use of IOUS to guide interventions during liver surgery is detailed. In this chapter, IOUS of the liver during open surgery (laparotomy) is described. The use of ultrasound during laparoscopy (laparoscopic ultrasound) for liver diseases is detailed in Chapter 17.

INDICATIONS

One of the earliest uses of IOUS during abdominal surgery was in hepatic surgery. Liver imaging remains one of the most common indications for IOUS, which serves both diagnostic and therapeutic purposes during liver surgery. The primary indications for the use of IOUS of the liver are to screen for metastatic lesions, both known and occult; to evaluate hepatic tumors for resectability; to assist the appropriate selection of interventions; and to provide image guidance for various procedures such as biopsy, ablation, and resection (Table 2).

The detection of metastatic disease to the liver from abdominal malignancies is important for staging and for decision making during surgical therapy. Despite improvements in other imaging techniques, IOUS remains the most accurate screening technique for metastatic disease of the liver (2–8). When combined with intraoperative inspection and palpation, the sensitivity of detection for liver metastases by IOUS exceeds 90% (9–11). While the limits of detection for hepatic metastasis remain around 5 to 10 mm for computed tomography (CT), magnetic resonance imaging (MRI), or positron emission tomography (PET), IOUS can detect lesions as small as 3 to 5 mm (12). IOUS, when used as a screening method, can expose otherwise unrecognized (occult) metastasis in 5% to 20% of patients with colorectal cancer (2,6,8,13–16). During operation in patients known to have metastatic tumors preoperatively, additional tumors will be found in up to 55% of patients (2,8,17–19). During planned resection or ablation of metastatic liver tumors (such as colorectal metastases), IOUS allows precise evaluation of

▶ **TABLE 1** Utility of Intraoperative Liver Ultrasound

Allows intraoperative imaging
Real-time imaging
Rapid use and acquisition of information
Highly sensitive and accurate
  - Defines intrahepatic anatomy
  - Detects lesions as small as 3 mm (e.g., occult lesions)
  - Determines relationship between lesions and vessels
Provides guidance for intraoperative procedures

the extent (size, number, location) of tumors, determination of resectability, and determination of the optimal procedure to be performed. In a number of studies, IOUS has been found to change the operative plan for liver tumors in 7% to 50% of operations (7,9,17,18,20,21). Thus, IOUS remains an important imaging technique for metastatic disease to the liver despite improvements in other imaging modalities.

The ease of use and accuracy of IOUS suggest a role for screening for liver metastases in patients with colorectal cancer. Approximately 5% to 20% of patients have synchronous metastases at the time of their index procedure (3,4,13,21–24). However, the role of routine versus selective liver screening with IOUS in these patients remains unanswered (25). If preoperative imaging of the liver is done routinely (usually by CT), the use of routine IOUS instead is recommended. On the other hand, if an oncologist typically obtains an abdominal CT scan for staging purposes despite the existence of an IOUS study, the cost effectiveness of routine IOUS may be questioned. Therefore, the incorporation of IOUS into practice will be determined based on local practice considerations.

IOUS also is excellent for staging during the management of other abdominal malignancies. Although the in-

▶ **TABLE 2** Indications for Intraoperative Ultrasound

Acquire new diagnostic information
  - Identify additional occult lesions
  - Screen for liver metastasis
  - Stage known primary malignancies
Localize nonpalpable lesions
Characterize hepatic tumors
  - Confirm known lesions
  - Determine intrahepatic position
  - Determine resectability
  - Detect vasculobiliary involvement
Guide hepatic interventions
  - Biopsy
  - Resection types
  - Resection guidance
  - Tumor ablation
Confirm completion of operation

cidence of liver metastases may not be as high as colorectal cancer, the presence of liver metastasis from other abdominal malignancies often significantly alters the planned procedure. Thus, selective screening may be the most appropriate use, evaluating the liver in those patients with T3 or T4 tumors or with clinically positive lymph nodes (13). Candidates for IOUS liver screening include patients with gastric, biliary, or pancreatic carcinoma; neuroendocrine tumor; gastrointestinal stromal tumor; and ovarian cancer. Thus, IOUS is an effective screening tool for both colorectal cancer and a variety of other abdominal malignancies.

The management of primary hepatic neoplasms is another prime indication for the use of IOUS. Hepatocellular carcinoma has become increasingly common in Western countries, and IOUS is essential for the detection of these tumors and their resection or ablation. Our Asian and European colleagues have developed substantial expertise in this area (1,26–32). Since hepatocellular carcinoma mostly occurs in the setting of a stiff liver (fibrosis or cirrhosis), tumors less than 5 cm in diameter are difficult to identify intraoperatively and can be found in only approximately 50% of cases by inspection and palpation alone (33,34). IOUS allows detection and accurate localization of these tumors (35,36). Furthermore, IOUS is more accurate than preoperative imaging in detecting the extent of the tumor, the presence of intrahepatic metastasis (so-called daughter nodules), invasion of surrounding vessels, or tumor thrombi (37–40).

IOUS is uniquely suited to aid the performance of a number of intraoperative procedures. Needle placement for biopsy of nonpalpable or deep lesions can be precisely guided under IOUS (41). Likewise, IOUS allows exact cannula placement for aspiration of cavitary lesions. Accurate targeting of hepatic tumors for ablative therapies (ethanol injection, cryotherapy, thermal ablation) is accomplished by IOUS, and the adequacy of treatment can be monitored in real time during the procedure (42–45). IOUS provides guidance for hepatic resections, including both anatomic and nonanatomic resections, especially when performing anatomic segmentectomies or subsegmentectomies. Its use has allowed the development of several novel approaches to liver surgery such as IOUS-guided systematic subsegmentectomy (28,32,45–52).

NORMAL HEPATIC ANATOMY

To take full advantage of IOUS, an in-depth understanding of hepatic anatomy is essential. The descriptions and definitions of hepatic anatomy have evolved substantially over time, most recently being influenced by the use of IOUS.

Surface features of the liver define one description of hepatic anatomy (Fig. 1). The falciform ligament and umbilical fissure divide the liver into a larger right portion of

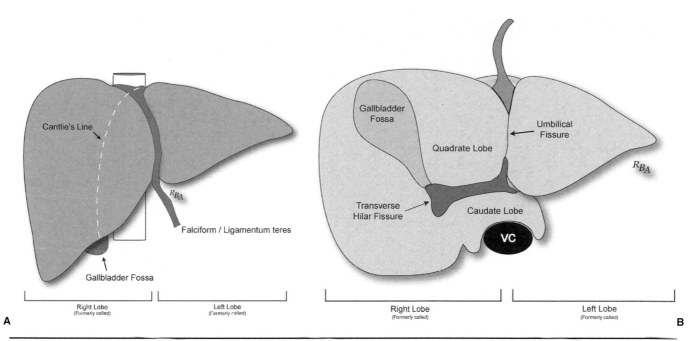

FIGURE 1. Surface features of the liver. **A:** Anterior surface. The falciform ligament visually divides the liver into two portions, formerly called the right lobe and left lobe. Cantlie's line runs from the middle of the gallbladder fossa to the left of the vena cava. This is the main portal scissura, which defines the course of the middle hepatic vein. **B:** Inferior surface. Like the falciform ligament, the umbilical fissure visually divides the liver into a formally called right and left lobe. Older nomenclature describes the quadrate lobe (now called segment 4), which is bounded by the gallbladder fossa, the transverse hilar fissure, and the umbilical fissure. The caudate lobe (segment 1) is the liver between the transverse hilar fissure and the vena cava (VC).

the liver (formerly called the right lobe) to the right of these structures and a smaller left portion (formerly called the left lobe). The portal structures enter the inferior surface of the liver forming the transverse hilar fissure. Anterior to this is the quadrate lobe, delimited on the left by the umbilical fissure and on the right by the gallbladder fossa. Posterior to the hilar fissure is the caudate lobe. While this nomenclature provides a good description of the liver based on surface features, its utility is inadequate for defining intrahepatic anatomy. Consequently, it is an insufficient descriptor for use in current hepatic surgery.

More useful is the so-called functional description of hepatic anatomy based on functional liver units defined by the portal pedicles and the hepatic veins. These functional units can be precisely defined by IOUS and individually resected as required by the disease process (53, 54). Initially defined by Cantlie in 1898, the functional units were refined and ultimately most completely described as the French system (55). This description defines eight segments, known as Couinaud's segments, based on their portal pedicles (Fig. 2; Table 3). The most recent refinement of this description was reported at the 2000 meeting of the International Hepatopancreatobiliary Association (IHPBA) in Brisbane, Australia (56).

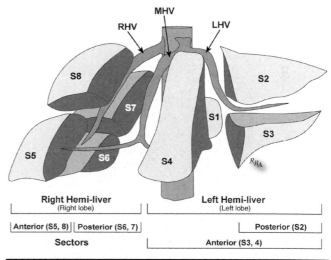

FIGURE 2. Segmental liver anatomy according to Couinaud. Each labeled segment (S1–S8) is supplied by a separate portal pedicle. The hepatic veins divide the liver into four sectors. The middle hepatic vein divides the liver in a right and left hemiliver (right and left lobe). The right hemiliver is composed of two sectors. The anterior sector (S5, S8) lies anterior to the right hepatic vein. The posterior sector (S6, S7) lies posterior to the right hepatic vein. The left hemiliver also is composed of two sectors. The anterior sector (S3, S4) lies anterior to the left hepatic vein. The falciform ligament/umbilical fissure lies between S3 and S4. The posterior sector (S2) lies posterior to the left hepatic vein. The bulk of S1 (caudate lobe) lies posterior to S4.

▶ **TABLE 3 Liver Segmental Anatomy**

Right Portal Vein	
Anterior branch	Anterior sector
Superior segment	Segment 8
Inferior segment	Segment 5
Posterior branch	Posterior sector
Superior segment	Segment 7
Inferior segment	Segment 6
Left Portal Vein	
Medial branches	Segment 4a/b
Lateral branches:	
First (superior) branch	Segment 2
Second (inferior) branch	Segment 3
Individual right and left portal branches	Segment 1 (caudate lobe)

Per Couinaud's description, the liver is divided into four sectors defined by the hepatic veins. The middle hepatic vein divides the liver in half, into a right and left hemiliver (also called the right and left lobe). The right hemiliver is composed of two sectors (referred to as sections in the IHPBA terminology). The anterior sector (section) is that liver between the middle and right hepatic veins. To the right (posterior) of the right hepatic vein is the posterior sector (section). These sectors are

further divided into a superior and inferior segment, each of which is supplied by an independent portal pedicle (Table 3). The main right portal pedicle divides into two parts: an anterior branch supplying the anterior sector and a posterior branch supplying the posterior sector. Each of these sectorial branches divides into a superior branch and an inferior branch. The inferior branch in the anterior sector supplies segment 5 and the superior branch supplies segment 8. Likewise, in the posterior sector, the inferior branch supplies segment 6 and the superior branch segment 7 (Fig. 3).

Although no external marking on the liver delineates the location of the right and left hemilivers, the line of division can be readily estimated. This line, also referred to as Cantlie's line, extends from the middle of the gallbladder fossa to the left side of the vena cava superiorly and defines the course of the middle hepatic vein (main portal scissura) (Fig. 1).

According to Couinaud's classification, the left hemiliver is divided into two sectors, anterior and posterior, by the left hepatic vein. The anterior sector is divided into two segments by the umbilical fissure (containing the portal pedicle): the medial segment (segment 4) to the right of the umbilical fissure/falciform ligament and

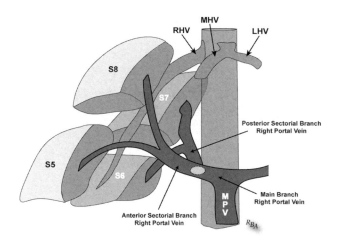

FIGURE 3. Right lobe segmental anatomy as defined by Couinaud (based on the right portal vein). The main portal vein (MPV) divides into a main right and left branch. The main branch of the right portal vein divides into the anterior and posterior sectorial branches. Each sectorial branch divides into a superior and inferior branch. The right anterior superior branch supplies segment 8 (S8). The right anterior inferior branch supplies segment 5 (S5). The right posterior superior branch supplies segment 7 (S7). The right posterior inferior branch supplies segment 6 (S6). The right hepatic vein (RHV) passes anterior to right posterior sectorial branch and posterior to the right anterior sectorial branch. MHV, middle hepatic vein; LHV, left hepatic vein.

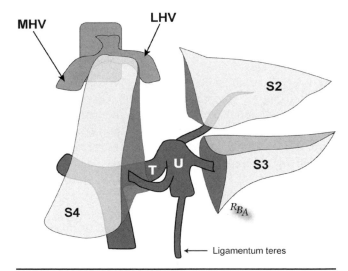

FIGURE 4. Left lobe segmental anatomy as defined by Couinaud (based on the left portal vein). The main portal vein divides into a main right and left branch. The left branch has a transverse portion (T) that runs at the base of segment 4 (S4). Upon entering the base of the umbilical fissure, it ascends and runs within the umbilical fissure. This is the umbilical portion (U) or ascending portion of the portal vein. The first branch off the umbilical portion of the vein is the posterior branch passing to the left and supplying segment 2 (S2). Two anterior branches supply the anterior sector. One runs to the left and supplies the lateral segment (S3). The other runs to the right and supplies the medial segment (S4). The left hepatic vein (LHV) runs anterior to the segment 2 portal pedicle and posterior to the segment 3 pedicle. MHV, middle hepatic vein.

the lateral segment (segment 3) to the left of the umbilical fissure/falciform ligament. Each of these segments also has an independent portal pedicle supplying it. The posterior sector contains only a single segment (segment 2) that is posterior to the left hepatic vein. It too is supplied by an independent portal pedicle. The IHPBA offers two alternative methods for describing the left hemiliver anatomy, which are similar to those of Couinaud. While it is common to refer to the left hemiliver segments in reference to its surface structures, this can result in confusion when communicating tumor locations or hepatic interventions. Rather than using the falciform ligament to denote the "medial" or "lateral" segments of the left hemiliver, the more accurate anatomic descriptions based on the segmental blood supply should be used (Fig. 4).

The final segment of the liver is segment 1 or the caudate lobe. This is an individual anatomic unit that receives its blood supply from both the right and left portal pedicles. Its hepatic venous drainage is through branches directly into the vena cava.

Although complex, a thorough understanding of the segmental anatomy of the liver is critical for interpreting IOUS and planning hepatic interventions. The ability to visualize these structures in three dimensions by IOUS will greatly facilitate one's skills as an ultrasonographer and hepatic surgeon.

INSTRUMENTATION AND TECHNIQUES

A number of probes are available for IOUS of the liver as described in detail in Chapters 3 and 13. When scanning the liver, a flat, side-viewing probe allows access to the limited space between the liver and diaphragm or anterior abdominal wall. A T-shaped, linear array or curvilinear array (convex) probe with a 7.5-MHz transducer is ideal for IOUS scanning of the liver (Fig. 5; see also Fig. 2 in Chapter 13). It provides a relatively large footprint providing wide images from the near fields, allowing efficient scanning of the liver parenchyma. The detail is superb and the depth of sound penetration is typically sufficient to examine the entire parenchyma. Occasionally, a 5-MHz probe is required for deeper sound penetration in patients with an enlarged liver, fatty infiltration, or cirrhosis (Fig. 6). For scanning superficial areas of the liver, the frequency can be increased (e.g., 10 MHz). Although not essential, color or power Doppler imaging can be helpful in a variety of circumstances, such as evaluating blood flow in the hepatic vasculature or determining the vascularity of hepatic tumors (see Figures 34 and 37 in Chapter 13).

IOUS liver scanning techniques (Table 4) are guided by several basic principles, many of which are outlined in Chapter 13. In addition, the liver examination should focus on answering several specific issues. The overriding goal is to develop a technique that works for the surgeon, covers the issues described below, and is followed fastidiously each time IOUS of the liver is performed.

Most often, IOUS examinations of the liver are performed by "contact scanning," placing the probe directly on the liver surface (Fig. 7). This allows for an excellent examination of the liver parenchyma and intrahepatic structures, but is not optimal for imaging masses or structures within 5 to 10 mm of the liver surface at the site of scanning (Fig. 8; see also Fig. 21 in Chapter 13). In addition, scanning an irregular liver surface (cirrhosis) is difficult with the contact scanning technique. In these circumstances, a "probe-standoff scanning" technique is required (Fig. 7). The liver can be immersed in saline, which serves as an acoustic coupling, and scanning can be done through the saline. Alternatively, a saline-filled glove or bag can be interposed between the probe and the liver surface to facilitate scanning in such situations. The difficulty in imaging superficial or surface lesions with IOUS reinforces the fact that intraoperative inspection and palpation and IOUS are complementary and that all of these must be performed to ensure complete evaluation of the liver (Fig. 9).

Transverse scanning is the basic technique for IOUS of the liver (Fig. 10). Longitudinal and oblique images are also important for defining intrahepatic structures and verifying the presence of lesions by displaying them in two or more planes. Sliding the probe over the liver surface in a cranial-to-caudal or side-to-side fashion is an appropriate and the most frequently used technique for IOUS liver scanning. Rotation (clockwise or counterclockwise) of the probe over a fixed point allows the surgeon to examine the area of interest in various planes (Fig. 11). Rocking or tilting the probe at a fixed point expands the field of view and allows examination of closely related structures (Fig. 12). When combined with saline immersion, rocking or tilting is particularly helpful for examining the superior segments of the liver at the dome and diaphragm (Figs. 13 and 14).

Liver scanning is carried out in several steps (Table 5). Before mobilization, the liver should be scanned to prevent artifacts, such as air (although usually not significant), that may result from the mobilization from obscuring the field of vision. For the purpose of screening the liver for tumors or lesions, IOUS scanning of the liver can be completed without mobilization of the liver in the majority of operations. Scanning is repeated following complete liver mobilization. The two major goals of liver scanning are (a) evaluation of the hepatic vasculature and (b) systematic scanning of the hepatic parenchyma. The initial scan should focus on the following:

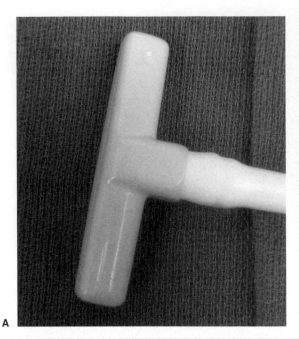
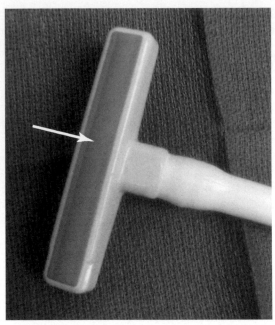

FIGURE 5. Intraoperative ultrasound T-probe (Aloka). **A:** Top view. **B:** Transducer (7.5 MHz linear) view (*arrow*).

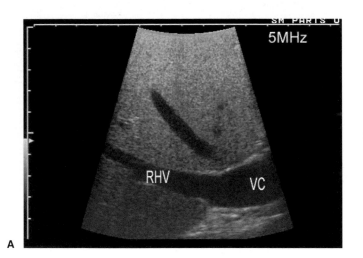
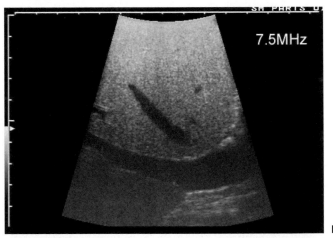
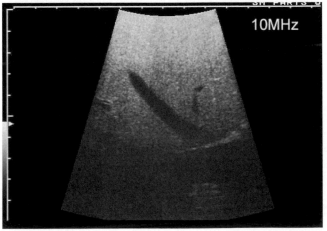

FIGURE 6. Diffuse fatty infiltration scanned by intraoperative ultrasound using 5-MHz **(A)**, 7.5-MHz **(B)** and 10-MHz **(C)** frequencies. To delineate deep areas of the liver, a lower frequency is required. Note the increased echogenicity of fatty liver with a fine granular pattern. RHV, right hepatic vein; VC, vena cava.

▶ **TABLE 4** Intraoperative Ultrasound Liver
Scanning Techniques

Probe placement
   Contact scanning
   Probe-standoff scanning
     ■ Saline immersion
     ■ Saline-filled glove
   Compression scanning
Probe movement
   Sliding across liver
   Rotating on an axis
   Rocking parallel to the scanning plane
   Tilting perpendicular to the scanning plane

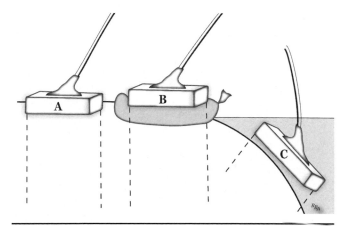

FIGURE 7. Probe placement for liver scanning. **A:** Contact scanning, directly on the liver surface. **B:** Probe-standoff scanning using a saline-filled bag or glove as an acoustic interface. **C:** Probe-standoff scanning using the saline immersion technique.

1. Delineation of the portal vein branches from the transverse portion of the portal vein to the terminal branches in both lobes. Vascular involvement by tumors should be identified. Attention also is paid to intrahepatic bile ducts.
2. Delineation of the hepatic vein branches from their entry into the vena cava to the terminal branches in both lobes. The surgeon should identify any anomalous hepatic veins, which are quite common. Vascular involvement by tumors should be identified.

3. The surgeon should systematically scan the entire liver parenchyma noting the primary or preoperatively known tumors and any other occult tumors or lesions. The liver should be scanned from various directions (e.g. from the inferior surface) as necessary to fully delineate any lesions (Fig. 15A).

(text continues on page 324)

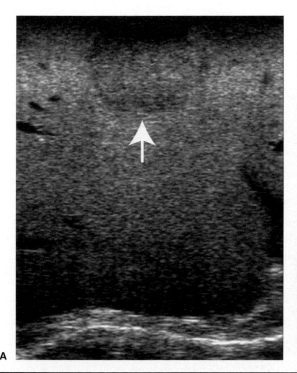
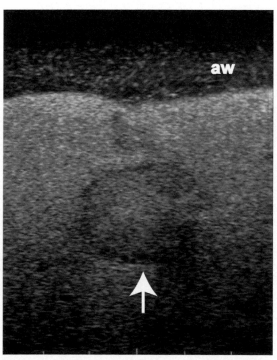

FIGURE 8. Examination of a liver mass (*arrows*) adjacent to the liver surface. **A:** Direct probe contact on liver surface. **B:** Probe-standoff technique using saline immersion demonstrating better imaging of this superficial lesion. Acoustic window (aw) using saline.

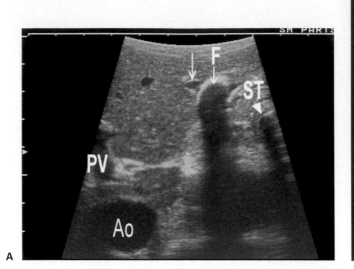

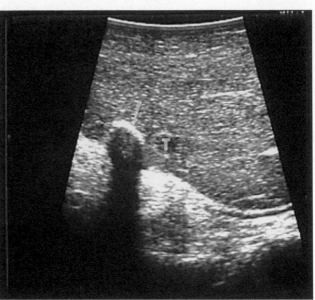

A   B

FIGURE 9. Intraoperative palpation and intraoperative ultrasound (IOUS) are complementary, and simultaneous palpation and scanning are useful to evaluate and characterize a lesion. **A:** A palpable tiny lesion in segment 3 appeared to be a cyst (*long arrow*). A surgeon's finger (associated with shadowing) is indicated by F and an arrow. PV, ascending portion of left portal vein; Ao, aorta; ST, stomach. Arrowhead designates a nasogastric tube in the stomach, causing shadowing. **B:** During a colon cancer operation, a lesion was palpated in segment 6. IOUS together with palpation showed this lesion (T) to be solid, highly suspicious of a metastasis. Surgeon's finger is indicated by an arrow.

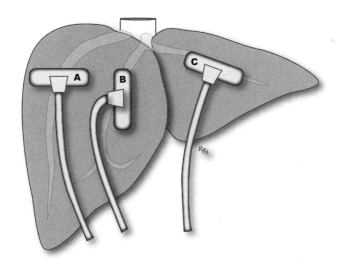

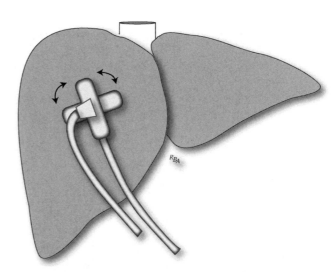

FIGURE 10. Basic probe positions for contact scanning of the liver. **A:** Transverse. **B:** Longitudinal. **C:** Oblique.

FIGURE 11. Rotating maneuver for liver scanning. Rotation of the probe on a fixed point allows examination of a structure in two planes.

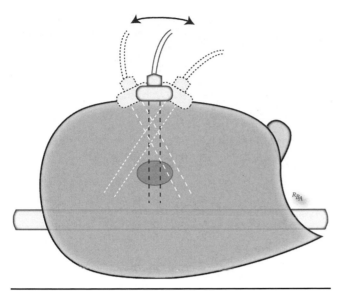

FIGURE 12. Rocking or tilting maneuver for liver scanning. Rocking or tilting the probe at a fixed point on the liver surface while maintaining contact allows examination of a wide area of liver around a point of interest.

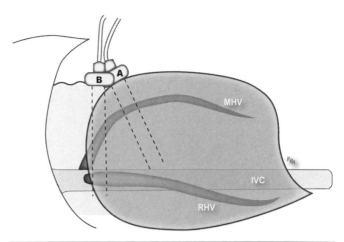

FIGURE 13. Rocking or tilting maneuver and saline immersion combined to allow examination of the superior portion of the liver. **A:** Direct probe contact allows examination of the central liver and the middle hepatic vein (MHV), but examination of the confluence of the hepatic veins with the inferior vena cava (IVC) using this method is sometimes difficult. **B:** Combining saline immersion with probe rocking or tilting at the same position allows excellent imaging of the confluence of the hepatic veins with the vena cava. The same maneuver is valuable for scanning the dome of the liver or the superior portion of segment 7. RHV, right hepatic vein.

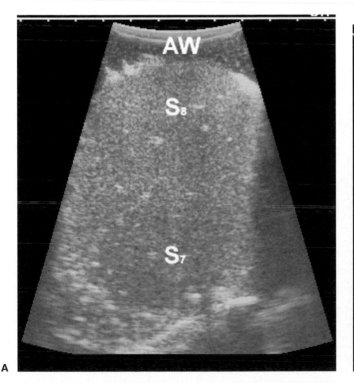

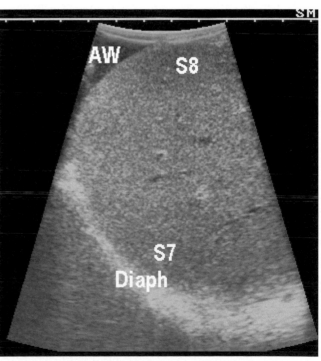

FIGURE 14. Intraoperative ultrasound scanning of superior portions of segments 7 and 8 (also segments 2 and 4) often requires rocking or tilting maneuvers with probe standoff and saline immersion. **A:** Transverse scanning of segments 7 (S_7) and 8 (S_8). **B:** Longitudinal scanning of segments 7 (S_7) and 8 (S_8). AW, acoustic window with saline for probe-standoff scanning; Diaph, diaphragm.

▶ **TABLE 5 Liver Scanning Steps**

Scan liver prior to mobilization
Repeat scanning after liver mobilization is performed
Identify portal branches and follow into segments
Identify hepatic vein junction with vena cava
- Follow to terminal branches
- Identify anomalous branches
Systematically scan liver parenchyma
- Note tumor location, size, and characteristics
- Note vasculobiliary involvement or thrombosis

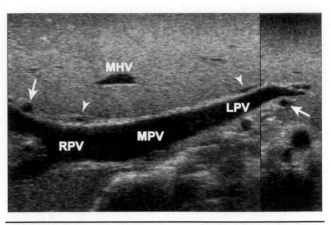

FIGURE 16. Transverse view of the hepatic hilum illustrating the main portal vein (MPV) as it branches into the right portal vein (RPV) and the left portal vein (LPV). The relationship of the middle hepatic vein (MHV) to the hepatic hilum is demonstrated. The hepatic arteries (*arrows*) and a portion of the bile ducts (*arrowheads*) can be seen.

4. The surgeon should establish the relationship between the portal and hepatic veins and all tumors noted on the systematic parenchymal scan, with special attention to their exact segmental locations.

IOUS scanning for liver screening can be performed as long as there is sufficient space for palpation of the liver. Usually it is not necessary to extend the skin incision just for screening. For ablation of tumors, liver mobilization generally is not required, and IOUS examination and guidance of ablation can be performed without mobilization. When the liver is mobilized for resection or other purposes, IOUS is repeated for the following reasons:

1. To repeat the systematic parenchymal scan with particular attention to the posterosuperior segment (segment 7) or other deeper portions of the liver that might not have been adequately seen on the initial survey (Fig. 15B).

2. To confirm the three-dimensional relationship of the tumors to the hepatic vasculature. The surgeon must understand the anatomic relationships as the liver is manipulated into position in preparation for resection.

Examination of the intrahepatic vasculature begins with contact scanning on the anterior surface of the liver at the level of the hepatic hilum. Initially, the liver is scanned in the transverse plane (Fig 16). The transverse

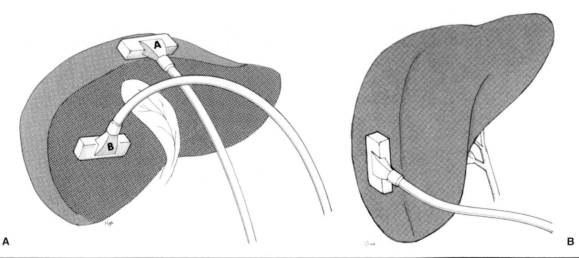

FIGURE 15. A: Intraoperative ultrasound (IOUS) scanning from the inferior surface of the liver. IOUS of the liver is most frequently performed from the anterior or diaphragmatic surface (A). An additional scanning from the inferior surface (B) is at times useful to better delineate certain lesions, particularly those in posterior or inferior positions of the liver. **B:** IOUS scanning after mobilization of the liver, showing scanning from the right lateral anterior surface of the liver. The spacial anatomy such as the relation of a lesion to vascular structures may change slightly after liver mobilization. Therefore, it is critical to rescan the liver after mobilization before resection or other hepatic procedures.

portion of the portal vein is identified and the right branch is examined. The main right branch is followed to its division into the anterior (segments 5 and 8) and posterior (segments 6 and 7) sectorial branches by sliding and rotating the probe (Fig. 17). Each sectorial branch is followed to its superior or inferior segmental branch (Fig. 18). This allows mapping of the entire inflow to the right lobe. Next, the transverse portion of the left portal vein is followed to the base of the umbilical fissure where the portal vein ascends anteriorly within the umbilical fissure. The ascending (or umbilical) portion of the left portal vein is followed to the right of the falciform ligament to identify the branches to the medial segment of the left lobe (segment 4). Following the vessels to the left of the falciform ligament identifies those branches to the lateral portion of the anterior or inferior segment of the left lobe (segment 3) and the posterior or superior segment of the left lobe (segment 2) that is posterior and superior to the left hepatic vein (Fig. 19).

The three major hepatic veins are initially identified by contact scanning at the superior-most portion (diaphragmatic surface) of the liver. This allows evaluation of their entry to the vena cava (Fig. 20). Each hepatic vein is followed peripherally to its terminal branches again by sliding and rotating the probe. Finally, the liver is scanned in the longitudinal (sagittal) plane and the vascular structures are reevaluated and confirmed. The retrohepatic vena cava can be evaluated along it full length in this fashion (Fig. 21). The aorta, which is located posterior to the left lobe, also is visualized in its longitudinal view (Fig. 22).

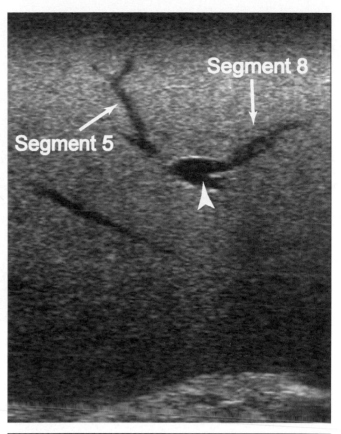

FIGURE 18. Right anterior sectorial portal vein branch (*arrowhead*). This gives rise to the anterior inferior segmental branches (segment 5) and the anterior superior segmental branches (segment 8).

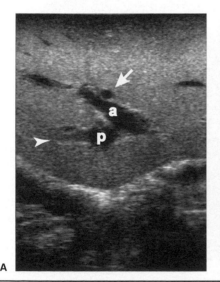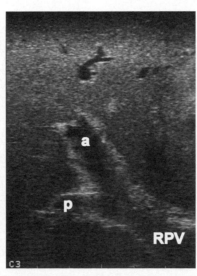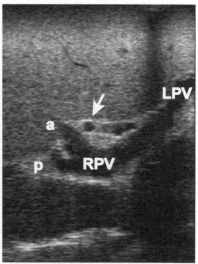

FIGURE 17. Right portal vein. **A:** Anterior (a) and posterior (p) sectorial branches. Segment 7 branch origin (*arrowhead*) off the posterior sectorial branch. **B:** Anterior and posterior sectorial branches as they arise from the main right portal vein (RPV). **C:** Right portal vein anterior and posterior sectorial branches as seen in a transverse view of the hepatic hilum. LPV, left portal vein. The arrows denote hepatic arteries.

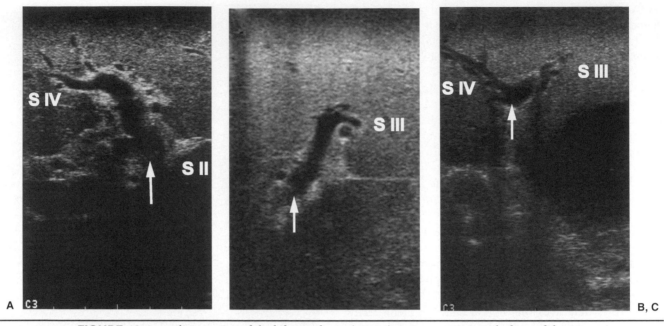

FIGURE 19. Ascending portion of the left portal vein (*arrows*). **A:** Arrow points to the base of the umbilical fissure, noting the origin of the ascending portion of the left portal vein. Branches to segment 2 (S II) can be seen to pass to the left of the umbilical fissure, whereas branches to segment 4 (S IV) pass to the right of the fissure. **B:** Origin of ascending portion of left portal vein at the base of the umbilical fissure (*arrow*) with a branch going to segment 3 (S III), to the left of the umbilical fissure. **C:** Terminal portion of ascending left portal vein (*arrow*) giving rise to branches to segments 3 (S III) and 4 (S IV).

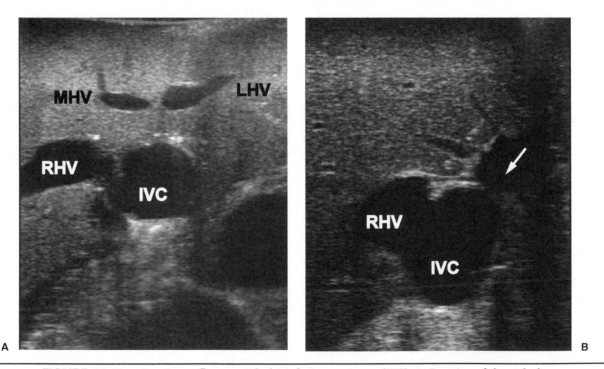

FIGURE 20. Hepatic vein confluence with the inferior vena cava (IVC). **A:** Junction of the right hepatic vein (RHV) with the IVC. The middle hepatic vein (MHV) and left hepatic vein (LHV) are seen just before they join into a common trunk. **B:** Junction of RHV with the IVC. The arrow demonstrates the common trunk of the MHV and LHV as it joins the IVC.

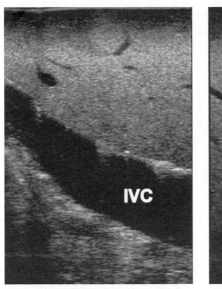
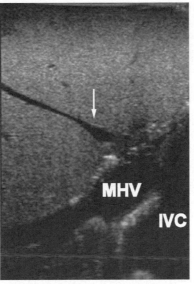
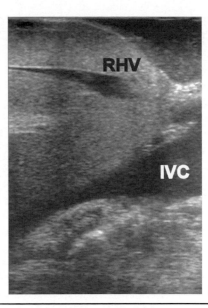

A   B, C

FIGURE 21. Longitudinal view of the inferior vena cava (IVC). **A:** View through central portion of the liver. **B:** Long view of middle hepatic vein (MHV) as it joins the IVC. A large branch (*arrow*) crossing from the right lobe of the liver drains into the MHV. **C:** Long view of right hepatic vein (RHV) as it drains into the IVC.

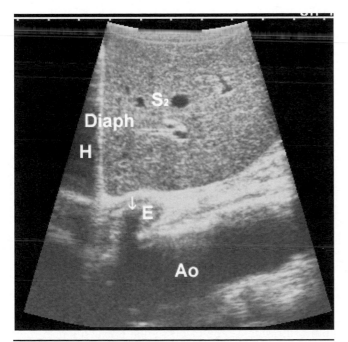

FIGURE 22. Longitudinal view of the aorta (Ao). The esophagus (E), the diaphragm (Diaph), and the heart (H) are also seen. S_2, segment 2 of the liver. An arrow indicates a nasogastric tube in the esophagus, causing shadowing.

After the intrahepatic vasculature is defined, systematic parenchymal scanning is performed to evaluate for parenchymal abnormalities, particularly hepatic masses. Lesions detected on preoperative studies are identified and evaluated. The presence of additional or occult lesions is sought. Systematic scanning is performed by contact scanning on the anterior or diaphragmatic liver surfaces. Beginning at the far left side of the liver, segments 2 and 3 are examined. The liver is scanned in a transverse plane, working cephalad to caudad, by sliding the probe. When the inferior edge of the liver is reached, the probe is moved a few centimeters (depending on the length of the footprint of the probe) to the patient's right and scanning commences from the superior to the inferior border. In this fashion, the entire extent of the liver parenchyma is viewed. After completing transverse scanning, sometimes (as needed) the probe is rotated 90 degrees and the liver rescanned in the longitudinal plane. Full delineation of segment 7 may require the rocking or tilting maneuver with a probe-standoff scanning technique (Fig. 14). Evaluation of the deepest portions of segments 6 and 7 may require scanning from the inferior or right lateral liver surfaces. Similarly, segment 1 may require scanning from the inferior surface (see Fig. 22 in Chapter 13).

Using this systematic approach to liver scanning, the goals outlined earlier can be accomplished. These techniques, coupled with an understanding of intrahepatic anatomy, will allow the surgeon to accurately localize any masses within the liver. Ultimately, this facilitates intraoperative decision making regarding the appropriate therapeutic approach.

NORMAL ULTRASOUND ANATOMY OF THE LIVER

One of the many advantages of IOUS is the ability to combine the surface features of the liver with the intrahepatic structures, as viewed by IOUS, to precisely define hepatic segmental anatomy. As described above, identification of both the portal and hepatic veins are critical to define the liver segments.

Normal liver parenchyma has a homogeneous echo pattern by IOUS. In general, the liver is more echogenic (brighter) than the adjacent right renal cortex during IOUS (Fig. 23). Less commonly, one can observe similar echogenicity between the liver and renal cortex.

Portal triads can be distinguished from hepatic veins based on their ultrasound appearance. The portal triad is invested by Glisson's capsule as it enters the liver parenchyma. Consequently, portal triads have an echogenic (bright white) border on IOUS. This contrasts with hepatic veins that tend to be thin walled and less echogenic (Fig. 24). Thus, hepatic veins typically lack this echogenic

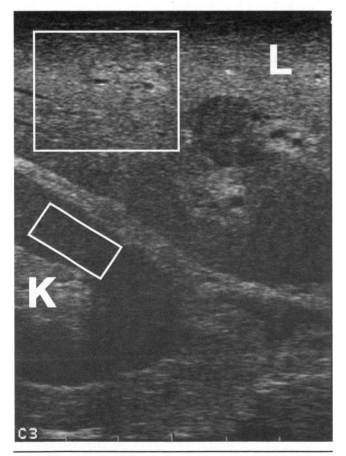

FIGURE 23. Normal liver echogenicity. The liver (L) parenchyma (outlined in the large box) is typically more echogenic than the renal (K) cortex (outlined in the small box).

rim, although larger veins can demonstrate some echogenicity, particularly when the ultrasound beam is perpendicular to the wall of a hepatic vein. If the nature of the structure is in question, it can be followed to either the main portal vein or vena cava depending on the type of structure it represents.

As noted previously, hepatic anatomy is described as sections (sectors) and segments that are defined by the intrahepatic vascular anatomy. In general, the portal vein branches are within the various segments (intrasegmental), whereas the hepatic veins are between segments (intersegmental). Initially, the vascular anatomy is defined by identifying the main portal vein at its division into the main right and left portal veins (Fig. 16; see also Fig. 23 in Chapter 13). This point is located at the hilum of the liver, at the base of segment 4. When viewed in the transverse plane, the portal vein is the largest tubular structure (in cross-section) within this portal triad and is the most posterior. Anterior to the main right and left portal veins lies the bile duct and hepatic artery (Fig. 25). More inferior in the hepatoduodenal ligament, the proper hepatic artery lies anterior to the portal vein toward the patient's left side. To the right of the proper hepatic artery and anterior to the portal vein is a second tubular structure, the bile duct (see Fig. 25 in Chapter 13 and Figs. 6 and 7 in Chapter 14). Color Doppler imaging is helpful to quickly distinguish the hepatic artery from the bile duct in the hepatoduodenal ligament or in the liver. Following the main right portal vein to the right, the portal triad divides into the anterior (segments 5 and 8) and posterior sectorial branches (segments 6 and 7) (Fig. 17). The anterior sectorial branch divides into a superior branch to segment 8 (Fig. 26) and an inferior branch to segment 5 (Fig. 18). Usually, there are two branches (ventral and dorsal) to segment 8 with a ventral branch frequently arising from a portion of the segment 5 pedicle. The segment 5 branch actually can consist of three to five branches entering the segment. Segment 7 usually has a single (superior) branch off the posterior sectorial branch that enters its substance (Fig. 17). One or two inferior branches off the posterior sectorial vessel supply segment 6 (Fig. 27). At the point where the main portal vein bifurcates, the left branch can be identified. It travels a transverse (parallel to the ultrasound probe) course that is much longer than that of the right portal vein (Fig. 28). Moving to the patient's left, the left portal vein then turns abruptly anteriorly (toward the probe) as it ascends into the umbilical fissure. Unlike the other branches of the portal veins, this portion of the left portal vein is intersegmental, running between segments 4 and 2/3. The portal triad at this location has the appearance of a tree with branches protruding to the right and left (Fig. 19). At the base of the portal vein (trunk of the tree), a branch to the patient's left supplies segment 2 (lateral superior branch). Toward the top

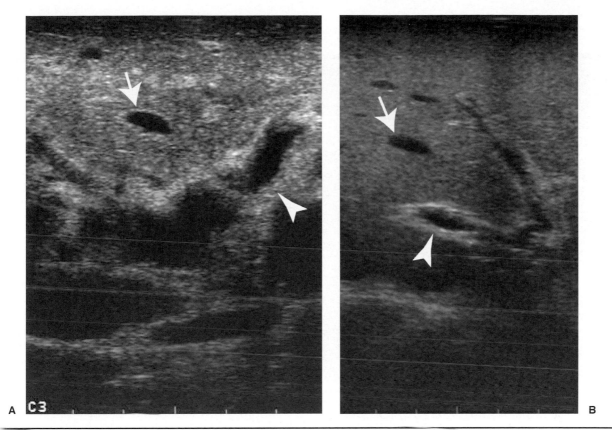

FIGURE 24. A,B: Echogenicity of portal veins and hepatic veins. Portal veins (*arrowheads*) have a thicker, more echogenic appearance compared to the thinner walled hepatic veins (*arrows*) with little echogenicity around their circumference.

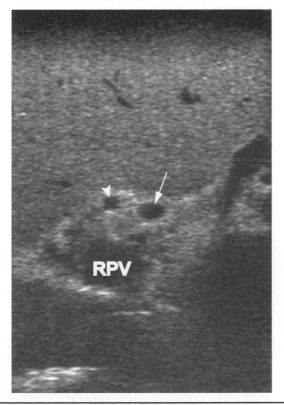

FIGURE 25. Relationship of the bile duct (*arrow*) and hepatic artery (*arrowhead*) anterior to the right portal vein (RPV) at the level of the hepatic hilum.

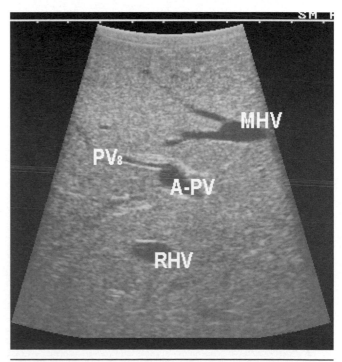

FIGURE 26. Anterior superior segment (segment 8) branch (PV_8) from the anterior branch of the right portal vein (A-PV). The middle hepatic vein (MHV) and the right hepatic vein (RHV) are also visualized.

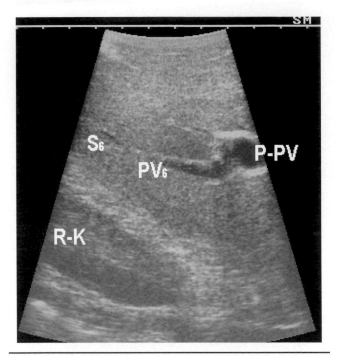

FIGURE 27. Posterior inferior segment (segment 6) branch (PV$_6$) from the posterior branch of the right portal vein (P-PV). Segment 6 (S$_6$) is located adjacent to the right kidney (R-K).

of the tree (close to the probe), one branch toward the right supplies segment 4 and one to the left supplies segment 3 (lateral inferior) (Fig. 19). Occasionally, branches off the transverse portion of the left portal vein are seen passing posteriorly to segment 1 (caudate lobe).

Portal venous anatomy is fairly constant with anomalies being uncommon. Occasionally the portal vein forms a trifurcation with separate right anterior and posterior sectorial branches coming off the main portal vein (Fig. 29A). These patients essentially lack a main right portal vein. In a similar fashion, the transverse portion of the left portal vein may be absent, resulting in an ascending left portal vein almost directly off the main portal vein bifurcation (Fig. 29B).

Three major hepatic veins—the right, middle, and left—drain the liver into the vena cava. In most cases, the right hepatic vein joins the vena cava separately while the middle and left veins join and enter the vena cava as a common orifice (more than 50% of the population) (Figs. 20 and 30). It is common to have variable hepatic venous anatomy. The three major hepatic veins can enter the vena cava separately. More than three major hepatic veins can be present. These variations include large right or left marginal veins that drain into the right or left he-

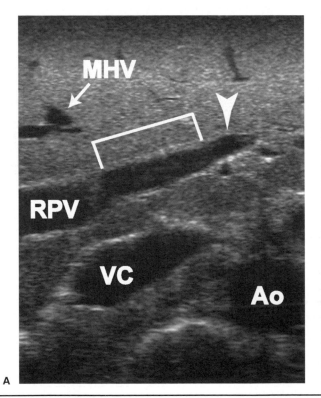

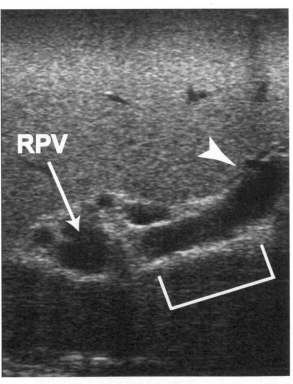

FIGURE 28. **A,B:** Transverse portion of the left portal vein (hypoechoic tubular structure demonstrated by the brackets) as it runs along the base of segment 4. The arrowheads indicate the point of transition between the transverse portion and the ascending portion of the left portal vein. Right portal vein (RPV), middle hepatic vein (MHV), vena cava (VC), and aorta (Ao) are shown.

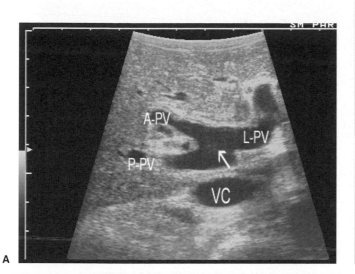

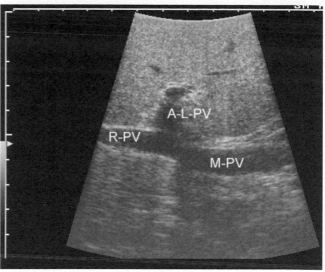

A   B

FIGURE 29. A: Portal vein trifurcation. The main portal vein, coming in the hepatic hilum (*arrow*), divides into the left portal vein (L-PV), right anterior portal vein (A-PV), and right posterior portal vein (P-PV), with the absence of a main right portal vein. VC, vena cava. **B:** Absence of the transverse portion of the left portal vein. The main portal vein (M-PV) divides directly into the ascending portion of the left portal vein (A-L-PV) and the main right portal vein (R-PV).

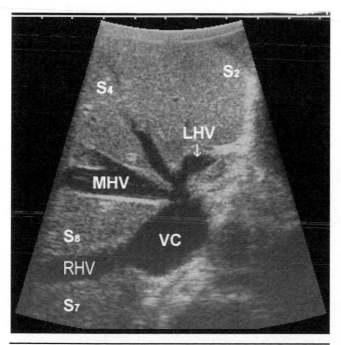

FIGURE 30. Three hepatic veins and the vena cava (VC). The right hepatic vein (RHV), middle hepatic vein (MHV), and left hepatic vein (LHV, *arrow*) are intersegmental and are landmarks of segmental anatomy. S_2, segment 2; S_4, segment 4; S_8, segment 8; S_7, segment 7.

patic veins. A large draining vein from the anterior sector (segments 5 and 8) frequently drains into the middle hepatic vein (Fig. 21). A large accessory right vein, the inferior right hepatic vein, may be present (approximately 20% of the population). This drains segment 6 directly into the vena cava, at the level just posterior to the main right portal vein (Fig. 31; see also Figure 23C in Chapter 13). Through the use of IOUS, these hepatic vein abnormalities can be readily identified.

The hepatic veins can be followed caudally into the liver parenchyma. As the probe is moved in this direction, the relationship of the hepatic veins and the portal veins can be captured together on the same image (Figs. 26 and 32). This facilitates identification of the hepatic segments and aids planning for hepatic resection.

IOUS can detect several ligaments associated with the liver. The ligamentum teres, a remnant of the obliterated umbilical vein, passes inferiorly to the falciform ligament toward the ascending portion of the left portal vein. It can be recognized as a thickened, hyperechoic band (Fig. 33). This structure separates segment 4 from segments 2/3. The ligamentum venosum, representing the ductus venosus remnant, is a thin, linear, hyperechoic band that runs almost parallel to the transducer. It appears to emanate from the left side of the left portal vein as it transitions from the transverse portion of the left portal vein to the ascending portion (Fig. 34).

(text continues on page 334)

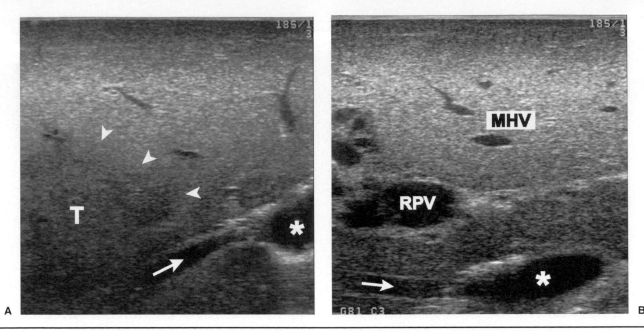

FIGURE 31. Inferior right hepatic vein (*arrows within the vein*) draining into the vena cava (*asterisk*). **A:** A tumor (T) lies directly anterior to the right inferior hepatic vein. Arrowheads mark the tumor border. **B:** Right inferior hepatic vein in relationship to the right portal vein (RPV) and the middle hepatic vein (MHV).

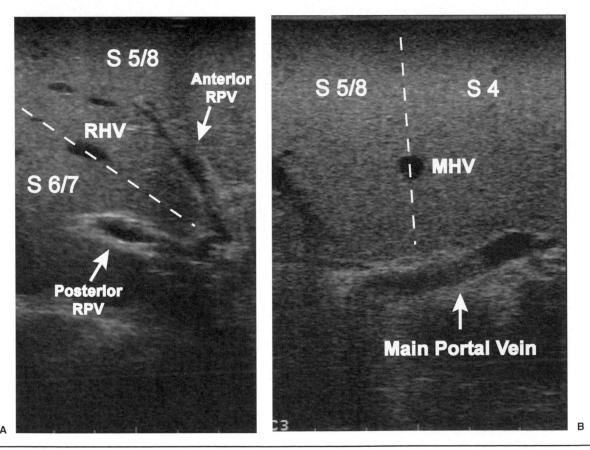

FIGURE 32. Intrahepatic relationship of hepatic veins and portal veins defines segmental anatomy. **A:** The right hepatic vein (RHV) lies between the anterior and posterior sectorial branches of the right portal vein (RPV). Anterior to the RHV are segments 5 and 8 (S 5/8). Posterior to the RHV are segments 6 and 7 (S 6/7). **B:** The middle hepatic vein (MHV) lies directly anterior to the transverse portion of the portal vein at the hepatic hilum. To the left of the MHV is segment 4 (S 4), to its right are segments 5 and 8 (S 5/8). The dotted lines divide the RHV in **A** and the MHV in **B**.

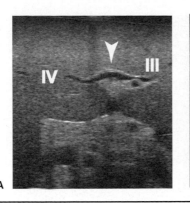
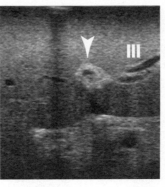
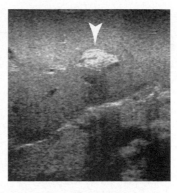

FIGURE 33. Ligamentum teres and its relationship to the left portal vein. **A:** Scanning from superior to inferior over the umbilical fissure, the terminal ascending portion of the left portal vein (*arrowhead*) can be seen with branches going into segments 3 (III) and 4 (IV). **B:** As the probe is moved more inferiorly, the junction of the ligamentum teres with the inferior most portion of the left portal vein can be identified (*arrowhead*). **C:** As the probe is moved closer to the inferior edge of the liver, the ligamentum teres (*arrowhead*) can be seen within the umbilical fissure.

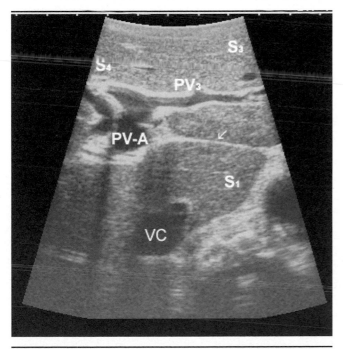

FIGURE 34. Ligamentum venosum and surrounding structures. The ligament venosum (*arrow*) separates segment 1 (S$_1$) and segment 2/3 (S$_3$). PV-A, ascending portion of left portal vein; PV$_3$, segment 3 branch; VC, vena cava; S$_4$, segment 4.

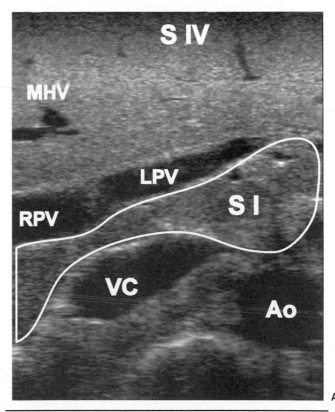

FIGURE 35. Segment 1 (caudate lobe). Intraoperative ultrasound identifies structures delineating the boundaries of the caudate lobe. **A:** Segment 1 (S I) is surrounded by the solid line. Anteriorly its boundary is the right (RPV) and left (LPV) portal veins at the hepatic hilum. Posteriorly its boundary is the vena cava (VC). Adjacent structures are the aorta (Ao), middle hepatic vein (MHV) and segment 4 (S IV). *(continued)*

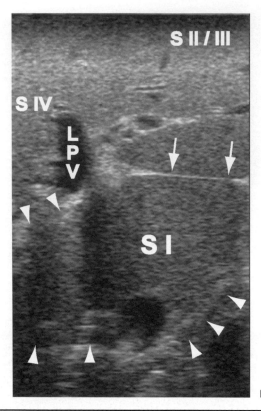

B

FIGURE 35. *(Continued)* **B:** The left side of segment 1 (S I) is delineated anteriorly by the ligamentum venosum (*arrows*) which separates segment 1 from segments 2 and 3 (S II / III). Toward the right, the anterior border is the left portal vein. Arrowhead*s* outline segment 1. Adjacent structures include the ascending portion of the left portal vein (LPV) and segment 4 (S IV).

The surrounding vascular structures and the ligamentum venosum identify the boundaries of segment 1 (caudate lobe) (Fig. 35). The transverse portion of the left portal vein denotes the anterior limit of segment 1. Further to the left of the portal vein is the thin hyperechoic ligamentum venosum that separates segment 1 from segments 2/3. Anterior to the ligamentum venosum are segments 2 and 3, whereas segment 1 lies posterior to this structure. This also is clearly visualized by longitudinal scanning (Fig. 36). Posterior to segment 1 is the vena cava, although occasionally segment 1 can extend posterior to the vena cava. Thus, segment 1 can be defined by these anatomic structures readily seen by IOUS.

ULTRASOUND CHARACTERISTICS OF HEPATIC PATHOLOGY

IOUS is useful for identifying and characterizing diffuse parenchymal changes within the liver (Table 6) (see Chapter 11). However, the most common use of IOUS is identification and characterization of mass lesions. Mass

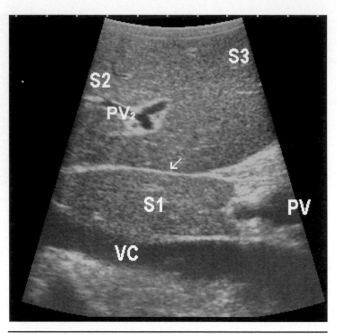

FIGURE 36. Segment 1 (S_1) in its longitudinal view. The ligamentum venosum (*arrow*) is anterior to S_1 and the vena cava (VC) is posterior to S_1. PV_2, segment 2 branch; S_2, segment 2; S_3, segment 3. PV (extrahepatic) main portal vein.

lesions may be cystic or solid, each being easily distinguished from the other by IOUS (see also Chapter 13 for more images of liver mass lesions). Several ultrasound features of a mass lesion can contribute to its characterization. The echogenicity and echo pattern of a lesion can suggest the nature of the mass. The ultrasound echogenicity is described in relationship to the surrounding hepatic parenchyma. Terms describing its appearance include *hyperechoic* (brighter, whiter), *isoechoic* (similar gray scale appearance), or *hypoechoic* (darker, blacker) in comparison with the surrounding liver tissue (Fig. 37). A

▶ **TABLE 6 Characteristics of Diffuse Liver Disease**

Steatosis (fatty liver)
Diffusely hyperechoic
Fine granular pattern
Poor sound transmission
Focal fatty sparing
Hypoechoic region in a fatty liver
"Geographic distribution"
No mass effect
Cirrhosis
Diffusely hyperechoic
Course pattern
Poor sound transmission
Regenerative nodule
Hypoechoic
No mass effect

mass may have mixed echo characteristics, referred to as heterogeneous (Fig. 38). The shape of the lesion and the nature of its borders may provide clues to the type of lesion. Shadowing may be seen lateral to the edges of the mass (lateral or edge shadowing) or directly behind the lesion (posterior shadowing) (Fig. 39). Alternatively, there may be enhancement (brighter echoes) posterior to the mass (posterior enhancement) (Fig. 40). Solid masses surrounded by a hypoechoic ring (halo, "bull's eye," or target pattern), are the typical appearance of malignant liver tumors (Fig. 41; see also Fig. 27 in Chapter 13). A le-

sion may have a mass effect, pushing surrounding vasculature aside (Fig. 42). It may invade the vessels (Fig. 43) or cause tumor thrombus formation within the lumen (Fig. 44; see also Fig. 37 in Chapter 13). Some mass lesions, such as focal fatty infiltration, may cause no mass effect, with the vessels passing through them unaltered. All of these characteristics can vary with the size of the mass. The smaller (less than 2 cm) or larger (more than 10 cm) the lesion, the more difficult the diagnosis based on ultrasound features alone.

(text continues on page 338)

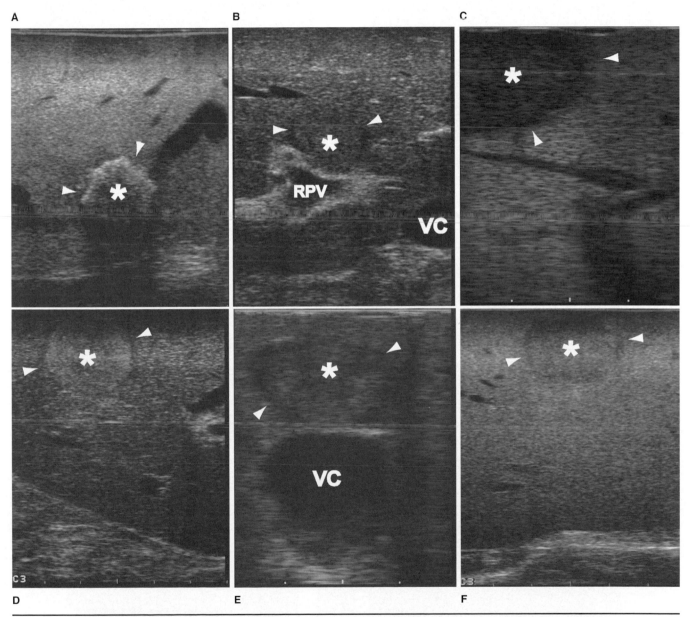

FIGURE 37. Echogenicity of liver masses. **A, D:** Hyperechoic masses. **B, E:** Isoechoic masses. These would be invisible without the hypoechoic ring surrounding the masses. **C, F:** Hypoechoic masses. The asterisk marks the central portion of the mass and the arrowheads the periphery. RPV, right portal vein; VC, vena cava.

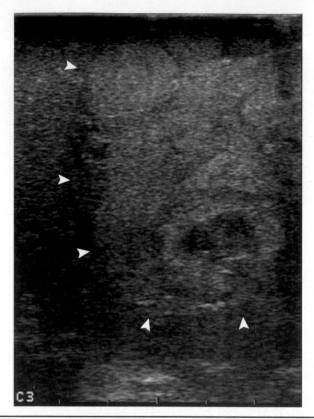

FIGURE 38. Heterogeneous liver mass. This mostly hyperechoic mass has hypo- and isoechoic regions mixed within its interior. Arrowheads mark the tumor's margins.

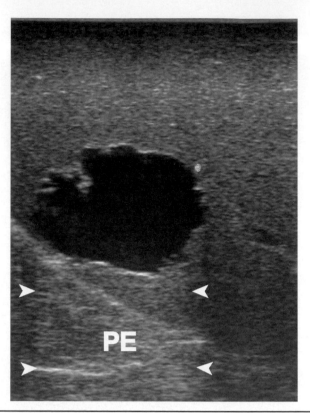

FIGURE 40. Posterior acoustic enhancement (PE, *between arrowheads*) deep to a mass (cyst).

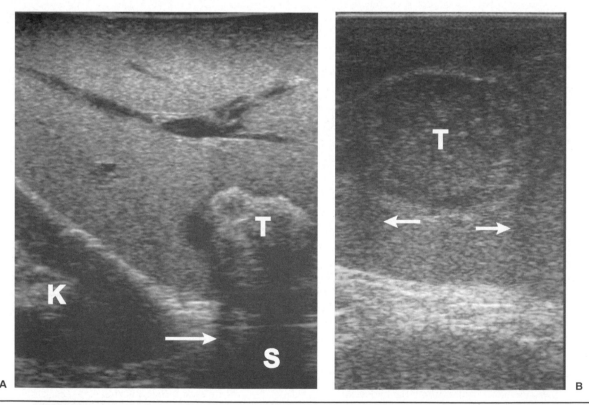

FIGURE 39. Tumor shadowing. **A:** This tumor (T) has two areas of posterior shadowing (*arrow and S*) resulting from sound wave attenuation. K, kidney. **B:** Lateral shadowing (*arrows*) is seen with this tumor (T).

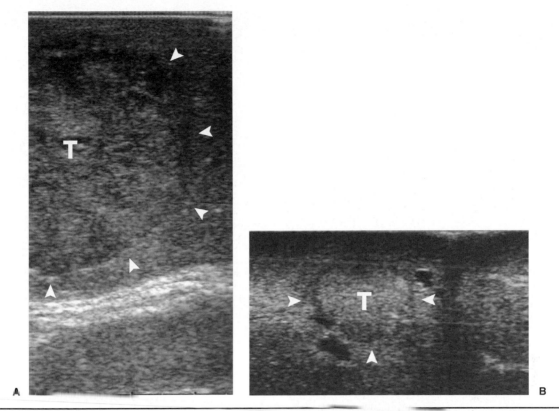

FIGURE 41. A,B: Tumor "halo." A hypoechoic ring (*arrowheads*) frequently surrounds malignant liver masses (T).

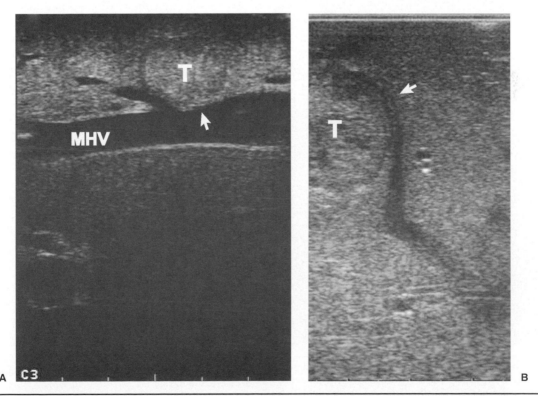

FIGURE 42. A,B: Tumor mass effect. Tumor (T) impinging (*arrow*) on hepatic veins. MHV, middle hepatic vein.

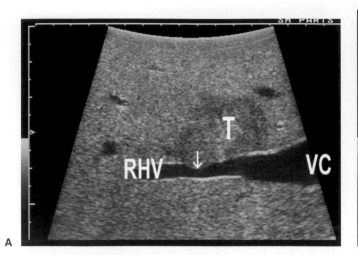
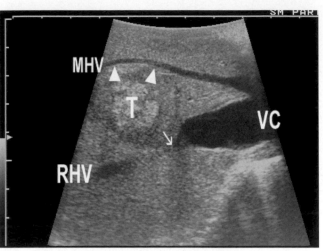

FIGURE 43. Vascular invasion of a malignant liver tumor. **A:** A tumor (T) (metastatic colon cancer) invading (*arrow*) the right hepatic vein (RHV). **B:** The same tumor (T) scanned from a different angle. The tumor was invading (*arrow*) the right hepatic vein (RHV) and displacing (*arrowheads*) the middle hepatic vein (MHV). VC, vena cava.

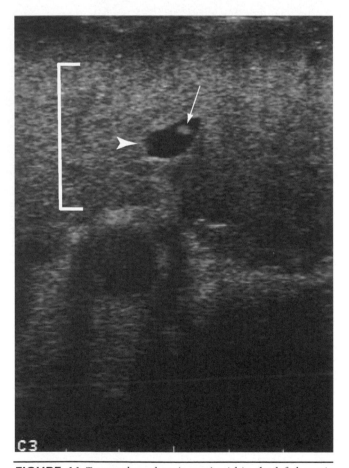

FIGURE 44. Tumor thrombus (*arrow*) within the left hepatic vein (*arrowhead*). It was caused by diffuse involvement by hepatocellular carcinoma (leading edge of tumor noted by bracket).

Cystic Liver Lesions

Cystic lesions of the liver have distinctive features on IOUS that allow definitive diagnosis based on ultrasound characteristics alone (Table 7). Simple cysts are round, anechoic (without echoes), and have sharp borders and posterior enhancement (Fig. 40; see also Fig. 30 in Chapter 13). Occasionally thin, linear, echoic structures can be seen running through cysts. These are septa within a cyst or a collection of several small cysts sharing common walls (Fig. 45). IOUS is so accurate that cysts as small as 1 to 3 mm can be detected. Multiple hepatic cysts can be seen as an isolated finding. However, polycystic liver disease is usually seen in the context of polycystic kidney disease (Fig. 46) (57,58).

If echogenic material other than a few thin septa is present in a cyst, the cyst is not simple but referred to as complex. Although simple cysts can develop hemorrhage or infection within, resulting in a complex sonographic image, this is rare. Alternative diagnoses include secondary cysts resulting from trauma, infection, or cystic neoplasms.

▶ **TABLE 7 Characteristics of Typical Cystic Liver Lesions**

Anechoic
Well-circumscribed borders
Posterior enhancement
Lateral shadowing
Occasional fine internal septa

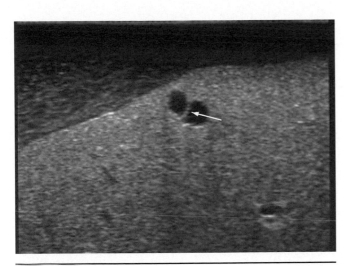

FIGURE 45. Septated liver cyst. *Arrow* indicates thin echogenic septum within this cyst.

Trauma can cause complex cystic lesions that result from hematoma in various stages of resolution. With time, these can evolve into lesions that appear to be primarily cystic, although some dependent debris or internal septa may be noted within. Cystic lesions resulting from infectious causes include pyogenic or amebic abscesses, candidiasis, and echinococcal (hydatid) disease. In most cases, these are unlikely to be discovered on IOUS for the first time without some preoperative indication of an infectious process. Pyogenic abscesses can have a typical rounded or ovoid appearance, but may have an irregular contour that can lead to confusion regarding the diagnosis (see Fig. 31 in Chapter 13). As these lesions develop an exudative collection, they usually have the appearance of a hypoechoic mass with posterior enhancement. However, more or less echogenicity may be present in the lesion depending on the stage of the abscess and the presence or absence of gas. Echogenic (hypo- or isoechoic) abscesses may mimic solid liver tumors. An acute abscess does not have a defined wall, whereas a chronic abscess may have an identifiable rind of tissue as the inflammatory process matures (59–61). Amebic abscesses have an appearance similar to and often indistinguishable from that of pyogenic abscesses (62). Amebic abscesses tend to occur close to the liver capsule (63). Suspicion of an amebic abscess should be raised in endemic areas. Serologic assays will confirm the diagnosis without the need for fluid aspiration. Candidal abscesses are uncommon but can be seen in seriously ill patients or those who are immunocompromised. A typical appearance would be multiple small (millimeter) lesions with an echogenic center and a hypoechoic rim (64,65). These can mimic target lesions, which are usually associated with malignant disease. Aspiration is often required to confirm the diagnosis. Hepatic cystic lesions in areas endemic for *Echinococcus* should be considered hydatid disease until this has been ruled out. In particular, a solitary hydatid cyst may be very difficult to distinguish from a simple hepatic cyst. Serologic testing should be done on these patients to determine whether they have had an echinococcal infection. Features of a single cyst that may help to determine an echinococcal origin include the presence of a multilayered or calcified wall or debris ("sand") within the cyst. Classically, though, hydatid cysts are multicystic lesions having a so-called cyst-within-a-cyst (honeycombed) appearance (66, 67). Finally, a complex cystic lesion may be a cystic neoplasm such as a biliary cystadenoma or adenocarcinoma. These lesions are multiseptated, have irregular cyst walls, and feature papillary projections within the cysts (68)

This discussion illustrates that the differential diagnosis for cystic liver lesions is sometimes complex (Table 8). As an initial step in the evaluation, patients from endemic areas should undergo serologic testing for amebic or echinococcal infections before any cyst intervention is considered. Once these infectious etiologic factors have been excluded from the diagnosis, percutaneous or intraoperative aspiration may be performed. This is often nec-

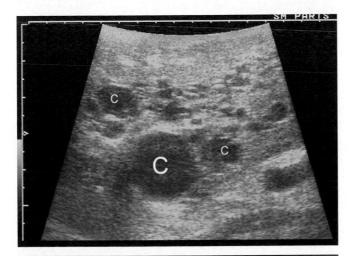

FIGURE 46. Polycystic liver disease. Numerous cysts are visualized, ranging from several millimeters to several centimeters (C).

▶ **TABLE 8 Cystic Liver Lesions**

Simple cyst
Polycystic liver disease
Resolving hematoma
Pyogenic abscess
Amebic abscess
Echinococcal disease
Cyst adenoma or adenocarcinoma

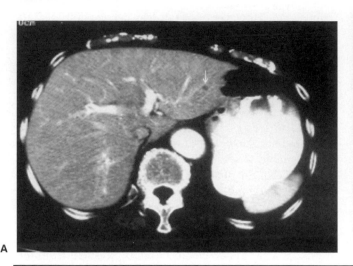

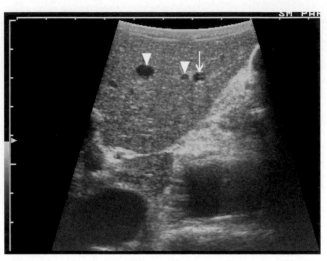

A   B

FIGURE 47. Intraoperative ultrasound (IOUS) diagnosis of a liver cyst. **A:** A preoperative computed tomography scan of a patient with rectal cancer showed a tiny lesion (*arrow*), but was insufficient to exclude or confirm metastasis. **B:** Intraoperatively the lesion was palpable but not visible. IOUS quickly diagnosed it to be a cyst (*arrow*). There was no need for intraoperative biopsy. Arrowheads denote peripheral portal vein branches. (This is the same case as Fig. 9A.)

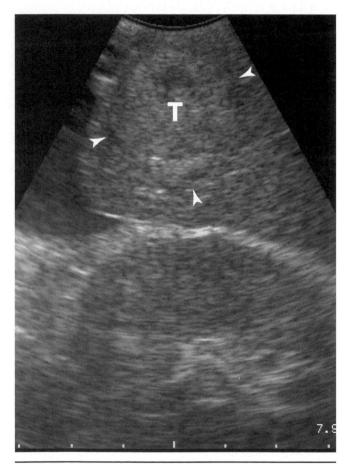

FIGURE 48. Isoechoic liver tumor (T). This tumor is identifiable due to the surrounding hypoechoic rim or halo (*arrowheads*).

▌ **TABLE 9 Common Solid Liver Lesions**

Benign	*Malignant*
Hemangioma	Metastatic disease
Focal nodular hyperplasia	Hepatocellular carcinoma
Adenoma	Intrahepatic cholangiocarcinoma
Regenerative nodule	
Focal fatty changes	

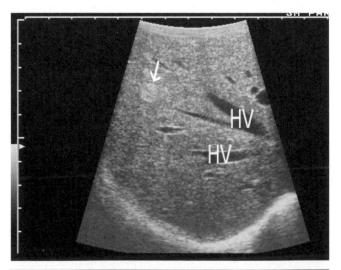

FIGURE 49. Small hemangioma. An 8 × 6 mm hyperechoic lesion (*arrow*) with a typical appearance of hemangioma. HV, hepatic veins.

essary to define the nature of complex cystic lesions and to distinguish them from solid lesions such as necrotic tumors.

On the other hand, the majority of cystic liver lesions encountered during IOUS or general surgical operations are simple cysts, which can be diagnosed by IOUS imaging without intervention (aspiration). The major advantage of IOUS is its capability of making the diagnosis of liver cysts and excluding solid tumors (e.g., metastases) when preoperative CT or ultrasound cannot characterize the liver lesions (Fig. 47).

Solid Liver Lesions

In general, IOUS can distinguish solid hepatic masses from cystic lesions without much difficulty. However, determining whether a solid mass is benign or malignant, based on IOUS characteristics alone, can be challenging. It is essential to place the finding of a mass lesion in the liver into the appropriate clinical context, as this will provide clues to its nature. Although a number of ultrasound characteristics for specific mass lesions have been described in an effort to identify them, biopsy is generally required for definitive diagnosis

The detectability of solid masses by IOUS depends on differences in contrast between the mass and the surrounding liver parenchyma. While hypo- and hyperechoic masses are readily seen, isoechoic masses may be difficult to discern from the surrounding liver (Figs. 37, 41, and 48). This is particularly true with smaller masses. Often, isoechoic masses can be detected only by the presence of a hypoechoic rim. In these difficult cases, secondary signs of a mass lesion may allow its detection. Distortion of surrounding structures, such as the bowing of vessels, can alert one to the presence of a mass (Fig. 42). Likewise, vascular invasion or thrombosis raises suspicion for a mass lesion (Figs. 43, 44). Any condition, such as hepatic steatosis, that increases the background echogenicity of the liver can make detection of hypoechoic mass lesions easier and detection of hyperechoic lesions more difficult.

Benign hepatic tumors are relatively uncommon, with the exception of hemangiomas, which are the most common benign liver tumors. Other benign liver masses include focal nodular hyperplasia, hepatic adenoma, regenerative nodules, and focal fatty changes. In Western countries, solid liver masses most commonly result from metastatic diseases; in the United States, metastatic tumors are 10 to 20 times more common than primary liver cancers. In other parts of the world, hepatocellular carcinoma is the most common solid hepatic tumor. Other solid malignancies in the liver, such as intrahepatic cholangiocarcinoma, are uncommon. Because ultrasound features of these benign and malignant lesions often overlap, all of these diagnoses must be considered in the differential (Table 9).

Benign Masses (Tumors)

Although the ultrasound features of many solid liver lesions share similarities, there are certain patterns that can help narrow the differential diagnosis. IOUS can generally provide better characterization of solid liver lesions than transabdominal ultrasound. Hemangiomas are benign, usually incidentally discovered, asymptomatic lesions. Although they can exhibit a variety of ultrasound appearances, most have fairly characteristic ultrasound features (69,70). They are well circumscribed, round, hyperechoic (bright) tumors (Fig. 49). Usually they are less than a few centimeters (less than 3 cm) in size. Posterior enhancement may be present. Most are single lesions, although occasionally several may be present. As hemangiomas increase in size, their echogenicity can change from homogeneous to heterogeneous (Fig. 50). Concurrently, their borders may become irregular, more scalloped than smooth. These changes make them more difficult to distinguish from malignant tumors. The primary issue with hemangiomas is distinguishing them from lesions requiring therapy. Although these tumors are highly vascular, blood flow through them is slow. Consequently, Doppler studies usually are not helpful in distinguishing them from other lesions. One method that may be helpful in diagnosing hemangiomas is to compress them with the probe during IOUS scanning. A reduction in echogenicity during compression suggests the diagnosis of hemangioma (71). When a definitive diagnosis cannot be made by these methods, needle biopsy is necessary. Studies have demonstrated the safety of this approach, even percutaneously, particularly if the biopsy is done through a section of normal hepatic parenchyma (72,73). Clearly, needle biopsy can be performed intraoperatively under IOUS guidance with almost no risk.

Focal nodular hyperplasia and hepatic adenomas are both benign focal liver masses. Distinguishing between them is important because adenomas require therapy due to their tendency to rupture and bleed, as well as their malignant potential (74). Adenomas tend to be single lesions, although both can present as multiple masses. Ultrasound characteristics range from hypo- to hyperechoic (more frequently hypoechoic). Others may be isoechoic and very difficult to distinguish from the surrounding liver. Finally, some lesions have a mixed pattern (75). Because both types of lesions have similar ultrasound appearances, even IOUS is not reliable in distinguishing between focal nodular hyperplasia and adenoma (Fig. 51) (76). The use of contrast-enhanced ultrasonography may improve the distinction between adenoma and focal

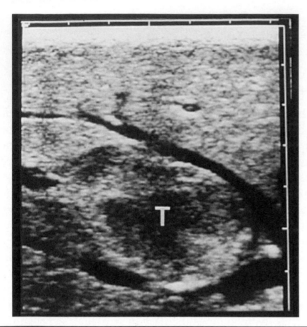

FIGURE 50. Large hemangioma (T). A 5 × 3 cm heterogeneous hemangioma, located between the middle and right hepatic veins. This shows a mixed hyper- and hypoechoic pattern, but there is no hypoechoic halo.

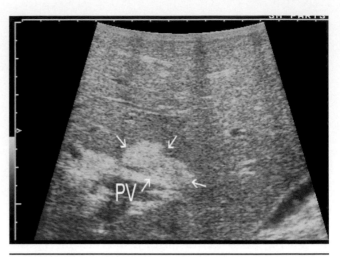

FIGURE 52. Focal fatty infiltration. A hyperechoic irregular lesion (*arrows*), 2 × 1 cm, located anterior to the portal vein (PV) in segment 4–5.

nodular hyperplasia (77,78). Ultimately, core needle biopsy is often necessary for definitive diagnosis.

Fatty changes in the liver can give the appearance of a mass lesion. Diffusely fatty liver (steatosis) causes increased echogenicity with a fine granular pattern. This

appears as an overall uniformly "bright" liver. This finding is important primarily because it can interfere with the IOUS examination. Steatosis attenuates sound waves resulting in less sound penetration, making examination of deeper structures difficult. Poor-penetration imaging can be overcome by using a lower frequency (e.g., 5 MHz) IOUS transducer (Fig. 6). In addition to diffuse fatty changes, the liver also can have isolated areas of fatty change. When these changes are focal and limited in scope, they can give the appearance of a mass lesion (Fig.

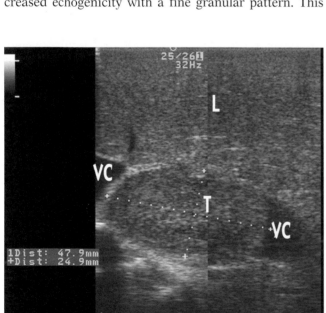

FIGURE 51. Focal nodular hyperplasia (CT). A 48 × 25 mm isoechoic tumor, which was located in segment 1, and was compressing the vena cava (VC), visualized in this longitudinal scanning. Intraoperative ultrasound–guided core needle biopsy showed this to be a focal nodular hyperplasia. L, segment 4 of the liver.

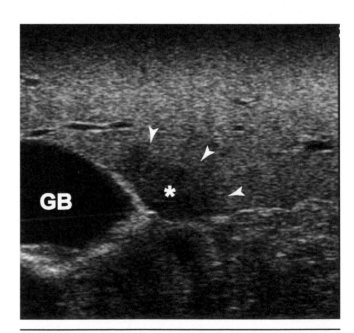

FIGURE 53. Diffuse fatty liver parenchyma with a focal area of sparing (*asterisk and arrowheads*) simulating a mass. These areas are often adjacent to the gallbladder (GB) and the portal structures in segment 4.

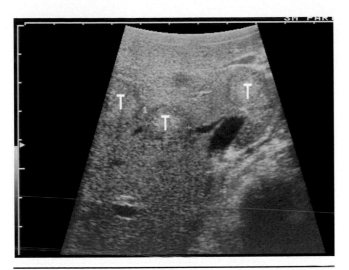

FIGURE 54. Multiple metastatic liver tumors. Three tumors (T) from colon cancer shows similar echo features with a hypoechoic rim.

52). Referred to as focal fatty infiltration, this appears as an echogenic "mass," often with irregular borders. Some of these lesions are more defined, described as "geographic" in appearance, meaning they may follow an anatomic plane and have sharply demarcated, angular borders. Some areas of focal fatty infiltration are rounded, nodular, or multifocal, rendering them indistinguishable from true hepatic tumors. Focal fatty changes are common in patients receiving corticosteroid therapy (79). On the other hand, in a liver with diffuse steatosis, areas may have focal sparing of the fatty infiltration, giving the impression of a mass lesion (Fig. 53). This appears as a relatively hypoechoic area within the hyperechoic fatty liver parenchyma (80). One clue to the nature of the perceived mass is the location of these findings. Areas of focal fatty change, particularly focal fatty sparing, are seen typically in segment 4 adjacent to the gallbladder, central portal structures, or along the falciform ligament (see Fig. 34 in

TABLE 11 Characteristics of Malignant Liver Tumors

Hypoechoic halo
  Target pattern
  Bull's-eye pattern
Mass effect on intrahepatic structures
Vascular or biliary invasion
Tumor thrombus

Chapter 11) (81). Another clue suggestive of focal fatty changes is the lack of secondary effects in and around the involved liver. In particular, the lack of vascular effacement or alterations in their course as vessels traverse these "masses" suggests that the area is one of fatty change rather than a true tumor.

Malignant Masses (Tumors)

In Western countries, most malignant liver tumors come from metastatic disease. Thus, IOUS is typically performed for liver screening in the context of a primary gastrointestinal malignancy. Solid tumors detected during IOUS should raise suspicion for metastatic disease until proven otherwise, especially if multiple lesions exist. Multiple metastases within the same liver may have different appearances between lesions. However, typically, multiple liver metastases from a single primary site have similar IOUS characteristics among the lesions (Fig. 54). Thus, a definitive histologic diagnosis of a single lesion or two is usually sufficient. If different appearing lesions are present, they may represent another process. Therefore, if a lesion will remain in the hepatic remnant following resection and any question regarding its nature remains, biopsy is appropriate to rule out malignancy.

Table 10 summarizes the ultrasound features of various liver tumors. Characteristic features suggestive of malignant liver tumors are listed in Table 11.

TABLE 10 Characteristic Ultrasound Features of Various Liver Tumors

Tumor Type	Shape	Boundary	Internal Echoes	Marginal Hypoechoic Zone	Posterior Echoes	Lateral Shadow
Metastatic carcinoma or cholangiocarcinoma	Cauliflower-like	Coarsely irregular	Vary	Present; thick	Attenuated or even	Absent
Metastatic sarcoma or carcinoid	Round	Sharp and smooth	Vary	Absent	Even or enhanced	Absent
Hepatocellular carcinoma	Round	Sharp and smooth	Vary; mosaic pattern	Present; thin	Enhanced	Occasionally present
Hemangioma	Round	Finely irregular	Echogenic or mixed	Absent	Even or enhanced	Absent

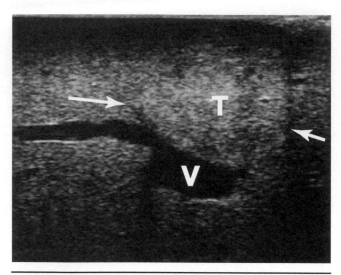

FIGURE 55. Isoechoic tumor (T) distinguishable from the surrounding liver parenchyma by the subtle hypoechoic ring or halo (*arrows*) and distortion of the adjacent vein (V).

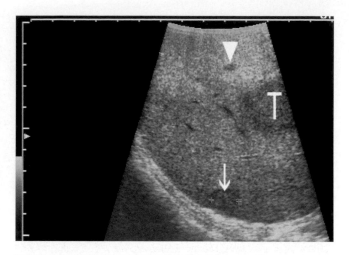

FIGURE 57. Hypoechoic occult metastatic tumors from colon cancer. In this intraoperative ultrasound (IOUS) image, one 2.5-cm tumor (T) was known preoperatively, whereas two other hypoechoic tumors, 12 mm (*arrow*) and 3 mm (*arrowhead*), were detected by IOUS for the first time.

Liver metastases can have a range of sonographic appearances (82). Echogenicity and echo pattern of metastatic tumors are dependent on the size of the tumor. Gastrointestinal metastases larger than 1 to 2 cm are frequently iso- to hyperechoic and surrounded by a hypoechoic ring or halo (target or bull's-eye lesion) (Figs. 41,

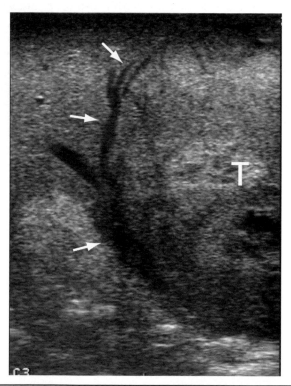

FIGURE 56. Vessel displacement (*arrows*) by a large metastatic tumor (T).

42, 48, and 55) (83). They produce a mass effect with distortion of surrounding structures. Occasionally vascular or biliary invasion can be seen; typically, however, these lesions push structures aside resulting in displacement of intrahepatic vessels (Figs. 42 and 56). The hyperechoic gastrointestinal metastatic lesions can be confused with hemangiomas. They differ in a number of ways. Unlike metastatic masses, hemangiomas lack mass effect and evidence of invasion, and in particular do not have the hypoechoic halo seen in metastases. If any uncertainty persists, core needle biopsy should be done. Hypoechoic gastrointestinal metastases also can occur. These are sometimes associated with mucin-producing metastasis and have been associated with a worse prognosis (84). When tumors become larger (more than 5 cm), they tend to demonstrate a heterogeneous echo pattern.

Smaller, potentially metastatic lesions identified in the liver by IOUS pose a difficult diagnostic problem. Lesions less than 1 to 2 cm in diameter tend to be hypoechoic and lack the features characteristic of a metastatic lesion (85). Despite this, they may retain the hypoechoic halo, which is highly suggestive of malignancy. In particular, IOUS-detected occult metastases are frequently less than 1 cm in diameter and show only a hypoechoic feature (Fig. 57; see also Fig. 26 in Chapter 13). Definitive diagnosis for such a small hypoechoic lesion generally requires biopsy. Metastatic lesions from nongastrointestinal primary sites may be identified during IOUS. Genitourinary metastases are more often hyperechoic, having a similar ultrasound appearance to larger gastrointestinal metastases. Other common malignancies, including breast cancer, lung cancer, neuroendocrine tumors, and sarcoma, tend to have

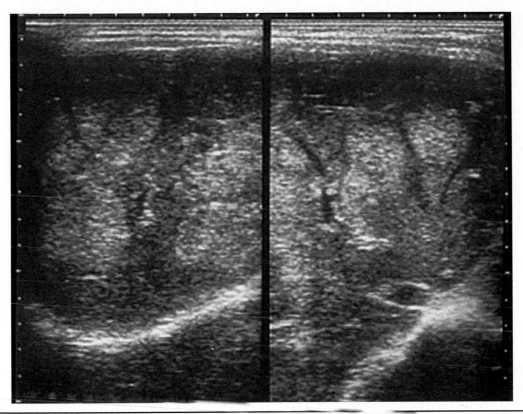

FIGURE 58. Diffuse liver involvement of metastatic tumor. This rectal cancer metastasis caused diffuse heterogeneous ill-defined changes of the liver with distortion of intrahepatic vascular structures.

hypoechoic metastases that can be associated with mass effect or invasive features. Finally, lymphomas can present as multiple small hypoechoic lesions.

Metastatic disease can have a number of uncommon presentations detectable by IOUS. Cystic metastases can be mistaken for simple or complex cysts. These metastases develop from mucin-producing primary lesions such as colon, pancreatic, or ovarian cancers. They appear as smooth-walled, anechoic lesions with posterior enhancement. Without evidence of interval enlargement on serial imaging studies or biopsy evidence of malignancy, they can be misinterpreted as benign. Central necrosis within a metastasis also can give the appearance of a cystic lesion. These masses have a hypoechoic interior with thickened, irregular walls or nodular projections. Often, debris can be identified within the cystic component. Calcified metastases are unusual, being seen in some colorectal, gastric, and ovarian metastases (86,87). Calcified metastases have a very echogenic appearance with posterior shadowing (Figs. 37 and 39). A metastatic deposit in a fatty liver can result in a confusing picture (88). These lesions appear hypoechoic in comparison with the increased echogenicity of the surrounding hepatic parenchyma. They may have posterior enhancement. Con-

sequently, metastatic lesions in this context may be mistaken for cysts during transabdominal ultrasound; however, such an error is rare with IOUS. Finally, not all metastases present as focal mass lesions. Diffuse metastatic involvement may be present from a variety of primary lesions, as well as diffuse hepatocellular carcinoma or lymphomatous involvement of the liver. In these cases, liver involvement can be difficult to recognize, as the ultrasound appearance is one of poorly defined, course changes throughout the involved liver parenchyma. These areas typically are seen as patchy regions (Fig. 44) or diffusely ill-defined heterogeneous regions (Fig. 58).

Hepatocellular carcinoma is the most common primary malignancy of the liver. IOUS has proved remarkably useful in detecting hepatocellular carcinomas with daughter nodules and planning operative therapy, particularly in the cirrhotic patient. IOUS can detect small tumors in the cirrhotic liver, including those missed preoperatively (33). Vascular invasion is common with hepatocellular carcinoma and is more detectable by IOUS than by preoperative imaging studies (89). The ultrasound characteristics of hepatocellular carcinomas can vary widely. Two primary forms of these tumors are recognized: nodular and diffuse. The nodular type is far

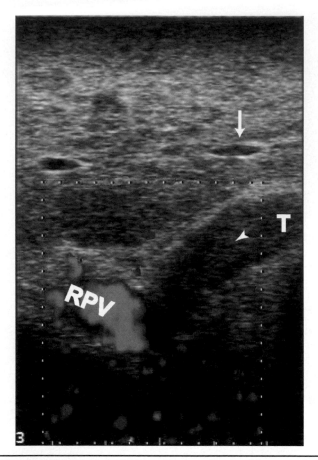

FIGURE 59. Tumor invasion with thrombosis of the main left portal vein. The arrowhead denotes the edge of the tumor thrombus (T) in the left portal vein. The arrow notes a small vein with echogenic tumor thrombus within it. The right portal vein (RPV) has flow indicated by color Doppler imaging. (See Color Plate 28.)

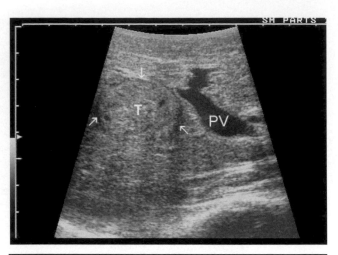

FIGURE 61. Hepatocellular carcinoma with a hypoechoic halo. A 32 × 22 mm isoechoic tumor (T) exhibiting a thin hypoechoic halo (*arrows*). PV, right anterior portal vein branch.

more common than the diffuse type. Nodular tumors may be single or multiple and are seen as discrete mass lesions. Diffuse tumors have infiltrative, indistinct borders making them often difficult to recognize. Diffuse tumors often blend in with the surrounding heterogeneous cirrhotic parenchyma on IOUS examination. Secondary signs such as vascular displacement or invasion should alert one to the possibility of diffuse hepatocellular carcinoma (Fig. 59). Nodular hepatocellular carcinomas typically have well defined boundaries and some echo characteristics that are suggestive of the diagnosis. A number of studies have evaluated the differing ultrasound charac-

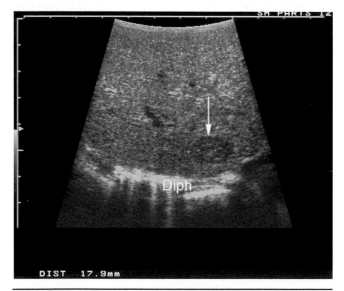

FIGURE 60. Small hypoechoic hepatocellular carcinoma. An 18-mm hepatocellular carcinoma (*arrow*) exhibiting a hypoechoic feature. Diph, diaphragm.

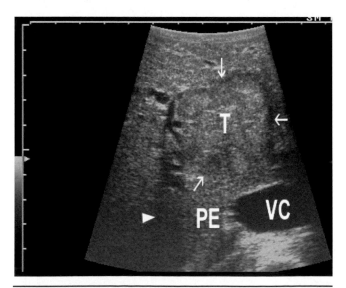

FIGURE 62. Larger (4.5 cm) hepatocellular carcinoma with some specific features: mosaic pattern (T) and thin hypoechoic rim (*arrows*). Posterior enhancement (PE) and lateral shadowing (*arrowhead*) are not so well visualized.

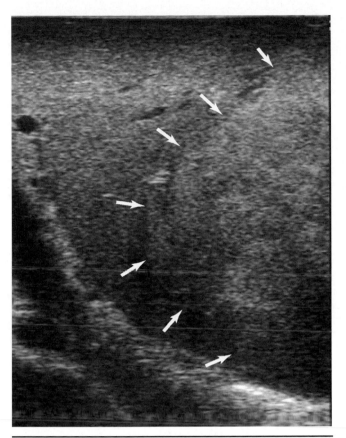

FIGURE 63. Large hepatocellular carcinoma (arrows define border) with hyperechoic, heterogeneous features.

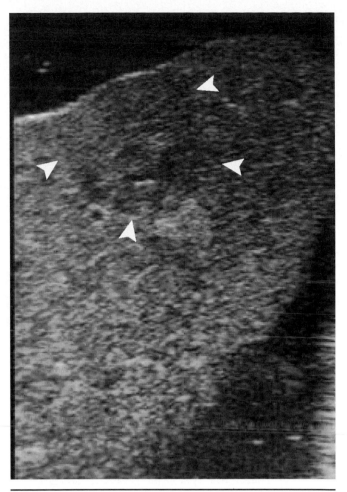

FIGURE 64. Regenerative nodule (*arrowheads*). These often appear as a small hypoechoic mass and can mimic small hepatocellular carcinomas. Intraoperative biopsy is required for diagnosis.

teristics of hepatocellular carcinomas and correlated these with pathologic findings. In general, hepatocellular carcinomas smaller than 2 cm in diameter tend to be uniformly hypoechoic (Fig. 60) (85,90). As hepatocellular carcinomas increase in size, their echogenicity changes (91). As their size increases, they become more echogenic and have a hypoechoic halo (Fig. 61). Tumors ranging from 2.1 to 5.0 cm are noted to have a mosaic pattern of internal echoes, a thin hypoechoic halo, posterior enhancement, and lateral shadowing (Fig. 62). These features are seen with much higher frequency in lesions in this size range than in those smaller than 2 cm (92). Finally, with further growth, hepatocellular carcinomas develop into hyperechoic lesions, often with heterogeneous features (Fig. 63) (93,94). Pathologic correlation suggests the increased echogenicity and heterogeneity is related to tumor hemorrhage or necrosis.

In the cirrhotic patient, other mass lesions should be considered in the differential diagnosis. Regenerative nodules may be apparent as discrete lesions on IOUS. They are often small and hypoechoic, mimicking small hepatocellular carcinomas (Fig. 64). It is frequently difficult to distinguish them from hepatocellular carcinoma based on IOUS characteristics alone (95). Hemangio-

mas can be present in the cirrhotic liver as hyperechoic masses. Hemangiomas less than 3 cm in size (hyperechoic) may be distinguished from hepatocellular carcinoma (hypoechoic); however, larger hemangiomas may be mistaken for hepatocellular carcinomas (96). The only reliable features to suggest hepatocellular carcinoma are the presence of a mass effect causing effacement or invasion of surrounding intrahepatic structures and/or a thin hypoechoic halo. Unfortunately, in many cases these features are absent and a definitive diagnosis is not possible. In these situations, core needle biopsy is necessary to establish the diagnosis.

In summary, cystic and solid masses in the liver can have varying and overlapping ultrasound appearances. This results in a broad differential diagnosis for a discovered lesion. However, by placing the finding of a mass lesion into the current clinical context for a particular patient, the differential diagnosis can be narrowed to a few suspect lesions. IOUS can provide an excellent character-

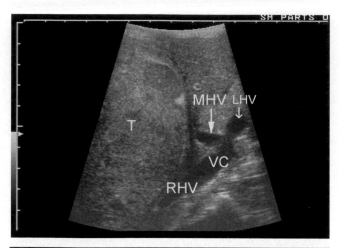

FIGURE 65. Resectable large hepatocellular carcinoma. A 12-cm tumor in the right lobe extending into segment 4. The tumor (T) was invading the right hepatic vein (RHV) and middle hepatic vein (MHV), but the vena cava (VC) and left hepatic vein (LHV) were intact. Ligation and transection of RHV and MHV appeared to be possible. Trissectionectomy was performed.

ization of these liver masses. Some general rules may help differentiate a malignant tumor from a benign one:

1. Effacement or invasion of intrahepatic structures is highly suggestive of a malignant lesion. This IOUS finding is especially valuable to determine the respectability of a tumor and to select the type of resection procedure to be performed (Figs. 65 and 66).
2. A hypoechoic ring (target or bull's-eye lesion) around a mass lesion is highly correlated with a malignant tumor, particularly if the patient is known to have a primary extrahepatic malignancy or in the presence of

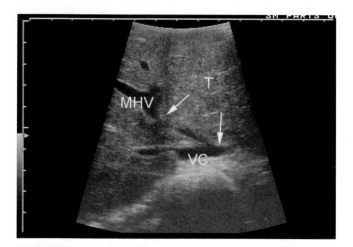

FIGURE 66. Unresectable metastatic liver tumor from a rectal cancer. An 8-cm tumor in segment 4. The tumor (T) was invading (*arrows*) the middle hepatic vein (MHV) and vena cava (VC). It was also invading the portal veins and bile ducts, and was judged to be unresectable.

a cirrhotic liver. This phenomenon is widely described in the literature and correlated with malignancy, but its sensitivity and specificity have not been well studied (83,97).

3. Multiple tumors in the setting of a primary extrahepatic malignancy should raise concern regarding metastatic disease.
4. Hyperechoic, well-circumscribed lesions smaller than 2 to 3 cm are suggestive of hemangiomas.
5. When the diagnosis of a hepatic mass lesion is in doubt, fine or core needle biopsy is necessary. IOUS can precisely guide such a biopsy.

ULTRASOUND GUIDANCE FOR HEPATIC INTERVENTIONS

Image-directed procedures are critical during hepatic surgery, and IOUS is the ideal means for assisting these procedures. IOUS facilitates needle placement for biopsy or treatment, probe positioning for ablation therapies, and image guidance for tissue dissection and hepatectomies (Table 12; see also Chapters 4 and 13 for more discussion of hepatic interventional IOUS).

Intraoperative Ultrasound–Guided Needle and Probe Placement

Needle or probe placement under direct ultrasound guidance allows for precise targeting of a lesion or vessel. Needle placement can be done with a needle guidance system that attaches to the probe (Fig. 67; see also Fig. 38 in Chapter 13) or by the freehand technique (see Chapters 4 and 13). The needle guidance system has the advantage of keeping the needle in the scanning plane and more reliably guiding the needle to the target. It has the disadvantage of requiring needle placement directly adjacent to the probe. This limits needle placement from re-

▶ **TABLE 12 Intraoperative Ultrasound Guidance for Hepatic Procedures**

Needle positioning
- Biopsy, aspiration, injection
- Catheter placement for cholangiography or drainage

Probe positioning
- Ethanol, cryoablation, or thermal ablation

Resectional procedures
- Margin determination and marking
- Parenchymal dissection and guidance

Special techniques
- Defining segmental anatomy
- Marking segmental inflow
- "Systematic subsegmentectomy"

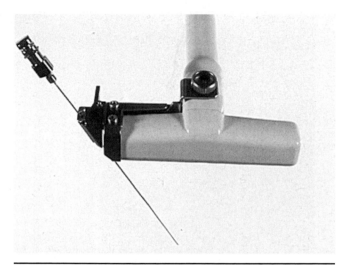

FIGURE 67. Needle guidance system for the intraoperative ultrasound probe.

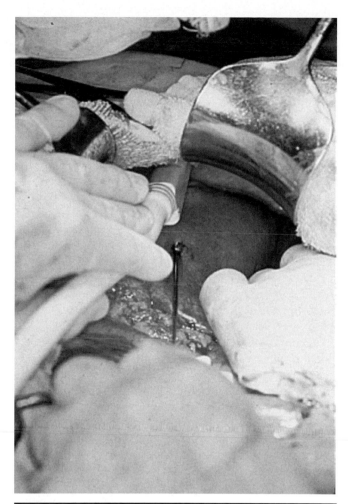

FIGURE 68. Freehand technique for intraoperative ultrasound–assisted needle guidance.

mote positions. Furthermore, depending on probe placement, a guidance system can be cumbersome or simply not usable due to limited space around the liver within the peritoneal cavity. An alternative approach is the freehand technique (Fig. 68). Although it can be more difficult to master, the freehand method is ultimately more versatile than the use of a guidance system. One of the keys to mastering ultrasound-guided procedures is to identify and maintain the needle in the scanning plane. The easiest way to accomplish this is to place the needle so that it lies in the long axis of the transducer (see Fig. 12 in Chapter 4). Needles appear as hyperechoic lines with or without posterior shadowing or reverberation artifacts (Fig. 69; see also Fig. 39 in Chapter 13). For the novice, superficial lesions can be punctured relatively easily by the freehand method, whereas deeper and/or smaller lesions are more easily targeted with a needle guidance system. With experience, more IOUS-guided procedures can be performed freehand.

Needle placement by IOUS is frequently required for diagnostic purposes. Aspiration of cyst fluid or drainage of an abscess can be performed by IOUS guidance. More commonly, biopsy of a lesion is required, and either fine needle aspiration or core needle biopsy can be used. If the question can be answered simply by demonstrating the presence of malignant cells, then fine needle aspiration is sufficient. In most cases a core needle biopsy is necessary to obtain histology to distinguish a malignant hepatic lesion from a benign one. This is particularly true if the possible diagnoses are hepatic adenoma, focal nodular hyperplasia, or hepatocellular carcinoma, or if the diagnosis is hepatocellular carcinoma as opposed to regenerative nodule, especially in the cirrhotic liver. Prac-

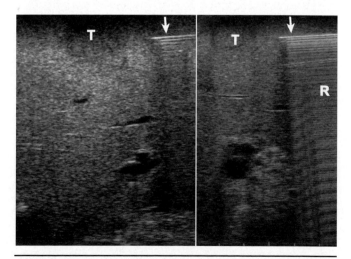

FIGURE 69. Needle guidance by intraoperative ultrasound. **A:** Needle (*arrow*) appears as a thin hyperechoic line, facilitating guidance into the tumor (T). **B:** Reverberation artifact (R) is frequently noted with highly reflective objects such as biopsy needles.

tically, because bleeding from a larger needle is not a major concern intraoperatively (achieving hemostasis is easy), IOUS-guided liver biopsy is almost always performed with a core needle. When using the core biopsy needle, one needs to remember that the final biopsy site is distal to the initial location of the tip of the needle. This should be taken into account during needle placement. Most core biopsy needles have an excursion during firing of approximately 1.5 to 2.5 cm. Therefore, the tip of the needle should be inserted this distance away from the final position of the lesion to be biopsied (Fig. 69A). To ensure that the lesion is adequately biopsied, a hyperechoic needle track can be seen within the lesion by IOUS (Fig. 70). In a similar fashion to needle guidance for biopsy, IOUS facilitates intraoperative cholangiography by identifying intrahepatic as well as extrahepatic bile ducts for cannulation for contrast injection. IOUS guidance allows for intrahepatic bile duct cannulation in order to perform transhepatic drainage catheter placement in the biliary system.

Accurate needle or probe placement for nonresectional tumor treatments requires IOUS guidance. Needle placement in a hepatocellular carcinoma for ethanol ablation can be directed by open IOUS (although the majority of ethanol injection therapies are performed percutaneously). As ethanol is instilled, IOUS can be used to monitor its dispersion throughout the lesion and assess its completeness in real time. Cryo- or thermal ablation techniques rely on IOUS for accurate probe placement and assessment of ablation adequacy (98). The cryotherapy probe is guided directly into the liver lesion under

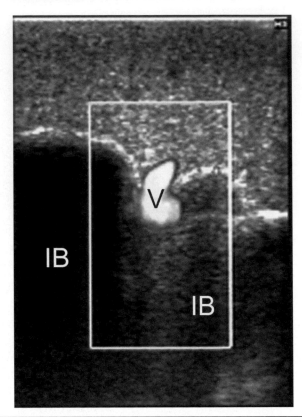

FIGURE 71. Following cryotherapy, a hypoechoic ablation zone is present representing the area of the "ice ball" (IB). There is a heat (cold) sink effect by an intrahepatic vessel (V, color Doppler imaging). (Courtesy of Dr. Maurice Arregui.)

IOUS control; multiple probes can be inserted at one time as needed for large ablations (99). During the cryotherapy, IOUS can be used to monitor the ablation zone in real time. This zone appears as a hyperechoic leading edge, which expands into the normal liver parenchyma. Posterior to this leading edge is acoustic shadowing, preventing further examination of structures within the ablation zone. This anechoic area of shadowing is the so-called ice ball, representing the area of ablation (Fig. 71). A sharp transition zone is readily apparent between the ice ball and normal liver on IOUS. This allows accurate assessment of ablation completeness, as the lesion of interest disappears within the leading edge of the ice ball.

Thermal ablation for unresectable liver tumors is a more recent development. Its success is critically dependent on the use of IOUS monitoring (100,101). In a similar fashion to cryotherapy, IOUS is important for probe guidance into the tumor. Real-time IOUS allows probe deployment monitoring to determine accurate placement of multiple retractable electrode needles within the lesion (Fig. 72; see also Fig. 46 in Chapter 4). Radiofrequency thermal ablation is technically more difficult to monitor by ultra-

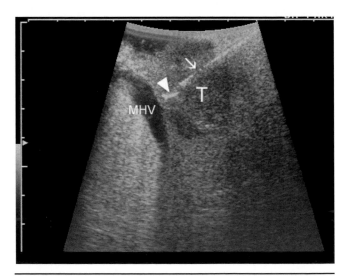

FIGURE 70. Hyperechoic needle and needle track. After intraoperative core needle biopsy of a tumor (T) adjacent to the middle hepatic vein (MHV), a needle is withdrawn. A needle track (*arrowhead*) often becomes hyperechoic due to air left behind. The withdrawn needle (*arrow*) is also seen.

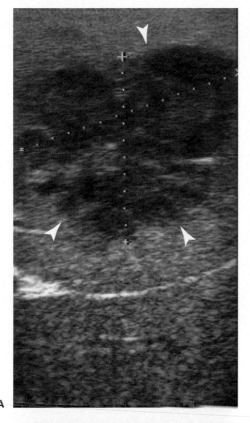

A

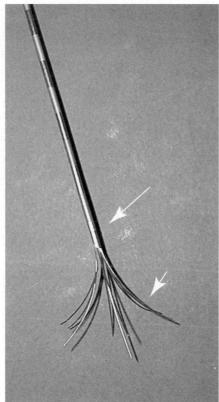

B

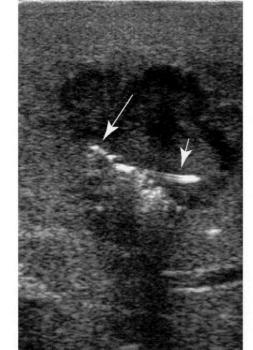

C

FIGURE 72. Radiofrequency probe placement by intraoperative ultrasound (IOUS) guidance. **A:** Hypoechoic hepatocellular carcinoma (*arrowheads*) for ablation. **B:** Radiofrequency probe (*long arrow*) with tines deployed (*short arrow*). **C:** IOUS guidance of radiofrequency probe into lesion with tines deployed. Arrows match those seen in **B**. Initial placement is critical as seen here the lesion becomes obscured by the needle and subsequent ablation.

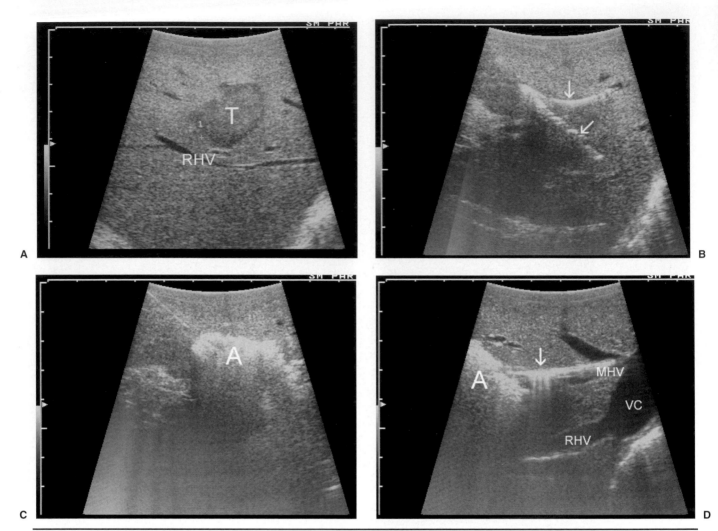

FIGURE 73. The process of radiofrequency thermal ablation of a liver tumor. **A:** A 28 × 19 mm metastatic colon tumor (T) in segment 5–8 between the right hepatic vein (RHV) and middle hepatic vein. **B:** Electrode-needles (*arrows*) were deployed. The tips of needles were guided by intraoperative ultrasound and located outside the tumor. **C:** Once ablation started, the ablated lesion (A) became hyperechoic, obscuring the tumor. **D:** Outgassing causes hyperechoic flowing echoes (*arrow*) in the draining vein. MHV, middle hepatic vein; RHV, right hepatic vein; VC, vena cava.

sound than cryotherapy, as the region of ablation is marked by diffuse, irregular, hyperechoic changes resulting from tissue gas formation. The gas causes hyperreflective changes in the area of interest obscuring the lesion during the ablation (see Fig. 47 in Chapter 4 and Fig. 49 in Chapter 13). Unlike cryotherapy, this ablation zone is not sharply demarcated due to the diffuse nature of the hyperechoic changes. This makes clear determination of ablation margins more difficult. Following completion of the ablation, the area remains hyperechoic with posterior shadowing for 10 to 20 minutes, obscuring tissue deep to the ablation zone. Precise probe placement at the beginning of the ablation is required for this procedure (Figs. 72 and 73; see also Figs. 50 and 51 in Chapter 13), as the IOUS determination

of the thermal ablation zone is a good, but not perfect approximation of its true extent (102)

IOUS-Guided Hepatic Incision and Resection

During hepatic resection, IOUS is used for a number of purposes. The simplest is to identify the lesion of interest and mark a resection margin around it. The margin site is located by IOUS and marked on the liver surface by scoring the capsule with the electrocautery. The scored capsule appears as a hypoechoic spot by IOUS, allowing verification of the surgical margin's position and width from the lesion prior to parenchymal transection (Fig. 74; see Fig. 44 in Chapter 13). Similarly, intrahepatic structures, such as the hepatic and portal veins, can be located and marked on the liver surface. During hepatic parenchymal dissection, IOUS can monitor the transection plane. This is performed by frequent IOUS examinations as the resection proceeds (Fig. 75; see also Figs. 42 and 43 in Chapter 13). The dissection plane is visualized as a hyperechoic line. In this fashion, the direction of the incision can be verified and its relationship to intrahepatic structures (lesions and vascular structures) identified prior to encoun-

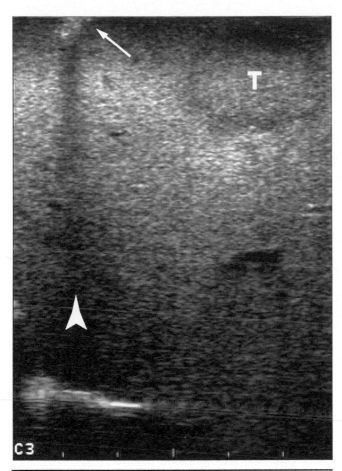

FIGURE 74. Intraoperative ultrasound (IOUS)–guided liver resection. The liver capsule is scored under IOUS guidance, resulting in a hyperechoic spot (*arrow*) and a hypoechoic line (shadowing) beneath the scored site (*arrowhead*). This allows an accurate determination of the resection margin from the tumor (T).

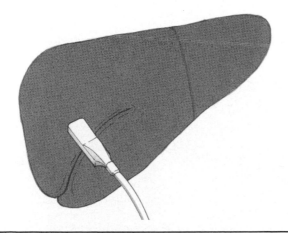

FIGURE 75. Intraoperative ultrasound (IOUS) guidance of liver resection by frequent scanning as the resection proceeds. IOUS is repeated over the dissection plane to visualize intrahepatic structures, particularly the relationship between dissection to a target lesion and the surrounding vascular structures.

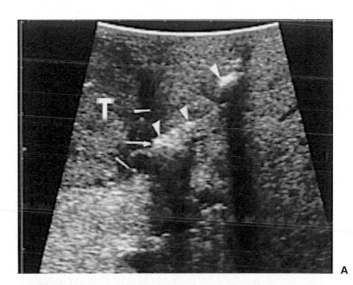

A

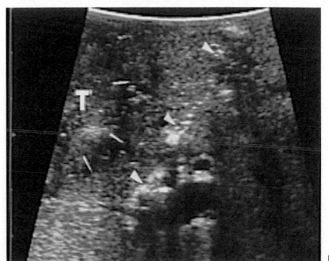

B

FIGURE 76. Correction of dissection direction by intraoperative ultrasound (IOUS) guidance. **A:** During resection of a metastatic colon cancer, IOUS was repeatedly used. In this sonogram, the dissection plane (*arrowheads*) was toward (*arrow*) the tumor (T, *thin arrowheads*). **B:** The direction of dissection was changed and IOUS was repeated. In this sonogram, the dissection plane (*arrowheads*) was away from the tumor (T, *thin arrowheads*), indicating an adequate margin.

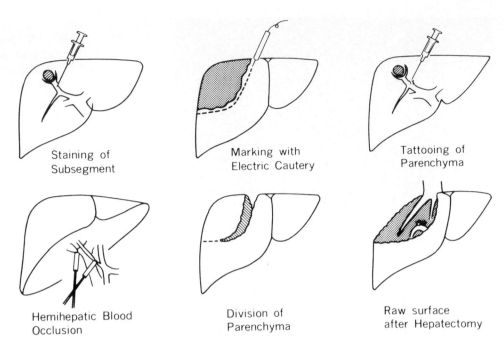

Staining of
Subsegment

Marking with
Electric Cautery

Tattooing of
Parenchyma

Hemihepatic Blood
Occlusion

Division of
Parenchyma

Raw surface
after Hepatectomy

FIGURE 77. Systematic subsegmentectomy. Operative steps for completion of subsegmentectomy. (Courtesy of Dr. Masatoshi Makuuchi.)

tering them during the dissection (Fig. 76). This approach allows constant monitoring of the transection plane and corrections in its direction or depth if needed.

Several specific hepatic resection techniques have been developed with the aid of IOUS. Without IOUS, these methods would be impossible. In particular, IOUS has allowed the marking and resection of individual anatomic segments and subsegments. This technique is called systematic subsegmentectomy, which employs IOUS-guided "staining" and "tattooing" techniques (Fig. 77) (49,89). Under IOUS guidance, a needle is used to puncture the portal vein supplying the area of the tumor and several milliliters of dye (e.g., indigo carmine) is injected (Fig. 78). This stains the hepatic parenchyma supplied by this portal pedicle and marks the area for resection (Fig. 79). The interface of the stained liver surface at its junction with unstained liver is scored with the electrocautery. A similar, counterstaining identification technique has been described to demarcate the hepatic segments (103). Likewise, the portal triad at the site of ligation can be tattooed by injecting blue dye into the

FIGURE 78. Subsegmental staining. The portal vein supplying the area for resection (*arrowhead*) is cannulated with a needle (*arrow* indicates needle tip) and the vein is injected with indigo carmine dye. (Courtesy of Dr. Masatoshi Makuuchi.)

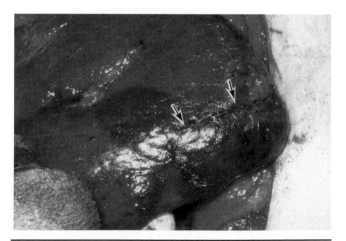

FIGURE 79. Staining of hepatic parenchyma. Anatomic resection of a part of segment 6. The stained area (*arrows*) is marked on the liver surface with an electrocautery. (Courtesy of Dr. Masatoshi Makuuchi.)

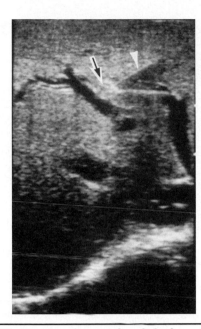

FIGURE 80. Tatooing the portal pedicle for subsegmentectomy. The portal pedicle supplying the subsegment for resection can be identified during the parenchymal transection by tattooing the adjacent liver parenchyma with blue dye. Dye is injected (*arrow*) through a needle guided into the liver parenchyma by intraoperative ultrasound in the proximity of the portal vein branch requiring ligation. A needle shaft with shadowing is indicated by the arrowhead. (Courtesy of Dr. Masatoshi Makuuchi.)

liver parenchyma just anterior to the vessels (Fig. 80) (1). This allows identification of the vessels for ligation as the parenchymal dissection proceeds. A similar method to identify the area supplied by a specific portal pedicle is to use IOUS to place a small occlusion balloon within the vessel. Balloon inflation in conjunction with hepatic artery control at the hilum will result in the characteristic ischemic color changes in the segment of interest. More recently, a "hooking" technique using IOUS has been described (46). Precise intrahepatic ligation sites can be identified for individual portal pedicles.

A common anatomic variant is an inferior right hepatic vein (draining vein of segment 6), which is present in approximately 20% of patients (Figs. 31 and 81) (104). IOUS recognition of this structure and mapping of the segments of the right lobe allows for four hepatectomy procedures with resection of the right hepatic vein and preservation of the inferior right hepatic vein (e.g., segment 7/8) resection while preserving segment 6 in situ (Fig. 82) (51,105). In a similar fashion, IOUS is useful during hepatectomy for living donor liver transplantation because it allows variant venous anatomy to be mapped during the dissection. This allows preservation and subsequent reconstruction of dominant or aberrant draining veins during the recipient operation (see Chapter 18 for ultrasound use for transplantation).

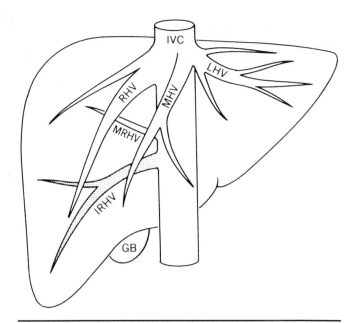

FIGURE 81. Inferior right hepatic vein (IRHV) in relationship to the vena cava (IVC), the right hepatic vein (RHV), a marginal right hepatic vein (MRHV), and the middle hepatic vein (MHV). (Courtesy of Dr. Masatoshi Makuuchi.)

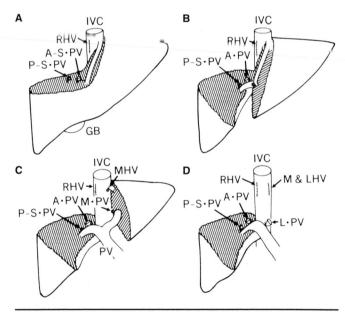

FIGURE 82. Four types of hepatectomies based on preservation of the inferior right hepatic vein. **A:** Resection of the right anterosuperior (A-S PV; segment 8) and posterosuperior (P-S PV; segment 7) segments. IVC, inferior vena cava; RHV, right hepatic vein; GB, gallbladder. **B:** Resection of the right anterior sector (A PV; segments 5 and 8) and the right posterosuperior segment (P-S PV; segment 7). **C:** Resection of the left medial (M PV; segment 4) and right anterior sector (A PV; segments 5 and 8) and the right posterosuperior segment (P-S PV; segment 7), an extended central bisegmentectomy. MHV, middle hepatic vein. **D:** Resection of the left lobe (L PV; segments 1–4), right anterior section (A PV; segments 5 and 8), and right posterosuperior segment (P-S PV, segment 7), an extended left trisegmentectomy. MHV, middle hepatic vein; LHV, left hepatic vein. (Courtesy of Dr. Masatoshi Makuuchi.)

Operative Techniques for Intraoperative Ultrasound–Guided Systematic Subsegmentectomy

Using IOUS-guided techniques, each subsegment (Couinaud's segment) can be anatomically resected. As an example, anatomic resection of segment 8 and segment 5 is described.

Segment 8 Subsegmentectomy

The round, falciform, and right coronary ligaments should be divided so that the right lobe is mobilized and the right hepatic vein is exposed. In about 90% of patients, segment 8 has two main portal vein branches: dorsal and ventral. The ventral branch and one to three branches of segment 5 forms a trunk in about 60% of patients. First, the dorsal branch is punctured under IOUS guidance and indigo carmine is injected. The stained dorsal area is then marked using an electrocautery. Second, the area of the ventral branch is marked in the same manner. Using these IOUS-guided staining methods, the margins of segment 8 are clarified. When only one portal branch is supplying the entire segment 8, this branch is punctured for staining (Fig. 78). Under hemihepatic clamp vascular occlusion of the left lobe, the liver parenchyma of the left margin, between segments 4 and 8, is divided. When the distal two thirds of the middle hepatic vein is exposed, vascular occlusion of the left lobe is removed. Subsequently, under hemihepatic vascular occlusion of the right lobe, the liver parenchyma of the caudal margin, between segments 5 and 8, is divided so that the perivascular connective tissue of the segment 5 portal vein branch is exposed. Division of the parenchyma is continued along the anterior portal vein. The IOUS-guided tattooing technique can be used as needed. Then the ventral and dorsal branches are exposed and divided, resulting in occlusion of the blood inflow to segment 8. After the proximal one third of the middle hepatic vein is exposed, the liver parenchyma of the right margin is dissected and the right hepatic vein is exposed from the caudal area to the cranial area, and its confluence with the inferior vena cava is confirmed. During dissection of the liver parenchyma, the middle and right hepatic veins and the anterior portal vein branches should be located using IOUS before deciding on the direction of the dissection. Finally, the rest of the parenchyma is divided, and the total resection of segment 8 is completed (Fig. 83).

Segment 5 Subsegmentectomy

Segment 5 usually has three to five portal vein branches, making it difficult to puncture all the branches. When total resection of this area is indicated, the ventral branch

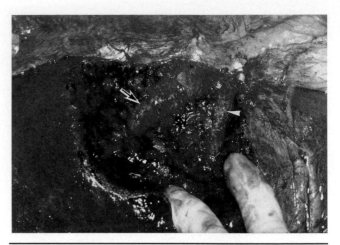

FIGURE 83. Segment 8 subsegmentectomy. This shows the raw surface of the liver after complete anatomic resection of segment 8. The right hepatic vein (*arrow*), middle hepatic vein (*arrowhead*), and two stumps of portal pedicles were exposed on the raw surface. (Courtesy of Dr. Masatoshi Makuuchi.)

of segment 8 and the branch of segment 6 should be punctured and injected with indigo carmine, which demonstrates the cranial and right borders of segment 5. This is the counterstaining identification technique method. The left margin can be identified by the hemihepatic occlusion technique of the left lobe vasculature. By dividing the liver parenchyma from the left margin of this area, the right branch of the middle hepatic vein is exposed and divided. The liver parenchymal dissection of the cranial border is then carried out. Subsequently, the portal vein branches of segment 5 are divided, beginning ventrally and moving dorsally until the main trunk of the anterior portal triad is totally exposed. Division of the right lateral margin completes the resection of segment 5.

In a similar fashion using IOUS, segment 6 and segment 7 subsegmentectomies can be accomplished. The left medial segment (segment 4) and the left lateral inferior and superior areas (segments 2 and 3) can be resected by conventional hepatectomy procedures. However, IOUS-guided systematic subsegmentectomy is possible when the superior or inferior part of segments 4, 2, 3, or another smaller area must be resected. When performing combined resection of two or more subsegments (e.g., segment 5 plus segment 6, segment 5 plus segment 4A), the same IOUS-guided techniques can be used to perform a complete anatomic resection of these areas.

ADVANTAGES AND LIMITATIONS

The primary advantage of IOUS is its flexibility and superb image quality (see Chapter 13). This results in an imaging technology that is highly accurate, easy to use, quick, and amenable to repeated use throughout a surgical procedure. Ultrasound is safe, and its real-time imaging capabilities make IOUS-guided procedures feasible, thereby ensuring greater safety for the patient and more precise performance of hepatic procedures.

Clear advantages have been described for IOUS in detecting and defining lesions within the liver compared to preoperative imaging techniques. When combined with intraoperative inspection and palpation, IOUS is the most sensitive means of detecting mass lesions in the liver. Identified lesions can be precisely localized in the liver and their relationship to intrahepatic structures, particularly vascular structures, clearly defined by multiple scanning planes. IOUS is accurate in detecting vascular invasion or tumor thrombus. For intraoperative interventions, no technique is as versatile and accurate as IOUS. Its use in the operating room provides the distinct advantage of real-time imaging, allowing precise guidance for a variety of procedures. This eliminates the need for blind procedures, thereby increasing the accuracy of intraoperative procedures and their safety. Finally, IOUS allows a number of procedures to be performed that would otherwise be impossible, such as systematic subsegmentectomy and radiofrequency thermal ablation.

IOUS of the liver has some specific limitations. Like other areas of ultrasound use, there is a learning curve. This can be readily overcome by practice and experience. Didactic and hands-on courses are available through the American College of Surgeons and other organizations to introduce one to the knowledge and skills required for IOUS. A period of mentoring with an experienced ultrasonographer will allow practice in conducting IOUS scanning, interpretation of the images, and the performance of ultrasound-guided procedures.

Limitations in imaging include the inability to detect smaller lesions, ducts, and vessels. IOUS cannot readily detect lesions less than 3 to 5 mm. Isoechoic lesions, even when larger, may be missed by IOUS. Determining the definitive diagnosis based on sonographic features alone also can be difficult or impossible. Interpretation of images may be incorrect, resulting in a false-negative or false-positive reading. When the IOUS characteristics of a lesion do not allow a definitive diagnosis, a biopsy is required.

CONCLUSIONS

IOUS has a critical role in hepatic surgery. It is highly sensitive for detecting small masses in the liver, allowing diagnosis of benign lesions as well as primary and secondary malignancies. This makes it a valuable screening tool in the operating room, particularly for the discovery of occult lesions. IOUS has an important role in defining hepatic segmental and intrahepatic anatomy. This facilitates the surgeon's understanding of the precise location of mass lesions within the liver, allowing the development and refinement of therapeutic strategies. Ultimately, IOUS can guide hepatic interventions such as biopsies, ablations, or resectional therapies. Currently, the use of IOUS is a standard, and hepatic surgery without IOUS is considered suboptimal. An in-depth knowledge of the information included here along with hands-on practice will be of significant benefit to the hepatic surgeon.

REFERENCES

1. Makuuchi M, Hasegawa H, Yamazaki S. Intraoperative ultrasonic examination for hepatectomy. Jpn J Clin Oncol 1981;11:367–390.
2. Machi J, Isomoto H, Yamashita Y, et al. Intraoperative ultrasonography in screening for liver metastases from colorectal cancer: comparative accuracy with traditional procedures. Surgery 1987:101:678–684.
3. Olsen AK. Intraoperative ultrasonography and the detection of liver metastases in patients with colorectal cancer. Br J Surg 1990;77:998–999.
4. Boldrini G, de Gaetano AM, Giovannini I, et al. The systematic use of operative ultrasound for detection of liver metastases during colorectal surgery. World J Surg 1987;11:622–627.
5. Gunven P, Makuuchi M, Takayasu K, et al. Preoperative imaging of liver metastases. Comparison of angiography, CT scan, and ultrasonography. Ann Surg 1985;202:573–579.
6. Clarke MP, Kane RA, Steele G Jr, et al. Prospective comparison of preoperative imaging and intraoperative ultrasonography in the detection of liver tumors. Surgery 1989;106:849–855.
7. Zacherl J, Scheuba C, Imhof M, et al. Current value of intraoperative sonography during surgery for hepatic neoplasms. World J Surg 2002;26:550–554.
8. Bloed W, van Leeuwen MS, Borel Rinkes IH. Role of intraoperative ultrasound of the liver with improved preoperative hepatic imaging. Eur J Surg 2000;166:691–695.
9. Parker GA, Lawrence W Jr, Horsley JS III, et al. Intraoperative ultrasound of the liver affects operative decision making. Ann Surg 1989;209:569–576; discussion 576–567.
10. Soyer P, Levesque M, Elias D, et al. Detection of liver metastases from colorectal cancer: comparison of intraoperative US and CT during arterial portography. Radiology 1992;183:541–544.
11. Knol JA, Marn CS, Francis IR, et al. Comparisons of dynamic infusion and delayed computed tomography, intraoperative ultrasound, and palpation in the diagnosis of liver metastases. Am J Surg 1993;165:81–87; discussion 87–88.
12. Clouse ME. Current diagnostic imaging modalities of the liver. Surg Clin North Am 1989;69:193–234.
13. Stone MD, Kane R, Bothe A Jr, et al. Intraoperative ultrasound imaging of the liver at the time of colorectal cancer resection. Arch Surg 1994;129:431–435; discussion 435–436.
14. Ravikumar TS, Buenaventura S, Salem RR, et al. Intraoperative ultrasonography of liver: detection of occult liver tumors and treatment by cryosurgery. Cancer Detect Prev 1994;18:131–138.
15. Machi J, Isomoto H, Kurohiji T, et al. Accuracy of intraoperative ultrasonography in diagnosing liver metastasis from colorectal cancer: evaluation with postoperative follow-up results. [see comments.]. World J Surg 1991;15:551–556; discussion 557.

16. Machi J, Isomoto H, Kurohiji T, et al. Detection of unrecognized liver metastases from colorectal cancers by routine use of operative ultrasonography. *Dis Colon Rectum* 1986; 29:405–409.

17. Jarnagin WR, Bach AM, Winston CB, et al. What is the yield of intraoperative ultrasonography during partial hepatectomy for malignant disease? *J Am Coll Surg* 2001;192: 577–583.

18. Kane RA, Hughes LA, Cua EJ, et al. The impact of intraoperative ultrasonography on surgery for liver neoplasms. *J Ultrasound Med* 1994;13:1–6.

19. Staren ED, Gambla M, Deziel DJ, et al. Intraoperative ultrasound in the management of liver neoplasms. *Am Surg* 1997;63:591–596; discussion 596–597.

20. Rifkin MD, Rosato FE, Branch HM, et al. Intraoperative ultrasound of the liver. An important adjunctive tool for decision making in the operating room. *Ann Surg* 1987;205: 466–472.

21. Solomon MJ, Stephen MS, Gallinger S, et al. Does intraoperative hepatic ultrasonography change surgical decision making during liver resection? *Am J Surg* 1994;168:307–310.

22. Russo A, Sparacino G, Plaja S, et al. Role of intraoperative ultrasound in the screening of liver metastases from colorectal carcinoma: initial experiences. *J Surg Oncol* 1989; 42(Suppl):249–255.

23. Stadler J, Holscher AH, Adolf J. Intraoperative ultrasonographic detection of occult liver metastases in colorectal cancer. *Surg Endosc* 1991;5:36–40.

24. Charnley RM, Morris DL, Dennison AR, et al. Detection of colorectal liver metastases using intraoperative ultrasonography. *Br J Surg* 1991;78:45–48.

25. Leen E, Angerson WJ, O'Gorman P, et al. Intraoperative ultrasound in colorectal cancer patients undergoing apparently curative surgery: correlation with two year follow-up. *Clin Radiol* 1996;51:157–159.

26. Raccuia SJ, Azoulay D. Clinical application of ultrasonography in liver surgery. *Ann Ital Chir* 1997;68:751–757.

27. Takigawa Y, Sugawara Y, Yamamoto J, et al. New lesions detected by intraoperative ultrasound during liver resection for hepatocellular carcinoma. *Ultrasound Med Biol* 2001;27:151–156.

28. Fan MH, Chang AE. Resection of liver tumors: technical aspects. *Surg Oncol* 2002;10:139–152.

29. Makuuchi M. Remodeling the surgical approach to hepatocellular carcinoma. *Hepatogastroenterology* 2002;49:36–40.

30. Makuuchi M, Imamura H, Sugawara Y, et al. Progress in surgical treatment of hepatocellular carcinoma. *Oncology* 2002;62 Suppl 1:74–81.

31. Regimbeau JM, Kianmanesh R, Farges O, et al. Extent of liver resection influences the outcome in patients with cirrhosis and small hepatocellular carcinoma. *Surgery* 2002; 131:311–317.

32. Torzilli G, Leoni P, Gendarini A, et al. Ultrasound-guided liver resections for hepatocellular carcinoma. *Hepatogastroenterology* 2002;49:21–27.

33. Sheu JC, Lee CS, Sung JL, et al. Intraoperative hepatic ultrasonography: an indispensable procedure in resection of small hepatocellular carcinomas. *Surgery* 1985;97:97–103.

34. Nagasue N, Suehiro S, Yukaya H. Intraoperative ultrasonography in the surgical treatment of hepatic tumors. *Acta Chir Scand* 1984;150:311–316.

35. Nagasue N, Kohno H, Chang YC, et al. Intraoperative ultrasonography in resection of small hepatocellular carcinoma associated with cirrhosis. *Am J Surg* 1989;158:40–42.

36. Salminen PM, Hockerstedt K, Edgren J, et al. Intraoperative ultrasound as an aid to surgical strategy in liver tumor. *Acta Chir Scand* 1990;156:329–332.

37. Makuuchi M, Hasegawa H, Yamazaki S. Development on segmentectomy and subsegmentectomy of the liver due to introduction of ultrasonography. *Nippon Geka Gakkai Zasshi* 1983;84:913–917 (in Japanese).

38. Makuuchi M, Hasegawa H, Yamazaki S. Intraoperative ultrasonic examination for hepatectomy. *Ultrasound Med Biol* 1983;Suppl 2:493–497.

39. Gozzetti G, Mazziotti A, Bolondi L, et al. Intraoperative ultrasonography in surgery for liver tumors. *Surgery* 1986;99: 523–530.

40. Hayashi N, Yamamoto K, Tamaki N, et al. Metastatic nodules of hepatocellular carcinoma: detection with angiography, CT, and us. *Radiology* 1987;165:61–63.

41. Castaing D, Emond J, Kunstlinger F, et al. Utility of operative ultrasound in the surgical management of liver tumors. *Ann Surg* 1986;204:600–605.

42. Machi J, Sigel B, Kurohiji T, et al. Operative ultrasound guidance for various surgical procedures. *Ultrasound Med Biol* 1990;16:37–42.

43. Machi J. Intraoperative and laparoscopic ultrasound. *Surg Oncol Clin North Am* 1999;8:205–226.

44. Wong SL, Edwards MJ, Chao C, et al. Radiofrequency ablation for unresectable hepatic tumors. *Am J Surg* 2001;182: 552–557.

45. Montorsi M, Santambrogio R, Bianchi P, et al. Perspectives and drawbacks of minimally invasive surgery for hepatocellular carcinoma. *Hepatogastroenterology* 2002;49:56–61.

46. Torzilli G, Takayama T, Hui AM, et al. A new technical aspect of ultrasound-guided liver surgery. *Am J Surg* 1999; 178:341–343.

47. Torzilli G, Makuuchi M. Ultrasound-guided liver subsegmentectomy: the peculiarity of segment 4. *J Am Coll Surg* 2001;193:706–708.

48. Makuuchi M, Hasegawa H, Yamazaki S, et al. The inferior right hepatic vein: ultrasonic demonstration. *Radiology* 1983;148:213–217.

49. Makuuchi M, Hasegawa H, Yamazaki S. Ultrasonically guided subsegmentectomy. *Surg, Gynecol Obstet* 1985;161: 346–350.

50. Makuuchi M, Hasegawa H, Yamazaki S, et al. The use of operative ultrasound as an aid to liver resection in patients with hepatocellular carcinoma. *World J Surg* 1987;11:615–621.

51. Makuuchi M, Hasegawa H, Yamazaki S, et al. Four new hepatectomy procedures for resection of the right hepatic vein and preservation of the inferior right hepatic vein. *Surg Gynecol Obstet* 1987;164:68–72.

52. Makuuchi M, Kosuge T, Takayama T, et al. Surgery for small liver cancers. *Semin Surg Oncol* 1993;9:298–304.

53. Lafortune M, Madore F, Patriquin H, et al. Segmental anatomy of the liver: a sonographic approach to the Couinaud nomenclature. *Radiology* 1991;181:443–448.

54. Solomon MJ, Stephen MS, White GH, et al. A new classification of hepatic territories using intraoperative ultrasound. *Am J Surg* 1992;163:336–338.

55. Couinaud C. *Le foie. Etudes anatomiques et chirurgicales.* Paris: Masson, 1957.

56. Anonymous. The Brisbane 2000 terminology of hepatic anatomy and resections. *HPB Surg* 2000;2:333–339.

57. Reynolds DM, Falk CT, Li A, et al. Identification of a locus for autosomal dominant polycystic liver disease, on chromosome 19p13.2–13.1. *Am J Hum Genet* 2000;67:1598–1604.

58. Qian Q, Li A, King BF, et al. Clinical profile of autosomal dominant polycystic liver disease. *Hepatology* 2003;37:164–171.

59. Sheen IS, Chien CS, Lin DY, et al. Resolution of liver abscesses: comparison of pyogenic and amebic liver abscesses. *Am J Trop Med Hyg* 1989;40:384–389.

60. Terrier F, Becker CD, Triller JK. Morphologic aspects of hepatic abscesses at computed tomography and ultrasound. *Acta Radiol Diagn (Stockh)* 1983;24:129–137.

61. Subramanyam BR, Balthazar EJ, Raghavendra BN, et al. Ultrasound analysis of solid-appearing abscesses. *Radiology* 1983;146:487–491.

62. Ralls PW, Colletti PM, Quinn MF, et al. Sonographic findings in hepatic amebic abscess. *Radiology* 1982;145:123–126.

63. Ralls PW, Barnes PF, Radin DR, et al. Sonographic features of amebic and pyogenic liver abscesses: a blinded comparison. *AJR Am J Roentgenol* 1987;149:499–501.

64. Ho B, Cooperberg PL, Li DK, et al. Ultrasonography and computed tomography of hepatic candidiasis in immunosuppressed patients. *J Ultrasound Med* 1982;1:157–159.

65. Maxwell AJ, Mamtora H. Fungal liver abscesses in acute leukaemia: a report of two cases. *Clin Radiol* 1988;39:197–201.

66. Gharbi HA, Hassine W, Brauner MW, et al. Ultrasound examination of the hydatic liver. *Radiology* 1981;139:459–463.

67. Lewall DB, McCorkell SJ. Hepatic echinococcal cysts: sonographic appearance and classification. *Radiology* 1985;155:773–775.

68. Choi BI, Lim JH, Han MC, et al. Biliary cystadenoma and cystadenocarcinoma: CT and sonographic findings. *Radiology* 1989;171:57–61.

69. Vilgrain V, Boulos L, Vullierme MP, et al. Imaging of atypical hemangiomas of the liver with pathologic correlation. *Radiographics* 2000;20:379–397.

70. Mirk P, Rubaltelli L, Bazzocchi M, et al. Ultrasonographic patterns in hepatic hemangiomas. *J Clin Ultrasound* 1982;10:373–378.

71. Choji K, Shinohara M, Nojima T, et al. Significant reduction of the echogenicity of the compressed cavernous hemangioma. *Acta Radiol* 1988;29:317–320.

72. Solbiati L, Livraghi T, De Pra L, et al. Fine-needle biopsy of hepatic hemangioma with sonographic guidance. *AJR Am J Roentgenol* 1985;144:471–474.

73. Caturelli E, Rapaccini GL, Sabelli C, et al. Ultrasound-guided fine-needle aspiration biopsy in the diagnosis of hepatic hemangioma. *Liver* 1986;6:326–330.

74. Closset J, Veys I, Peny MO, et al. Retrospective analysis of 29 patients surgically treated for hepatocellular adenoma or focal nodular hyperplasia. *Hepatogastroenterology* 2000;47:1382–1384.

75. Hung CH, Changchien CS, Lu SN, et al. Sonographic features of hepatic adenomas with pathologic correlation. *Abdom Imaging* 2001;26:500–506.

76. Shamsi K, De Schepper A, Degryse H, et al. Focal nodular hyperplasia of the liver: radiologic findings. *Abdom Imaging* 1993;18:32–38.

77. Dill-Macky MJ, Burns PN, Khalili K, et al. Focal hepatic masses: enhancement patterns with SH U 508A and pulse-inversion US. *Radiology* 2002;222:95–102.

78. von Herbay A, Vogt C, Haussinger D. Pulse inversion sonography in the early phase of the sonographic contrast agent levovist: differentiation between benign and malignant focal liver lesions. *J Ultrasound Med* 2002;21:1191–1200.

79. Dietrich CF, Schall H, Kirchner J, et al. Sonographic detection of focal changes in the liver hilus in patients receiving corticosteroid therapy. *Z Gastroenterol* 1997;35:1051–1057.

80. Caturelli E, Squillante MM, Andriulli A, et al. Hypoechoic lesions in the "bright liver": a reliable indicator of fatty change. A prospective study. *J Gastroenterol Hepatol* 1992;7:469–472.

81. Aubin B, Denys A, Lafortune M, et al. Focal sparing of liver parenchyma in steatosis: role of the gallbladder and its vessels.[comment]. *J Ultrasound Med* 1994;14:77–80.

82. Marchal G, Tshibwabwa-Tumba E, Oyen R, et al. Correlation of sonographic patterns in liver metastases with histology and microangiography. *Invest Radiol* 1985;20:79–84.

83. Marchal GJ, Pylyser K, Tshibwabwa-Tumba EA, et al. Anechoic halo in solid liver tumors: sonographic, microangiographic, and histologic correlation. *Radiology* 1985;156:479–483.

84. Gruenberger T, Jourdan JL, Zhao J, et al. Echogenicity of liver metastases is an independent prognostic factor after potentially curative treatment. *Arch Surg* 2000;135:1285–1290.

85. Itai Y, Ohtomo K, Ohnishi S, et al. Ultrasonography of small hepatic tumors. *Radiat Med* 1987;5:14–19.

86. Hale HL, Husband JE, Gossios K, et al. CT of calcified liver metastases in colorectal carcinoma. *Clin Radiol* 1998;53:735–741.

87. Paley MR, Ros PR. Hepatic calcification. *Radiol Clin North Am* 1998;36:391–398.

88. Konno K, Ishida H, Sato M, et al. Liver tumors in fatty liver: difficulty in ultrasonographic interpretation. *Abdom Imaging* 2001;26:487–491.

89. Makuuchi M, Takayama T, Kosuge T, et al. The value of ultrasonography for hepatic surgery. *Hepatogastroenterology* 1991;38:64–70.

90. Sheu JC, Sung JL, Chen DS, et al. Ultrasonography of small hepatic tumors using high-resolution linear-array real-time instruments. *Radiology* 1984;150:797–802.

91. Sheu JC, Chen DS, Sung JL, et al. Hepatocellular carcinoma: US evolution in the early stage. *Radiology* 1985;155:463–467.

92. Makuuchi M, Hasegawa H, Yamazaki S, et al. Ultrasonic characteristics of the small hepatocellular carcinoma less than five centimeters in diameter, mosaic pattern of internal echoes and posterior echo enhancement. *Acta Hepatol Jpn* 1981;22:1740.

93. Ebara M, Ohto M, Shinagawa T, et al. Natural history of minute hepatocellular carcinoma smaller than three centimeters complicating cirrhosis. A study in 22 patients. *Gastroenterology* 1986;90:289–298.

94. Cottone M, Marceno MP, Maringhini A, et al. Ultrasound in the diagnosis of hepatocellular carcinoma associated with cirrhosis. *Radiology* 1983;147:517–519.

95. Kanematsu M, Hoshi H, Yamada T, et al. Small hepatic nodules in cirrhosis: ultrasonographic, CT, and MR imaging findings. *Abdom Imaging* 1999;24:47–55.

96. Caturelli E, Pompili M, Bartolucci F, et al. Hemangioma-like lesions in chronic liver disease: diagnostic evaluation in patients. *Radiology* 2001;220:337–342.

97. Wernecke K, Henke L, Vassallo P, et al. Pathologic explanation for hypoechoic halo seen on sonograms of malignant liver tumors: an in vitro correlative study. *AJR Am J Roentgenol* 1992;159:1011–1016.

98. Onik G, Kane R, Steele G, et al. Society of gastrointestinal radiologists Roscoe E. Miller award. Monitoring hepatic cryosurgery with sonography. *AJR Am J Roentgenol* 1986;147:665–669.

99. Gaitini D, Kopelman D, Soudak M, et al. Impact of intraoperative sonography on resection and cryoablation of liver tumors. *J Clin Ultrasound* 2001;29:265–272.

100. Machi J, Uchida S, Sumida K, et al. Ultrasound-guided radiofrequency thermal ablation of liver tumors: percutaneous, laparoscopic, and open surgical approaches. *J Gastrointest Surg* 2001;5:477–489.

101. Machi J, Oishi AJ, Mossing AJ, et al. Hand-assisted laparoscopic ultrasound-guided radiofrequency thermal ablation of liver tumors: a technical report. *Surg Laparosc Endosc Percut Tech* 2002;12:160–164.

102. Leyendecker JR, Dodd GD, 3rd, Halff GA, et al. Sonographically observed echogenic response during intraoperative radiofrequency ablation of cirrhotic livers: pathologic correlation. *AJR Am J Roentgenol* 2002;178:1147–1151.

103. Takayama T, Makuuchi M, Watanabe K, et al. A new method for mapping hepatic subsegment: counterstaining identification technique. *Surgery* 1991;109:226–229.

104. Nakamura S, Tsuzuki T. Surgical anatomy of the hepatic veins and the inferior vena cava. *Surg Gynecol Obstet* 1981;152:43–50.

105. Baer HU, Dennison AR, Maddern GJ, et al. Subtotal hepatectomy: a new procedure based on the inferior right hepatic vein. *Br J Surg* 1991;78:1221–1222.

Intraoperative Ultrasound of the Pancreas and Other Abdominal Organs

Junji Machi, Nicholas Zyromski, and Lawrence P. McChesney

Pancreatic surgery is generally associated with higher morbidity and mortality among general surgical operations. In spite of various preoperative imaging studies, accurate diagnosis or localization of pancreatic disease is often difficult until the time of surgery. Exploration of the pancreas requires meticulous tissue dissection, which may increase operative time and risk. Two imaging modalities have been employed during pancreatic operations to assist in such an exploration: intraoperative pancreatography and intraoperative ultrasound (IOUS). Although intraoperative pancreatography provides useful information in certain situations (e.g., pancreatic trauma), its clinical usefulness is limited. IOUS, on the other hand, offers a wider scope of information and is easily repeated during various pancreatic operations. In addition, IOUS can be used during laparotomy to assess for diseases of other abdominal and retroperitoneal organs, such as the gastrointestinal tract, the spleen, and the adrenal gland.

Real-time B-mode ultrasound was first introduced during pancreatic surgery in 1980 by Lane et al. and Sigel et al. (1,2). Since then, Machi and Sigel have used IOUS in the operative management of pancreatitis, pancreatic tumors (3–16), and diseases of other abdominal organs (17–21). This chapter reviews our experience and literature, and describes instrumentation and techniques, indications, clinical results, ultrasound images, advantages and limitations of IOUS of the pancreas and other intraabdominal and retroperitoneal organs during open surgery (laparotomy). Laparoscopic ultrasound of the pancreas and other organs are described in Chapter 17.

INSTRUMENTATION AND TECHNIQUES (Table 1)

Instrumentation

Real-time B-mode imaging or color/power Doppler imaging systems with frequency around 7.5 MHz are most frequently used for IOUS scanning of the pancreas and other abdominal organs (10–17). While superficial areas of the pancreas and other abdominal organs can be scanned with higher frequency (e.g., 10 MHz), deeper regions of the abdomen or retroperitoneum sometimes require lower frequency (e.g., 5 MHz). Chapter 13 describes the details of the scanner and the probe for IOUS as well as basic scanning techniques. When the operative field is limited or the region of interest is deeply located (e.g., obese patient), the use of a cylindrical (pencil-like) end-viewing probe may be needed. Otherwise, in the majority of operations, the pancreas and other abdominal organs can be examined with a flat side-viewing T- or I-shaped probe.

Scanning Techniques

Scanning of the pancreas can be performed at any time; however, acquiring new information that helps decide the type of operation to be performed necessitates that IOUS be used early in the course of the operation, even immediately after laparotomy and prior to any tissue dissection.

There are two approaches for IOUS scanning of the pancreas: indirect scanning through other structures and direct scanning of the exposed organ. Before performing surgical tissue dissection, the pancreas can be scanned indirectly through the stomach, duodenum, mesocolon, or gastrocolic or hepatogastric ligaments (Fig. 1). Particularly in a nonobese patient without marked abdominal fatty tissue, this indirect scanning is quite effective. The scanning is usually quick and convenient because tissue dissection is not needed. Direct scanning of the pancreas requires dissection to enter the lesser sac and exposure of the anterior surface of the pancreas. Most often, the best images of the pancreas are obtained by direct scanning (Fig. 2). During these scanning maneuvers, contact scanning and probe-standoff scanning should be appropriately used. When the pancreas is imaged through other structures or when deep areas of interest are imaged,

▶ **TABLE 1** Intraoperative Ultrasound Scanning
Techniques of the Pancreas and
Other Organs

1. 5–10 MHz (7.5 MHz) flat side-viewing T- or I-shaped probe
2. Scanning immediately after laparotomy and repeat scanning thereafter
3. Appropriate use of contact scanning and probe-standoff scanning with saline immersion
4. Pancreas: indirect and indirect scanning, longitudinal and transverse scanning
5. Delineation of intraabdominal and retroperitoneal vascular structures: color or power Doppler imaging
6. Localization of islet cell tumors: IOUS scanning with palpation after pancreas mobilization
7. Gastrointestinal tract: instillation of saline in the lumen
8. Spleen: saline immersion method, avoid splenic injury
9. IOUS-guided techniques for needle placement and tissue dissection

IOUS, intraoperative ultrasound.

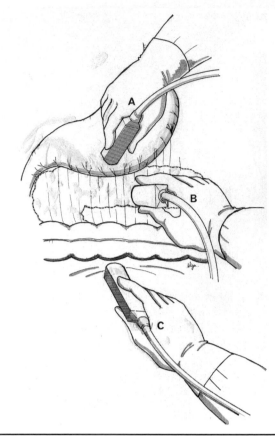

FIGURE 1. Indirect scanning of the pancreas through the stomach **(A)**, gastrocolic ligament **(B)**, and mesocolon **(C)**, using a cylindrical end-viewing probe. A flat probe can also be used.

contact scanning is usually used. On the other hand, when the surface or superficial areas of the exposed pancreas are imaged, probe standoff with saline immersion should be applied (Fig. 3).

For complete examination, the pancreas is examined thoroughly from the head to tail, generally from the anterior (ventral) side, using both longitudinal and transverse scanning (Fig. 4). Longitudinal scanning is conducted by placing the probe along the long axis of the pancreas and visualizing the main pancreatic duct in a longitudinal section (Fig. 5). The normal main pancreatic duct is almost always visualized by IOUS. In transverse scanning, a cross-section (transverse section) of the pancreas and the duct is delineated. For systematic examination of the entire organ, sliding and at times rotating, tilting, and rocking maneuvers are employed (Fig. 6). For the examination of the pancreatic head and uncinate process, scanning is also carried out from the right lateral or anterolateral side in addition to the anterior side. Mobilization of the duodenum (Kocher's maneuver) is rarely needed to scan the pancreatic head. This scanning approach is the same technique as scanning for distal biliary tract (Fig. 7) (see Chapter 14): the intrapancreatic bile duct and the periampullary region are best seen by this scanning. Throughout the IOUS examination of the pancreas, surrounding structures including blood vessels, such as the celiac artery branches, portal tributaries, aorta, mesenteric artery, vena cava, and renal vessels, are observed (Fig. 5).

Additional techniques should be used with special attention to the entire pancreas for IOUS of islet cell tumors, which are often small and multiple. For a combina-

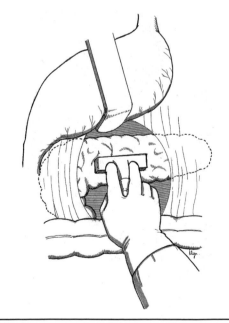

FIGURE 2. Direct scanning of the exposed pancreas after transection of the gastrocolic ligament, using a flat T-shaped side-viewing probe.

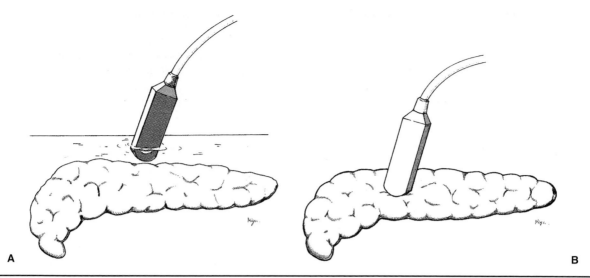

FIGURE 3. Probe-standoff scanning of the pancreas with saline immersion **(A)** and contact scanning of the pancreas **(B)**, using a cylindrical probe. A flat probe can also be used.

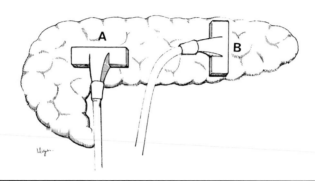

FIGURE 4. Longitudinal **(A)** and transverse **(B)** scanning of the pancreas using a flat T-shaped probe.

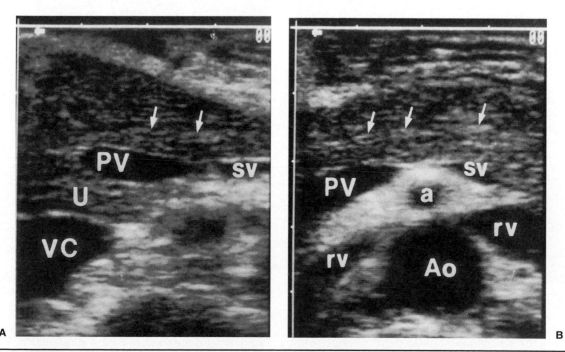

FIGURE 5. Longitudinal views of the normal pancreas along the course of the pancreatic duct. **A:** Pancreatic head and neck including uncinate process (U). The normal pancreatic duct (*arrows*) is delineated. PV, portal vein; SV, splenic vein; VC, vena cava. **B:** Pancreatic body. The duct (*arrows*) is delineated. Ao, aorta; a, superior mesenteric artery; rv, left renal vein.

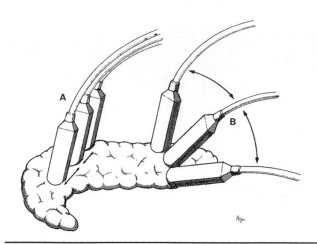

FIGURE 6. Probe manipulations to scan the pancreas, including sliding **(A)** and rocking maneuvers **(B)** . Although a cylindrical probe is shown here, the same probe maneuvers can be performed with a flat probe.

tion of thorough inspection and palpation and IOUS, the pancreas should be fully mobilized. The initial scanning can be performed before pancreas mobilization, and this may localize a tumor. However, because islet cell tumors (except for insulinoma) are often multiple, especially in multiple endocrine neoplasia (MEN) syndrome (type 1),

IOUS should be repeated after mobilization and palpation of the pancreas. After an extended Kocher maneuver and reflection of the spleen and the splenic flexure of the colon, the exposed pancreas is scanned using contact and probe standoff techniques (Figs. 3 and 8). It is helpful to scan the pancreas while palpation is performed simultaneously (Fig. 9). The entire pancreas is imaged both longitudinally and transversely. When a tumor is detected, its relation to the pancreatic duct is examined (Fig. 10). Particularly for gastrinomas, which are frequently located in extrapancreatic regions, IOUS scanning is extended to surrounding structures such as the gastrointestinal tract, especially the duodenum, hepatoduodenal ligament, mesocolon, mesenterium, and perivascular areas.

IOUS scanning of the gastrointestinal tract usually requires instillation of saline solution into its lumen (e.g., via nasogastric tube) in order to appropriately distend the wall (17–20). In addition, probe standoff is needed to image the anterior (superficial) wall of the gastrointestinal tract in order to keep it in the focal zone of the IOUS probe (Figs. 11 and 12).

The basic techniques for IOUS scanning of other intraabdominal and retroperitoneal organs or structures are the same as those of scanning of the pancreas or hepatobiliary systems. The appropriate use of contact scanning and probe-standoff scanning is important. The

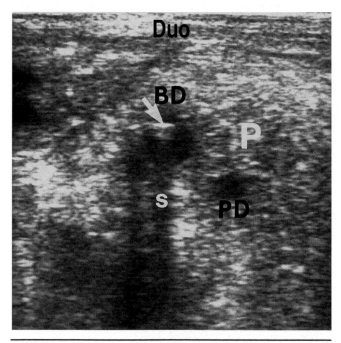

FIGURE 7. Pancreatic head demonstrated by scanning from the right anterolateral side. The distal bile duct (BD) and the pancreatic duct (PD) are seen within the pancreas (P). Transduodenal scanning is performed through the duodenum (Duo). A bile duct calculus (*arrows*) is present with acoustic shadowing (S).

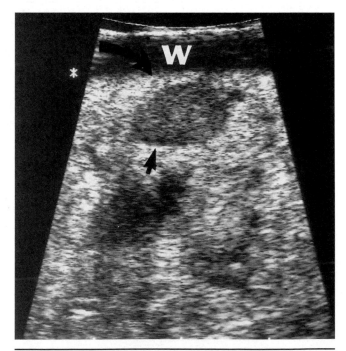

FIGURE 8. Probe-standoff scanning of the pancreas. An insulinoma (*small straight arrow*) is located near the pancreatic surface (*curved arrow*) and is clearly visualized. W indicates an acoustic window created by saline immersion for standoff scanning.

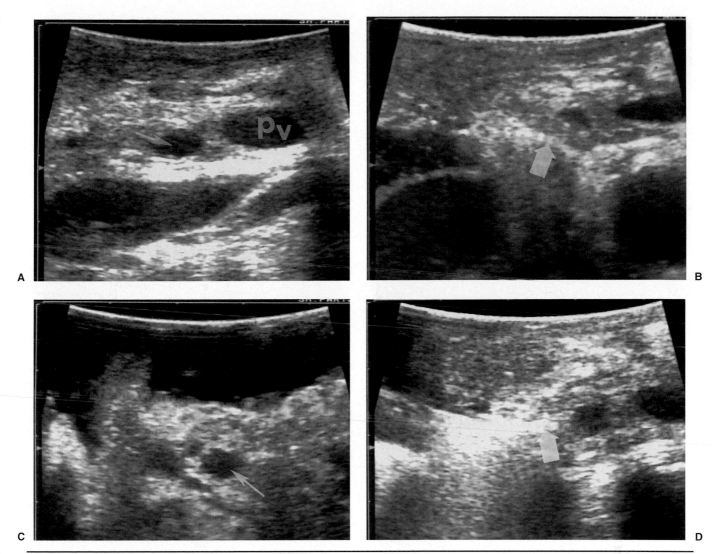

FIGURE 9. Pancreatic cyst, its palpation and needle aspiration. **A:** A 6 × 4 mm cyst (*arrow*) was detected in the head of pancreas by intraoperative scanning from the anterior side. **B:** After mobilization of the pancreatic head, the surgeon's inserted a finger (*arrow*) behind the pancreas to palpate the cyst. **C:** Scanning of the same cyst (*arrow*) for the posterolateral side. **D:** A curved needle (*arrow*) was guided by IOUS toward the cyst for aspiration. (Reproduced with permission from Yahara T, Machi J, McCarthy L. Negative intraoperative ultrasonography suggests islet cell hyperplasia in an adult patient with hyperinsulinemia. *Surg Rounds* 2002;25:30–32.)

organ or the region of interest should be scanned longitudinally and transversely and from various directions, using sliding, rotating, tilting, and rocking maneuvers. Because of its posterior (dorsal) location, the spleen is at times difficult to image, particularly when the operative field is limited. The saline immersion method is used for probe-standoff scanning and even for contact scanning, especially in the performance of tilting or rocking maneuvers. Care should be taken not to injure the spleen by excessive probe manipulation during IOUS scanning.

Intraoperative Color or Power Doppler Imaging

Intraoperative color or power Doppler imaging possesses several advantages, which are described in Chapter 13. In particular, quick delineation of vascular structures and distinction of vessels from other hypoechoic or anechoic areas by this modality are useful during pancreatic and other abdominal surgery (see Figs. 33, 35, and 36 in Chapter 13).

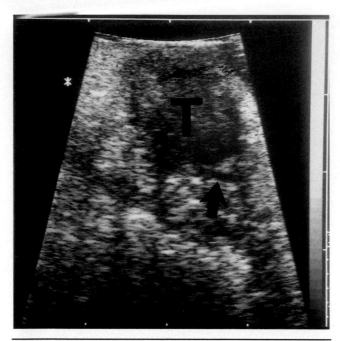

FIGURE 10. Scanning of an 18 mm insulinoma (T) in the pancreatic body, showing its relation to the main pancreatic duct (*arrow*).

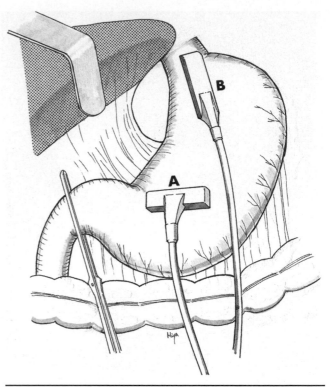

FIGURE 11. Scanning of the stomach antrum to body using a T-shaped probe **(A)** and scanning of the stomach cardia using an I-shaped probe **(B)** . The stomach is appropriately distended with saline solution.

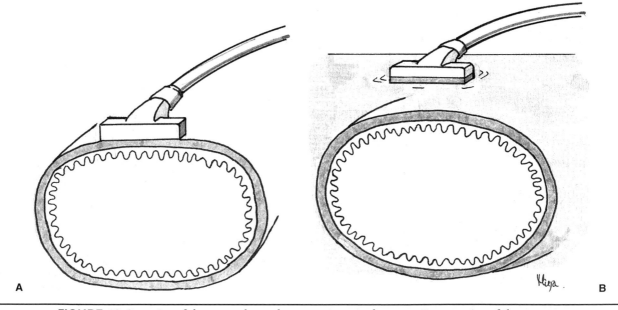

FIGURE 12. Scanning of the stomach or other gastrointestinal tract. **A:** For scanning of the posterior (deep) wall, contact scanning is performed by placing the probe on the anterior wall. **(B):** For scanning of the anterior (superficial) wall, probe-standoff scanning is performed by positioning the probe away from the wall with saline immersion.

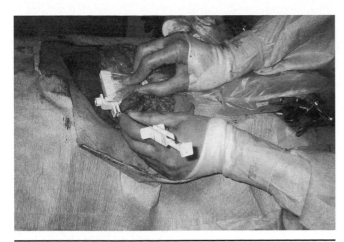

FIGURE 13. Intraoperative core needle biopsy of the pancreatic head under intraoperative ultrasound guidance using a needle guidance system attached to the probe.

Guidance Techniques

IOUS-guided techniques are used mainly for needle placement and for tissue dissection (see Chapter 13). A needle guidance system that is attachable to the IOUS probe is commercially available and is valuable in guiding a needle precisely into a target (Fig. 13); this helps prevent injuries to the pancreatic duct or vascular structures. For large targets, IOUS-guided needle placement procedures can be performed in a freehand fashion. A needle is best inserted into tissue from one lateral end side of the probe and advanced parallel to the scanning plane so that the entire shaft of the needle is displayed (Fig. 9) (see Chapter 4).

During pancreatic surgery, the procedure that most frequently involves IOUS guidance for tissue dissection is pancreatotomy for opening of the pancreatic duct as illustrated in Figure 45 of Chapter 13. The ultrasound probe is positioned over the pancreatic duct in a longitudinal manner and an exploratory needle is introduced into the center of the duct. Needle placement in the duct should be clearly demonstrated on the ultrasound image and is confirmed by aspiration of succus pancreaticus. Once proper needle placement is assured, the pancreatic tissue is incised along the needle until the duct is open (9). The same technique can be used to open pancreatic cysts, to approach small pancreatic tumors (e.g., enucleation of islet cell tumors), or to open abdominal abscesses.

NORMAL ULTRASOUND ANATOMY

Normal ultrasound anatomy of the pancreas and other abdominal organs is also described in Chapters 11 and 12. A few IOUS images of the pancreas are presented in

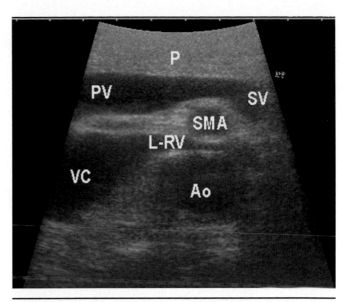

FIGURE 14. Normal pancreas (neck to body) and vascular structures. The echogenicity of the pancreas (P) is similar to that of retroperitoneal fatty tissue. PV, portal vein; SV, splenic vein; SMA, superior mesenteric artery; VC, vena cava; Ao, aorta; L-RV, left renal vein.

Figure 24 of Chapter 13. The normal pancreas appears as a homogeneous, echogenic structure lying in front of the portal and splenic veins (Fig. 14). The uncinate process may extend from the pancreatic head behind the portal-mesenteric vein (Fig. 5). The normal main pancreatic duct is visualized as a tubular structure, 2 to 3 mm in diameter, in the center of the pancreas (Fig. 5). The echo-

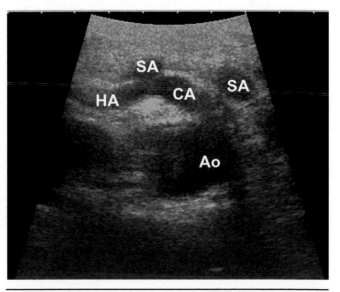

FIGURE 15. Transverse view of the aorta (Ao), from where the celiac artery (CA) and its branches are demonstrated. HA, common hepatic artery; SA, splenic artery.

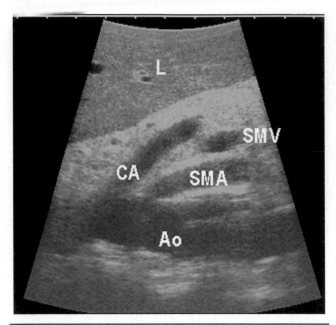

FIGURE 16. Longitudinal view of the aorta (Ao), from where the celiac artery (CA) and the superior mesenteric artery (SMA) are coming off. SMV, superior mesenteric vein. The scanning is performed using the liver (L) as an acoustic window.

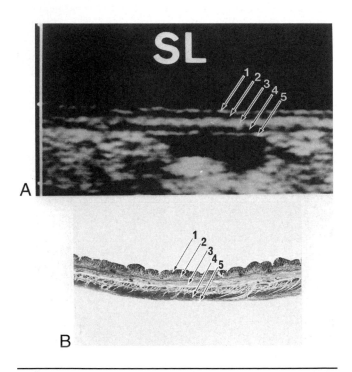

FIGURE 17. Normal ultrasound five-layer structure of the stomach wall (**A**) with its histologic structure (**B**). SL, stomach lumen. 1, the mucosal surface; 2, mucosa and muscularis mucosae; 3, submucosa; 4, muscularis propria; 5, serosa and subserosa.

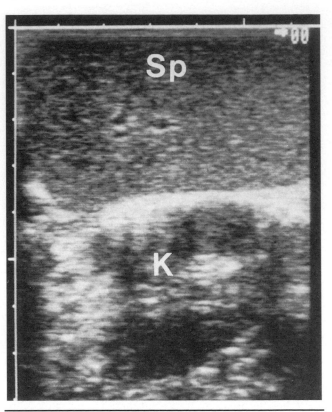

FIGURE 18. Normal spleen (Sp) demonstrated by contact scanning with the probe positioned under the left diaphragm. K, a part of the left kidney.

genicity of the pancreas increases gradually with aging: it becomes almost the same as the surrounding fatty retroperitoneal tissue in the elderly, and therefore the border of the pancreas becomes unclear. In such a circumstance, the pancreas is recognized by surrounding organs (stomach, duodenum) and vascular structures. Identification and delineation of intraabdominal and retroperitoneal vascular structures are particularly important (Fig. 5; see also Fig. 24B in Chapter 13). Figures 15 and 16 demonstrate transverse and longitudinal views of the celiac artery and other major vessels. Figure 17 demonstrates the normal five-layer structures of the gastric wall. Figure 18 demonstrates the normal spleen, showing a homogeneous echo texture. The spleen is normally slightly more echogenic than the liver.

INDICATIONS AND CLINICAL RESULTS

Pancreas

Pancreatic surgery has emerged as one of the important applications of IOUS (1–16,22–32); relevant surgical diseases of the pancreas include acute and chronic pancre-

▶ **TABLE 2** Indication for Intraoperative
Ultrasound of the Pancreas

1. Evaluation of complications of pancreatitis
2. Evaluation of pancreatic cancer and pancreatic cystic lesion
3. Localization or detection of islet cell tumor
4. Guidance of pancreatic surgical procedures

▶ **TABLE 4** Results of Intraoperative
Ultrasound During Operations
for Pancreatic Diseases

Disease	Number of Operations	IOUS Useful
Pancreatitis (mostly chronic)	194	144 (74.2%)
Pancreatic cancer	148	115 (77.7%)
Islet cell tumor	17	14 (82.4%)
Pancreatic cystic lesions and other neoplasms	14	11 (78.6%)
Total	373	284 (76.1%)

IOUS, intraoperative ultrasound.

atitis, pancreatic cancer, pancreatic cystic lesion, pancreatic islet cell tumor, and other rare neoplasms. From our experience during operations for these diseases (2–17), four indications for IOUS have been identified as listed in Table 2. New information obtained by IOUS for each pancreatic disease is summarized in Table 3. We have performed IOUS during 373 open operations for various pancreatic diseases. As summarized in Table 4, IOUS provided useful information to assist in the performance of pancreatic surgery in 76% of operations.

Pancreatitis

Chronic pancreatitis causes various complications including pancreatic duct dilatation, pseudocyst, intrapancreatic bile duct stenosis, and splenic or portal vein thrombosis. IOUS can provide accurate imaging information with which to diagnose, localize, or exclude these complications. Primary diagnosis of the complications of pancreatitis is usually made by preoperative imaging. However, IOUS can also diagnose previously unknown problems during the operation; in particular, IOUS may detect additional lesions or areas of disease when only a

▶ **TABLE 3** New Information Provided by
Intraoperative Ultrasound during
Pancreatic Surgery

1. Pancreatitis
   Detection, exclusion, or localization:
      Dilated pancreatic duct, pseudocyst, abscess
      Intrapancreatic bile duct stenosis, portal or splenic vein
         thrombosis
   Decision on internal drainage procedure
2. Pancreatic cancer
   Diagnosis of pancreatic cancer
   Determination of the extent of tumor spread (staging) and
      resectability
      Cancer invasion to blood vessel (particularly portal system),
         lymph node metastasis, liver metastasis
3. Pancreatic cystic lesion
   Distinction of simple cyst from cystic neoplasm
   Delineation of the lesion in relation to the duct and vessels
4. Islet cell tumor
   Localization of tumor, detection or exclusion of multiple tumors:
      Insulinoma, gastrinoma, other tumor (rare)

single lesion or area has been known preoperatively. For example, small pseudocysts may be identified only by IOUS during a pancreaticojejunostomy (Puestow's operation) for preoperatively diagnosed, dilated pancreatic duct. More commonly, IOUS is used to precisely localize a lesion. Because of chronic dense inflammation, even dilated pancreatic ducts or relatively large pseudocysts may be nonpalpable intraoperatively. The exact location of such lesions is quickly and readily demonstrated by IOUS, and if needed, an exploratory needle can be inserted under IOUS guidance for confirmation. By clearly delineating the pancreatic duct or pseudocyst, IOUS facilitates decisions regarding the type of operation to be performed. Prior to initiating a planned operation, the size of the duct can be accurately measured by IOUS, thus helping to decide whether pancreaticojejunostomy or, alternatively, pancreatic resection should be performed. Depending on IOUS findings regarding the exact location of a pseudocyst and its relation to the gastrointestinal tract, the site for internal drainage (i.e., stomach, duodenum, or jejunum) can be determined. IOUS is also helpful in excluding pathologic processes at sites where focal abnormality is suspected by preoperative studies or at operation. Pancreatic swelling may suggest the presence of a pseudocyst. IOUS discerns whether such a mass is cystic or solid due to inflammation. IOUS is less frequently beneficial during operations for acute pancreatitis because acute tissue inflammation with necrosis obscures ultrasound images. However, when surgical exploration makes it difficult to identify lesions or structures such as vascular and biliary systems, IOUS may be helpful. In particular, detection, localization, or exclusion of abscesses is often facilitated by IOUS.

We have performed IOUS procedures in 194 operations for pancreatitis: 173 for chronic pancreatitis and 21 for acute pancreatitis. Eighty-two of the chronic pancreatitis operations were for pseudocysts, and 11 of the acute pancreatitis operations were for abscesses. Of the 194 operations for pancreatitis, IOUS was deemed to be useful in 144 (74.2%). The main benefits provided by IOUS were acquisition of new imaging information to help guide surgical management early during operation and guidance of surgical procedures. On the basis of IOUS findings during 173 operations for chronic pancreatitis, previously planned surgical procedures were altered in 38 operations (22.0%): pancreatic resection was changed to internal drainage of the pancreatic duct in 12 operations, or vice versa in 8 operations, and the internal drainage sites (i.e., stomach, duodenum, or jejunum) of pseudocysts were changed in 18 operations.

Pancreatic Cancer

During pancreatic cancer surgery, IOUS is indicated for tumor diagnosis and staging. IOUS can assist in the diagnosis of pancreatic cancer by assessing the cause of obstructive jaundice and by guiding intraoperative biopsy. Patients often undergo laparotomy for obstructive jaundice without a preoperative tissue diagnosis. IOUS can quickly reveal the absence of bile duct calculi as a cause of jaundice. Even when a mass is palpable in the head of the pancreas, there is often uncertainty whether it is a tumor or a localized (focal) pancreatitis. At times, a definitive mass cannot be palpated because of the small size of the tumor or the presence of pancreatitis associated with a cancer. IOUS can generally distinguish pancreatic cancer from chronic pancreatitis, although such a distinction may be sometimes difficult based on IOUS images alone. A small cancer causing bile duct obstruction can be delineated in the pancreatic head or periampullary region. A palpable or even nonpalpable mass of the pancreas can be biopsied (when indicated) with the guidance of IOUS to establish a tissue diagnosis.

A more common use of IOUS in pancreatic cancer is to help determine the extent of spread and the resectability. Surgical exploration can promptly detect peritoneal dissemination and superficially located liver metastases; however, surgical exploratory evaluation of vessel invasion of tumor necessitates extensive tissue dissection. IOUS demonstrates the relationship of a tumor to blood vessels, particularly the superior mesenteric-portal vein, and can provide information of resectability based on vessel invasion prior to extensive tissue dissection. The superior accuracy of IOUS has been shown in diagnosing portal vein invasion of pancreatic cancer in comparison with preoperative studies (13–16,28,31). Liver metastasis is also more accurately diagnosed with IOUS than with preoperative studies or surgical exploration. Diagnosis of occult liver metastasis is of particular importance in avoiding noncurative major pancreatic resection. Regional lymph nodes, including nonpalpable ones, can be detected. Not only peripancreatic nodes but also paraaortic, periceliac, mesenteric, and other remote nodes are examined by IOUS prior to extensive tissue dissection. Lymph nodes that are suspicious for metastasis by IOUS may be selected and biopsied intraoperatively to determine the staging and resectability.

We have performed IOUS in 148 operations for pancreatic cancer. IOUS was considered to be useful in 115 (77.7%), mainly in determining the tumor extent and the resectability. In 50 operations, we compared the accuracy of IOUS in diagnosing portal vein invasion with preoperative studies, which included transabdominal ultrasound, computed tomography, and the portal venous phase of superior mesenteric arteriography (16). After preoperative studies and IOUS, in all operations surgical exploration of the portal vein and microscopic examination of specimens when resected were performed. Gross or microscopic examination confirmed the presence of portal vein invasion in 21 operations and the absence of invasion in 29 operations. The diagnostic capability of IOUS was significantly better than that of the combination of preoperative studies in terms of specificity, positive predictive value, and overall accuracy, as shown in Table 5.

Pancreatic Cystic Lesions

In addition to pseudocysts, various cystic lesions occur in the pancreas and include simple cyst, serous cystadenoma, mucinous cystadenoma or cystadenocarcinoma, and intraductal papillary mucinous tumor. The clinical and ultrasound features of these cystic lesions are also described in Chapter 20.

During laparotomy, IOUS can distinguish a simple cyst from other cystic lesions. When a simple cyst is delineated without multicystic features or a solid component, it is managed by IOUS-guided aspiration without resection. On the other hand, differentiation of cystic neoplasms (e.g., serous versus mucinous, etc.) is often difficult, even with IOUS imaging. IOUS can be used to demonstrate the lesion in relation to the pancreatic duct and vascular structures, to guide aspiration for cystic

▶ **TABLE 5 Comparison of Preoperative Studies and Intraoperative Ultrasound in Diagnosing Portal Vein Invasion by Pancreatic Cancer**

Factor	Preoperative Studies (%)	IOUS (%)
Sensitivity	76.2	90.5
Specificity	58.6	89.7 ($p < 0.05$)
Positive predictive value	57.1	86.4 ($p < 0.05$)
Negative predictive value	77.3	92.9
Overall accuracy	66.0	90.0 ($p < 0.01$)

IOUS, intraoperative ultrasound.

fluid analysis and biopsy for diagnosis, and to assist in resection of the cystic lesion. The extension of intraductal papillary tumor can be determined by IOUS, allowing for an adequate margin of resection.

Islet Cell Tumors

Pancreatic islet cell tumors are relatively uncommon but may pose surgically difficult problems. The metabolic effects of these hormonally active tumors are serious and in some cases life threatening. Many of these tumors (except insulinomas) are malignant. Although a wide variety of islet cell tumors occur, the two most common are insulinomas and gastrinomas. Insulinomas are generally benign, solitary, and intrapancreatic small neoplasms. Most measure less than 2 cm. On the other hand, more often gastrinomas are multiple and associated with MEN. Many gastrinomas are extrapancreatic. It is critical to precisely localize and completely resect these tumors at the time of surgery.

Preoperative localization of islet cell tumors has been performed by a variety of techniques, including standard noninvasive imaging studies, such as transabdominal ultrasound, computed tomography (CT), and magnetic resonance imaging (MRI), and invasive imaging methods, such as selective angiography, venous sampling with and without stimulation for elevated hormone, and endoscopic ultrasound (33–38). Recently, scintigraphy with radiolabeled analogs of somatostatin and positron emission tomography has been used with some success (39,40). Even with these preoperative studies, however, these tumors may remain elusive. Not infrequently, the surgeons need to attempt to find and remove them without precise knowledge of their location. Between 20% and 60% of insulinomas and between 30% and 50% of gastrinomas are not imaged prior to surgery (33–35,41–51). The greatest morbidity and mortality in operations for pancreatic islet cell tumors occur when precise localization cannot be made and extensive blind pancreatic resection is performed.

IOUS has had a major influence on the surgical management of islet cell tumors, especially insulinomas. In many cases, IOUS is capable of localizing tumors that have not been detected by preoperative imaging and are not visible or palpable at surgery (34,35,41–51). Because of their characteristic hypoechoic nature, islet cell tumors as small as 3 to 4 mm can be delineated by IOUS. IOUS decreases operating time by confirming the suspected location of the lesion and by showing its relationship to the major vessels and the pancreatic duct. When an IOUS scan shows a tumor that has not been localized preoperatively and is not palpable at surgery, a potential surgical failure can be turned into a success. IOUS also

may diagnose multiple islet cell tumors or may exclude previously suspected multiple tumors.

Islet cell tumors within the pancreatic parenchyma can be detected by IOUS with a high degree of accuracy; however, extrapancreatic tumors are more difficult to detect. Therefore, IOUS is more effective for insulinoma than gastrinoma because most insulinomas are located within the pancreas. The detectability (localization capability) of preoperative studies, IOUS, and intraoperative palpation for insulinoma and gastrinoma is summarized in Table 6 (41,43–45,47,49). A combination of surgical exploration with inspection and palpation and IOUS provides the best means to detect and localize islet cell tumors; more than 90% to 95% of tumors can be detected utilizing this intraoperative combination. For this reason, some recommend that routine, extensive preoperative localization studies not be performed except for reoperations for recurrent or persistent disease. For malignant islet cell tumors, IOUS can be used to determine the extent of disease, particularly liver metastasis.

The resection of islet cell tumors is also facilitated with the assistance of IOUS. Once the tumor has been identified, its distance to the margins of the pancreas and its relationship to the pancreatic duct and adjacent vital structures can be ascertained; such information may be used to plan the extent of resection. If enucleation of the tumor is to be performed, IOUS can be used to find the most direct route through the least amount of surrounding pancreas; the enucleation is carried out by intermittent scanning until the tumor can be directly visualized.

Guidance of Pancreatic Procedures

Guidance of various pancreatic procedures is a useful application of IOUS. IOUS can assist needle placement for intraoperative biopsy of tumors or aspiration of cystic

▶ **TABLE 6** Detectability (Localization) of Islet Cell Tumors by Various Methods

Method	Tumor Type	Detectability (%)
Preoperative ultrasound:		15–59
Computed tomography		36–60
Arteriography		53–75
Intraoperative palpation	Insulinoma	42–88
	Pancreatic gastrinoma	91
	Extrapancreatic gastrinoma	100
Intraoperative ultrasound	Insulinoma	83–100
	Pancreatic gastrinoma	95
	Extrapancreatic gastrinoma	58

lesions. Under IOUS guidance, a needle can be inserted into the exact location of the target lesion and inadvertent injury to blood vessels or the pancreatic duct can be prevented. For small islet cell tumors, enucleation after localization is facilitated with the use of IOUS guidance. During pancreaticojejunostomy for chronic pancreatitis, IOUS-guided pancreatotomy is generally performed quickly and safely despite the duct often being nonpalpable due to inflammation (see Chapter 13). In a similar manner, opening of a pseudocyst for drainage can be performed with relative ease using IOUS for guidance.

When a patient with advanced pancreatic cancer has significant pain, intraoperative celiac ganglion block can be performed under IOUS guidance. Tissue dissection around the celiac artery is not required. The aorta and the celiac artery are identified, and alcohol is injected on both sides of the aorta using a long needle guided by IOUS.

Gastrointestinal Tract (Table 7)

The most common use of IOUS during surgery for gastrointestinal cancer (i.e., colorectal cancer, gastric cancer) is to screen the liver for metastasis or to evaluate metastatic liver tumors (see Chapter 15). In addition, IOUS can be used to evaluate the depth of tumor invasion, vascular invasion, and lymph node metastasis, all of which are important factors in determining the cancer stage (15–20,52,53).

> **TABLE 7 Indications for Intraoperative Ultrasound of Other Abdominal Organs**

Gastrointestinal tract
Localization of small gastrointestinal cancer (tumor)
Determination of the staging and resectability: gastric and esophageal cancer
Depth of tumor invasion, vascular invasion, lymph node and liver metastasis
Spleen
Evaluation of preoperatively suspected lesions
Guidance of needle placement
Localization of accessory spleen
Adrenal gland
Localization and detection of small adrenal tumors
Evaluation of large or malignant adrenal tumors
Retroperitoneum
Evaluation of primary retroperitoneal sarcomas
Detection of suspicious metastatic retroperitoneal lymph nodes
Localization and guidance of procedures for recurrent retroperitoneal or pelvic cancers
Abdominal abscess
Localization, needle guidance and drainage assistance
Abdominal vascular surgery
Localization of veins during shunts for portal hypertension
Post-reconstruction assessment

On high-resolution ultrasound images, the wall of the gastrointestinal tract exhibits a five-layer appearance, which corresponds to the layered structures obtained on histologic examination. IOUS can demonstrate distortion or destruction of the normal five-layer configuration as a result of cancer invasion. Thus, the depth of tumor invasion and intramural lateral tumor extension can be determined by IOUS (18–20,53). This IOUS information is similar to that provided by endoscopic ultrasound (see Chapter 20). IOUS can localize early gastric cancers that are sometimes not palpable during the operation. Nonpalpable colonic cancers can also be localized by IOUS (54).

During surgery for gastric cancer, dissection of perigastric lymph nodes is usually not difficult. However, dissection of lymph nodes remote to the stomach, in particular paraaortic lymph nodes, is technically more difficult and time consuming. Therefore, diagnosis of metastases to these lymph nodes by an imaging study is helpful for surgeons. For this reason, we evaluated the accuracy of IOUS in diagnosing paraaortic lymph node metastasis in 30 gastric cancer operations (20). The sensitivity, specificity, and overall accuracy of IOUS in diagnosing paraaortic lymph node metastasis were 100%, 84.6%, and 90.9%, respectively. IOUS was significantly superior to preoperative ultrasound and CT.

Vascular invasion of gastrointestinal cancer such as aortic invasion of esophageal cancer can also be assessed by IOUS. Most gastrointestinal cancer operations can be completed without the use of IOUS; however, IOUS can provide useful and at times critical findings, such as lymph node or liver metastases and vascular invasion, which may determine the resectability of these cancers. Prelaparotomy laparoscopy with laparoscopic ultrasound for esophagogastric cancers has became popular to obtain similar information; this is discussed in Chapter 17.

Spleen

The use of IOUS of the spleen is uncommon. The main indication is to evaluate preoperatively suspected or questionable splenic lesions, to guide needle placement for aspiration or biopsy, and to localize an accessory spleen. Preoperative studies, such as CT, may at times show lesions in the spleen in patients with abdominal malignancy. During laparotomy, IOUS can quickly distinguish cystic from solid splenic lesions; cystic lesions can be observed or aspirated under IOUS guidance. If indicated, splenic abscesses can be drained under IOUS guidance in a manner similar to liver abscess drainage. Lymphoma, leukemia, or metastatic tumors may involve the spleen. IOUS-guided biopsy can be performed for these solid tumors. Radiofrequency thermal ablation of metastatic splenic tumors is also feasible under IOUS guidance, similar to ablation of metastatic liver tumors. Although an accessory spleen is usually detected by preoperative imaging methods, its intraoperative localization is sometimes difficult during reoperation for recurrent hematologic disorders. IOUS can promptly localize an accessory spleen, even deep in abdominal tissues, thereby facilitating accessory splenectomy.

Adrenal Gland

The majority of adrenal operations are currently performed laparoscopically, and laparoscopic ultrasound has appeared to be a useful adjunct (see Chapter 17). When open adrenal surgery is performed, IOUS can also be utilized. Although cystic lesions can be readily distinguished from solid adrenal tumors, differentiation of various tumors by IOUS imaging alone is difficult. IOUS is helpful in quickly localizing small adrenal tumors (e.g., aldosteronoma) and in demonstrating surrounding structures, particularly vascular structures, so as to facilitate tissue dissection directly to the tumor. For large and particularly malignant adrenal tumors, IOUS may demonstrate tumor invasion into surrounding structures and help determine the resectability. IOUS can also be used to identify bilateral or multicentric adrenal tumors.

Retroperitoneum

For primary retroperitoneal tumors, mostly sarcomas, IOUS may be used to evaluate for local invasion as well as for lymph node and liver metastasis. More frequently, IOUS is used to evaluate retroperitoneal or pelvic lymph nodes during cancer surgery of hepatobiliary, pancreas, gastrointestinal tract, and other abdominal organs. Particularly, lymph nodes that are not easily dissected (e.g., paraaortic lymph nodes, retropancreatic lymph nodes) can be assessed quickly; if suspicious nodes are detected by IOUS, these are selectively biopsied for histologic examination. In such instances, IOUS-guided needle biopsy can be performed.

Gastrointestinal, renal, or other abdominal cancers may recur in the retroperitoneum or pelvis. Surgical resection is indicated in selected patients with such recurrence. Because of adhesions and disrupted anatomy from previous surgeries, localization and surgical exploration of recurrent tumors is often difficult and time consuming. IOUS is helpful in such a circumstance, an example of which is reoperation for recurrent rectal cancer in the pelvis after previous resection and radiation. After intraoperative localization or detection of such tumors, IOUS can be used to determine the resectability and to guide needle biopsy when indicated. Retroperitoneal and pelvic recurrent cancers can also be treated by radiofrequency ablation under IOUS guidance as well as transabdominal ultrasound guidance (55).

Abdominal Abscess

Most intraabdominal and retroperitoneal abscesses are currently managed by CT or ultrasound-guided percutaneous drainage. However, when open surgical drainage is required (due to lack of percutaneous access), surgical exploration and dissection may be difficult due to inflammation or previous surgery. IOUS facilitates precise localization, exploratory needle aspiration, and appropriate drainage of such abscesses (17,21).

Abdominal Vascular Surgery

There are two principal types of abdominal vascular surgery for IOUS that may be of assistance: bypass procedures for aortoiliac and renovascular diseases, and portal systemic shunt for decompression of portal hypertension. Post-reconstruction assessment after bypass operations can be performed by IOUS to detect or exclude intimal flaps, anastomotic strictures, or thrombi (see Chapter 8). During operation for portal hypertension, especially splenorenal and mesocaval shunt, initial IOUS is of particular help in identifying veins such as the splenic, renal, and mesenteric veins and the vena cava. Precise localization of these veins can minimize tissue dissection, which is often associated with bleeding due to portal hypertension. After shunt procedures, IOUS can be repeated to assess the integrity of the vascular anastomosis.

Other Organs or Pathologic Processes

In a similar fashion to other abdominal cancers, during gynecologic cancer operation, particularly for ovarian cancer, IOUS can be used to evaluate for local tumor extension as well as lymph node and liver metastasis. Foreign bodies in the abdomen can be localized and their removal facilitated by IOUS.

Whenever laparotomy is performed for pathologic processes or diseases that might be difficult to access or detect intraoperatively, it would be a good idea to have IOUS available so that the surgeon can use it when appropriate.

ULTRASOUND IMAGES OF PATHOLOGIC PROCESSES

Images of pathologic lesions of the pancreas and other abdominal organs are also shown in Chapters 11 and 12.

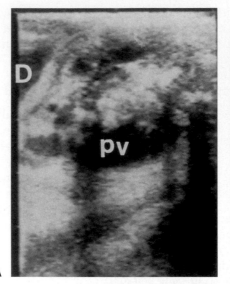
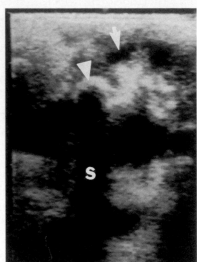

FIGURE 19. **A:** Pancreatic head. Chronic pancreatitis showing hyperechogenicity with significant calcifications. D, duodenum; PV, portal vein. **B:** Pancreatic body. The ductal lumen (*arrow*) was seen. There was a large pancreatic duct calculus (*arrowhead*) accompanied by an acoustic shadow (S).

Pancreatitis

Sonographically, chronic pancreatitis is characterized by increased echogenicity of pancreatic parenchyma, frequently associated with calcifications (Fig. 19). At times, calcifications are so intense that deep penetration of sound becomes limited. In such instances, the pancreas should be imaged from different locations and angles.

In chronic pancreatitis, the pancreatic ducts may be normal in size but are more often dilated (Fig. 20). The lumen of the ducts is usually anechoic, and its diameter can be quickly and easily measured. At times, the ducts are associated with a combination of strictures and dilatations, thus producing a "chain of lakes" appearance.

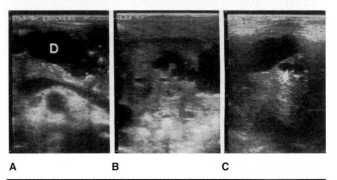

FIGURE 20. Chronic pancreatitis with dilated pancreatic ducts. **A:** Pancreatic neck showing the significantly dilated main pancreatic duct (D). **B and C:** Pancreatic body to tail showing a "chain of lakes" appearance. An arrow indicates a dilated duct branch.

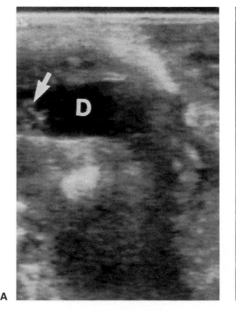
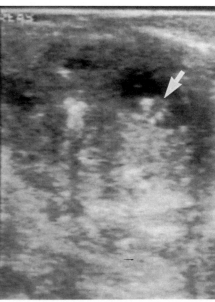

FIGURE 21. A pancreatic duct calculus (*arrow*) in a dilated pancreatic duct (D) with chronic pancreatitis. **A:** Longitudinal section of the pancreas. **B:** Transverse section of the pancreas. This particular calculus was not associated with an acoustic shadow.

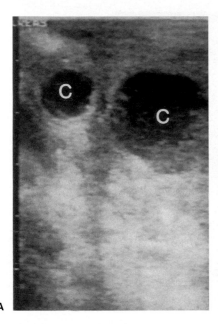

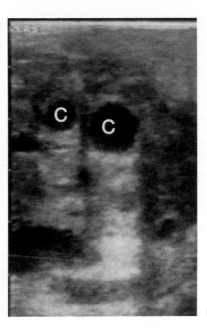

A   B

FIGURE 22. Multiple pancreatic pseudocysts. Cysts were associated with posterior enhancement. **A:** Two preoperatively known pseudocysts (C) in the head of the pancreas were localized by intraoperative ultrasound (IOUS). **B:** Two additional pseudocysts (C) were detected by IOUS in the body of the pancreas. These are 8 mm and 4 mm in size.

Pancreatic duct calculi are occasionally present in the ducts. These calculi are sonographically similar to bile duct calculi and are hyperechoic, but they may or may not be associated with acoustic shadows (Figs. 19 and 21). When the pancreatic ducts are full of calculi (although such situations are uncommon), delineation of the duct lumen and its measurement may become difficult on IOUS examination.

Pancreatic pseudocysts are readily detected on IOUS due to their anechoic appearance and associated posterior enhancement (Fig. 22). Pseudocysts as small as 2 to 3 mm can be detected. At times, pseudocysts contain de-

bris or sludge (Fig. 23). The size, the distance between multiple cysts, and the relation to blood vessels can be determined; such information helps in the performance of drainage procedures (Figs. 24 and 25). The relation of pseudocysts to the stomach and duodenum can be delineated (Figs. 26 and 27). This information is valuable in selecting the stomach, duodenum, or jejunum as the preferred site for internal drainage.

In contradistinction to chronic pancreatitis, acute pancreatitis shows an overall hypoechoic appearance or a mixed echo pattern due to edema or associated necrotic

(text continues on page 378)

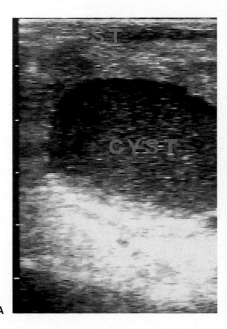

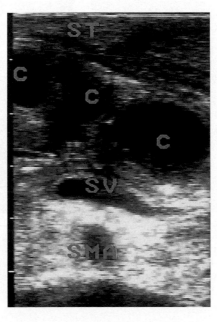

A   B

FIGURE 23. Multiple pancreatic pseudocysts. Scanning was performed through the stomach (ST). **A:** A large pseudocysts (CYST) containing debris showing intracystic echoes. **B:** Smaller pseudocysts (C) with little debris. SV, splenic vein; SMA, superior mesenteric artery.

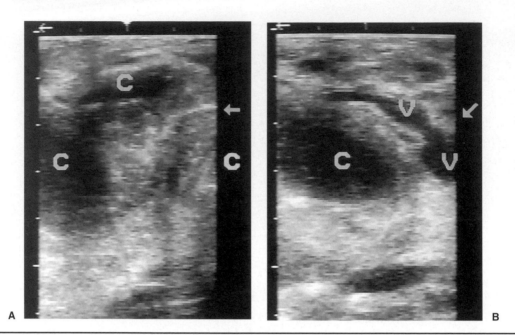

FIGURE 24. The relation of blood vessels to pancreatic pseudocysts for internal drainage. **A:** After cystotomy of a large pseudocyst, a finger (*arrow*) was inserted in the cyst to determine its relation to other cysts (C) in order to drain one cyst to another. These cysts were in the pancreatic body. **B:** In the pancreatic head, another cyst (C) was present. However, there was an intervening vein (V), detected by intraoperative ultrasound. Therefore, this cyst was drained separately.

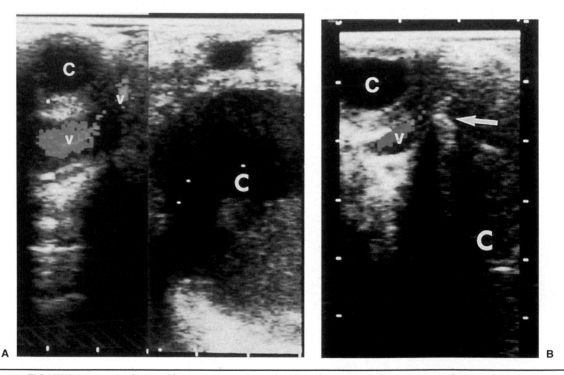

FIGURE 25. A vein detected by intraoperative color Doppler imaging between pseudocysts during an operation for chronic pancreatitis. **A:** Color Doppler imaging demonstrated a venous branch (v) between a preoperatively known large pseudocyst (C) and an intraoperative ultrasound–detected small pseudocyst (C). (See Color Plate 29.) **B:** After cystotomy of the large cyst, a metal probe (*arrow*) was introduced into the large cyst to examine the relation of the two cysts to the intervening vein (v). (See Color Plate 30.)

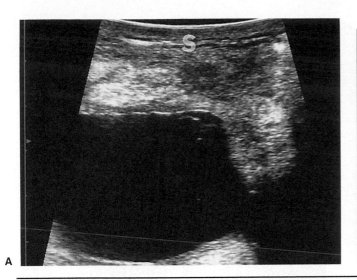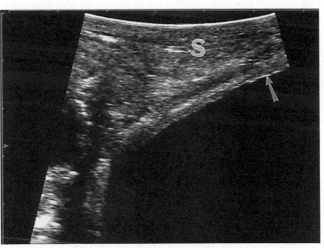

FIGURE 26. The relation of a pseudocyst to the stomach (S) for internal drainages. **A:** There were thick tissues between the stomach and cyst. It was not a good location for drainage. **B:** The site of cyst-gastrostomy was selected (*arrow*) where the stomach was in direct contact with the cyst wall.

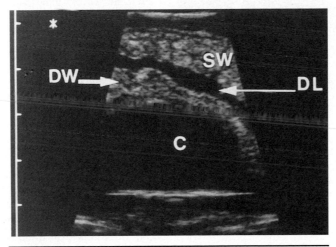

FIGURE 27. Pancreatic pseudocyst and its relation to the duodenum. The anatomic relation of the cyst (C) to the duodenal wall (DW), duodenal lumen (DL), and stomach wall (SW) was clearly understood. On the basis of this intraoperative ultrasound finding, cystoduodenostomy was performed for internal drainage.

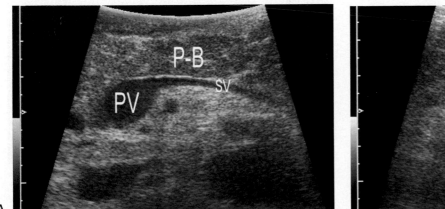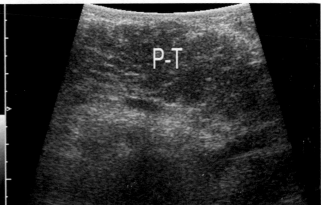

FIGURE 28. Acute pancreatitis. Hypoechoic, heterogeneous, and swollen pancreatic body (**A:** P-B) to tail (**B:** P-T). It was not so severe pancreatitis. PV, portal vein; SV, splenic vein.

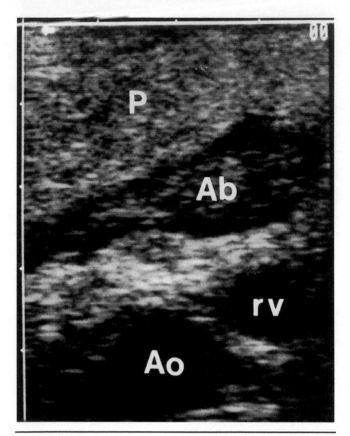

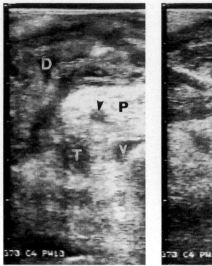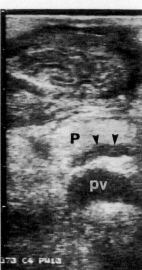

FIGURE 30. A small hypoechoic periampullary cancer diagnosed by intraoperative ultrasound. Preoperative studies failed to identify a tumor. **A:** Scanning through the duodenum (D) demonstrated a 9 × 11 mm hypoechoic tumor (T). P, pancreatic head; V, portal vein, which was partially compressed by compression maneuver of the probe. **B:** A mildly dilated pancreatic duct (*arrowheads*) at the neck of the pancreas (P). PV, portal vein.

FIGURE 29. A pancreatic abscess associated with acute pancreatitis. Intraoperative ultrasound revealed multiple abscesses including a relatively small abscess (Ab) behind the pancreas (P). It was difficult to locate this abscess by surgical exploration alone. Ao, aorta; rv, left renal vein.

and hemorrhagic tissue (Fig. 28). Anatomy is distorted, and images of structures are frequently indistinct. Pancreatic abscesses are cystic, but usually less well defined, and contain debris (Fig. 29). Because of these features, abscesses, especially small ones, are more difficult to identify with IOUS than are pseudocysts.

Pancreatic Cancer

Pancreatic cancers are usually relatively hypoechoic as compared with normal pancreatic tissue, especially when small, although large tumors show a mixed pattern. Pancreatic head or periampullary cancers are at times associated with chronic pancreatitis because of duct obstruction. In such instances, there is a greater difference in echogenicity between cancer (hypoechoic) and pancreatitis (hyperechoic), and this facilitates the detection of small pancreatic tumors. With IOUS, pancreatic tumors as small as 1 cm are readily detectable (Fig. 30). Ampullary adenomas are also hypoechoic; therefore, the dis-

tinction between adenoma and carcinoma is generally difficult sonographically (Fig. 31).

Portal vein or superior mesenteric vein invasion is one of the most important findings that IOUS may provide. When there is a distinct distance between a detected tumor and the vein, the absence of vessel invasion is obvious on IOUS examination (Figs. 30 and 32). When the vein is surrounded (encased) by a tumor, causing a stric-

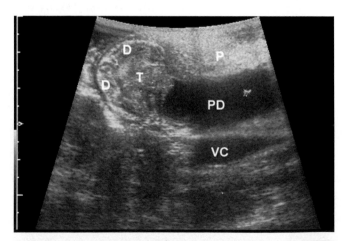

FIGURE 31. Ampullary adenoma (T), 16 × 15 mm, obstructing the pancreatic duct (PD), which was markedly dilated. Ultrasonically it cannot be distinguished from carcinoma. P, pancreatic head; D, duodenal wall; VC, vena cava.

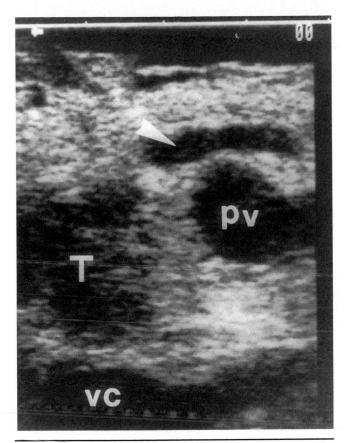

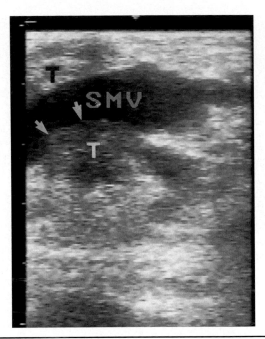

FIGURE 34. Portal vein invasion of a pancreatic cancer. The growth (*arrows*) of the tumor (T) was diagnosed at the junction of the superior mesenteric vein (SMV) to the portal vein. The tumor was 5 cm in size, and only a part of the tumor was displayed in this image.

FIGURE 32. Pancreatic head cancer without invasion to the portal vein. The tumor (T) was hypoechoic, 2 × 2. 5 cm in size, and was away from the portal vein (PV). An arrowhead indicates dilated pancreatic duct secondary to cancer. VC, vena cava.

ture (Fig. 33), or when tumor growth (Fig. 34) or a tumor thrombus (Fig. 35) is visualized within the venous lumen on IOUS images, the diagnosis of portal vein invasion is highly likely. On the other hand, when the vein is abutted by the tumor, the wall of the vein (which is echogenic)

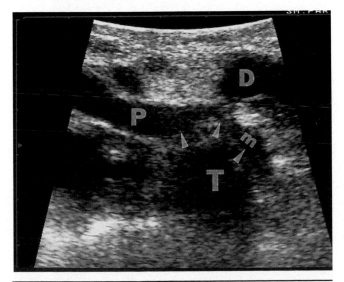

FIGURE 33. Pancreatic cancer with invasion to the portal vein. Intraoperative ultrasound scanning was performed along the course of the portal vein (P) and superior mesenteric vein (m). The tumor (T) was causing a significant stricture of the veins (*arrowheads*). D, dilated pancreatic duct.

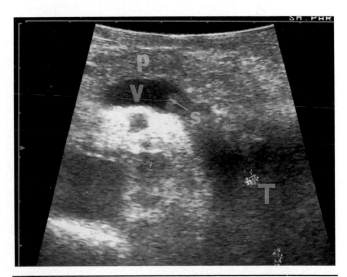

FIGURE 35. Pancreatic body cancer with a tumor thrombus. From the tumor (T) of the body of pancreas, a tumor thrombus in the splenic vein (S) was extending (*arrow*) to the portal vein (V). P, pancreatic neck.

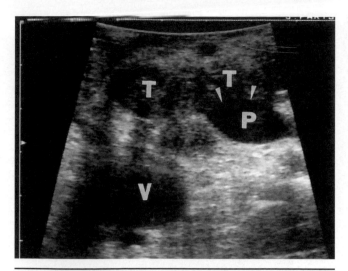

FIGURE 36. Pancreatic cancer with portal vein invasion. The anterior wall of the portal vein (P) was distorted (*arrowheads*) by the hypoechoic tumor (T), strongly suggesting the vein invasion. Surgical dissection and exploration confirmed this diagnosis of portal vein invasion. V, vena cava.

should be carefully examined. Abutment of a tumor to the intact echogenic wall of the vein suggests that tumor invasion is not likely. However, when the echogenic vessel wall is distorted or destroyed by a hypoechoic tumor, a diagnosis of portal vein invasion is likely (Fig. 36). The

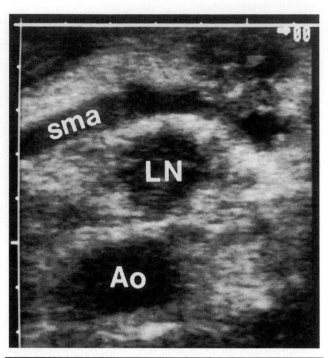

FIGURE 37. Metastatic lymph node from a pancreatic cancer. Intraoperative ultrasound scanning before tissue dissection showed this 2 cm hypoechoic roundish lymph node (LN) near the superior mesenteric artery (sma). This was ultrasonically diagnosed as a metastatic superior mesenteric lymph node, and was confirmed by intraoperative biopsy. Ao, aorta.

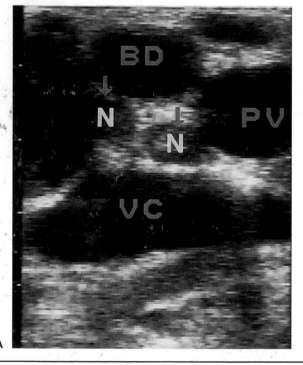

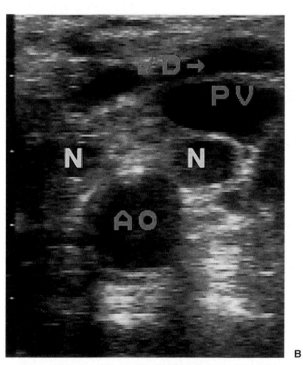

FIGURE 38. Suspicious lymph nodes for metastases from pancreatic cancer. **A:** Retropancreatic lymph nodes (N, *arrows*). BD, dilated bile duct; PV, portal vein; VC, vena cava. **B:** Periaortic lymph nodes (N). D with arrows, dilated pancreatic duct; PV, portal vein; Ao, aorta. When intraoperative ultrasound detects such nodes, intraoperative biopsy is needed.

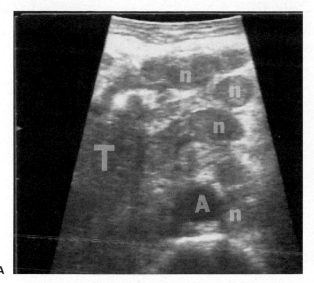

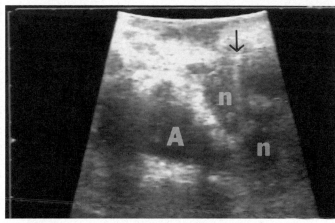

FIGURE 39. Intraoperative ultrasound (IOUS)–guided celiac ganglion block in a patient with unresectable pancreatic cancer causing pain. **A:** Multiple metastatic periaortic and periceliac lymph nodes (n). T, pancreatic tumor; A, aorta. **B:** Under IOUS guidance, a needle (*arrow*) was inserted (without any tissue dissection) toward the left side of the aorta (A) at the level of the celiac artery. Alcohol injection was performed on both sides of the aorta.

same diagnostic criteria of IOUS can be used to determine cancer invasion or involvement of arteries such as the hepatic artery.

Obstruction by tumor and proximal dilatation of the bile duct and the pancreatic duct are readily visualized by IOUS (Figs. 30, 32, and 33). Liver metastasis from pancreatic cancer most frequently demonstrates a hypoechoic or mixed pattern, although a hyperechoic appearance may be seen on rare occasions. IOUS can detect peripancreatic or remote lymph nodes as small as 3 to 4 mm. Metastatic nodes are more likely to be large (long axis more than 10 to 15 mm), roundish (the ratio of the short axis to the long axis greater than 0.5), have a well-defined border, and be diffusely hypoechoic or mixed in their echo patterns (Fig. 37). Although a final diagnosis is made by histologic examination, IOUS helps to identify suspicious lymph nodes (Fig. 38) and to select them for biopsy during operation. IOUS-guided celiac ganglion block for pancreatic cancer pain control is shown in Figure 39.

Pancreatic Cystic Lesions and Other Neoplasms

Besides pancreatic pseudocysts, IOUS can delineate other cystic diseases of the pancreas as well as their relation to surrounding structures. Figures 9 and 40 show a simple pancreatic cyst that was aspirated under IOUS guidance. Figure 41 shows a cystadenoma demonstrating a microcystic and solid pattern (see Fig. 36 in Chapter 13). Figure 42 shows a cystadenocarcinoma demonstrat-

ing a macrocystic pattern. There are many other uncommon pancreatic neoplasms; a solid cystic papillary tumor is shown in Figure 43.

Islet Cell Tumors

A pancreatic islet cell tumor usually (more than 90% of the time) appears as a distinct, round, homogeneous, hypoechoic mass within the pancreas (Figs. 8, 10, and 44). On occasion (less than 10% of the time) it may be iso-

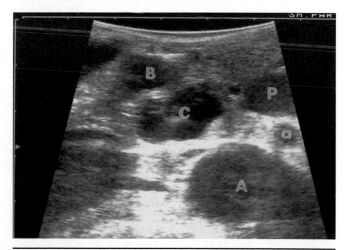

FIGURE 40. A simple pancreatic cyst (C), 2 × 1 cm in size, in the head of pancreas. B, bile duct; P, portal vein; a, superior mesenteric artery; A, aorta.

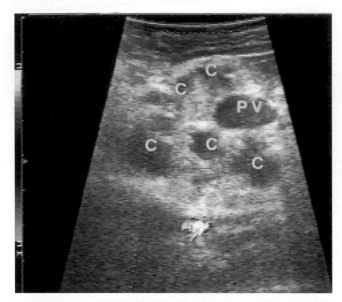

FIGURE 41. Cystadenoma of the pancreas. The tumor contained multiple small cystic (C) and tumorous (T) components. The portal vein (PV) was partly encased but not invaded by the tumor (see Fig. 36 in Chapter 13 for color Doppler image of the same lesion).

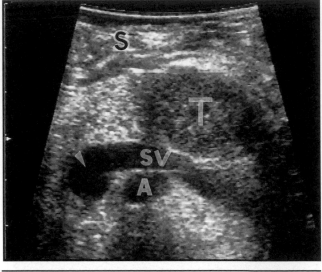

FIGURE 43. Solid cystic papillary tumor of the body of pancreas. Indirect intraoperative scanning through the stomach (S) showed a solid hypoechoic heterogeneous tumor, difficult to distinguish from an adenocarcinoma sonographically. A histology after resection made this diagnosis. SV, splenic vein; A, superior mesenteric artery; (*arrowhead*) portal vein.

echoic with a hypoechoic rim. Large islet cell tumors, such as nonfunctioning tumors, may exhibit a heterogeneous mixed echo pattern, at times associated with cystic areas due to tumor necrosis. Some islet cell tumors show increased vascularity as compared with the adjacent pan-

creas if color Doppler imaging is used (Fig. 45); others do not show increased flow. If a possible lesion is encountered, the probe should be rotated while keeping the lesion in view so as to ensure that it is a true lesion (Fig. 46). Extrapancreatic gastrinomas are also usually hypoechoic

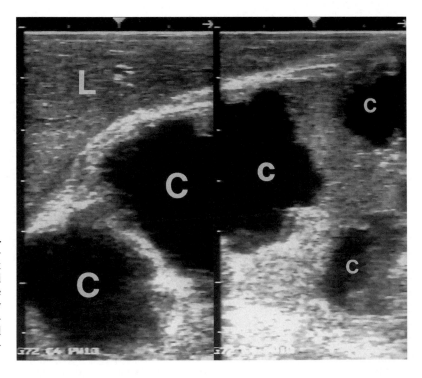

FIGURE 42. Cystadenocarcinoma of the pancreas. Transhepatic scanning through the left lateral segment of the liver (L) demonstrated large multicystic (C) tumor in the head of the pancreas. Although a diagnosis of malignancy could not be made by intraoperative ultrasound alone, the macrocystic feature and growth pattern suggested mucinous cystadenocarcinoma.

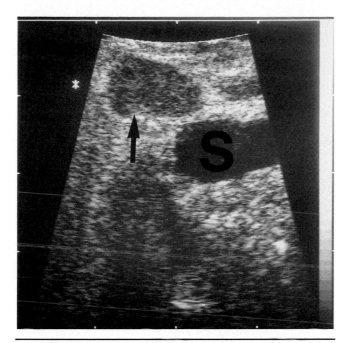

FIGURE 44. Intrapancreatic gastrinoma. A hypoechoic homogeneous solid tumor (*arrow*) with a well-defined border within the pancreas, typical appearance of islet cell tumor. S, splenic vein.

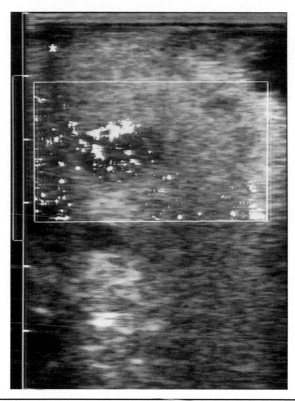

FIGURE 45. Intraoperative color Doppler imaging of a 1-cm gastrinoma demonstrated increased blood flow (bright areas) in the tumor, indicating hypervascularity.

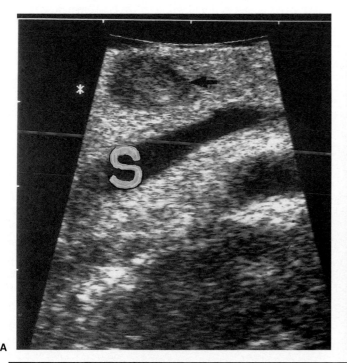

A

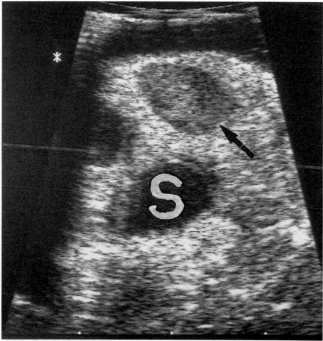

B

FIGURE 46. Insulinoma scanned by rotating the intraoperative ultrasound probe. **A:** Longitudinal scanning of the body of pancreas demonstrated a hypoechoic tumor (arrow). S, splenic vein. **B:** After rotating the probe 90 degrees, transverse view of the pancreas showed the same round tumor (*arrow*).

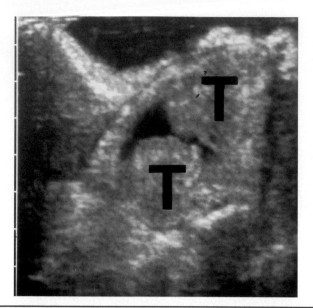

FIGURE 47. Extrapancreatic gastrinoma. Intraoperative ultrasound demonstrated two relatively hypoechoic tumors (T) within the wall of duodenum.

in comparison with surrounding tissues (Fig. 47). IOUS of the liver and peripancreatic and retroperitoneal lymph nodes should also be part of every abdominal exploration for pancreatic islet cell tumors. This is especially true if it is likely, as with gastrinomas, that the tumor has malignant potential. Metastatic islet cell tumors involving the liver can vary from hypoechoic (more frequent) to hyperechoic (less frequent) compared to the adjacent paren-

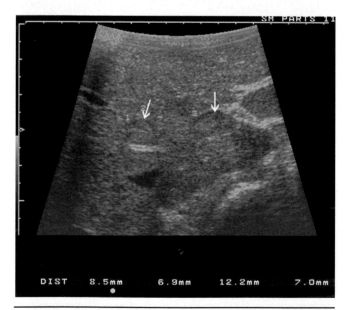

FIGURE 48. Multiple metastatic liver tumors from malignant nonfunctioning islet cell tumor. Two small tumors (*arrows*), 9 × 7 mm and 12 × 7 mm, in segment 4B exhibited an isoechoic feature with a hypoechoic rim.

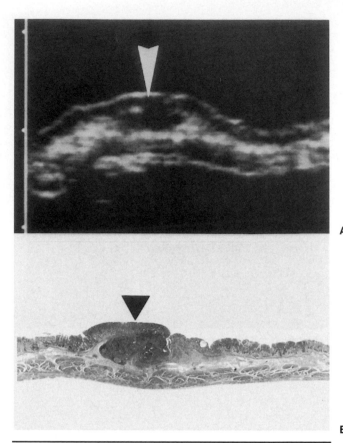

FIGURE 49. Early gastric cancer. **A:** Intraoperative ultrasound demonstrating a hypoechoic tumor (*arrowhead*) invading the third hyperechoic submucosal layer. **B:** Corresponding histology of this early cancer.

chyma (Fig. 48; see also Fig. 51 in Chapter 13). In a few instances, a tumor is isoechoic; in such instances, the tumor is generally detectable due to its having a thin, hypoechoic rim or by changes related to compression on dynamic scanning.

Gastrointestinal Tumors

High-frequency ultrasound images of gastrointestinal tumors such as gastric cancer, esophageal cancer, and rectal cancer are shown in Chapters 19 and 20. These chapters also describe ultrasound and histologic features of five-layer gastrointestinal wall structure in some detail. Figure 49 demonstrates early gastric cancer which was not palpable and was localized by IOUS. Figure 50 demonstrates gastric cancer invading the distal esophagus. IOUS images of metastatic lymph nodes from gastric cancer are shown in Figure 51.

Spleen

IOUS images of splenic cysts and solid tumors are similar to those of liver cysts and tumors. Figure 52 demon-

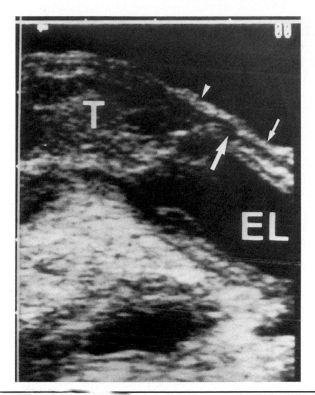

FIGURE 50. Gastric cancer invading the lower esophagus. Intraoperative ultrasound demonstrating invasion of a tumor (T) of gastric cardia into the esophagus: a large arrow indicates destruction of esophageal layered structure by cancer invasion. A small arrow indicates the normal five layers of esophagus. EL, esophageal lumen; (*arrowhead*) the level of esophagogastric junction.

strates splenic involvement by an abdominal lymphoma. IOUS-guided radiofrequency ablation of a metastatic splenic tumor from rectal cancer is shown in Figure 53. A small accessory spleen that is hypoechoic as compared with surrounding fatty tissue is shown in Figure 54.

Adrenal Gland

Small adrenal tumors such as aldosteronoma or cortical adenoma are hypoechoic, homogeneous, and well defined (Fig. 55). Large adrenal tumors, particularly adrenal carcinomas, tend to be heterogeneous and may be associated with secondary changes such as cystic degeneration or calcification (Fig. 56).

Retroperitoneum

Primary retroperitoneal tumors such as liposarcoma and malignant fibrous histiocytoma are large at the time of surgery and show a heterogeneous echo pattern, often with a cystic component (Fig. 57). Retroperitoneal hematoma sometimes resembles retroperitoneal tumors even with IOUS imaging.

Metastatic lymph nodes are relatively large, round, and hypoechoic (as already described): pancreatic cancer metastasis in Figure 37 and gastric cancer metastasis in Figure 51. Figure 58 shows multiple retroperitoneal lymph node involvement by lymphoma. Metastatic carci-

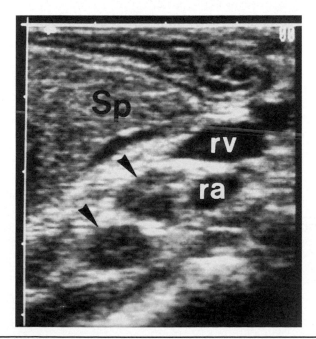

FIGURE 51. Metastatic paraaortic lymph nodes from gastric cancer. Sagittal paraaortic intraoperative ultrasound scanning detected two hypoechoic lymph nodes (*arrowheads*) during gastric cancer operation. Sp, spleen; ra, left renal artery; rv, left renal vein.

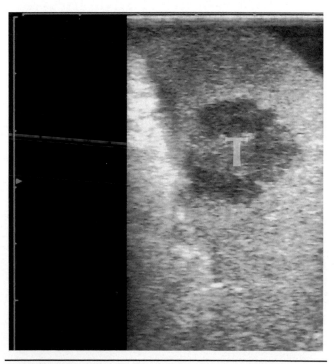

FIGURE 52. Splenic lymphoma. A 2-cm hypoechoic tumor (T) was detected in the spleen in a patient with abdominal (retroperitoneal) lymphoma.

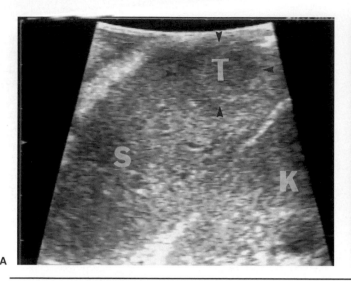

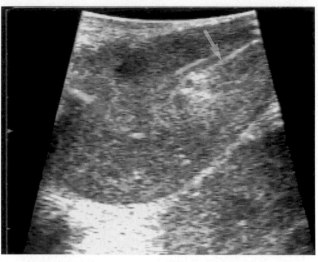

FIGURE 53. Splenic metastatic tumor from a rectal cancer. **A:** Intraoperative ultrasound (IOUS) was used to localize a metastatic tumor (T, *arrowheads*) in the spleen (S) as well as multiple liver metastases. K, left kidney. **B:** An electrode-cannula (*arrow*) was inserted into the tumor under IOUS guidance for radiofrequency thermal ablation.

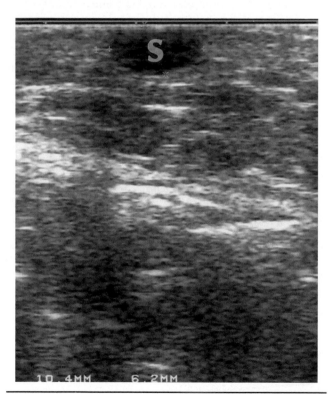

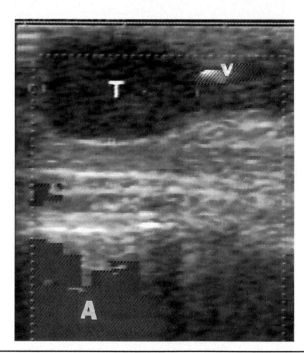

FIGURE 55. Adrenal adenoma. During laparoscopic adrenalectomy for hyperaldosteronism, a left adrenal tumor (T), 18 × 12 mm, which was hypoechoic, was readily localized by intraoperative ultrasound (laparoscopic ultrasound). Color Doppler imaging showed an adrenal vein (V). A, aorta.

FIGURE 54. Accessory spleen. During an operation for recurrent immune thrombocytopenia purpura, an accessory spleen (S), 10 × 6 mm, which was hypoechoic, was readily localized by IOUS.

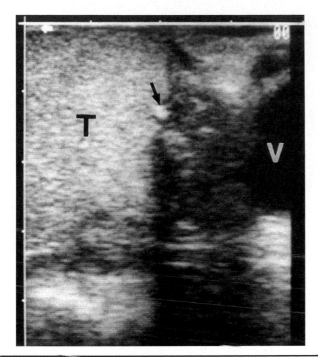

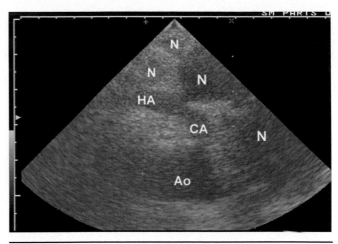

FIGURE 58. Multiple retroperitoneal lymphadenopathy due to lymphoma. A minilaparotomy was performed for excisional biopsy of retroperitoneal lymph nodes. A small intraoperative ultrasound cylindrical sector probe was used to localize nodes (N). Ao, aorta; CA, celiac artery; HA, hepatic artery.

FIGURE 56. Large adrenal tumor with calcification. It was a 6-cm hyperechoic liposarcoma (T) of the right adrenal gland. An arrow indicates one of calcifications associated with shadowing. An intraoperative ultrasound scan showed the relation of the tumor to the inferior vena cava (V).

larger. Figure 60 shows pelvic recurrence of a rectal cancer that was difficult to detect by surgical exploration; IOUS quickly localized this tumor and demonstrated its relation to iliac vessels.

noid lymph nodes treated by IOUS-guided radiofrequency thermal ablation are shown in Figure 59.

Recurrent cancer in the retroperitoneum or the pelvis exhibits similar characteristics to the primary cancer: hypoechoic when small and mixed echo pattern when

Abdominal Abscess

Intraabdominal and retroperitoneal abscesses show varying appearances on IOUS. They can exhibit a typical cystic feature (see Fig. 38 in Chapter 4); in such circum-

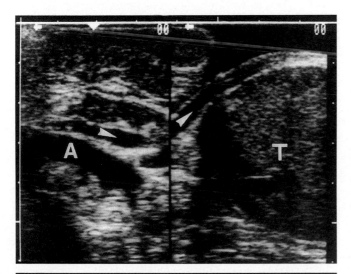

FIGURE 57. Retroperitoneal malignant fibrous histiocytoma. A large tumor (T) exhibited a hypoechoic heterogeneous feature. The course of a surrounding artery is indicated by arrowheads. A, aorta.

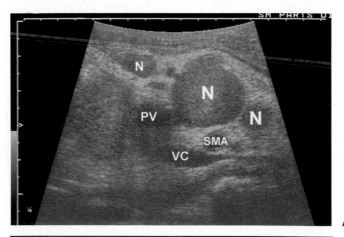

A

FIGURE 59. Multiple metastatic retroperitoneal and mesenteric lymph nodes from carcinoid tumor. **A:** Multiple small and large mesenteric lymph nodes (N). These were hypoechoic, round, and well marginated. PV, portal vein; VC, vena cava; SMA, superior mesenteric artery. *(continued)*

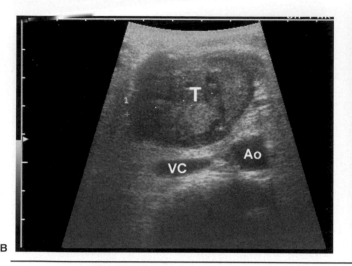

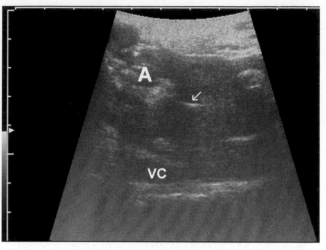

FIGURE 59. *(Continued)* **B:** A 46 × 36 mm metastatic retroperitoneal lymph node. This tumor (T) was located just anterior to the vena cava (VC) and aorta (Ao). **C:** For the purpose of cytoreductive palliation for symptomatic carinoid, intraoperative ultrasound–guided radiofrequency ablation was performed. This shows hyperechoic changes of ablation (A) of the tumor. An arrow indicates one electrode-needle. VC, vena cava.

stances, IOUS detection of abscesses is relatively easy. Identification of abscesses may be difficult when abscesses show internal echoes, irregular borders and lack of posterior enhancement (Figs. 29 and 61).

Abdominal Vessel

Figure 62 demonstrates an anastomotic stricture with thrombus formation detected by IOUS after a portacaval shunt.

ADVANTAGES AND LIMITATIONS (Table 8)

General advantages and limitations of IOUS are described in Chapter 13. IOUS is particularly useful during pancreatic surgery because a suitable alternative intraoperative imaging method is usually not available. Intraoperative pancreatography or cystography may be used, but these radiographic contrast studies are applicable only to special situations. Therefore, IOUS may be viewed as the

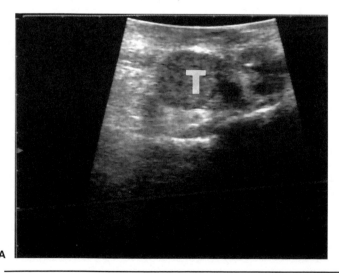

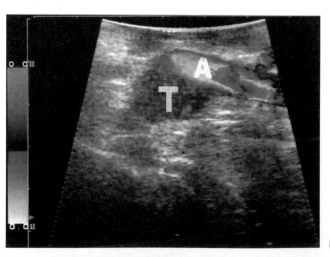

FIGURE 60. Pelvic recurrent cancer in a patient with previous surgery and radiation for a rectal cancer. During laparotomy, surgical exploration was difficult to identify this recurrent cancer. **A:** Intraoperative ultrasound scanning readily localized this nonpalpable tumor (T). **B:** Tumor was located adjacent to the right iliac artery (A), demonstrated by color Doppler imaging. (See Color Plate 31.)

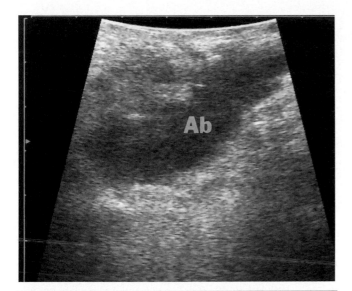

FIGURE 61. Retroperitoneal abscess. Although preoperative computed tomographic scan showed abscesses, intraoperative exploration was difficult. Intraoperative ultrasound (IOUS) was helpful in localizing and draining abscesses. This abscess (Ab) did not exhibit a typical cystic appearance (such as anechoic, smooth border, posterior enhancement) but was detected by IOUS

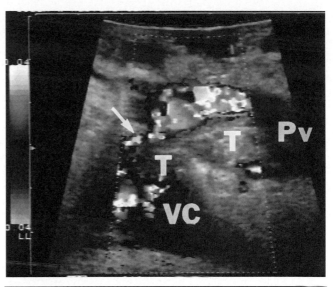

FIGURE 62. Anastomotic stricture and thrombus formation of a portacaval shunt. Intraoperative ultrasound demonstrated a stricture (*arrow*) at the anastomosis between the portal vein (Pv) and vena cava (VC). Intraoperative color Doppler imaging was valuable to recognize the significance of stricture and the extent of thrombus formation (T). (See Color Plate 32.)

primary intraoperative imaging technique for the pancreas. The speed, safety, accuracy, and capability to guide procedures are major advantages of IOUS during pancreatic surgery (3–17).

IOUS examination at the outset of operations for pancreatitis or pancreatic cancer usually takes less than 10 to 15 minutes. It is much shorter than the time required to obtain similar information by surgical exploration with extensive tissue dissection. For example, diagnosis of portal vein invasion of cancer can be made with IOUS assessment in about 5 minutes, whereas it may take 30 minutes or more with surgical exploration alone. Therefore, IOUS reduces overall operating time. Possible complications resulting from surgical dissection for exploration can be decreased with the use of IOUS. IOUS enables the detection or diagnosis of diseases that cannot be provided by surgical exploration even after tissue dissection, such as detection or localization of unrecognized or nonpalpable pseudocysts during operation for pancreatitis, diagnosis of occult liver metastasis during operation for pancreatic cancer, or precise localization of occult islet cell tumors. Accurate intraoperative diagnosis of IOUS permits more appropriate surgical management and thereby reduces the likelihood of postoperative disease recurrence or future problems.

IOUS is generally more accurate than preoperative studies in the diagnosis of complications of pancreatitis, in determining the extent of pancreatic cancer, and in lo-

calizing islet cell tumors. The ability to guide various procedures is a unique advantage of IOUS. Blind needle placement for biopsy of tumors or aspiration of cystic lesions or the ducts entails risks such as bleeding, infection, and fistula formation. With the use of IOUS-guided needle placement, such complications can be avoided. Compared with blind procedures, we have found IOUS-guided pancreatic incision to be especially useful in opening the ducts, cysts, and abscesses. Intraoperative

▶ **TABLE 8** **Advantages and Limitations of Intraoperative Ultrasound of the Pancreas and Other Abdominal Organs**

Advantages
1. Primary intraoperative imaging method: no alternative
2. Speed, safety, repeatability
3. Valuable and accurate information during surgery for pancreatitis, pancreatic cancer, islet cell tumor, pancreatic cystic lesion, gastrointestinal cancer, retroperitoneal tumor, abdominal abscess, and other diseases
4. Ability to guide various procedures
5. Facilitation of learning laparoscopic ultrasound

Limitations
1. Limited capability in detecting tumors, abscesses, fistulas
2. IOUS scanning and image interpretation are generally somewhat difficult as compared with IOUS of the liver and the biliary tract

IOUS, intraoperative ultrasound.

color Doppler imaging possesses several advantages, which are summarized in Chapter 13. Pancreatic diseases that have been evaluated by IOUS are also currently examined by laparoscopic ultrasound. Laparoscopic ultrasound of the pancreas has the capability of providing similar information to open IOUS because the two methods have basically the same image resolution; this is described in detail in Chapter 17. Advantages of IOUS for other abdominal diseases are similar to those for pancreatic diseases. IOUS can provide valuable and sometimes otherwise unobtainable information during operations for gastrointestinal cancer, splenic disease, adrenal tumor, retroperitoneal tumor, abdominal abscess, and other diseases.

Limitations of IOUS are related to the size of detectable tumors, abscesses, or other diseases and to detection or localization of a pancreatic fistula or a communication between the duct and pseudocyst. Pancreatic cancers smaller than 5 to 6 mm and islet cell tumors smaller than 3 to 4 mm usually cannot be detected, even with high-frequency (e.g., 7.5-MHz) IOUS. Liver metastases smaller than 4 to 5 mm are also undetectable. Small abdominal abscesses are at times difficult to identify. Pancreatic fistulas and duct–pseudocyst communications, particularly small ones, are often difficult to delineate with IOUS (Fig. 63). Radiologic contrast studies are more suitable for visualization of these conditions. The employment of a higher frequency instrument may decrease these limitations of IOUS. For example, intraportal endovascular ultrasound using a 20-MHz transducer has been shown to be highly accurate in the diagnosis of portal vein invasion by cancer (56). However, although the resolution is improved, the sound penetration decreases with higher frequency systems. Therefore, one should always consider this trade-off in performing IOUS. Generally, IOUS of the pancreas and some other organs is somewhat more difficult than IOUS of the liver and biliary tract in terms of scanning technique and image interpretation. Surgeons may need more experience in order to have expertise in IOUS of these organs.

CONCLUSIONS

Accurate imaging information is valuable in performing successful pancreatic operations. The applications for intraoperative radiographic contrast studies are limited for pancreatic evaluation, whereas IOUS has become the primary intraoperative imaging modality during pancreatic surgery because of its wide applicability. IOUS has provided useful information in more than 75% of the pancreatic operations in our experience. During operation for chronic pancreatitis, IOUS helps to detect, localize, or exclude complications of pancreatitis, including dilated pancreatic ducts, pseudocysts, and abscesses. During op-

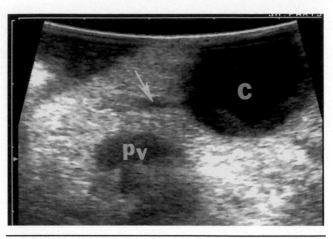

FIGURE 63. Pancreatic duct–pseudocyst communication diagnosed by intraoperative ultrasound (IOUS). The communication of a normal-size pancreatic duct (*arrow*) with a pseudocyst (C) was clearly seen. PV, portal vein. Generally, such a communication is often difficult to identify by IOUS.

eration for pancreatic cancer, IOUS can help to determine the extent of tumor and thereby its resectability. IOUS is presently the standard imaging modality during operations for islet cell tumors such as insulinoma and gastrinoma. In addition, IOUS can be used to guide various procedures such as needle placement for biopsy or aspiration and pancreatic incision for opening the pancreatic duct for drainage. IOUS can also provide valuable information during surgery for a variety of other abdominal diseases. Appropriate use of IOUS can eliminate unnecessary tissue dissection, reduce operating time, and may reduce operative complications and recurrence of diseases. IOUS-guided procedures are much safer and quicker than blind methods. We believe that these advantages outweigh the limitations of IOUS, and we encourage surgeons to routinely use IOUS during pancreatic operations and to selectively use IOUS during other abdominal operations. Laparoscopic ultrasound has become available, and this new technique is an important adjunct during laparoscopic exploration, particularly for pancreatic and other abdominal cancers. Information obtained by IOUS during open pancreatic surgery and other abdominal surgery regarding techniques, indications, images, advantages, and limitations presented in this chapter will be useful for surgeons in the performance of laparoscopic ultrasound of the pancreas and other abdominal organs.

REFERENCES

1. Lane RJ, Glazer G. Intraoperative B-mode ultrasound scanning of the extra-hepatic biliary system and pancreas. *Lancet* 1980;II(8190):334–337.
2. Sigel B, Coelho JCU, Spigos DG, et al. Ultrasound and the pancreas. *Lancet* 1980;II(8207):1310–1311.

3. Sigel B, Coelho JCU, Donahue PE, et al. Ultrasonic assistance during surgery for pancreatic inflammatory disease. *Arch Surg* 1982;117:712–716.
4. Sigel B, Coelho JCU, Machi J, et al. The application of real-time ultrasound imaging during surgical procedures. *Surg Gynecol Obstet* 1983;157:33–37.
5. Sigel B, Machi J, Ramos JR, et al. The role of imaging ultrasound during pancreatic surgery. *Ann Surg* 1984;200:486–493.
6. Sigel B, Machi J, Kikuchi T, et al. The use of ultrasound during surgery for complications of pancreatitis. *World J Surg* 1987;11:659–663.
7. Machi J, Sigel B. Overview of benefits of operative ultrasonography during a ten year period. *J Ultrasound Med* 1989;8:647–652.
8. Machi J, Sigel B, Kurohiji T, et al. Operative ultrasound guidance for various surgical procedures. *Ultrasound Med Biol* 1990;16:37–42.
9. Machi J, Sigel B, Kodama I, et al. Ultrasound-guided pancreatotomy for opening the pancreatic duct. *Surg Gynecol Obstet* 1991;173:59–60.
10. Machi J, Sigel B. Intraoperative ultrasonography (Ultrasonography of small parts). *Radiol Clin North Am* 1992;30:1085–1103.
11. Machi J, Sigel B. Intraoperative ultrasonography. In: Trede M, Carter DC, eds. *Surgery of the Pancreas.* Edinburgh London: Churchill Livingstone, 1993;147–151.
12. Machi J, Sigel B, Kurohiji T, et al. Operative color Doppler imaging for general surgery. *J Ultrasound Med* 1993;12:455–461.
13. Machi J, Sigel B, Zaren HA, et al. Operative ultrasonography during hepato-biliary and pancreatic surgery. *World J Surg* 1993;17:640–646.
14. Machi J, Sigel B. Operative ultrasound in general surgery. *Am J Surg* 1996;172:15–20.
15. Machi J, Sigel B. Intraoperative Ultrasound. *Probl Gen Surg* 1997;14:94–106.
16. Machi J. Intraoperative and laparoscopic ultrasound. *Surg Oncol Clin North Am* 1999;8:205–226.
17. Machi J. *Operative Ultrasonography—Fundamentals and Clinical Applications* (In Japanese). Tokyo: Life Science, 1987.
18. Machi J, Takeda J, Sigel B, et al. Normal stomach wall and gastric cancer: evaluation with high-resolution operative ultrasound. *Radiology* 1986;159:85–87.
19. Machi J, Takeda J, Kakegawa T, et al. The detection of gastric and esophageal tumor extension by high-resolution ultrasound during surgery. *World J Surg* 1987;11:664–671.
20. Kodama I, Machi J, Tanaka M, et al. The value of operative ultrasonography in diagnosing tumor extension of carcinoma of the stomach. *Surg Gynecol Obstet* 1992;174:479–484.
21. Machi J, Sigel B, Beitler JC, et al. Ultrasonic examination during surgery for abdominal abscess. *World J Surg* 1983;7:409–415.
22. Jakimowicz JJ, Carol EJ, Jurgens PTHJ. The preoperative use of real-time B-mode ultrasound imaging in biliary and pancreatic surgery. *Dig Surg* 1984;1:55–60.
23. Rifkin MD, Weiss SM. Intraoperative sonographic identification of nonpalpable pancreatic masses. *J Ultrasound Med* 1984;3:409–411.
24. Smith SJ, Vogelzang RL, Donovan J, et al. Intraoperative sonography of the pancreas. *AJR* 1985;144:557–562.
25. Telander RL, Charboneau JW, Haymond MW. Intraoperative ultrasonography of the pancreas in children. *J Pediatr Surg* 1986;21:262–266.
26. Plainfosse MC, Bouilot JL, Rivaton F, et al. The use of operative sonography in carcinoma of the pancreas. *World J Surg* 1987;11:654–658.
27. Printz H, Klotter HJ, Nies C, et al. Intraoperative ultrasonography in surgery for chronic pancreatitis. *Int J Pancreatol* 1992;12:233–237.
28. Serio G, Fugazzola C, Iacona C, et al. Intraoperative ultrasonography in pancreatic cancer. *Int J Pancreatol* 1992;11:31–41.
29. Back MR, Sadra M, Dempsy ME, et al. Intraoperative ultrasound assessment in management of complex pancreatic pseudocysts. *Surg Endosc* 1997;11:1126–1128.
30. Kubota K, Noie T, Sano K, et al. Impact of intraoperative ultrasonography in surgery for cystic lesions of the pancreas. *World J Surg* 1997;21:72–77.
31. Sugiyama M, Hagi H, Atomi Y. Reappraisal of intraoperative ultrasonography for pancreatobiliary carcinomas: assessment of malignant portal venous invasion. *Surgery* 1999;125:160–165.
32. Kaneko T, Nakao A, Inoue S, et al. Intraoperative ultrasonography by high-resolution annular array transducer for intraductal papillary mucinous tumours of the pancreas. *Surgery* 2001;129:55–65.
33. Shawker TH, Doppman JL, Dunnick NR, et al. Ultrasonic investigation of pancreatic islet cell tumors. *J Ultrasound Med* 1982;1:193–200.
34. Galiber AK, Reading CC, Charboneau JW, et al. Localization of pancreatic insulinoma: comparison of pre- and intraoperative US with CT and angiography. *Radiology* 1988;166:405–408.
35. Gunther RW, Klose KJ, Ruckert K, et al. Localization of small islet-cell tumors. Preoperative and intraoperative ultrasound, computed tomography, arteriography, digital subtraction angiography, and pancreatic venous sampling. *Gastrointest Radiol* 1985;10:145–152.
36. Krudy AG, Doppman JL, Jensen RT, et al. Localization of islet cell tumors by dynamic CT: comparison with plain CT, arteriography, sonography, and venous sampling. *AJR* 1984;143:585–589.
37. Doppman JL, Nieman L, Miller DL, et al. Insulinomas: localization with selective intraarterial injection of calcium. *Radiology* 1991;178:237–241.
38. Wank SA, Doppman JL, Miller DL, et al. Prospective study of the ability of computed axial tomography to localize gastrinomas in patients with Zollinger-Ellison syndrome. *Gastroenterology* 1987;92:905–912.
39. Kvols LK, Brown ML, O'Connor MK, et al. Evaluation of a radiolabeled somatostatin analog (I-123 octreotide) in the detection and localization of carcinoid and islet cell tumors. *Radiology* 1993;187:129–133.
40. Ahlstrom H, Eriksson B, Bergstrom M, et al. Pancreatic neuroendocrine tumors: diagnosis with PET. *Radiology* 1995;195:333–337.
41. Angelini L, Bezzi M, Tucci G, et al. The ultrasonic detection of insulinomas during surgical exploration of the pancreas. *World J Surg* 1987;11:642–647.
42. Cromack DT, Norton JA, Sigel B, et al. The use of high-resolution intraoperative ultrasound to localize gastrinomas: an initial report of a prospective study. *World J Surg* 1987;11:648–653.
43. Klotter HJ, Ruckert K, Kummerle F, et al. The use of intraoperative sonography in endocrine tumors of the pancreas. *World J Surg* 1987;11:635–641.
44. Grant CS, Van Heerden J, Charbonneau WJ, et al. Insulinoma. The value of intraoperative ultrasonography. *Arch Surg* 1988;123:843–848.
45. Norton JA, Cromack DT, Shawker TH, et al. Intraoperative ultrasonographic localization of islet cell tumors. A prospective comparison to palpation. *Ann Surg* 1988;207:160–168.
46. Doppman JL, Shawker TH, Miller DL. Localization of islet cell tumors. *Gastroenterol Clin North Am* 1989;18:793–804.
47. Norton JA, Shawker TH, Doppman JL, et al. Localization and surgical treatment of occult insulinomas. *Ann Surg* 1990;212:615–620.
48. Zeiger MA, Shawker TH, Norton JA. Use of intraoperative ultrasonography to localize islet cell tumors. *World J Surg* 1993;17:448–454.
49. Huai JC, Zhang W, Niu Ho, et al. Localization and surgical treatment of pancreatic insulinomas guided by intraoperative ultrasound. *Am J Surg* 1998;175:18–21.
50. Boukhman MP, Karam JM, Shaver J, et al. Localization of insulinoma. *Arch Surg* 1999;134:818–823.

51. Hiramoto JS, Feldstein VA, LaBerge JM, et al. Intraoperative ultrasound and preoperative localization detects all occult insulinomas. *Arch Surg* 2001;136:1020–1026.

52. De Manzoni G, Macri A, Borzellino G, et al. The value of in vitro ultrasonography in the intraoperative staging of gastric cancer. *Surg Endosc* 1994;8:765–769.

53. Demirci S, Cetin R, Yerdel MA, et al. Value of high-resolution intraoperative ultrasonography in the determination of limits of horizontal tumor spread during surgery for gastric malignancy. *J Surg Oncol* 1995;59:56–62.

54. Luck AJ, Thomas ML, Roediger WEW, et al. Localization of the nonpalpable colonic lesion with intraoperative ultrasound. *Surg Endosc* 1999;13:526–527.

55. Machi J, Oishi AJ, Furumoto NL, et al. Sonographically guided radio frequency thermal ablation for unresectable recurrent tumors in the retroperitoneum and the pelvis. *J Ultrasound Med* 2003;22:507–513.

56. Kaneko T, Nakao A, Inoue S, et al. Intraportal endovascular ultrasonography in the diagnosis of portal vein invasion by pancreatobiliary carcinoma. *Ann Surg* 1995;222:711–718.

Laparoscopic Ultrasound of the Liver, Pancreas, and Other Abdominal Organs

Junji Machi and Bruce D. Schirmer

Intraoperative ultrasound (IOUS) was well established for use during open surgery before the advent of the laparoscopic revolution. The latter, which began in approximately 1989, has had a rapid increase in use in the practice of surgery, particularly general surgery. Prior to that time, the use of laparoscopy was limited to diagnosis and basic therapy by gynecologists, and only a few general surgeons and hepatologists employed laparoscopy in the assessment of intraabdominal conditions. Incorporation of ultrasound with laparoscopy did not occur with significant frequency until the early to mid-1990s, when general surgeons had adopted laparoscopy as the standard for cholecystectomy and assessment of intraabdominal malignancy. Although laparoscopic ultrasound (LUS) is also used in many other laparoscopic operative settings, it has been in relation to these two operative situations that LUS has found its most rapid application and popularity. This chapter outlines the specific aspects of LUS that differ from those of both percutaneous transabdominal ultrasound and open IOUS. The equipment, operative setup, trocar placement, and techniques are discussed for evaluation of the various abdominal organs, particularly the liver and pancreas. The value and technique of hand-assisted LUS is described. Indications for LUS that are associated with improvements in diagnosis or management of abdominal lesions are presented. Clinical applications and results are described together with ultrasound images of abdominal pathologic processes. Advantages of LUS and recommendations for getting started in the performance of LUS are briefly discussed in the conclusions section of this chapter. Because LUS of the biliary system (particularly calculous diseases and cholecystectomy) is detailed in Chapter 14, this chapter focuses on the liver, pancreas, and other abdominal organs. (See also Chapter 13 for discussion of instrumentation, techniques, advantages, and indications of LUS as well as IOUS.)

EQUIPMENT AND ITS ADVANTAGES

LUS equipment differs from that of IOUS equipment used in intraoperative open surgery in several important aspects. The LUS probe, due to the limitations of the trocar size, must be of a long and cylindrical shape to reach the recesses of the abdominal cavity through the access of the trocar sites. Most standard LUS probes pass through a 10-mm trocar. The LUS transducer, usually a linear or curvilinear (convex) array transducer, is located on the side near the tip of the long probe (side-viewing probe) (see Figs. 2 and 40 in Chapter 13). The probe shaft is rigid or flexible. Steering of the flexible probe is similar to that of a bronchoscope or a gastrointestinal endoscope. The flexible probes are more adaptable to scanning over the surface of larger convex-shaped organs such as the dome of the liver, whereas rigid probes require probe-standoff scanning to achieve visualization of such areas. The convex transducer allows for a combination of a relatively focused field of examination and some depth of sound penetration for areas where scanning movement is limited. Lately, rigid probes with end-viewing sector or convex transducers have become available (see Figs. 3 and 41 in Chapter 13).

One major advantage in performing LUS, as with open IOUS, is that the abdominal wall and its potential for image distortion is eliminated. The LUS probe can be placed directly on the organ to be imaged, eliminating any potential artifact that would be conveyed by the abdominal wall. Placement of the probe directly on the organ also allows one to use a transducer with a higher frequency. Since depth of sound penetration need not be great, a higher frequency transducer, normally 7.5 MHz or even higher, can be used for LUS. The images obtained from the high-frequency transducer give a better resolution and offer greater diagnostic accuracy than those obtained by the transabdominal ultrasound with a lower frequency transducer (3 to 5 MHz). This is why IOUS or LUS, whether via a laparotomy or laparoscopic approach, will yield a higher incidence of small lesions when assessing abdominal organs. Thus, LUS for laparoscopic procedures to determine disease stage of a variety of tumors is essential to optimize the detection of potential metastatic lesions or other preoperatively unrecognized diseases.

OPERATIVE SETUP

The operative setup for LUS is similar to that for IOUS. The optimal situation is to have the ultrasound monitor in the same line of vision as the monitor for the laparoscopic telescope. Any other arrangement makes it difficult to coordinate both LUS probe manipulation and laparoscopic manipulation of tissues to assist in the ultrasound process. The ultrasound machine and screen are typically placed adjacent to the laparoscopic tower with its monitor (see Fig. 8 in Chapter 13). This is easily done for any operating room without built-in overhead booms for equipment. Should the latter be available, the ultrasound machine is optimally designed to be incorporated in the overhead boom and the image displayed on the monitors. A convenient way to visualize both laparoscopic and ultrasound images simultaneously is to employ a screen-splitting device for a single monitor, i.e., "picture-in-picture" (see Fig. 8 in Chapter 13). This allows optimal proximity of visualization of both the laparoscopic and the ultrasound images, and is particularly helpful during LUS-guided therapeutic procedures such as biopsy. However, the surgeon must balance the loss of size of image with that of the convenience of having both laparoscopic and ultrasound images displayed side by side.

Sterilization of LUS probes can be performed via two different approaches. Cold gas sterilization of equipment is one possibility. The advantage of this method is that the probe is completely sterile and easier to manipulate during the procedure because no covers are involved. The disadvantage is that the probe may only be used for one procedure per day, since the gas sterilization process is an overnight process. Lately, a new chemical sterilization (e.g., Steris, Sterrad) has become possible for LUS probes, which can be sterilized in 30 to 60 minutes (see Fig. 4 in Chapter 13). Using a sterile probe cover is the alternative approach (see Fig. 5 in Chapter 13.). This allows the probe to be used in multiple cases per day or without prior planning. The disadvantage is the necessity of applying the cover to the probe intraoperatively, as well as the awkwardness of having the probe cover on and the potential for the cover tearing, causing intraoperative contamination. However, once the team becomes experienced in their application and use, the process becomes more routine. Similarly, experience in handling the cov-

ered probe has minimized the incidence of cover tearing and contamination.

TECHNIQUES

Trocar Placement

The technique of LUS scanning is similar in many ways to that of open IOUS scanning (see Chapter 13). The same principle of scanning images in two or more planes to rule out artifact and determine their three-dimensional configuration still applies. The major difference in the laparoscopic approach is that the location of introduction of the ultrasound probe is limited by the location of the trocars. The laparoscopic surgeon should plan trocar placement in such positions that allow for appropriate scanning of the organ or organs in question. The surgeon should not hesitate to place additional trocars for successful and thorough LUS scanning.

The scanning techniques of LUS for each organ depend strongly on the type of LUS probes (i.e., side viewing versus front viewing, rigid versus flexible probes) and the location of trocar insertion sites. The location and number of trocars for LUS probe insertion differ, depending on the target organ, the intraperitoneal condition of the patient, the type of LUS probes, and the operator's preference (1–3).

During laparoscopic cholecystectomy, 10-mm umbilical and subxiphoid trocars can usually be used for introduction of an LUS probe for evaluation of the bile ducts. On the other hand, for LUS examination of the liver, pancreas, or other organs, first the umbilical port can be made for laparoscopic exploration, and the second trocar site for LUS can be selected depending on the intraperitoneal condition as determined by laparoscopy. Umbilical, subxiphoid, right and left subcostal ports are frequently used for LUS probe insertion (Fig. 1). A flexible probe requires fewer trocars. For example, for scanning the liver, umbilical, and subxiphoid, right and/or left subcostal trocars may be needed with the rigid probe (3) (see Fig. 19A in Chapter 13), whereas only umbilical and right subcostal trocars may be sufficient with the flexible probe. An end-viewing rigid LUS probe provides different images from those of a side-viewing LUS probe, and it is especially helpful for needle guidance (4) (see Fig. 41 in Chapter 13). LUS scanning techniques of abdominal organs using a side-viewing LUS probe are described below.

Scanning of the Liver (Table 1)

The basic steps of LUS scanning of the liver are the same as those of open IOUS: delineation of vascular structures and systematic scanning of the entire liver (see Chapter

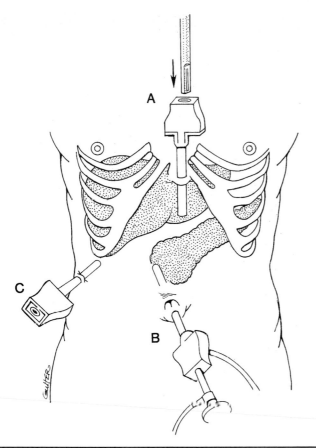

FIGURE 1. Placement of trocars for laparoscopic ultrasound scanning of the liver, pancreas and other abdominal organs. (A) Subxiphoid, (B) umbilical, and (C) right subcostal ports are frequently used.

▶ **TABLE 1** Laparoscopic Ultrasound Scanning Technique of the Liver

1. Umbilical, subxiphoid, and subcostal trocar ports
2. The basic laparoscopic ultrasound scanning steps: similar to open intraoperative ultrasound
3. Contact scanning more often than probe-standoff scanning
4. Delineation of vascular structures: segmental anatomy
5. Systematic scanning of the entire liver
6. Can divide the falciform ligament as needed

15). Ideally, the liver is imaged in its transverse views. However, particularly with the rigid probe, imaging is often difficult, and the longitudinal (sagittal) and oblique sections of the liver are more frequently obtained. The transverse sections of the liver are more easily visualized with the flexible probe.

LUS scanning of the liver is typically started with the insertion of the LUS probe through the right subcostal port. During this subcostal scanning, the LUS probe is best visualized by a laparoscope introduced from the umbilical port. First, the probe is advanced and placed on the anterior surface of the liver near the hepatic hilum, where the transverse section of the liver is obtained (Fig. 2). Here, the transverse portion of the portal vein is readily identified. Anterior to the portal vein are the bile duct and the hepatic artery. The branches of the right portal vein are then followed. This is achieved by withdrawal (toward the patient's right side) and a "sliding" maneuver

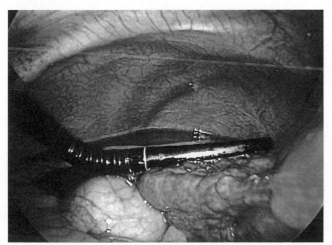

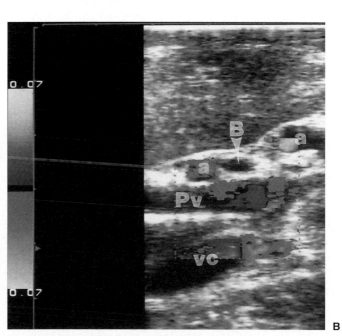

FIGURE 2A. **A:** Transverse laparoscopic ultrasound (LUS) scanning of the liver at the hepatic hilum. A flexible LUS probe is inserted via the right subcostal port and placed on the anterior surface of the liver in a transverse fashion. The liver is cirrhotic. **B:** Laparoscopic ultrasound image of the hepatic hilum in the transverse view. Color Doppler imaging showing blood flow in the portal vein (Pv), hepatic artery (a), and vena cava (vc). The bile duct (B, *arrowhead*) can be readily distinguished from the artery because of the absence of blood flow. (See Color Plate 33.)

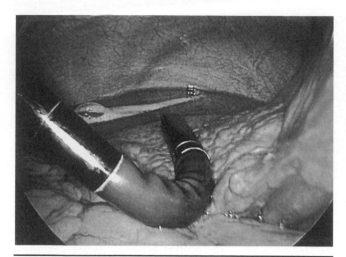

FIGURE 3. Longitudinal laparoscopic ultrasound (LUS) scanning of the liver at the segment 5 to 4 areas. A flexible LUS probe is placed on the anterior surface of the liver in a longitudinal fashion.

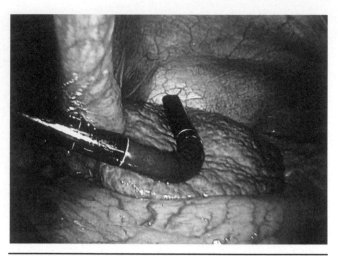

FIGURE 4. Longitudinal laparoscopic ultrasound (LUS) scanning of the left lobe (lateral segment). A LUS probe is moved to the left side of the falciform ligament and placed in a longitudinal fashion.

of the probe on the liver surface. The anterior and posterior branches and subsequently the segmental branches are visualized. The left portal vein is then followed from the hilum. The ascending (umbilical) portion of the portal vein and subsequently the branches to the medial segment (segment 4) and the lateral segments (segments 2 and 3) are visualized. Three hepatic veins are also seen by scanning from the subcostal port. The probe is moved cephalad (superiorly) near the dome of the liver, from where the entries of the right, middle, and left hepatic veins into the inferior vena cava are delineated. The demonstration of the portal vein, hepatic vein, and their branches is important to understand the segmental anatomy of the liver and the exact location of lesions whenever detected.

After visualization of the intrahepatic vessels, the entire liver is scanned in a systematic fashion. This is accomplished by placing the probe on the anterior and superior (diaphragmatic) surfaces of the liver in a transverse or longitudinal manner (Fig. 3) and sliding the probe sequentially. For the right lobe of the liver, scanning can be started from the medial portion. After the sweep scan of each path, the probe is moved to the next path (about 3 cm apart), and scanning is continued to visualize the entire right lobe. The deep areas of the posterior segments (segments 6 and 7) are at times not delineated clearly because of a limited sound penetration with a high-frequency transducer. In such an instance, the probe is positioned on the inferior surface of the liver, and scanning of these areas is performed in an upward manner. The caudate lobe (segment 1) is delineated by scanning from the anterior surface mostly; however, if it is not, it too can be imaged from the inferior surface. The

left lobe of the liver is scanned in a similar fashion. Most parts of the medial segment (segment 4) of the left lobe are imaged from the right side of the falciform ligament. For the scanning of the lateral segments, the probe should be moved to the left side of the ligament (Fig. 4). However, because of the presence of the falciform ligament, the superior areas of the lateral segments (segment 2) may not be sufficiently scanned from the right subcostal port, especially with the rigid probe. In this situation, the falciform ligament can be divided so that the

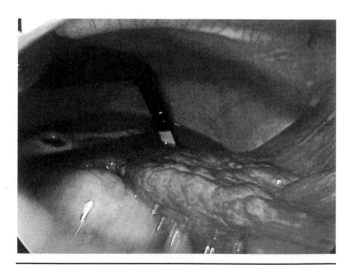

FIGURE 5. Laparoscopic ultrasound probe-standoff scanning with a saline immersion technique. Saline is introduced in the right subphrenic space, and the probe is placed over the dome of the liver. An upward flexion of the probe from this location enables visualization of the superior portion of the right lobe, particularly segment 7.

▶ **TABLE 2** **Laparoscopic Ultrasound Scanning Technique of the Pancreas**

1. Right subcostal and umbilical ports: scanning of the body to tail
2. Subxiphoid port: scanning of the head
3. Longitudinal and transverse scanning
4. Delineation of surrounding vascular structures
5. Appropriate use of contact and probe-standoff scanning

probe can be brought to the segment 2 area, or another port (such as the left subcostal, umbilical or subxiphoid port) can be used.

When the rigid probe is used, the scanning of the entire liver from one port is difficult or impossible; therefore, the second or third port (e.g., umbilical, subxiphoid, or left subcostal port) should be placed and used for complete examination (3). Even with the flexible probe, scanning from another port may help to more readily delineate the different areas of the liver. Contact scanning is the principal technique used during the LUS examination of the liver. However, the probe-standoff technique is also valuable during scanning from any port (Fig. 5). In order to perform the saline immersion method for the probe-standoff scanning, it is helpful to position the patient in a Trendelenburg position so that more of the saline solution stays in the upper abdomen.

Scanning of the Pancreas (Table 2)

The basic steps of LUS screening of the pancreas are similar to those of open IOUS: longitudinal and transverse scanning from the anterior surface particularly for imaging the pancreatic body and tail, and scanning from the right side for imaging the pancreatic head (see Chapter 16). Usually, the right subcostal and umbilical ports can be used for longitudinal and transverse scanning of the pancreas, and the subxiphoid port can be used for scanning of the pancreatic head (3) (see Fig. 19B in Chapter 13). The pancreas is visualized through organs or tissues such as the stomach (Figs. 6 and 7) and exposure of the anterior surface of the pancreas is not frequently required.

Commonly, LUS scanning is started from the right subcostal port, and this is performed through the stomach or the ligaments. With subcostal scanning, the longitudinal section of the pancreas (longitudinal to the course of the pancreas or the main pancreatic duct) is obtained (Fig. 7). The normal main pancreatic duct is almost always detected. The duct is followed from the head to the tail of the pancreas and the entire gland is sweep-scanned by sliding and sometimes rotating the probe. On the right side, sometimes the pancreatic head, particularly the periampullary region, may not be adequately visualized by the subcostal scanning; therefore, this region should be subsequently examined by the subxiphoid scanning. On the left side, along with the pancreatic tail, the left kidney and the spleen are delineated. Various vascular structures, including the aorta and its branches, the vena cava, the renal vein, and the portal system, are identified.

The transverse sections of the pancreas are then imaged (Fig. 8). Scanning from the umbilical port is necessary if the rigid probe is used to image the transverse sections. This scanning is technically similar to the longitudinal scanning. Scanning of the pancreatic head from

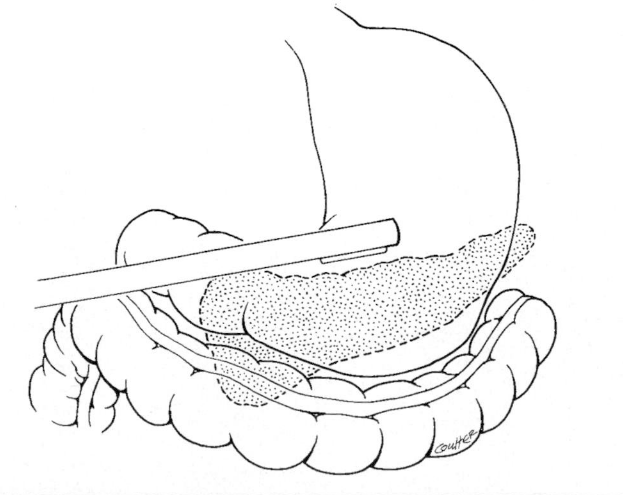

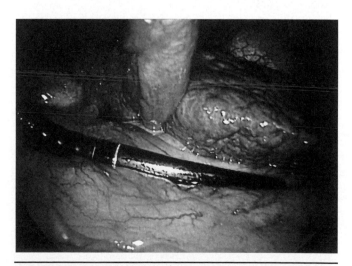

FIGURE 6. Transgastric laparoscopic ultrasound scanning of the pancreas. Without any tissue dissection, immediately after peritoneal insufflation, the pancreas can be scanned in this manner.

FIGURE 7. Longitudinal laparoscopic ultrasound (LUS) scanning of the pancreas. A LUS probe is inserted via the right subcostal port and placed over the pancreatic region. The pancreatic head to tail can be scanned in its longitudinal view.

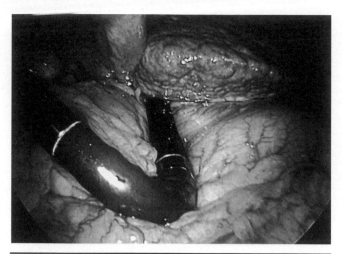

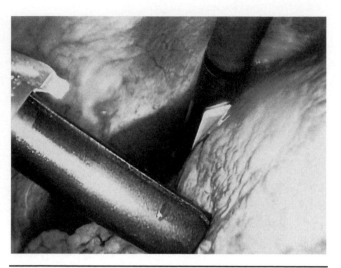

FIGURE 8. Transverse laparoscopic ultrasound (LUS) scanning of the pancreas. A flexible LUS probe which is inserted via the right subcostal port is flexed so that the transverse section (cross-section) of the pancreas is visualized.

FIGURE 9A. This shows both end-viewing laparoscopic ultrasound (LUS) probe and side-viewing LUS probes. The end-viewing probe is inserted via the right subcostal port, the side-viewing probe via the subxiphoid port, and both are imaging the segment 5 to 6 areas.

the subxiphoid port is essentially the same as the subxiphoid scanning of the distal bile duct (see Chapter 14). The LUS probe is positioned right lateral or anterolateral to the pancreatic head. The probe is slid as long as space permits. The rotating maneuver is especially valuable during the subxiphoid scanning from the superior (cephalad) portion of the pancreatic head to the uncinate process. Blood vessels such as the portal system, vena cava, hepatic artery, and gastroduodenal artery are iden-

tified. The intrapancreatic portion of the bile duct in its transverse section is readily detected in the pancreatic head. Frequently, the junction of the bile duct and the pancreatic duct is delineated at the ampulla.

Scanning of the Retroperitoneum and Other Abdominal Organs

The basic scanning methods of LUS of the retroperitoneum and other organs are similar to those of IOUS (see Chapter 16), using various LUS scanning techniques already described. Scanning the retroperitoneum is generally more difficult than scanning the solid organs, due

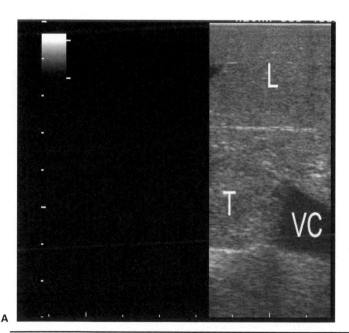

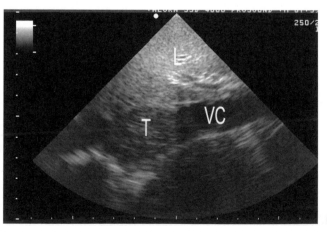

A   B

FIGURE 9B. **A:** A rectangular image obtained by a side-viewing linear array probe. Longitudinal view of the liver (L), showing compression of the vena cava (VC) by a tumor (T) in the caudate lobe. **B:** A sector image obtained by an end-viewing sector probe. The compression of the vena cava (VC) by the same tumor (T) was delineated.

in large part to the irregularities of the tissue surface and the lack of easy access of the probe to many areas of the retroperitoneum without the presence of intervening gas-filled loops of bowel. Rotation of the patient to the right side may allow for displacement of much of the small intestine to the right and may aid in exposing the retroperitoneal area at the base of the small bowel mesentery.

Throughout the examination of the liver, pancreas, and other abdominal organs from various ports, it is critical to understand the orientation and the direction of images on the monitor screen. At times, exactly the same area is imaged from completely opposite directions utilizing the different ports. Therefore, it is important to always maintain the left side of the image on the monitor screen toward the patient's right side or toward the patient's head. Maintaining orientation is accomplished by using the right–left direction function of the ultrasound machine and changing the direction of the image as needed.

The difference of ultrasound images provided by side-viewing and end-viewing LUS probes is shown in Figure 9A and 9B: a rectangular image versus a sector image. Figure 2B shows a color Doppler imaging of normal anatomy demonstrating a transverse section of the hepatic hilar area. Sonograms of the normal anatomy obtained by LUS should be essentially the same as those obtained by IOUS during open surgery (see Chapters 13 to 16 for sonograms of the liver, pancreas, retroperitoneum, and other abdominal organs).

HAND-ASSISTED LAPAROSCOPIC ULTRASOUND (Table 3)

In the last few years, hand-assisted laparoscopic surgery has been developed as a promising hybrid of laparoscopic surgery and open surgery. Hand-assisted laparoscopy can provide direct tactile feedback and improved hand–eye coordination by the surgeon. It still appears to preserve most of the advantages of fully laparoscopic procedures. This new technique has been applied successfully to a variety of surgical operations, particularly more complex procedures such as gastrointestinal operations or solid organ surgeries (5). During these operations, hand-assisted LUS can be used. Technically, hand-assisted LUS scanning is easier than conventional LUS because open IOUS probes can be used (5,6).

▶ **TABLE 3** **Hand-Assisted Laparoscopic Ultrasound**

1. Take advantage of LUS and open IOUS
2. Hand-access device and trocar placement
3. Use of open IOUS probe (not LUS probe)
4. Scanning and needle guidance easier than conventional LUS

LUS, laparoscopic ultrasound; IOUS, intraoperative ultrasound.

Usually, the patient is placed in a lithotomy position, and the surgeon stands between the patient's legs. The location of a hand-access device and a 10-mm trocar for laparoscopy is determined based on the location of the organ and the target lesion to be scanned and operated on. For example, during liver tumor evaluation or surgery, when tumors are located in the right lobe of the liver, the medial segment of the left lobe, or in both lobes, the hand-access device is placed at the right mid- or lower abdomen, and the 10-mm trocar is placed in the periumbilical region to the left mid- or lower abdomen (Fig. 10). When liver tumors are located in the lateral segment of the left lobe, the hand-access device is placed at the central portion of the abdomen, and the 10-mm trocar is placed at the left lower abdomen. After laparoscopic exploration is performed in the usual fashion, a 7- to 8-cm skin incision is made with the abdomen insufflated, and the hand-access device is placed at the predetermined location in the abdomen.

A conventional open IOUS probe (but not an LUS probe) is used for the scanning of the liver or other organs. A small 5- to 10-MHZ side-viewing linear array or curvilinear array (convex) T-shaped IOUS probe is preferable. The probe is introduced into the peritoneal cavity along with the surgeon's left hand. Under laparoscopic visualization, hand-assisted LUS examination is performed for the entire liver or other organs in the same manner as IOUS during open surgery. Hand-assisted LUS-guided biopsy or ablation of tumors can be performed in a manner similar to open IOUS-guided procedures (6) (see Chap-

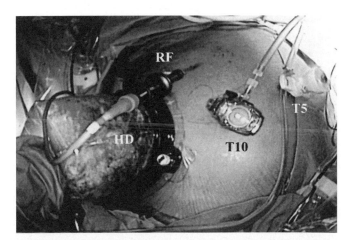

FIGURE 10. Placement of a hand-access device (HD) and trocars for hand-assisted laparoscopic ultrasound (LUS). The LUS probe is brought into the peritoneal cavity with the surgeon's left hand. T10, 10-mm trocar; T5, 5-mm trocar; RF, a radiofrequency ablation cannula used for hand-assisted LUS-guided ablation of a liver tumor for this particular operation. (Reproduced with permission from Machi J, Oishi AJ, Mossing A, et al. Hand-assisted laparoscopic ultrasound–guided radiofrequency thermal ablation of liver tumors: a technical report. *Surg Laparosc Endosc Percutan Tech* 2002;12:160–164.)

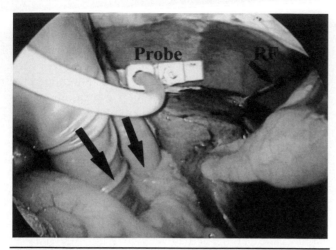

FIGURE 11. During hand-assisted laparoscopic surgery of the liver, the Pringle's maneuver can be performed by surgeon's fingers (*two long arrows*). An intraoperative ultrasound probe and a radiofrequency ablation cannula (RF; *arrow*) are also seen. (Reproduced with permission from Machi J, Oishi AJ, Mossing A, et al. Hand-assisted laparoscopic ultrasound–guided radiofrequency thermal ablation of liver tumors: a technical report. *Surg Laparosc Endosc Percutan Tech* 2002;12:160–164.)

ters 4 and 13; see also Fig. 48 in Chapter 13). When a hepatic inflow occlusion (Pringle's maneuver) is needed during liver tumor ablation or resection, the surgeon can compress the hepatoduodenal ligament with his or her fingers (Fig. 11).

Hand-assisted LUS takes advantages of benefits of both LUS and open IOUS. Ultrasound scanning is much easier and may be more accurate with an open IOUS probe than a conventional LUS probe. Because an ultrasound guidance system that is attached to an IOUS probe is available, hand-assisted LUS guidance of a needle or a cannula is technically easier and more precise than conventional LUS guidance. Open IOUS probes are less costly and more available than LUS probes. Hand-assisted laparoscopic operations are becoming additional useful surgical techniques in which hand-assisted LUS can be a valuable adjunct for surgeons.

INDICATIONS

The indications for LUS are, ideally, the same as those for IOUS during open surgery. In fact, these indications may be even more imperative and essential if the operative strategy is to use a laparoscopic approach, and diagnosis is thereby not facilitated by intraoperative palpation of organs and structures. In such circumstances, where the comparable open operative approach would allow ready diagnosis by palpation, the laparoscopic approach must rely on the use of information obtained via LUS for successful performance of the procedure.

TABLE 4 Indications for Laparoscopic Ultrasound for Malignant Tumors

1. Adjunct to laparoscopic exploration: compensation for the limitation of laparoscopy
2. Evaluation of hepatobiliary, pancreatic, and esophagogastric tumors (localization, characterization, detection, staging, resectability)
3. Screening of liver metastasis
4. Guidance of laparoscopic procedures: biopsy, ablation, resection

The organs or areas for which LUS is most indicated for intraoperative assessment are solid abdominal organs, biliary tree, and retroperitoneum. The liver, bile duct, gallbladder, pancreas, spleen, adrenal, and retroperitoneum compose the organs most frequently assessed using LUS (7–18).

Indications for Abdominal Malignant Tumors (Table 4)

LUS is indicated whenever laparoscopic exploration is performed for abdominal malignant tumors (10–18). Laparoscopy has been shown to more correctly predict the resectability of abdominal tumors than preoperative studies. Because of the known limitations of diagnostic laparoscopy, LUS has been introduced as an adjunct to laparoscopy. During the last decade, a number of studies have reported the value of LUS for abdominal malignant tumors, in particular hepatobiliary, pancreatic, and gastrointestinal tumors. LUS has demonstrated a capability of providing tumor staging information in addition to that derived from laparoscopic visual exploration alone. Laparoscopic inspection is effective to detect peritoneal dissemination and metastasis to the liver surface but not to evaluate structures or organs under the surface. LUS can compensate for this limitation of laparoscopy. LUS delineates tumors deep in the parenchyma of organs, especially solid organs such as the liver. The retroperitoneal structures are visualized without tissue dissection. First, local tumor invasion to other structures, particularly blood vessels, can be evaluated by LUS. Second, liver metastasis and lymph node metastasis are assessed in a manner similar to IOUS at open surgery.

Studies on malignant liver tumors showed that LUS demonstrated liver tumors that had been imperceptible to laparoscopic inspection in 20% to 40% of patients (Table 5). Additional information regarding the resectability, such as major vascular invasion or lymph node metastasis, was obtained by LUS in 10% to 30% (19–26). Similar results were reported by studies of laparoscopy with LUS on pancreatic cancer (27–36), biliary cancer (36–39), and gastroesophageal cancer (40–46).

▶ **TABLE 5** Value of Laparoscopic Ultrasound for Malignant Tumors

1. Detects liver tumors imperceptible to laparoscopic inspection in 20%–40% of patients
2. Provides other information (e.g., vascular invasion) in 10%–30%
3. Overall, laparoscopy with laparoscopic ultrasound establishes unresectability in 20%–50% of patients who have been considered to have potentially resectable tumors, thereby decreasing unnecessary or nontherapeutic laparotomies to less than 10%

▶ **TABLE 6** Laparoscopic Ultrasound for Various Abdominal Diseases

1. Biliary tract
    Staging and resectability of biliary cancer
    Evaluation of gallbladder polyp
2. Esophagus, stomach, intestine
    Staging and resectability of gastroesophageal cancer
    Assistance of gastrointestinal resection
3. Adrenal gland
    Localization and assistance of resection of adrenal tumor
    Evaluation of malignant adrenal tumors
4. Spleen
    Evaluation of splenic lesions: cystic vs solid
    Localization of accessory spleen
5. Retroperitoneum and other abdomen
    Evaluation and biopsy guidance of tumors or lymph nodes
    Assistance of drainage of abscess or fluid collections, removal of foreign body

Overall, LUS provided more staging information than did laparoscopy alone, and laparoscopy with LUS established unresectability in 20% to 50% of patients who had been considered to have potentially resectable tumors preoperatively. In these studies, because of better staging by laparoscopy together with LUS, the predicted resectability was higher than 90% to 95%, which was confirmed by subsequent laparotomy. Laparoscopic exploration prior to planned laparotomy will be increasingly utilized for various abdominal malignancies, and LUS is capable of improving the staging accuracy, thereby decreasing unnecessary or nontherapeutic laparotomies. The efficacy of these indications for LUS is further described below.

Currently, laparoscopic cancer surgery (e.g., laparoscopic colectomy for colon cancer) is being investigated. Once patients undergo laparoscopic (not open) resection of primary abdominal cancers, LUS will likely have an important role in determination of accurate staging, especially in screening of the liver for metastasis (47,48).

LUS is indicated to guide various laparoscopic procedures, just as IOUS does with open procedures. LUS can be used to guide a needle into a tumor or lymph node for biopsy (49). Nonresectional treatments for liver tumors, such as laparoscopic cryoablation or radiofrequency thermal ablation, have been developed recently for use with LUS guidance; in these operations, ablation probe or cannula placement is guided by LUS, and the treatment process is monitored by LUS images (50–54). LUS-guided laparoscopic liver resection has also been reported (55,56).

Other Indications (Table 6)

A number of additional applications have been suggested in recent reports on LUS during laparoscopic surgery or exploration. These include, but are not limited to, evaluation and biopsy guidance of uncertain liver lesions or liver tumors of unknown cause, evaluation of gallbladder polyps, localization of intrahepatic stones, detection and drainage assistance of pancreatic pseudocysts or other abdominal fluid collections (57–59), localization and assistance of resection of pancreatic islet cell tumors (60–

64), assistance during surgery of liver cysts (65), assistance during adrenal tumor resections (66–69), guidance of gastric tumor resection (70), and evaluation of retroperitoneal tumors or lymph nodes (71,72). LUS is capable of guiding a variety of laparoscopic procedures, the number of which seems to be increasing yearly.

Laparoscopic technology continues to advance rapidly, and laparoscopic surgery continues to apply to larger numbers and various types of abdominal diseases. With more laparoscopic procedures being performed, the application and utility of LUS during laparoscopic surgery are expected to increase.

CLINICAL APPLICATIONS, RESULTS, AND ULTRASOUND IMAGES OF PATHOLOGY

An important application of LUS is the accurate staging of intraabdominal solid tumors. LUS staging of tumors may involve scanning of any or all of the solid organs of the abdomen in a diligent search for evidence of metastatic disease. Therapeutic applications of LUS have been increasing as well. Organ-specific applications of LUS are discussed with some clinical results and LUS images of pathology.

Liver (Table 7)

For the liver, the most common applications for LUS include screening for the presence of hepatic metastatic disease during a staging laparoscopy; determining the characteristics, size, and location of tumors seen by preoperative imaging studies such as computed tomography

▶ **TABLE 7 Laparoscopic Ultrasound of the Liver**

1. Evaluation, staging, and resectability for primary and metastatic tumors
2. Evaluation of tumor of unknown cause
3. Guidance of biopsy, ablation, and resection of liver tumors
4. Localization of intrahepatic stones
5. Assistance of liver cyst drainage

(CT) or transabdominal ultrasound to assess for malignant potential (Fig. 12); determining the relationship of a hepatic tumor to major hepatic vascular structures in terms of resectability; and guiding biopsy, ablation, and resection of tumors performed laparoscopically.

Open IOUS is the most accurate method for staging hepatic tumors, both primary and metastatic, to determine resectability (see Chapter 15). Many hepatic tumors are unresectable due to bilobar distribution, extrahepatic metastases, cirrhosis, or major vascular involvement. Preoperative imaging methods such as transabdominal ultrasound, CT, or magnetic resonance imaging have an accuracy of only 50% to 80% in predicting resectability.

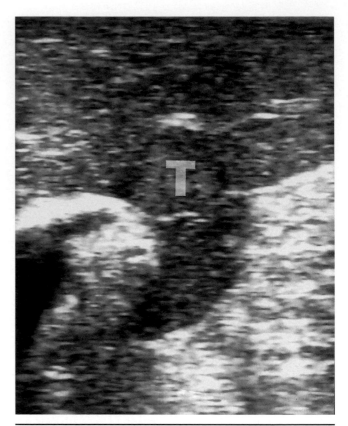

FIGURE 13. A metastatic liver tumor (T) from a colon cancer, detected by laparoscopic ultrasound. It was 12 × 10mm in size, isoechoic with a hypoechoic rim, and was located in segment 2.

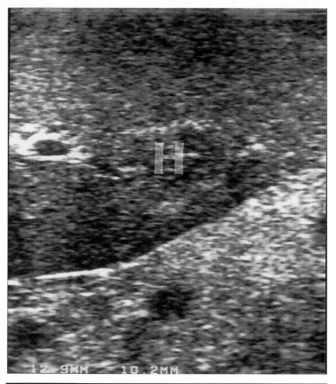

FIGURE 12. Laparoscopic ultrasound (LUS) characterization of a hepatic hemangioma (H). In this patient with a history of a breast cancer, preoperative computed tomography showed a possible metastatic liver tumor. LUS demonstrated a hypoechoic tumor, 13 × 10 mm, with a hyperechoic rim in segment 3. This LUS finding was suggestive of a hemangioma (but not a malignant tumor), which was confirmed by LUS-guided biopsy.

Even CT portography is not as accurate as IOUS in predicting resectability. The experiences with open IOUS have demonstrated that approximately 10% of hepatic tumors are detected only with IOUS. Using laparoscopy and LUS, the experienced surgeon can have the same diagnostic capability in evaluating hepatic tumors as with the traditional approach of laparotomy and IOUS (see Chapter 13). Comparative studies with preoperative imaging methods have demonstrated a superior accuracy of LUS in detecting and evaluating liver tumors (73–76). Figures 13 and 14 show metastatic liver tumors from colorectal cancers detected by LUS.

Primary hepatic tumors have the highest incidence, relative to all types of abdominal tumors involving solid organs, of being restaged or reclassified when laparoscopy with LUS is performed. John et al. (19) found that staging laparoscopy disclosed findings in 46% of patients deemed to have resectable primary hepatic tumors preoperatively (by standard imaging procedures) that resulted in their being restaged into an unresectable category. LUS detected additional tumors in 33% of the patients. LUS is also highly efficient and sensitive for screening for metastases from colorectal carcinoma dur-

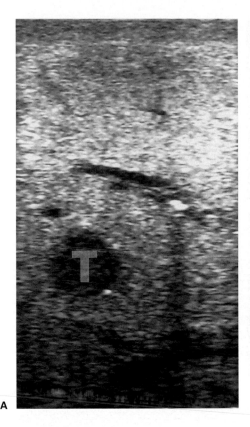

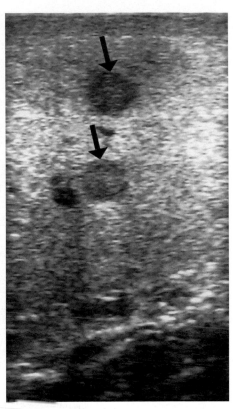

FIGURE 14. Multiple metastatic tumors. Preoperative computed tomography showed five tumors, but LUS detected three more tumors. **A:** A preoperatively known metastatic liver tumor (T), 10 mm in size, hypoechoic, in segment 5-6. **B:** LUS detected two tumors (*arrows*), 7 mm and 6 mm, hypoechoic, in segment 4.

ing laparoscopic exploration or laparoscopic colon resection. In patients with known liver malignancy, primary or metastatic, LUS findings led to a determination of unresectability and an unnecessary laparotomy was avoided in 25% of patients (20). Figures 15 and 16 show hepatocellular carcinomas with daughter nodules (intrahepatic metastases) and the extent of the tumor. Figure 17 demonstrates an unresectable hepatocellular carcinoma due to major intrahepatic vascular invasion.

Whenever liver lesions or tumors are detected by LUS, LUS-guided biopsy can be performed. Technically, LUS-guided needle placement is usually easier with an end-viewing LUS probe than with a side-viewing LUS probe (Figs. 18 and 19). Primary and metastatic tumors of the liver can be ablated using several forms of energy. Radiofrequency thermal ablation has become the most popular method of ablation in the past several years. The approach to hepatic tumor ablation can be via open surgery, laparoscopic, hand-assisted laparoscopic, or percutaneous under ultrasound guidance (6,51,53) (see Chapters 4 and 13). LUS guidance of the radiofrequency probe is essential to achieve accurate ablation of the tumor. Several studies have demonstrated the safety and local control efficacy of LUS-guided radiofrequency ablation for primary and metastatic liver tumors: major complications are less than 10%, and local tumor recurrence is about 10% (50–53). Siperstein et al. have the largest expe-

rience with laparoscopic ablation with a local recurrence rate of 12% with minimal morbidity (52). Figures 20 and 21 demonstrate radiofrequency ablation of liver tumors performed under LUS guidance and hand-assisted LUS guidance, respectively.

Hepatic resections for tumor, when done therapeutically for cure, require the removal of the tumor with an adequate margin to prevent local recurrence. In such situations, IOUS is essential to guide resection. Though used most frequently during laparotomy for open hepatic resection, there are increasing numbers of centers with accumulating experiences of using a laparoscopic approach for successful hepatic resection of tumors for cure. These tumors have, to date, usually been located in the lateral segments of the left lobe (segments 2 and 3) or the anterior segments of the right lobe. They have most frequently been benign, but malignant primary and metastatic tumors have also been resected laparoscopically. LUS has been uniformly used by surgeons using a laparoscopic approach for hepatic resection to guide resection margins (55,56).

A laparoscopic approach has been used to drain liver cysts as well. When such cysts are beneath the liver surface precluding laparoscopic visual detection, LUS is needed for their localization and for selection of opening sites for drainage (65).

(text continues on page 406)

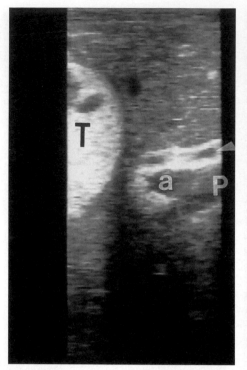

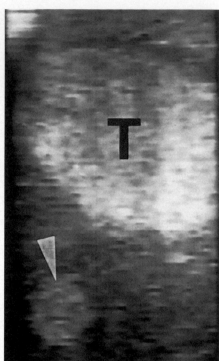

FIGURE 15. Hepatocellular carcinoma located in segment 5–8. **A:** A 4-cm hyperechoic tumor (T) in its relation to the anterior branch (a) of the right portal vein (P). **B:** A daughter nodule (*arrowhead*) of the main tumor (T) was detected by laparoscopic ultrasound. Both were located in segment 5–8 (anterior segment) and were resectable.

A

B

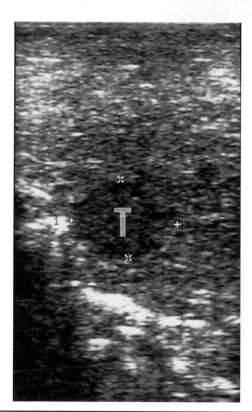

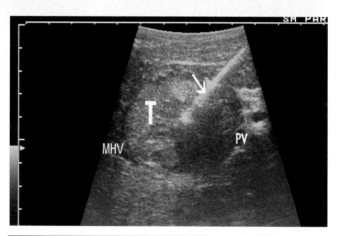

FIGURE 17. Unresectable hepatocellular carcinoma due to vascular invasion. A 5.5-cm tumor (T) in segment 5, extending to segments 4 and 8. The tumor invaded the middle hepatic vein (MHV) and the portal vein (PV). An arrow indicates a biopsy needle guided by hand-assisted laparoscopic ultrasound. The tumor was ablated.

FIGURE 16. An intrahepatic metastasis of hepatocellular carcinoma in the contralateral lobe. The main large tumor was in the right lobe. Laparoscopic ultrasound identified a 16 × 12 mm, hypoechoic daughter nodule (T) in segment 3. One other nodule was also detected. These findings established unresectability of this hepatocellular carcinoma. All tumors were ablated.

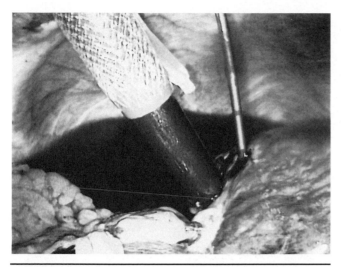

FIGURE 18. End-viewing laparoscopic ultrasound (LUS)–guided needle or cannula placement. It is easier to guide a needle (maintain a needle in the scanning plane) with an end-viewing LUS. This picture shows LUS guidance of an ablation cannula; biopsy needle guidance is basically the same.

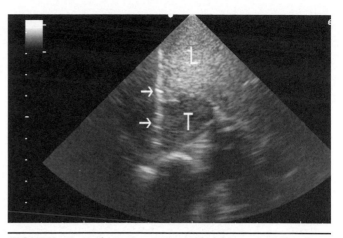

FIGURE 19. End-viewing LUS guided biopsy needle placement. The sector image showing a hyperechoic needle (*arrows*) through the liver parenchyma (L) into the tumor (T) in the caudate lobe. This was the same tumor shown in Figure 9B. Histologically, it was a focal nodular hyperplasia; therefore, surgical resection was avoided.

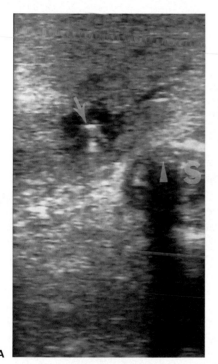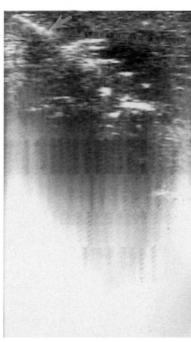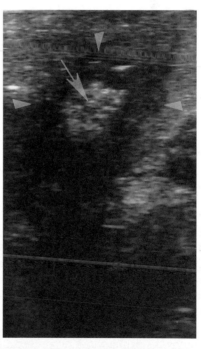

A   B, C

FIGURE 20. Laparoscopic ultrasound–guided radiofrequency thermal ablation of a small hepatocellular carcinoma. **A:** A 9-mm hypoechoic tumor was located in segment 3, adjacent to the stomach (S). An arrow indicates an ablation cannula-needle in the tumor prior to ablation. Arrowhead denotes nasogastric tube with shadowing. **B:** During ablation, the ablated lesion became hyperechoic. An arrow indicates a shaft of the cannula. **C:** Several minutes after completion of ablation. The ablated lesion (approximately 2.5 cm) is indicated by arrowheads. Arrow denotes remaining hyperechoic gas in the center of the ablated lesion.

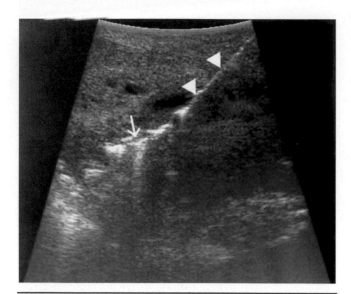

FIGURE 21. Hand-assisted laparoscopic ultrasound (LUS)–guided radiofrequency thermal ablation of a large metastatic tumor. An ablation cannula is clearly visualized in its entire shaft (*arrowheads*) because of easier guidance by hand-assisted LUS. The image was obtained soon after beginning of ablation, and the ablation lesion was becoming hyperechoic (*arrow*). (Reproduced with permission from Machi J, Oishi AJ, Mossing A, et al. Hand-assisted laparoscopic ultrasound–guided radiofrequency thermal ablation of liver tumors: a technical report. *Surg Laparosc Endosc Percutan Tech* 2002;12:160–164.)

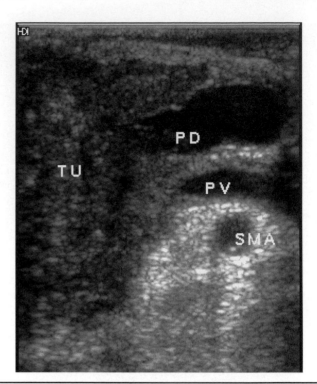

FIGURE 22. Resectable pancreatic head cancer. A longitudinal laparoscopic ultrasound view of the pancreas showed a large pancreatic head tumor (TU) causing pancreatic duct obstruction with distal duct dilation (PD). However, the portal vein (PV) was away from the tumor without cancer invasion. SMA, superior mesenteric artery. The tumor was resected by a Whipple procedure. (Courtesy of Dr. Maurice Arregui.)

Pancreas (Table 8)

LUS, which is performed during prelaparotomy laparoscopy, is useful for staging of cancer and determination of resectability of pancreatic carcinoma where visual laparoscopic examination has not ruled out resectability. Liver metastasis and local invasion such as involvement of the portal vein or superior mesenteric artery can often be more accurately judged by LUS than preoperative studies (27–36).

Laparoscopy with LUS has been used for tumors of the head, but also for tumors of the body and tail of the pancreas, in which the resectability rate is very low and operative palliation is not required for biliary or gastrointestinal obstruction. A complete staging laparoscopy with LUS includes visualizing the peritoneal surfaces for metastases, examining the primary tumor for direct invasion of nearby structures (especially blood vessels), and imaging areas of

regional lymph nodes and the liver for metastatic deposits. If this laparoscopic staging procedure with LUS shows resectable disease, then the operation proceeds to open laparotomy and resection for tumors of the proximal pancreas (pancreatoduodenectomy) (Fig 22). If the tumors are in the distal pancreas, then the potential for a laparoscopic distal pancreatectomy, usually with splenectomy, is also afforded to the operating surgeon with advanced laparoscopic operative skills. Should the laparoscopy show unresectable disease, confirmed by biopsy (at times LUS-guided biopsy), then laparotomy is avoided. Laparoscopy with LUS disclosed unresectable pancreatic cancer in 19% to 59% of patients who were thought to have resectable disease on preoperative imaging (27–29). Figures 23 and 24 show portal vein invasion of pancreatic cancer, and Figure 25 shows a metastatic liver tumor; these LUS findings suggest unresectability of pancreatic cancer.

Effective palliative measures for pancreatic cancer are available without the need for open surgery. Biliary and gastrointestinal bypass procedures can be provided by percutaneous or endoscopic approaches, or a laparoscopic operative approach as well. For patients with unresectable cancer causing pain, LUS-guided celiac ganglion block can be performed (Fig. 26; see also Fig. 39 in

▶ **TABLE 8 Laparoscopic Ultrasound of the Pancreas**

1. Staging and resectability for pancreatic carcinoma
2. Guidance of pancreatic biopsy
3. Assistance of pancreatic tumor resection
4. Assistance of pancreatic pseudocyst drainage
5. Localization and assistance of resection of islet cell tumors such as insulinoma

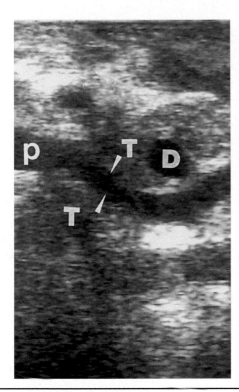

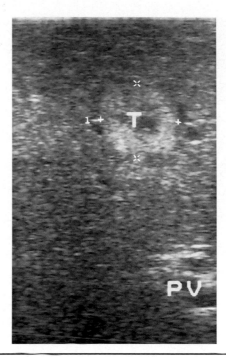

FIGURE 25. Metastatic liver tumor from a pancreatic head cancer. Prelaparotomy laparoscopic ultrasound demonstrated a metastatic tumor (T), 1.2 × 1.3cm, in segment 5–8, indicating unresectability of cancer. PV, the anterior branch of the right portal vein

FIGURE 23. Unresectable pancreatic head cancer. A transverse laparoscopic ultrasound view of the pancreas showed a pancreatic head tumor (T) surrounding and invading (*arrowheads*) the portal vein (P) to the superior mesenteric vein, indicating unresectability of cancer. D, cross-section of dilated pancreatic duct.

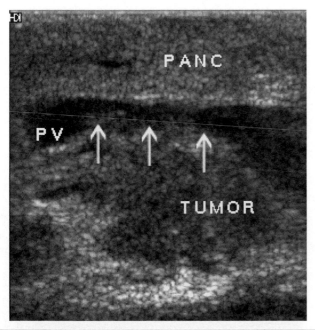

FIGURE 24. Unresectable pancreatic head cancer. Laparoscopic ultrasound showed a growth or invasion (*arrows*) of a pancreatic head–uncinate tumor to the portal vein (PV), indicating unresectability of cancer. (Courtesy of Dr. Maurice Arregui.)

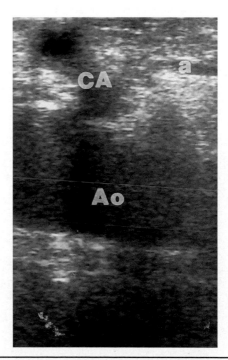

FIGURE 26. Celiac ganglion block can be performed during laparoscopy under laparoscopic ultrasound (LUS). This LUS image shows a longitudinal view of the aorta (Ao) with its branches, the celiac artery (CA), and superior mesenteric artery (a). The celiac ganglion block is performed on both sides of the aorta at the level of the celiac artery.

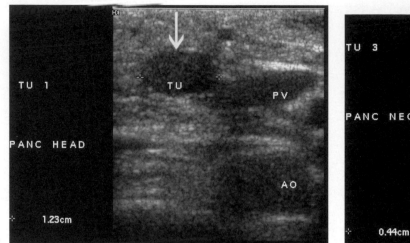 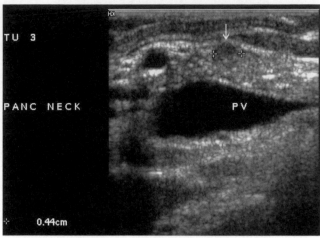

FIGURE 27. Multiple islet cell tumors localized and detected by laparoscopic ultrasound (LUS) in a patient with a multiple endocrine neoplasm syndrome. **A:** A tumor (TU, *long arrow*), 1.2 cm in size, localized in the head of the pancreas. PV, portal vein; AO, aorta. **B:** Another tumor (*short arrow*), 0.4 cm in size, detected by transgastric LUS in the neck of the pancreas. (Courtesy of Dr. Maurice Arregui.)

Chapter 16). Thus, by combining staging laparoscopy with LUS as well as these approaches for palliation, unnecessary laparotomy can be avoided in a high percentage of patients with unresectable pancreatic cancer.

LUS can be helpful for the localization of benign tumors of the pancreas, particularly islet cell tumors such as insulinomas (60–64). Here, resection or enucleation using a laparoscopic approach follows careful LUS localization of the tumor. During laparoscopy for other islet cell tumors such as gastrinoma, LUS may diagnose or exclude multiple tumors (Fig. 27). Resection of these tumors is also assisted by repeated LUS scanning during the course of tissue dissection. Figure 28 demonstrates an acinar cell adenoma, which was resected laparoscopi-

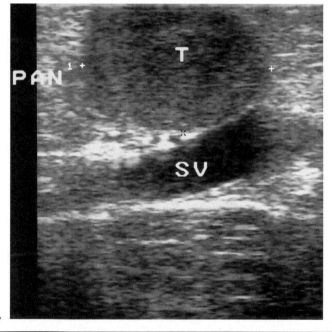 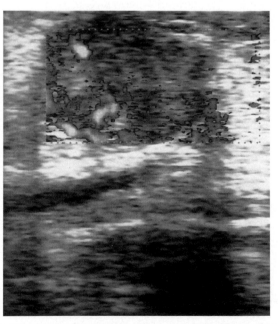

FIGURE 28. Acinar cell adenoma. **A:** A preoperatively known tumor (T), 2.2 × 1.5 cm, was localized by laparoscopic ultrasound in the tail of pancreas (PAN). It was a well-defined hypoechoic homogeneous tumor, suggesting a benign feature. SV, splenic vein. **B:** Power Doppler imaging demonstrated intratumoral blood vessels. Laparoscopic distal pancreatectomy was performed. (See Color Plate 34.)

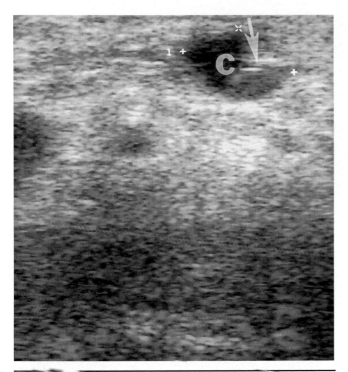

FIGURE 29. Laparoscopic ultrasound (LUS)–guided needle aspiration of a pancreatic cyst. A 1.2 × 0.8 cm cyst (C) that was not visualized from the pancreatic surface was localized by LUS. A needle (*arrow*) was inserted into the cyst under LUS guidance for aspiration.

cally. Various pancreatic cystic lesions or neoplasms are evaluated by LUS in a similar fashion to open IOUS (see Chapter 16).

Management of pancreatitis, both laparoscopic-directed drainage of pseudocyst and drainage of pancreatic necrosis or abscess, can be aided by LUS assessment of the location and extent of the pseudocyst or abscess (57–59). Particularly, LUS can aid in selecting the most appropriate site of opening of pseudocysts. LUS-guided needle placement is also valuable for biopsy of pancreatic solid lesions and aspiration of pancreatic cystic lesions (Fig. 29).

Biliary Tract

LUS can be used in the assessment of patients with tumors of the porta hepatis, for staging and resectability (36–39). These may be primary bile duct cancers, metastatic tumors involving nodes in the porta hepatis, or gallbladder cancer as the most common tumor types found in this area (see Chapter 14). Tumors of the bile ducts or gallbladder often present with jaundice and as advanced tumors. Staging laparoscopy and LUS along with other preoperative imaging studies to evaluate the level of bile duct involvement are helpful in determining resectability of the lesions. This is especially true for carcinomas of the proximal bile duct, referred to as Klatskin tumors. For

Klatskin tumors, the usual determinant of resectability is cancer involvement into the liver parenchyma, and so laparoscopy and LUS less frequently change resectability for these tumors. For example, Van Delden et al. (37) found a change in tumor stage in 23% of patients with bile duct tumors and avoidance of unnecessary laparotomy in 9% of patients with tumors of the proximal bile duct. However, for carcinomas of the distal extrahepatic bile duct, staging laparoscopy with LUS is more helpful. Tumors of the gallbladder also present with a high incidence of metastatic involvement, and staging of these tumors with a laparoscopic approach including LUS is quite helpful in yielding a high rate of unresectability.

Esophagus, Stomach, and Intestinal Tract

LUS is helpful in staging tumors of the stomach and esophagus as well (40–46). In these types of tumors, however, the incidence of findings that restage the patient or cause changes in therapy in terms of resectability or surgical management is lower than that in either hepatic or pancreatic tumors. Studies have shown the incidence of findings at laparoscopy combined with LUS that avoided unnecessary laparotomy for gastric or distal esophageal cancers as being between 5% and 16% (42). During laparoscopic resection of gastrointestinal tumors that are not visible by laparoscopy (e.g., subserosal tumors), LUS can be used for localization and to guide resection.

Adrenal Gland

LUS has been increasingly reported as being helpful for the localization of the adrenal gland, especially on the left side, during laparoscopic adrenalectomy (66–69). The lo-

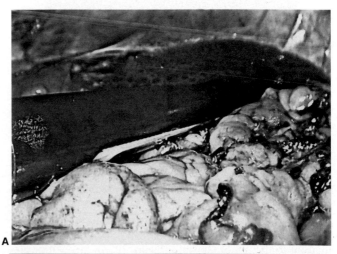

A

FIGURE 30A. Laparoscopic ultrasound scanning of the left upper retroperitoneum for localization of a left adrenal tumor.

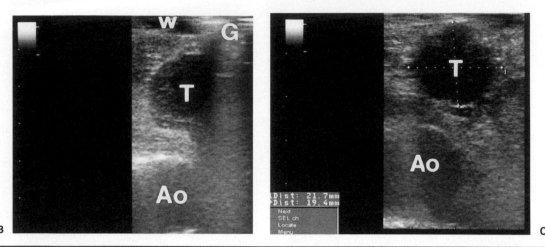

FIGURE 30. *(Continued)* A small left adrenal tumor (aldosteronoma) localized by laparoscopic ultrasound (LUS). **B:** LUS scanning soon after peritoneal insufflation localized a hypoechoic tumor (T). Probe-standoff scanning was performed with saline immersion. The aorta (Ao) was seen medial-posterior to the tumor. W, acoustic window using saline; G, gas causing a posterior artifact. **C:** During laparoscopic tissue dissection, LUS was repeated. The tumor (T), 2.2 × 1.9cm, was then located more superficially.

calization of adrenal tumors, particularly small tumors, early in the course of operation (e.g., immediately after insufflation) can facilitate laparoscopic tissue dissection, thereby decreasing the operating time (Fig 30; see also Fig. 55 in Chapter 16). By repeating LUS scanning, tissue dissection may be guided. LUS delineates surrounding structures such as vascular structures, including the renal and adrenal vessels, splenic vessels, aorta and vena cava, the kidney, spleen, pancreas, and gastrointestinal tract, which may also help to avoid injuries to these structures (Fig 31). For malignant adrenal tumors, local tumor invasion as well as liver and lymph node metastasis can be assessed to determine the resectability (Fig 32).

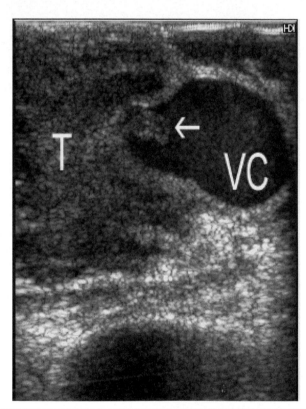

FIGURE 32. Malignant right adrenal tumor with a tumor thrombus. Laparoscopic ultrasound showed a large metastatic adrenal tumor (T) from a lung cancer, causing a tumor thrombus (*arrow*) in the inferior vena cava (VC). (Courtesy of Dr. Maurice Arregui.)

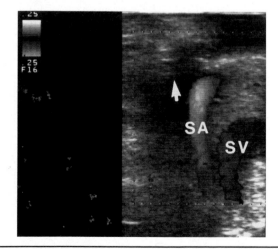

FIGURE 31. Laparoscopic ultrasound color Doppler imaging demonstrated the splenic artery (SA) and the splenic vein (SV) adjacent to the tumor shown in Figure 30. An arrow indicates the direction of the adrenal tumor posteriorly and inferiorly.

Spleen

When laparoscopic splenectomy is performed, LUS may not be needed in most operations; however, if splenectomy is for a malignant disease, LUS may be used to determine the extent of spread of a tumor. LUS is more frequently performed to evaluate preoperatively identified splenic lesions. LUS can distinguish cystic from solid lesions readily, and characterize solid tumors (Figs. 33 and 34). At times, preoperatively unrecognized splenic lesions can be identified by LUS (Fig. 35). Accessory spleens can be localized quickly by LUS to facilitate laparoscopic accessory splenectomy (see Fig. 54 in Chapter 16).

Retroperitoneum and Other Abdominal Pathology

When laparoscopic exploration or surgery is performed for malignant retroperitoneal tumors or any other abdominal tumors, LUS together with laparoscopy is useful for tumor staging and for determination of resectability,

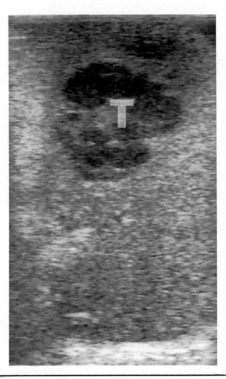

FIGURE 34. Splenic solid tumor (lymphoma). In a patient with suspected lymphoma, laparoscopic ultrasound showed a hypoechoic, heterogeneous, 2-cm, solid tumor (T) in the midportion of the spleen.

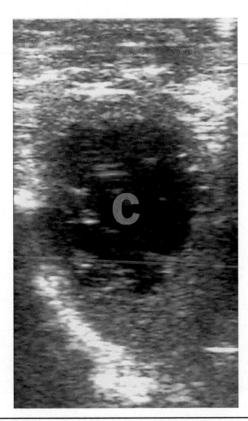

FIGURE 33. Complex splenic cyst. Preoperative computed tomography resulted in detection of a lesion in the spleen but with poor characterization. During laparoscopic cholecystectomy for symptomatic gallstones, laparoscopic ultrasound (LUS) was performed. With LUS the lesion was diagnosed as a complex cyst (C), 2.5 cm, in the upper portion of the spleen; therefore, no further treatment was required.

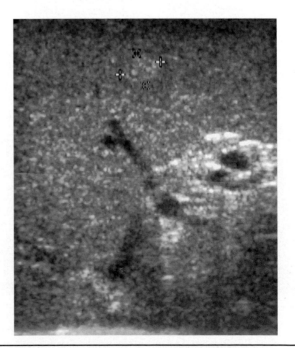

FIGURE 35. Occult splenic lesions detected by laparoscopic ultrasound (LUS). During laparoscopic resection of a recurrent gastrointestinal stromal tumor, LUS identified a 5 × 4 mm hyperechoic lesion (*cursors*) in the spleen. It was too small to characterize by LUS.

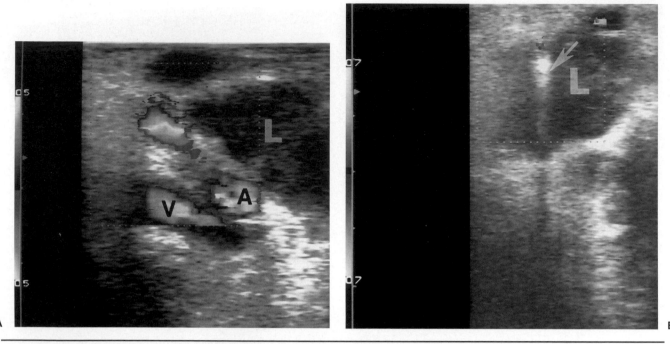

FIGURE 36. Retroperitoneal lymphoma. **A:** Laparoscopic ultrasound (LUS) (color Doppler imaging) quickly localized multiple enlarged lymph nodes (L) in the retroperitoneum and demonstrated their relation to vascular structures such as the splenic artery (A) and vein (V). (See Color Plate 35.) **B:** LUS-guided core needle biopsy of a lymph node. LUS was used to guide a needle (*arrow*) into a lymph node (L), avoiding injury to blood vessels.

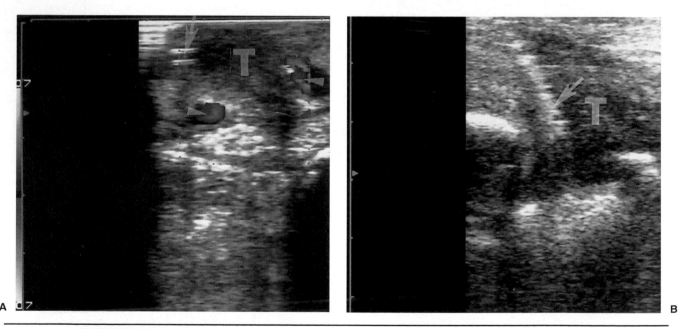

FIGURE 37. Recurrent pelvic lymphoma. **A:** A large tumor (T) surrounding the left ureter was localized by laparoscopic ultrasound (LUS) (color Doppler imaging) in the left side of the pelvis. An arrow indicates a stent in the ureter. Arrowheads indicate ileac vessel branches. (See Color Plate 36.) **B:** LUS-guided core needle biopsy. Under LUS guidance, a needle (*arrow*) was inserted into the tumor (T) after selecting the safe location for biopsy to avoid injury to the ureter or blood vessels.

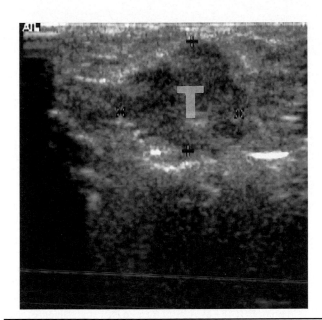

FIGURE 38. Recurrent gastrointestinal stromal tumor. During laparoscopic resection, laparoscopic ultrasound allowed quick localization of this 1.3 × 1.4 cm hypoechoic tumor (T) in the left upper abdomen and facilitated laparoscopic tissue dissection.

in a manner similar to LUS for hepatobiliary and pancreatic cancers. If solid tumors or enlarged lymph nodes are detected, LUS-guided needle biopsy can be performed. For example, when laparoscopy is performed for a patient with suspected lymphoma, lymph nodes or masses can be biopsied under LUS guidance (Figs. 36 and 37). Recurrent abdominal or retroperitoneal cancers can be localized and biopsied by LUS, particularly when laparoscopic exploration and tissue dissection are difficult due to previous surgery (Fig. 38). LUS can be a valuable method during laparoscopic abdominal abscess drainage and foreign body removal.

CONCLUSIONS

LUS is a new form of IOUS that represents a merger of technologies of laparoscopy and IOUS. In addition to the indication for LUS during laparoscopic cholecystectomy for calculous diseases, LUS is indicated during laparoscopic explorations and operations for malignant abdominal diseases, particularly hepatobiliary, pancreatic, and gastroesophageal cancers. There are many other applications of LUS reported for benign and malignant diseases of various organs, including the adrenal gland, spleen, and retroperitoneum. Diseases and organs for which LUS is indicated are essentially similar to those for open IOUS.

There are advantages and limitations of LUS (see Table 6 in Chapter 13). The major advantage is that LUS can compensate for the limitation of laparoscopy, provid-

ing more diagnostic information and thereby improving the accuracy. Prelaparotomy laparoscopic exploration with LUS for malignant diseases is becoming popular, especially to avoid nontherapeutic laparotomy. LUS guidance capability is indispensable during minimally invasive laparoscopic procedures such as biopsy, ablation, and resection. New ultrasound technologies are currently incorporated in LUS as well as in open IOUS. For example, color or power Doppler imaging enhances the capability of LUS (77) (see Chapter 13). Three-dimensional ultrasound has become available for use during LUS (78). Furthermore, an LUS technique has been expanded to thoracoscopic procedures; intraoperative thoracoscopic ultrasound has been reported to assist pulmonary nodule resection (79,80).

Although LUS is potentially capable of providing the same diagnostic information as open IOUS, the actual diagnostic accuracy of LUS may not be as high as that of open IOUS due to a more demanding technical aspect of LUS and a strong dependency of LUS examination on the laparoscopic surgeon's competency in scanning. Laparoscopic surgeons who are interested in learning LUS are encouraged to master open IOUS at the same time; the ability to perform IOUS greatly facilitates the learning curve for LUS. In addition, whenever laparoscopy is performed for abdominal diseases or pathologic lesions that might be difficult to access, localize, or diagnose by laparoscopy alone, it is highly recommended that LUS be available in the operating room so that the surgeon can utilize it liberally. In this manner, the surgeon will become more experienced with LUS and may even find a new application for LUS.

REFERENCES

1. Jakimowicz J. Laparoscopic intraoperative ultrasonography, equipment and techniques. *Semin Laparosc Surg* 1994;1: 52–61.
2. Bezzi M, Merlino R, Orsi F, et al. Laparoscopic sonography during abdominal laparoscopic surgery: technique and imaging findings. *AJR Am J Roentgenol* 1995;165:1193–1198.
3. Machi J, Schwartz, JH, Zaren HA, et al. Technique of laparoscopic ultrasound examination of the liver and pancreas. *Surg Endosc* 1996;10:684–689.
4. Hozumi M, Ido K, Hiki S, et al. Easy and accurate targeting of deep-seated hepatic tumors under laparoscopy with a forward-viewing convex-array transducer. *Surg Endosc* 2003; 17:1256–1260.
5. Cuschieri A. Laparoscopic hand-assisted surgery for hepatic and pancreatic disease. *Surg Endosc* 2000;14:991–996.
6. Machi J, Oishi AJ, Mossing A, et al. Hand-assisted laparoscopic ultrasound-guided radiofrequency thermal ablation of liver tumors: a technical report. *Surg Laparosc Endosc Percutan Tech* 2002;12:160–164.
7. Jakimowicz JJ. Review: intraoperative ultrasonography during minimal access surgery. *J R Coll Surg (Edinb)* 1993;38: 231–238.
8. Stiegmann GV, McIntyre RC Jr. Laparoscopic ultrasonography: has it extended the horizon? *Gastrointest Endosc Clin North Am* 1995;5:869–878.

9. Liu JB, Feld RI, Barbot DJ, et al. Laparoscopic ultrasound: its role in laparoscopic surgery. *Semin Laparosc Surg* 1996;3:50–58.
10. Callery MP, Strasberg SM, Doherty GM, et al. Staging laparoscopy with laparoscopic ultrasonography: optimizing resectability in hepatobiliary and pancreatic malignancy. *J Am Coll Surg* 1997;185:33–39.
11. Thompson DM, Tetik C, Arregui ME. Laparoscopic ultrasound. *Probl Gen Surg* 1997;14:107–116.
12. Kolecki R, Schirmer B. Intraoperative and laparoscopic ultrasound. *Surg Clin North Am* 1998;78:251–271.
13. Machi J. Intraoperative and laparoscopic ultrasound. *Surg Oncol Clin North Am* 1999;8:205–226.
14. Nieveen van Dijkum EJ, de Wit LT, van Delden OM, et al. Staging laparoscopy and laparoscopic ultrasonography in more than 400 patients with upper gastrointestinal carcinoma. *J Am Coll Surg* 1999;189:459–465.
15. Tsioulias GJ, Wood TF, Chung MH, et al. Diagnostic laparoscopy and laparoscopic ultrasonography optimize the staging and resectability of intraabdominal neoplasms. *Surg Endosc* 2001;15:1016–1019.
16. Goudas LA, Brams DM, Birkett DH. The use of laparoscopic ultrasonography in staging abdominal malignancy. *Semin Laparosc Surg* 2000;7:78–86.
17. Rau B, Hunerbein M, Schlag PM. Is there additional information from laparoscopic ultrasound in tumor staging? *Dig Surg* 2002;19:479–483.
18. Cuesta MA, Meijer S, Borgstein PJ, et al. Laparoscopic ultrasonography for hepatobiliary and pancreatic malignancy. *Br J Surg* 1993;80:1571–1574.
19. John T, Greig J, Crosbie JL, et al. Superior staging of liver tumors with laparoscopy and laparoscopic ultrasound. *Ann Surg* 1994;220:711–719.
20. Barbot DJ, Marks JH, Feld RI, et al. Improved staging of liver tumors using laparoscopic intraoperative ultrasound. *J Surg Oncol* 1997;64:63–67.
21. Lo CM, Lai EC, Liu CL, et al. Laparoscopy and laparoscopic ultrasonography avoid exploratory laparotomy in patients with hepatocellular carcinoma. *Ann Surg* 1998;227:527–532.
22. Rahusen FD, Cuesta MA, Borgstein PJ, et al. Selection of patients for resection of colorectal metastases to the liver using diagnostic laparoscopy and laparoscopic ultrasonography. *Ann Surg* 1999;230:31–37.
23. Farnagin WR, Bodniewicz F, Dougherty E, et al. A prospective analysis of staging laparoscopy in patients with primary and secondary hepatobiliary malignancies. *J Gastrointest Surg* 2000;4:34–43.
24. Catheline JM, Turner R, Champault G. Laparoscopic ultrasound of the liver. *Eur J Ultrasound* 2000;12:169–177.
25. Figueras J, Valls C. The use of laparoscopic ultrasonography in the preoperative study of patients with colorectal liver metastases. *Ann Surg* 2000;232:721–723.
26. Montorsi M, Santambrogio R, Bianchi P, et al. Laparoscopy with laparoscopic ultrasound for pretreatment staging of hepatocellular carcinoma: a prospective study. *J Gastrointest Surg* 2001;5:312–315.
27. Murugiah M, Paterson-Brown S, Windsor JA, et al. Early experience of laparoscopic ultrasonography in the management of pancreatic carcinoma. *Surg Endosc* 1993;7:177–181.
28. Bemelman WA, De Wit LT, van Delden OM, et al. Diagnostic laparoscopy combined with laparoscopic ultrasonography in staging of cancer of the pancreatic head region. *Br J Surg* 1995;82:820–824.
29. John TG, Greig JD, Carter DC, et al. Carcinoma of the pancreatic head and periampullary region. Tumor staging with laparoscopy and laparoscopic ultrasound. *Ann Surg* 1995;221:156–164.
30. van Delden OM, Smits NJ, Bemelman WA, et al. Comparison of laparoscopic and transabdominal ultrasonography in staging of cancer of the pancreatic head region. *J Ultrasound Med* 1996;16:207–212.
31. Minnard EA, Conlon KC, Hoos A, et al. Laparoscopic ultrasound enhances standard laparoscopy in the staging of pancreatic cancer. *Ann Surg* 1998;228:182–187.
32. Catheline JM, Turner R, Rizk N, et al. The use of diagnostic laparoscopy supported by laparoscopic ultrasonography in the assessment of pancreatic cancer. *Surg Endosc* 1999;13:239–245.
33. Pietrabiassa A, Caramella D, Di Candio G, et al. Laparoscopy and laparoscopic ultrasonography for staging pancreatic cancer: critical appraisal. *World J Surg* 1999;23:998–1003.
34. Schachter PP, Avni Y, Shimonov M, et al. The impact of laparoscopy and laparoscopic ultrasonography on the management of pancreatic cancer. *Arch Surg* 2000;135:1303–1307.
35. Menack MJ, Spitz JD, Arregui ME. Staging of pancreatic and ampullary cancers for resectability using laparoscopy with laparoscopic ultrasound. *Surg Endosc* 2001;15:1129–1134.
36. Vollmer CM, Drebin JA, Middleton WD, et al. Utility of staging laparoscopy in subsets of peripancreatic and biliary malignancies. *Ann Surg* 2002;235:1–7.
37. van Delden OM, De Wit LT, Van Dijkum EJMN, et al. Value of laparoscopic ultrasonography in staging of proximal bile ducts tumors. *J Ultrasound Med* 1997;16:7–12.
38. Weber SM, DeMatteo RP, Fong Y, et al. Staging laparoscopy in patients with extrahepatic biliary carcinoma. Analysis of 100 patients. *Ann Surg* 2002;235:392–399.
39. Tilleman EH, de Castro SM, Buscho OR, et al. Diagnostic laparoscopy and laparoscopic ultrasound for staging of patients with malignant proximal bile duct obstruction. *J Gastrointest Surg* 2002;6:426–431.
40. Bemelman WA, van Delden OM, Van Lanschot JJB, et al. Laparoscopy and laparoscopic ultrasonography in staging of carcinoma of the esophagus and gastric cardia. *J Am Coll Surg* 1995;181:421–425.
41. Hunerbein M, Rau B, Schlag PM. Laparoscopy and laparoscopic ultrasound for staging of upper gastrointestinal tumors. *Eur J Surg Oncol* 1995;21:50–55.
42. Anderson DN, Campbell S, Park KGM. Accuracy of laparoscopic ultrasonography in the staging of upper gastrointestinal malignancy. *Br J Surg* 1996;83:1424–1428.
43. Finch MD, John TG, Garden OJ. Laparoscopic ultrasonography for staging gastroesophageal cancer. *Surgery* 1997;121:10–17.
44. Stein HJ, Kraemer SJM, Feussner H, et al. Clinical value of diagnostic laparoscopy with laparoscopic ultrasound in patients with cancer of the esophagus and cardia. *J Gastrointest Surg* 1997;1:167–173.
45. Romijn MG, Van Overhagen H, Spillenaar Bilgen EJ, et al. Laparoscopy and laparoscopic ultrasonography in staging of oesophageal and cardial carcinoma. *Br J Surg* 1998;85:1010–1012.
46. Wakelin SJ, Deans C, Crofts TJ, et al. A comparison of computerized tomography, laparoscopic ultrasound and endoscopic ultrasound in the preoperative staging of oesophagogastric carcinoma. *Eur J Radiol* 2002;41:161–167.
47. Foley EF, Kolecki RV, Schirmer BD. The accuracy of laparoscopic ultrasound in the detection of colorectal cancer liver metastases. *Am J Surg* 1998;176:262–264.
48. Hartley JE, Kumar H, Drew PJ, et al. Laparoscopic ultrasound for the detection of hepatic metastases during laparoscopic colorectal cancer surgery. *Dis Colon Rectum* 2000;43:320–324.
49. Santambrogio R, Bianchi P, Pasta A, et al. Ultrasound-guided interventional procedures of the liver during laparoscopy. Technical considerations. *Surg Endosc* 2002;16:349–354.
50. Siperstein AE, Rogers SJ, Hansen PD, et al. Laparoscopic thermal ablation of hepatic neuroendocrine tumor metastases. *Surgery* 1997;122:1147–1155.
51. Bilchik AJ, Rose DM, Allegra DP, et al. Radiofrequency ablation; a minimally invasive technique with multiple applications. *Cancer J* 1999;5:356–361.
52. Siperstein A, Garland A, Engle K, et al. Local recurrence after laparoscopic radiofrequency thermal ablation of hepatic tumors. *Ann Surg Oncol* 2000;7:106–113.
53. Machi J, Uchida S, Sumida K, et al. Ultrasound-guided radiofrequency thermal ablation of liver tumors; percutane-

ous, laparoscopic and open surgical approaches. *J Gastrointest Surg* 2001;5:477–489.

54. Lezoche E, Peganini AM, Feliciotti F, et al. Ultrasound-guided laparoscopic cryoablation of hepatic tumors: preliminary report. *World J Surg* 1998;22:829–836.
55. Cuesta MA, Meijer S, Paul MA, et al. Limited laparoscopic liver resection of benign tumors guided by laparoscopic ultrasonography: report of two cases. *Surg Laparosc Endosc Percutan Tech* 1995;5:396–401.
56. Linden BC, Humar A, Sielaff TD. Laparoscopic stapled left lateral segment liver resection: technique and results. *J Gastrointest Surg* 2003;7:777–782.
57. Schachter PP, Avni Y, Gvirtz G, et al. The impact of laparoscopy and laparoscopic ultrasound on the management of pancreatic cystic lesions. *Arch Surg* 2000;135:260–264.
58. Pertsemlidis D, Edye M. Diagnostic and interventional laparoscopy and intraoperative ultrasonography in the management of pancreatic disease. *Surg Clin North Am* 2001;81:363–377.
59. Schachter PP, Shimonov M, Czerniak A. The role of laparoscopy and laparoscopic ultrasound in the diagnosis of cystic lesions of the pancreas. *Gastrointest Endosc Clin North Am* 2002;12:759–767.
60. Gagner M, Pomp A, Herrera MF. Early experience with laparoscopic resections of islet cell tumors. *Surgery* 1996;120:1051–1054.
61. Sussman LA, Christie R, Whittle DE. Laparoscopic excision of distal pancreas including insulinoma. *Aust N Z J Surg* 1996;66:14–16.
62. Spitz JD, Lilly MC, Tetik C, et al. Ultrasound-guided laparoscopic resection of pancreatic islet cell tumors. *Surg Laparosc Endosc Percutan Tech* 2000;10:168–173.
63. Lo CY, Lo CM, Fan ST. Role of laparoscopic ultrasonography in intraoperative localization of pancreatic insulinoma. *Surg Endosc* 2000;14:1131–1135.
64. Iihara M, Kanbe M, Okamoto T, et al. Laparoscopic ultrasonography for resection of insulinomas. *Surgery* 2001;130:1086–1091.
65. Schachter P, Sorin V, Avni Y, et al. The role of laparoscopic ultrasound in the minimally invasive management of symptomatic hepatic cysts. *Surg Endosc* 2001;15:364–367.
66. Heniford BT, Iannitti DA, Hale J, et al. The role of intraoperative ultrasonography during laparoscopic adrenalectomy. *Surgery* 1997;122:1068–1074.
67. Lucas SW, Sptiz JD, Arregui ME. The use of intraoperative ultrasound in laparoscopic adrenal surgery. *Surg Endosc* 1999;13:1093–1098.

68. Brunt LM, Bennett HF, Teefey SA, et al. Laparoscopic ultrasound imaging of adrenal tumors during laparoscopic adrenalectomy. *Am J Surg* 1999;178:490–495.
69. Pautler SE, Choyke PL, Pavlovich CP, et al. Intraoperative ultrasound aids in dissection during laparoscopic partial adrenalectomy. *J Urol* 2002;168:1352–1355.
70. Cugat E, Hoyuela C, Rodriguez-Santiago JM, et al. Laparoscopic ultrasound guidance for laparoscopic resection of benign gastric tumors. *J Laparoendosc Adv Surg Tech A* 1999;9:63–67.
71. van Delden OM, de Wit LT, Hulsmans F-JH, et al. Laparoscopic ultrasonography of abdominal lymph nodes: correlation with pathologic findings. *J Ultrasound Med* 1998;17:21–27.
72. Yang WT, Cheung TH, Ho SS, et al. Comparison of laparoscopic sonography with surgical pathology in the evaluation of pelvic lymph nodes in women with cervical cancer. *AJR Am J Roentgenol* 1999;172:1521–1525.
73. Goletti O, Buccianti P, Chiarugi M, et al. Laparoscopic sonography in screening metastases from gastrointestinal cancer: comparative accuracy with traditional procedures. *Surg Laparosc Endosc Percutan Tech* 1995;5:176–182.
74. Feld RI, Liu JB, Nazarian L, et al. Laparoscopic liver sonography: preliminary experience in liver metastases compared with CT portography. *J Ultrasound Med* 1996;15:289–295.
75. Foroutani A, Garland AM, Berber E, et al. Laparoscopic ultrasound vs triphasic computed tomography for detecting liver tumors. *Arch Surg* 2000;135:933–938.
76. Milsom JW, Jerby BL, Kessler H, et al. Prospective, blinded comparison of laparoscopic ultrasonography vs. contrast-enhanced computerized tomography for liver assessment in patients undergoing colorectal carcinoma surgery. *Dis Colon Rectum* 2000;43:44–49.
77. Jakimowicz JJ, Stuiltiens GN. Laparoscopic intraoperative ultrasonography, color Doppler, and power flow application. *Semin Laparosc Surg* 1997;4:110–119.
78. Harms J, Feussner H, Baumgartner M, et al. Three-dimensional navigated laparoscopic ultrasonography. First experiences with a new minimally invasive diagnostic device. *Surg Endosc* 2001;15:1459–1462.
79. Hida Y, Kato H, Nishibe T, et al. Value of intraoperative intrathoracic ultrasonography during video-assisted thoracoscopic pulmonary resection. *Surg Laparosc Endosc Percutan Tech* 1996;6: 472–475.
80. Santambrogio R, Montorsi M, Bianchi P, et al. Intraoperative ultrasound during thoracoscopic procedures for solitary pulmonary nodules. *Ann Thorac Surg* 1999;68:218–222.

Ultrasound Use in Organ Transplantation

Lawrence P. McChesney, Thomas Walsh, and Sara Goddu

Solid organ transplantation has advanced over recent years from a therapy of experimentation to the standard of care for end-organ diseases of the kidney, liver, pancreas, heart, lung, and intestines. In the year 2002, organ transplants were performed 24,898 times with patient and graft survival rates of 75% to 95%, far exceeding the survival rates of the patients without transplantation (1,2). This increased effectiveness has been attributed to improved technical aspects of the operation, better immunosuppression, and specialized patient care in the pre- and posttransplantation periods. Graft losses have been reduced significantly. Today the most common cause for graft loss after the first year is death with a functioning graft.

One of the factors that have contributed to increased graft survival is the ability to identify graft dysfunction and its causes(s) while it is still reversible. Biochemical markers provide functional evaluation, but anatomic evaluation is required to accurately determine the cause of graft dysfunction. The ability to evaluate a transplant organ by a noninvasive approach is required. In this chapter, the application, instrumentation, and techniques of ultrasound for various transplant organs, including kidney, pancreas, liver, and heart, are described.

APPLICATION OF ULTRASOUND FOR ORGAN TRANSPLANTATION (Table 1)

Although various imaging modalities can be used for organ transplantation, ultrasound provides most of the required diagnostic information in a timely manner and with acceptable sensitivity and specificity (Table 1). Ultrasound evaluation of the transplant organ can be obtained within the transplant clinic and can easily be repeated for follow-up evaluation. Ultrasound can also be used for accurate guidance to obtain tissue for histologic diagnosis. Overall, ultrasound provides relevant information in the investigation of organ dysfunction, resulting in early intervention with improved outcomes.

Ultrasound is helpful in the evaluation of the organ donor as well. Echocardiography of the donor heart provides initial selection criteria. Ultrasound also provides guidance for percutaneous biopsy of the liver for donor selection.

INSTRUMENTATION AND TECHNIQUES

Abdominal organs are imaged with the use of a 3.5- to 5.0-MHz transducer. This allows for adequate sound penetration and resolution. Many times in the postoperative course, identifying a window for scanning access of the appropriate view is difficult; in such cases, removal of the operative dressing is usually required.

Renal transplants are placed in the pelvis, either intraperitoneally or retroperitoneally. They are typically palpable in the iliac fossa. Placement of the ultrasound transducer directly over the palpable kidney provides an excellent window for imaging the vasculature and the ureter, and for obtaining resistive indices.

A common site for implantation of the pancreas allograft is in the iliac fossa. With the utilization of portal drainage, the pancreas is placed beneath the transverse mesocolon. Therefore, familiarity with the technique used by the transplantation surgeon is helpful. When the graft is placed in the iliac fossa, the body and tail are positioned along the lateral gutter of the abdomen. This provides an optimal window for viewing the pancreas while avoiding intervening bowel.

Implantation of the transplant liver is accomplished via a bisubcostal incision with or without a xiphoid incision. Although imaging through the anterior abdominal wall (subcostal scanning) is possible, right intercostal scanning often provides the best window for the evaluation of the hilar structures and visualization of a possible hematoma of the right hepatic fossa.

> **TABLE 1** Application and Advantages of
> Ultrasound for Organ Transplantation

1. Evaluation of graft dysfunction and other posttransplantation complication:
   a. Readily available, noninvasive, repeatable, and highly accurate
   b. Relevant information allowing for early intervention (with improved outcomes)
2. Guidance of biopsy for histologic diagnosis:
   Safe and precise needle guidance
3. Evaluation and biopsy guidance of donor organs
4. Evaluation of organ recipients

RENAL TRANSPLANTATION (Table 2)

Renal transplantation both from cadaveric and living donors is the most frequent solid organ transplant. In 2002, 14,775 renal transplantation procedures were performed. Of those, half may be expected to result in an episode of dysfunction within the first year. That potentially accounts for 7,000 ultrasound examinations being done for the evaluation of renal transplant dysfunction. Ultrasound has the advantage of being readily available, noninvasive, and associated with high sensitivity/specificity in evaluating renal transplant dysfunction. The workup for renal allograft dysfunction includes evaluation of vascular inflow/outflow, ureteral obstruction/stenosis/leak, extrarenal mass effect such as a hematoma/lymphocele, and measurement of the vascular resistance in the substance of the kidney.

Vascular Thrombosis and Ureter Complications

Two percent of renal transplants will develop vascular thrombosis, with venous thrombosis occurring more often than arterial (3). Thrombosis predominately occurs within the first 48 hours following implantation. The clinical presentation of venous thrombosis initially involves development of markedly bloody urine with the onset of acute oliguria. Pain over the allograft is present, as well as ipsilateral lower extremity edema from adja-

> **TABLE 2** Ultrasound for Renal Transplantation

1. Evaluation of renal graft dysfunction
2. Evaluation of posttransplantation complications:
   a. Vascular (arterial and venous) thrombosis
   b. Ureter obstruction/stenosis: hydroureter, hydronephrosis
   c. Hematoma, lymphocele
3. Evaluation of acute rejection: measurements of resistive indices
4. Guidance of biopsy of transplant kidney

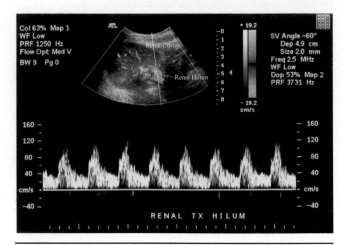

FIGURE 1. Ultrasound with Doppler spectrum of the transplant kidney demonstrating excellent flow in the renal artery and renal vein. (See Color Plate 37.)

cent iliac vein thrombosis/stenosis. However, hematuria can also occur secondary to bleeding from the anastomosis of the ureter to the bladder or from Foley catheter–related injury.

Arterial thrombosis produces acute anuria from the transplant kidney. Other causes of oliguria can be preservation injury to the graft or development of acute tubular necrosis. Ultrasound of the transplant kidney confirms inflow in the transplant renal artery as well as outflow in the transplant renal vein (Fig. 1). Urgency in making the diagnosis is required if salvage of the graft is to be possible.

If the creatinine does not reach normal levels, investigation of obstruction/stenosis of the transplant ureter should be performed. Stenosis/necrosis occurs in 2% of renal transplants (4). Ultrasound reveals the presence of hydroureter and dilatation of the renal pelvis (Fig. 2).

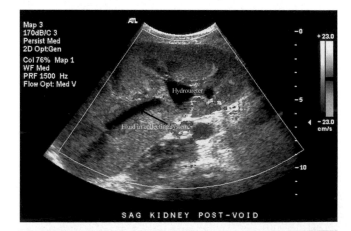

FIGURE 2. Hydroureter is sometimes difficult to visualize. However, the identification of dilated renal pelvis and calyces are suggestive of ureteral obstruction/stenosis.

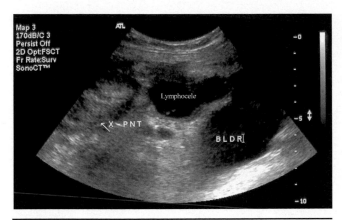

FIGURE 3. Lymphocele is seen as a hypoechoic fluid collection adjacent to the transplant kidney. Mass effect of the collection results in impairment of regional perfusion and/or ureteral obstruction.

Prompt diagnosis allows for the insertion of a ureteral stent or revision of the ureteral anastomosis.

Hematoma and Lymphocele

Peritransplantation hemorrhage in the immediate postoperative period can result in a mass effect, which reduces renal perfusion and subsequent urine output in the extraperitoneal transplant kidney. Ultrasound identifies a hematoma, thereby allowing for evacuation. In the third to twelfth weeks posttransplantation, the development of a lymphocele also produces a mass effect resulting in deterioration of renal function (Fig. 3) (5). Ipsilateral edema of the lower extremity and or scrotal/labial edema are presenting signs. Ultrasound readily provides the diagno-

sis of a lymphocele. Evacuation of the lymphocele by creation of a peritoneal window is an effective treatment and results in improvement of renal function.

Acute Rejection

Acute rejection of the allograft most frequently occurs in the first 90 days following transplantation. The relevant ultrasound findings in cases of acute rejection include absence of vascular impairment, absence of hydroureter, and absence of extrarenal mass such as lymphocele. Rejection produces intercellular edema resulting in a swollen kidney and increased vascular resistance. Vascular resistance in the transplant kidney is noted by the measurement of resistive indices (peak systolic pressure − end diastolic pressure/peak systolic pressure). This measurement is obtained in the arcuate arteries, preferably at the superior pole, middle, and inferior pole of the kidney (Fig. 4). A normal resistive index value is 0.4 to 0.7. An increased resistive index in the kidney would be supportive of the diagnosis of rejection (Fig. 5) (6). However, any process that increases interstitial edema produces an increased resistive index. Therefore, increased resistive index is not specific to allograft rejection.

Ultrasound also guides the successful performance of a core biopsy of the transplant kidney in more than 95% of attempts, thus allowing for accurate histologic diagnosis of rejection. Biopsy of an arterialized organ has the potential to cause bleeding from the biopsy site. However, experience has found the procedure to be safe when precautionary measures are taken (Fig. 6). Complications such as extrarenal hematoma or hematuria occurs in less than 5% of cases under such precautions.

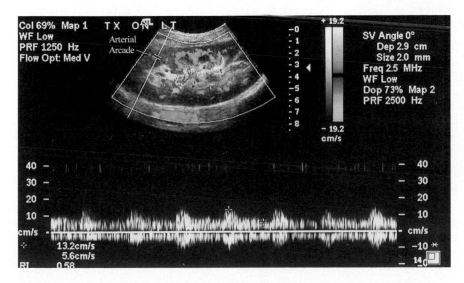

FIGURE 4. Vascular resistive index (RI) is obtained from the arcuate arterials within the cortex of the kidney. In this sonogram, the RI is 0.58. (See Color Plate 38.)

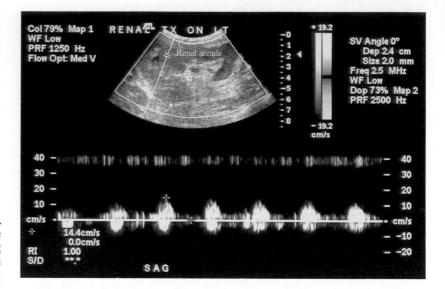

FIGURE 5. Interstitial edema from multiple sources increases vascular resistance resulting in loss of diastolic flow in the renal arcade. In this sonogram the resistive index (RI) is 1.00.

PANCREAS TRANSPLANTATION (Table 3)

Pancreas transplantation is performed for the management of diabetes with complications that have failed medical management. Of patients referred for pancreas transplantation, 87% have chronic renal failure secondary to the diabetes. These patients are candidates for combined pancreas and renal transplantation. Success rates have improved significantly over the last several years, with more than 95% patient and more than 90% pancreas graft survival in some programs. Successful pancreas transplantation not only relieves the patient of the need for exogenous insulin but also normalizes glycosylation of proteins, with the reversal of complications such as neuropathies and stabilization of retinopathy.

Surgical Techniques of Pancreas Transplantation

The anatomic placement of the pancreas graft is dependent on the route of venous drainage. Systemic drainage can be achieved by placing the graft in the iliac fossa, thereby allowing the graft portal vein to drain into the recipient iliac or caval system (Fig. 7). Some data support positioning the transplant pancreas to allow venous drainage to the recipient portal venous system. This can be achieved by placing the anastomosis of the donor portal vein into a branch of the superior mesenteric vein. This positions the graft high in the abdomen and typically under the transverse mesocolon.

Arterial blood flow to the pancreas is from the splenic artery, gastroduodenal artery, and superior mesenteric artery. Because these arteries share origins with the vascular supply to the liver and both donor organs are to be used for transplantation, reconstruction of the arterial supply to the pancreas graft is required (Fig. 8). The pan-

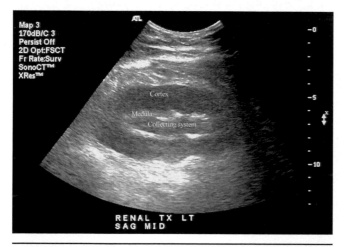

FIGURE 6. Ultrasound demonstrates a clear image of the transplant kidney without intervening structures, allowing for accurate guidance for percutaneous biopsy. This technique subsequently reduces complications and increases success in obtaining tissue.

▶ **TABLE 3 Ultrasound for Pancreas Transplantation**

1. Evaluation of posttransplantation complications:
   a. Fluid collections: abscess, duodenal segment leak
   b. Ultrasound-guided aspiration
   c. Vascular thrombosis
2. Evaluation of pancreatic graft dysfunction: acute rejection, preservation injury, reflux pancreatitis, or duct stenosis:
   Detection of fluid collection, pancreatic duct dilatation
3. Guidance of biopsy of transplant pancreas

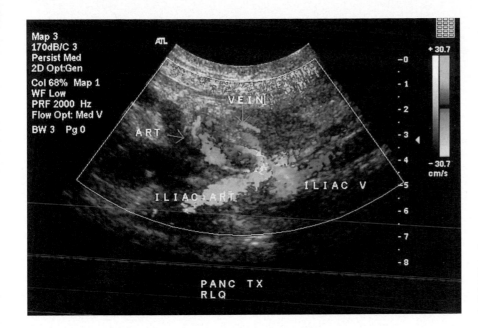

FIGURE 7. Ultrasonic depiction of the portal vein flow into the iliac vein and adjacent arterial flow via the reconstructed arterial conduit of the pancreas graft. (See Color Plate 39.)

creas has an extensive collateral circulation, and therefore only two of the three inflows are required for adequate arterialization of the pancreas graft. Using the donor common, internal, and external iliac arteries, reconstruction is carried out. This is achieved by the anastomosis of the donor internal iliac artery to the graft splenic artery and the donor external iliac artery to the orifice of the graft superior mesenteric artery. This allows for a long donor common iliac artery to be used for anastomosis to the recipient iliac artery. Because of the frequent calcification of iliac arteries in diabetes patients, this extension graft is helpful to reach a soft portion of the recipient iliac artery for an end-to-side anastomosis.

The approach utilized to obtain exocrine drainage has undergone considerable change over the years. The pancreas is implanted with the attached duodenum to provide a conduit for exocrine drainage. Anastomosis of the transplant duodenum to the urinary bladder provides a safe and reliable method of exocrine drainage. However, significant complications, such as reflux pancreatitis, dehydration, metabolic acidosis secondary to bicarbonate loss, and increased rates of urinary tract infections, may

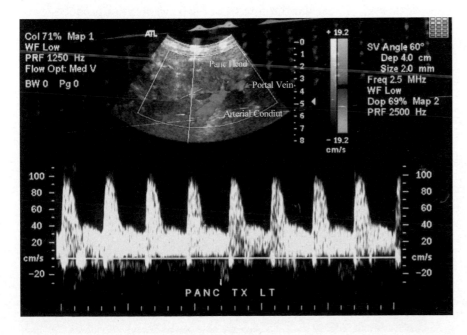

FIGURE 8. Ultrasound with Doppler spectrum depicting the arterial reconstruction and arterial inflow to the transplant pancreas. (See Color Plate 40.)

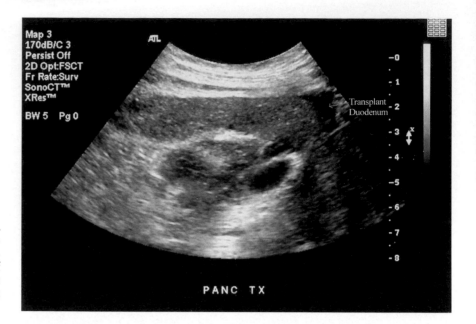

FIGURE 9. In this ultrasound, the duodenum attached to the head of the transplant pancreas is hypoechoic suggestive of peripancreatic fluid collection. Peristalsis identifies the structure as the transplant duodenum.

occur. Enteric drainage of the exocrine material has been found in many programs to be more advantageous than bladder drainage. We have not seen an increase in the rate of anastomotic complications or decreased graft survival with enteric drainage.

Fluid Collections

Fluid collections adjacent to the pancreas graft are common and usually resolve spontaneously. Persistent fluid collection surrounding the pancreas graft results from abscess collection or duodenal segment leak. Aspiration of the fluid collection under ultrasound guidance helps to differentiate the high amylase content of a duodenal segment leak from a lymphocele (Fig. 9) (7).

Vascular Complications

Thrombosis of the vascular supply to the transplant pancreas occurs with an incidence of 10% to 15%. Ultrasound is reliable in the evaluation of such complications. Transplant pancreas portal vein thrombosis occurs much more frequently than graft arterial thrombosis (Fig. 10) (8). Modification in the technique of venous anastomosis, such as complete mobilization of the recipient iliac vein or anastomosis directly to the side of the inferior vena cava, has markedly reduced the incidence of venous thrombosis.

When exocrine drainage is provided by the anastomosis of the transplant duodenum to the recipient bladder, vascular thrombosis of the pancreas graft produces gross hematuria. In the enteric-drained graft, hematuria is ab-

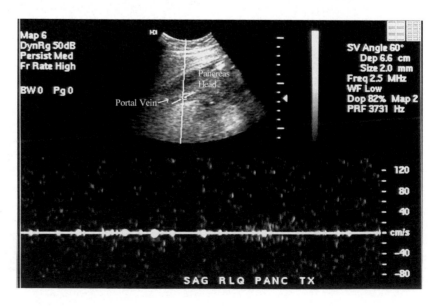

FIGURE 10. Ultrasound of the transplant pancreas showing the absence of flow in the portal vein of the transplant pancreas.

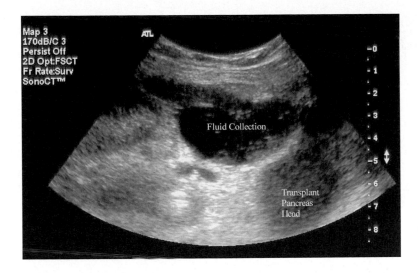

FIGURE 11. Hypoechoic mass consistent with peripancreatic fluid collection.

sent but a markedly increased serum amylase is seen accompanied by pain over the graft. Diagnosis is made by urgent ultrasound evaluation of the vascular grafts.

Pancreas Graft Dysfunction

Edematous pancreatitis and hyperamylasemia have several causes in the transplanted pancreas and are not specific to a single etiologic factor. Dysfunction of the transplant pancreas secondary to rejection, preservation injury, or reflux pancreatitis produces an increased serum amylase and a decreased exocrine amylase. Bladder drainage of the transplant pancreas allows for measurement of the amylase content in the urine. A reduction of urinary amylase is suggestive of rejection of the transplant pancreas. Increases in serum amylase have also been found to be a reliable marker for graft dysfunction. Continuous elevation of the serum glucose does not occur until loss of more than 90% of the islet cell mass has occurred and is not a useful marker for early graft dysfunction. Therefore, increased serum amylase should result in urgent ultrasound evaluation of the transplanted pancreas.

Ultrasound examination can reveal the presence of peripancreatic fluid and abnormalities in the vascular supply (Fig. 11). The visualization of an increase in the diameter of the pancreatic duct suggests ductal stenosis or duodenal obstruction as the cause of hyperamylasemia (9).

Biopsy of the Pancreas Graft

Ultrasound provides accurate guidance to obtain core biopsy of the transplant pancreas. Previously, biopsy of the pancreas was thought to be associated with a high rate of complications. Currently, core biopsy of the pancreas

with ultrasound guidance is successful in more than 95% of attempts, with a less than 1% complication rate (Fig. 12) (10). The histologic findings combined with the ultrasound findings can separate immunologic acute cellular rejection from pancreatitis of other causes.

LIVER TRANSPLANTATION (Table 4)

Ultrasound has become an essential tool for the treatment of patients with end-stage liver disease as well as following liver transplantation. Assessment of the patency of the portal vein during liver transplant evaluation, guidance in the performance of donor liver biopsy, and identification of complications after transplantation are some of the vital applications of ultrasound.

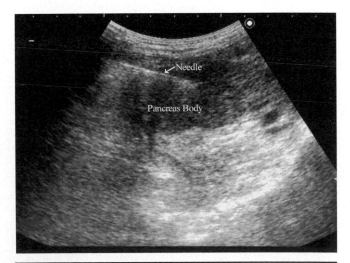

FIGURE 12. Ultrasound guidance of percutaneous biopsy of the transplant pancreas. A hyperechoic needle is clearly seen entering the pancreatic parenchyma.

▶ **TABLE 4** Ultrasound for Liver Transplantation

1. Evaluation and needle guidance for end-stage liver disease: ascites, portal hypertension, and hepatic malignancy
2. Guidance of donor liver biopsy
3. Evaluation of posttransplantation complications:
   a. Bleeding (hematoma).
   b. Vascular thrombosis.
   c. Biliary complications.
4. Evaluation of hepatic graft dysfunction
5. Assistance in living donor transplantation
6. Intraoperative ultrasound during transplantation

End-Stage Liver Disease

Treatment of patients with end-stage liver disease prior to transplantation requires attending to the complications of cirrhosis such as ascites, portal hypertension, and hepatic malignancies. Ascites not responsive to diuretic therapy may be due to complicating factors such as portal vein obstruction or spontaneous bacterial peritonitis. Absence of flow in the protal vein on Doppler ultrasound is suggestive of portal vein thrombosis/obstruction. The identification of an intraportal thrombus separates this entity from stasis of flow secondary to severe portal hypertension or reversal of flow. The ability to obtain ascitic fluid under ultrasound guidance for microbiological evaluation secures the diagnosis of spontaneous bacterial peritonitis allowing for appropriate antibiotic use. Diuretic-resistant ascites is initially managed by large-volume paracentesis. Ultrasound is helpful in selecting the appropriate anatomic site for paracentesis, thereby preventing catastrophic visceral or vascular injury (Fig. 13).

Identification and characterization of an intrahepatic mass are best performed by triple-phase computed tomography. However, once the lesion is identified, follow-up monitoring is readily achieved with ultrasound. (Fig. 14) (11).

Portal hypertension in the cirrhotic patient is usually secondary to sinusoidal portal hypertension. However, the identification of presinusoidal hypertension due to thrombosis of the portal or splenic vein is needed for appropriate management.

During the evaluation of the potential liver transplant candidate, confirmation of the patency of the portal system by Doppler ultrasound again ensures a reliable vascular inflow for the liver graft (Fig. 15). Postsinusoidal portal hypertension is commonly secondary to Budd–Chiari syndrome or obstruction of venous outflow from the liver and may be diagnosed by Doppler ultrasound demonstrating absence of flow in the hepatic veins.

Liver Donor Evaluation

In 2002, transplantation programs in the United States were responsible for the performance of 5,328 liver transplantation procedures. Donor grafts from living donors accounted for 358 transplants (1). Over the last 10 years the number of liver transplants has increased by 75%; however, the number of cadaveric donors increased only by 37%. The waiting list for liver transplantation has increased from 2,217 candidates in 1992 to 17,408 in 2002, representing a 685% increase. Because of this disparity, the criteria as to what is an acceptable donor organ have expanded. One of the most accurate determinants of a usable donor liver is revealed by liver biopsy. Donor liver biopsy previously had been obtained only during the time of procurement. However, in many programs a biopsy on the donor liver is performed in the early stages so as to limit expended resources should the organ be deemed unusable. Ultrasound provides a safe and accurate means

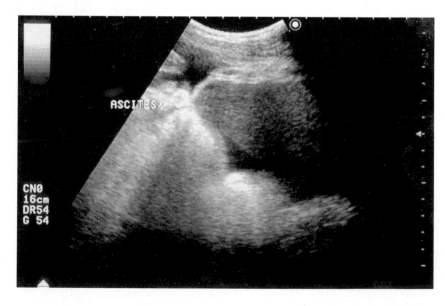

FIGURE 13. Ultrasonic detection and evaluation of the anechoic/hypoechoic ascites in relation to adjacent visceral structures.

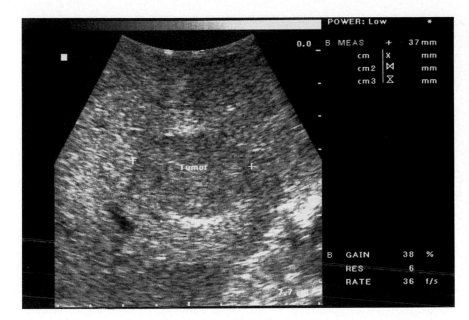

FIGURE 14. Transabdominal ultrasound demonstrating a hepatic adenoma (Tumor), which is 37 mm in diameter.

to guide a biopsy to obtain donor tissue well in advance of the donor operation. This allows a more efficient placement of the donor organ, selection of recipient needs, and efficiency in cold ischemia times.

Bleeding Complications

Ultrasound provides essential information in the postoperative management of liver transplantation patients. Liver transplantation is performed in patients with ongoing coagulopathy. This coagulopathy is not reversed immediately following implantation of the donor liver. Fifteen percent of posttransplantation patients have ongoing bleeding necessitating a return to the operating room. Ultrasound in the posttransplantation phase provides the ability to evaluate the significance or amount of abdominal hematoma and thus to determine the need for operative evacuation.

Vascular Thrombosis

Vascular thrombosis occurs in 5% of liver transplants. Hepatic artery thrombosis occurs much more frequently than portal vein thrombosis. The transplant biliary tree is solely dependent on the donor hepatic artery as its only blood supply. Thrombosis of the hepatic artery within the early posttransplantation period results in extrahepatic biliary necrosis and subsequent biliary sepsis. Therefore,

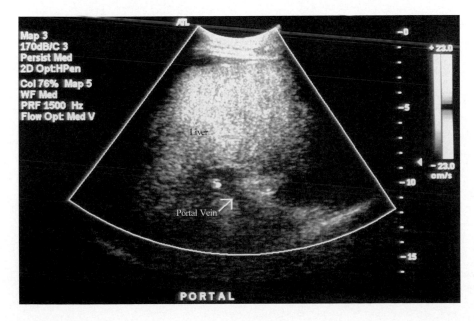

FIGURE 15. In the evaluation of this potential liver transplantation candidate, ultrasound identified absence of portal vein flow. However, subsequent carbon dioxide contrast ultrasound revealed a patent portal vein with sluggish flow.

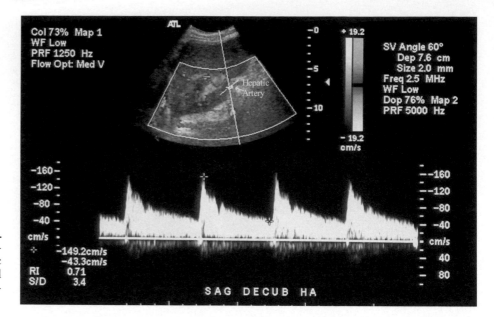

FIGURE 16. Ultrasound with Doppler spectrum demonstrating hepatic artery flow high in the hilum, beyond the arterial anastomosis in the transplant liver.

hepatic artery thrombosis within the first week of transplantation is an indication for emergent retransplantation (Fig. 16). Portal vein thrombosis results in production of massive ascites in excess of a liter per hour. Diagnosis and emergent thrombectomy is facilitated by bedside ultrasound evaluation of the transplant portal vasculature (12).

Biliary Complications

Bile duct complications occur in 14% of liver transplants. Ultrasound can identify fluid collections in the porta hepatis suggestive of a bile leak. Ultrasound can also iden-

tify intrahepatic ductal dilatation (Fig. 17). Timely ultrasound diagnosis and correction of biliary complications allows for prolonged graft survival and decreases the need for retransplantation (13).

Hepatic Dysfunction

Postoperative hepatic dysfunction is identified by abnormalities of liver function tests. The cause of the hepatic dysfunction is further evaluated by ultrasound and histologic examinations. The ultrasound examination includes the elimination of vascular compromise, biliary obstruction, and perihilar fluid collections. Ultrasound also provides a safe guidance for biopsy of the liver.

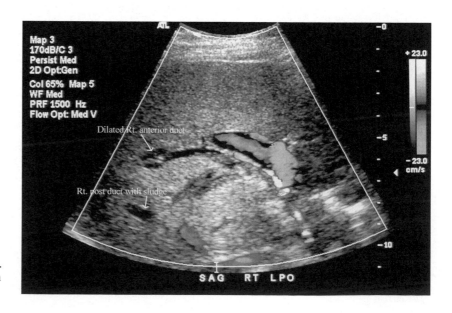

FIGURE 17. Intrahepatic bile duct dilatation indicative of distal bile duct obstruction.

Living Donor Liver Transplantation

Liver transplantation utilizing a living donor was first performed by Henri Bismuth and subsequently championed by Christopher Brolesch and the team at the University of Chicago. This methodology utilizes the living donor left lateral segments (segments 2–3) to replace the entire hepatic mass of infants and children. This technique was found to be safe for the donor and provided transplantation for the infant at an earlier stage. The techniques learned from left lateral segment living donor liver grafts combined with advancements in hepatobiliary surgical techniques have provided the incentive for adult-to-adult living donor liver transplantation. Intraoperative ultrasound provides assistance in living donor surgery by defining the vascular anatomy. Experience has shown the need to include anastomosis of an accessory right hepatic vein to prevent graft congestion and subsequent loss. Intraoperative ultrasound allows for confirmation of the existence of an accessory vein and determination of its size prior to resection (14,15).

HEART TRANSPLANTATION (Table 5)

Echocardiography is an important modality in all phases of the cardiac transplantation process including evaluation of potential cardiac transplant recipients, evaluation of donor heart function, intraoperative monitoring of the cardiac graft, and long-term assessment of cardiac graft function.

In the United States, 2,197 cardiac transplantation procedures were performed in the year 2002. Patient/graft survivals for orthotopic heart transplants are 85% to 90% at 1 year, 70% at 5 years, and 45% to 50% at 10 years after transplantation.

Heart Organ Recipients

In evaluating potential recipients for heart transplantation, two-dimensional echocardiography with color flow Doppler imaging, spectral Doppler imaging, and, more recently, tissue Doppler examination is the single most useful modality. Echocardiography can provide data on right and left ventricular systolic function, cardiac chamber size, myocardial mass, and quantitative evaluation of valvular disease. Blood pool Doppler and tissue Doppler allow for the evaluation of left ventricular hemodynamics, including pulmonary artery systolic pressure, prediction of left atrial pressure, and a qualitative evaluation of left ventricular diastolic function. These data are useful in predicting the etiologic progression of heart failure and in providing useful information for long-term prognosis in patients with end-stage heart failure.

Heart Organ Donors

In the evaluation of organ donors, echocardiography determines overall systolic function, left ventricular wall thickness, chamber size, and presence of valvular insufficiency. In organ donors who have sustained chest trauma, echocardiography is the most sensitive method for detecting evidence of cardiac contusion.

Intraoperative Use

During implantation of the donor heart, intraoperative transesophageal echocardiography (TEE) is used to evaluate the function of the newly implanted donor heart. During this time, intraoperative TEE assesses both left ventricular and right ventricular systolic function. Patients who have increased pulmonary vascular resistance experience significant right ventricular dilation and impairment of right ventricular systolic function in the early postoperative period. TEE is used in conjunction with hemodynamic data to guide therapy aimed at reducing the pulmonary vascular resistance, including the manipulation of inotropic support or the addition of inhaled nitric oxide. The appearance of mitral or tricuspid insufficiency is associated with pulmonary hypertension and high pulmonary vascular resistance, which can be detected early with TEE. The aortic and pulmonary artery anastomosis can also be evaluated by TEE for kinking or stenosis, which may lead to graft dysfunction without prompt correction.

Posttransplantation Assessment in Adults

The tools used for the ongoing assessment of the cardiac allograft following orthotopic heart transplantation include endomyocardial biopsy for surveillance of rejection, echocardiography, radionuclide angiography, and coronary angiography. Echocardiography provides the single best assessment of overall graft function among the modalities currently available. However, despite the strong correlation between left ventricular systolic and diastolic echocardiographic findings of dysfunction and acute cellular rejection, in the adult population the rela-

▶ **TABLE 5 Ultrasound for Heart Transplantation**

1. Echocardiography in all phases of cardiac transplants process
2. Evaluation of heart transplant recipient
3. Evaluation of donor heart
4. Intraoperative ultrasound use during heart transplantation
5. Posttransplantation assessment: acute rejection of allograft
6. Pediatric posttransplantation assessment
7. Guidance of endomyocardial biopsy
8. Evaluation of coronary allograft arteriopathy: intravascular ultrasound

tionship has not been sufficiently reliable as to make a definitive diagnosis (16,17). Because of this limitation, percutaneous endomyocardial biopsy has become the "gold standard" for the diagnosis of acute cellular rejection.

Posttransplantation Assessment in Children

In the pediatric population, echocardiographic parameters of rejection are used more commonly. This is particularly true in infant recipients in whom routine surveillance endomyocardial biopsy would pose a substantial risk of injury to the neonatal heart. Changes in left ventricular wall thickness or mass, an increase in left ventricular systolic dimension, and a decrease in fractional shortening have been noted during significant rejection (18). An algorithm based on multiple echocardiographic measurements of left ventricular systolic function has been used as primary rejection surveillance in infants, leading to infrequent right ventricular endomyocardial biopsy.

Endomyocardial Biopsy

In experienced hands, biopsies of the right ventricular side of the inner ventricular septum result in a complication rate of less than 0.4%. However, fluoroscopic-guided endomyocardial biopsy results in significant cumulative radiation exposure for both the operator and the patient. Fluoroscopic guidance gives poor delineation of the three-dimensional structures of the right heart, making it difficult to avoid injury to the tricuspid apparatus. Echocardiography has been used to guide the placement of a *bioptome* through the tricuspid valve, away from the tricuspid valve apparatus and against the right ventricular side of the inner ventricular septum, decreasing the incidence of cardiac injury during biopsy (19). This technique is particularly useful in adults with very small right ventricular cavities or in children.

Recent reports suggest that endomyocardial biopsies performed for routine surveillance beyond 6 to 12 months after orthotopic heart transplantation have an extremely low yield (20). This has prompted centers to discontinue the practice of performing routine surveillance endomyocardial biopsies beyond 1 year after transplantation. Therefore, echocardiography has now assumed an increased role in surveillance for the onset of late graft dysfunction. A significant decline in left ventricular systolic function detected on echocardiogram, with or without symptoms, is now regarded as an indication for endomyocardial biopsy.

Coronary Allograft Arteriopathy

Coronary allograft arteriopathy represents the most important biologic barrier to long-term survival of heart transplant recipients. This entity represents a diffuse form of coronary artery disease whose hallmark is proliferation of the intimal layer of the coronary vessels and accelerated atherosclerosis with obliteration of the small- to medium-sized coronary artery. Significant arteriopathy is seen in approximately 50% of patients between 3 and 5 years after transplantation. Its cause is multifaceted, consisting of injury to the vasculature by preexisting coronary atherosclerosis in the donor, and further injury associated with the process of brain death, cold ischemia, and graft implantation. Changes in the vasculature manifest secondary to the traditional coronary risk factors of posttransplantation and acceleration of the atherosclerotic process, as well as proliferation of the intimal layers due to the process of chronic rejection (21). Traditional evaluation of cardiac allograft arteriopathy with coronary angiography only yields significant angiographic findings when the arteriopathy is so advanced as to be demonstrated on a coronary angiogram. Intravascular ultrasound (IVUS) has provided a new tool by which coronary allograft arteriopathy can be detected at a much earlier stage and its extent can be better quantitated. Advancing a 3-Fr 40-MHz catheter-type ultrasound transducer through a 6-Fr coronary guiding catheter at the time of the patient's annual coronary angiography can easily facilitate IVUS. The intimal layer of multiple segments of the coronary vasculature can be imaged and the extent and severity of arteriopathy quantitated. This technique has been used by the Multicenter Intravascular Ultrasound Transplant Study Group to document the incidence and progression of transplant coronary artery disease over a 1-year period (21). This study has provided important insights into the progression of transplant coronary artery disease. However, therapeutic options beyond good immunosuppression and control of traditional risk factors are very limited. At present, the use of IVUS is regarded mainly as a tool in the ongoing investigation of the biology of transplant coronary heart disease.

CONCLUSIONS

Solid organ transplantation has made great strides to become the standard of care for end-organ disease. Improvements in survival are a result of improved early detection of complications. Ultrasound is the single most applicable tool to diagnosis or assist in the diagnosis of these complications. In renal transplantation, the identification of fluid collections, vascular complications, and/or urological complications allows for correction and long-term graft survival. In pancreas transplantation, the ability to accurately diagnose acute rejection in time for reversal of the immunologic insult has changed the survival rate of a transplant from 40% to 90% or more. In liver transplantation, the ability to detect vascular thrombosis allows for emergent intervention to alter precipitous loss of a life-sustaining graft. The use of intraoperative ultrasound to tailor the living liver donor operation and initial monitoring of hepatic venous outflow will see expanded application. Ultrasound-based techniques used in a cardiac transplantation center's echocardiographic laboratory provide valuable tools in the management of heart failure, the evaluation of potential candidates for orthotopic heart transplantation, the selection of donor hearts, the long-term assessment of cardiac allograft function, and as a powerful research tool in the field of cardiac transplantation. The goal of the routine use of echocardiography in the diagnosis of acute cellular rejection in the transplanted heart has not been realized, but combined techniques of two-dimensional echocardiography, spectral Doppler, and tissue Doppler have added substantially to our understanding of the changes in structure and function that occur in the transplanted heart.

REFERENCES

1. http://www.optn.org/latestData/rptData.asp
2. Pedi VR, First MR. Diagnosis and treatment of renal dysfunction episodes. In: Normal DJ, Turka LA, eds. *Primer on transplantation*, 2nd ed. Mt. Laurel, NJ: American Society of Transplantation, 2001:459–466.
3. Brennan DC. Immediate postoperative management of the kidney transplant recipient. In: Normal DJ, Turka LA, eds. *Primer on transplantation*, 2nd ed. Mt. Laurel, NJ: American Society of Transplantation, 2001:440–447.
4. Cranston D. Urological complications after renal transplantation. In: P.J. Morris, ed. *Kidney transplantation: principles and practice*, 4th ed. Philadelphia: WB Saunders, 1994:330–338.
5. Rosenthal JT. The transplant operation and its surgical complications. In: Danovitch G, ed. *Handbook of kidney transplantation*, 2nd ed. Boston: Little, Brown, and Co., 2000:178–179.
6. Jakobsen JA, Brabrand K, Egge TS, et al. Doppler examination of the allografted kidney. *Acta Radiologica* 2003;44:3–13.
7. Pozniak MA, Propeck PA, Kelcz F, et al. Imaging of the pancreas transplant. *Radiol Clin North Am* 1995;33:581–594.
8. Dachman AH, Newmark GM, Thistlethwaite JR, et al. Imaging of the pancreatic transplantation using portal venous and enteric exocrine drainage. *AJR Am J Roentgenol* 1998;171:157–163.
9. Ciancio G, Montalvo B, Roth D, et al. Allograft pancreatic duct dilatation following bladder drained simultaneous pancreas-kidney transplantation: clinical significance. *J Pancreas* 2000;1:4–12.
10. Klassen DK, Weir MR, Cangro CB, et al. Pancreas allograft biopsy: safety of percutaneous biopsy: results of a large experience. *Transplantation* 2002;73:553–555.
11. Libbrecht L, Bielen D, Verslype C, et al. Focal lesions in cirrhotic explant livers: pathological evaluation and accuracy of pretransplant imaging examinations. *Liver Transplantation* 2002; 8:749–761.
12. Nishida S, Kato T, Levi D, et al. Effect of protocol Doppler ultrasonography and urgent revascularization on early hepatic artery thrombosis after pediatric liver transplantation. *Arch Surg* 2002;137:1279–1283.
13. Shaw AS, Ryan SM, Beese RC, et al. Ultrasound of non-vascular complications in the post liver transplant patient. *Clin Radiol* 2003;58:672–680.
14. Huang TL, Chen TY, Chen CL, et al. Hepatic outflow insults in living-related liver transplantation by Doppler sonography. *Transplant Proc* 2001;33:3464–3465.
15. Gondolesi GE, Florman S, Matsumoto C, et al. Venous hemodynamics in living donor right lobe liver transplantation. *Liver Transplantation* 2002;8:809–813.
16. Valantine HA, Fowler MB, Hunt SA, et al. Changes in Doppler echocardiographic indexes of the left ventricular function as potential markers for acute cardiac rejection. *Circulation* 1987;76:V86–V92.
17. Gill EA, Borrego C, Bray BE, et al. Left ventricular mass increases during cardiac allograft vascular rejection. *J Am Coll Cardiol* 1995;25:922–926.
18. Boucek MM, Mathis CM, Boucek CM, et al. Prospective evaluation of echocardiography for primary rejection surveillance after infant heart transplantation: comparison with endomyocardial biopsy. *J Heart Lung Transplant* 1994;3:66–73.
19. Williams GA, Kaintz RP, Habermehl KK, et al. Clinical experience with two-dimensional echocardiography to guide endomyocardial biopsy. *Clin Cardiol* 1985;8:137–140.
20. Sethi GK, Kosaraju S, Arabia FA, et al. Is it necessary to perform surveillance endomyocardial biopsies in heart transplant recipients? *J Heart Lung Transplant* 1995;14:1047–1051.
21. Yeung AC, Davis SF, Hauptman PJ, et al. Incidence and progression of transplant coronary artery disease over 1 year: results of a multicenter trial with use of intravascular ultrasound. Multicenter Intravascular Ultrasound Transplant Study Group. *J Heart Lung Transplant* 1995;14:S215–S220.

Anorectal Ultrasound

Theodore J. Saclarides

Anorectal ultrasound has emerged as an invaluable tool for the assessment of a variety of conditions involving the rectum and anus. Its advantages over other imaging modalities include the fact that it is mobile and hence can be used in the office, the operating room, or at the patient's bedside. In comparison with magnetic resonance imaging (MRI), for example, it is far less expensive and the learning curve is such that minimal training is required to master the technique. Its chief advantage over other imaging modalities is the fact that it can be placed in close proximity to the area of interest within the rectum and anus. As such, fine anatomic detail and spacial resolution are far more easily obtained. It should be stressed that this is a focused examination of the anus and rectum and is not meant to serve as a screening test for other diseases of the pelvis, such as prostate cancer.

INDICATION

Anorectal ultrasound can be used for diagnosis of both malignant and benign conditions (Table 1). With respect to the former, ultrasound can determine the depth of tumor penetration and may also determine which rectal cancers are appropriate for transanal excision because of their superficial nature. Similarly, if full-thickness penetration or suspicious lymph nodes are seen, one may advise preoperative chemotherapy and radiation. If a lesion of intermediate thickness is imaged (invasion into the muscularis propria but not beyond), one may advise prompt low anterior resection without neoadjuvant therapy. With respect to tumors of the anal canal, one can determine whether local excision is appropriate or if radiation and chemotherapy is required because of involvement of the sphincter muscles. In addition, surveillance of the anastomosis and operative site can be performed with anorectal ultrasound, and is especially indicated for patients who have undergone transanal excision of a tumor. With respect to benign conditions of the anus,

anorectal ultrasound has emerged as an extremely important tool in the evaluation of patients with fecal incontinence. It is considered by many to be the initial test in the workup because it immediately identifies patients who have a surgically correctable abnormality. Anorectal ultrasound can also be used in the evaluation of patients with complex anal fistula, anal pain without an identifiable source, and perianal abscess.

EQUIPMENT

A high-frequency radial ultrasound system (e.g., B&K) is the equipment frequently employed for anorectal ultrasound (Table 2). This system provides a 360-degree cross-sectional image of the rectum and anus. Scanning can be performed with either the 7- or the 10-MHz transducer. Sound waves at the higher frequency will not penetrate as deeply; however, delineation of the superficial anatomy is enhanced. Consequently, many physicians choose the 10-MHz transducer for scanning within the anal canal and the 7-MHz transducer for scanning within the rectum whereby visualization of metastatic lymph nodes deep within the mesorectum is improved. The author has chosen the 10-MHz transducer for all scanning because this frequency optimizes superficial imaging while still permitting detection of metastatic nodes if present. The ultrasound probe is approximately 25 cm in length and is easily inserted through the anal canal into the rectum. Centimeter markings on the outside of the probe are useful as spatial reference points. The transducer rotates at approximately 4 cycles per second and is covered with either a latex balloon for imaging within the rectum or a hard plastic cap for imaging within the anal canal (Fig. 1). Whichever end is chosen must be filled with water in order to establish acoustic coupling between the ultrasound transducer and the tissue being imaged. The entire assembly is then covered with a latex condom, which facilitates cleaning and sterilization and shortens the time interval between examinations.

Chapter 19

▶ TABLE 1 Indication for Anorectal Ultrasound

Malignant:
  Determine if transanal excision is appropriate
  Determine which tumors should be treated with neoadjuvant
    therapy
  Surveillance of anastomosis at excision site
Benign:
  Fecal incontinence workup
  Assess complex anal fistulae and abscesses
  Evaluate patients with anorectal pain

▶ TABLE 2 Equipment and Technique
of Anorectal Ultrasound

	Equipment	Technique
Rectal	7- or 10-MHz, latex balloon	Proctoscopy first to localize lesion Scan cephalad to caudad Focus on rectal wall then mesorectum
Anus	10-MHz, plastic cap	Identify puborectalis as the upper limit Next, image the internal then the external sphincter

TECHNIQUE

Preparation for anorectal ultrasound is accomplished with a small-volume enema administered 1 hour before the examination. A formal bowel preparation is not necessary. Patients may be positioned in either the left lateral or the lithotomy position; the choice is determined by examiner preference. A consistent approach for each sonographer is recommended to facilitate anatomic orientation during retrospective image review. Generally, no sedation is required. When imaging tumors within the upper rectum, proctoscopy with a specially designed, commercially available proctoscope is performed first to locate the lesion. Once the tumor is visualized, the ultrasound probe is inserted under direct vision through the scope up to the tumor, at which point the proctoscope is withdrawn over the shaft of the ultrasound probe. For cancers in the middle and lower rectum, this proctoscope is not needed because digital examination can usually direct the physician to the proper quadrant within the rectum. It is also not necessary to scope large cancers regardless of their location because the ultrasound image of a large lesion is obvious and not likely to be misleading. Imaging of tumors is generally started several centimeters above the lesion, and the probe is then withdrawn in a proximal-to-distal direction in order to detect metastatic lymph nodes that, if present, will more frequently be located above the tumor rather than below. Once the tumor is seen and imaged, close-up views are selected to delineate the various layers of the bowel wall and to determine the depth of penetration by the tumor. Once this is accomplished, the examiner may switch to standard views in order to scan the tissue and mesentery outside of the rectum for lymph nodes or tumor deposits.

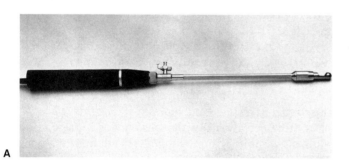

A

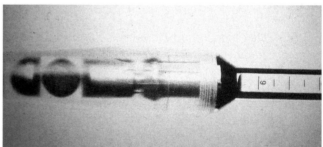

B

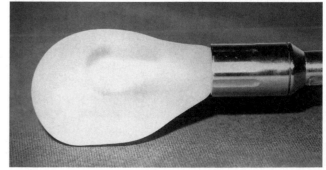

C

FIGURE 1. A: High-frequency radial ultrasound with a rotating transducer at the tip. B: Plastic cap covering the rotating transducer for imaging in the anal canal. C: Water-filled balloon covering the transducer for imaging in the rectum.

▶ **TABLE 3** Normal Ultrasound Anatomy

Male:
   Seminal vesicles, prostate
Female:
   Cervix, vagina, small bowel
Both genders:
   Anococcygeal ligament, pelvic floor
   Anal canal:
      Puborectalis
      Internal anal sphincter (hypoechoic)
      External anal sphincter (hypoechoic)

NORMAL ULTRASOUND ANATOMY OF THE PELVIS AND RECTAL WALL

Certain anatomic landmarks assist the sonographer during anorectal ultrasound (Table 3). When scanning within the rectum in the posterior quadrant, one sees the anococcygeal ligament as a hypoechoic triangle. Anteriorly, the vagina and prostate can be seen quite easily; the former is a hypoechoic crescent-shaped space lined by a hyperechoic membrane. As one descends toward the pelvic floor, the striated muscle fibers of the puborectalis muscle can be seen as a horseshoe-shaped accumulation of hyperechoic muscle fibers. The open end of this horseshoe is oriented anteriorly toward the vagina and prostate (Fig. 2). As one descends into the anal canal, the in-

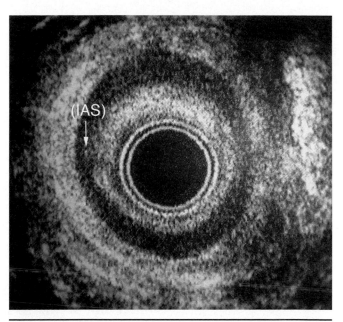

FIGURE 3. The internal anal sphincter (*arrow,* IAS) is a dark hypoechoic band.

ternal sphincter muscle can be seen as a well-demarcated hypoechoic band (Fig. 3). The external sphincter, in contrast, is hyperechoic and the muscle fibers are more loosely arranged (Fig. 4).

There are gender differences that are important for anorectal scanning. For example, in the male pelvis, the seminal vesicles are visualized as paired, wing-shaped, hypoechoic structures anteriorly that fan out into the lateral spaces on either side of the rectum (Fig. 5). These should not be confused with metastatic lymph nodes.

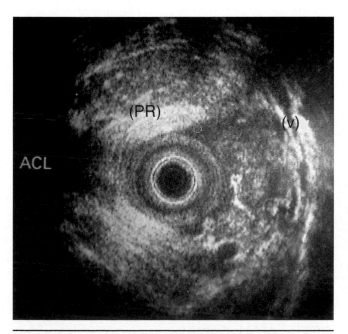

FIGURE 2. The anococcygeal ligament (ACL) is seen posteriorly and the vagina (V) anteriorly as a hypoechoic crescent-shaped space. The puborectalis (PR) is seen as a horse-shoe–shaped accumulation of hyperechoic muscle fibers.

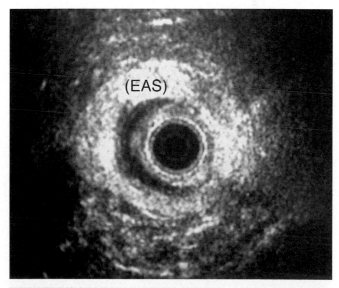

FIGURE 4. The external anal sphincter (EAS) consists of loosely arranged hyperechoic bands.

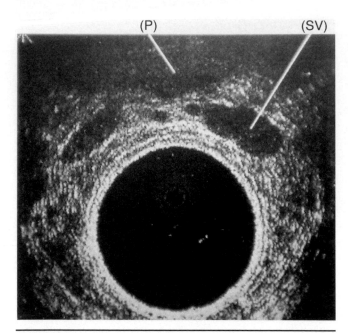

FIGURE 5. The seminal vesicles (SV) and prostate (P).

Caudally within the male pelvis, the prostate is seen as a well-defined structure anteriorly. In women, the cul-de-sac may descend further into the pelvis than in males, and in this area peristalsing loops of small bowel or ovaries may be visualized. The cervix may be seen as a circular or oval-shaped structure with mixed echogenicity and, immediately below this, the vagina will be visualized (Fig. 6).

Close-up images of the rectal wall demonstrate alternating white and dark lines; there has been controversy as to what each of these lines represents. It is currently

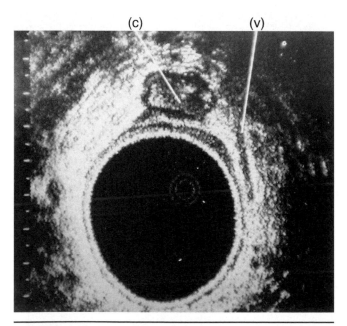

FIGURE 6. The cervix (C) and vagina (V).

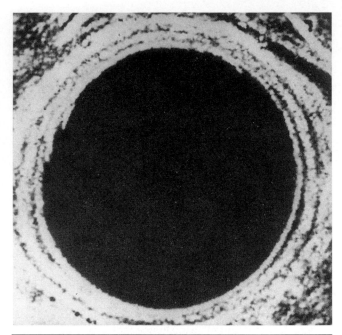

FIGURE 7. The sonographic layers of the rectal wall. Inner white, balloon interface; first dark, mucosa; middle white, submucosa; second dark, muscularis propria; outer white, interface with perirectal fat.

believed that the innermost white (hyperechoic) line represents the interface between the water-filled balloon and the mucosa. The innermost dark (hypoechoic) line represents the mucosa. The middle white line represents the submucosa, and in terms of cancer staging, this line is of paramount importance because its disruption implies tumor invasion through the submucosa. The second dark band is the muscularis propria. If this band is thickened or expanded in the area of the tumor relative to the muscularis at other areas, then tumor infiltration of the muscularis is presumed. The outermost white (hyperechoic) line is the interface between the muscularis propria and the extrarectal fat (Fig. 7) (1). This does not represent a serosa because the rectum lacks such a layer for the majority of its course through the pelvis. When the examiner exercises patience and diligence, occasionally the muscularis propria may be witnessed as two distinct hypoechoic layers that represent the circular and longitudinal muscle layers. Therefore, in such instances the normal sonographic appearance of the rectal wall would consist of seven rather than five layers (see also Chapter 20).

NORMAL ANATOMY OF THE ANAL CANAL

It is important to have a full understanding of the normal anatomy of the various portions of the anal canal. The anal canal has arbitrarily been divided into upper, middle, and lower portions, and the sonographic appearance of each of these regions is quite different. In the *upper* anal canal, one can see the puborectalis muscle as a horseshoe-shaped conglomeration of hyperechoic striated fibers. The open end of the horseshoe is directed anteriorly. Striated muscle (hyperechoic) will not be visualized anteriorly in the upper anal canal; this should not be mistakenly diagnosed as a sphincter injury. External to the puborectalis muscle is the anococcygeal ligament posteriorly and the vagina anteriorly. Also at the upper end of the anal canal, one can visualize the internal sphincter as a uniform tight circle of hypoechoic tissue. In the *middle* anal canal, the internal anal sphincter reaches its greatest thickness. Normally, the internal sphincter has a thickness of 2 mm; however, with advancing age, the internal sphincter will become thicker, not because of increased muscle mass but presumably because of the presence of more connective tissue in the muscle. At this level one can also visualize portions of the external anal sphincter that are striated hyperechoic fibers found in a more loosely arranged configuration. Although the external sphincter does not demonstrate the compactness of the internal sphincter, it nevertheless can be easily imaged and should form a complete circle. In the *lower* anal canal, the internal anal sphincter has descended to its full extent beyond which the external anal fibers can be seen more caudally. In the distal-most portion of the anal canal, one can see only the external anal sphincter.

In addition to determining whether or not the internal and external anal sphincters are intact, one can measure their thickness in cross-section as well as their height in a craniocaudad direction. With regard to the thickness of the external sphincter, it is fairly uniform laterally and posteriorly; however, anteriorly, especially in women, there can be attenuation of these muscle fibers. If one places a finger inside the vagina and gently and ever so slightly compresses the tissue toward the probe, one can measure the thickness of the perineal body. Its normal thickness is approximately 1 cm. Certainly, if the muscle fibers are attenuated anteriorly, this could explain and contribute to fecal incontinence. The height of the external sphincter can also be measured as one arbitrarily chooses a reference point on the centimeter gradations on the ultrasound probe as the starting point and measures the length over which the fibers form a complete circle. The height of the sphincter complex should be approximately 3 cm. Anything less should be considered abnormal, especially in a patient who is experiencing symptoms of fecal incontinence.

ULTRASOUND IN MALIGNANT DISEASE

The usefulness of anorectal ultrasound for rectal cancer is based on its capability to determine depth of penetration with a reliable degree of certainty. As such, it may se-

lect those tumors that are candidates for transanal excision by way of their superficial nature. Alternatively, it may be used to select tumors that require preoperative radiation and chemotherapy based on their transmural penetration/fixation to extrarectal viscera or involvement of regional lymph nodes. If ultrasound demonstrates that the tumor has penetrated partially into the muscularis propria but not beyond and there are no suspicious lymph nodes, then one may proceed directly with a transabdominal resection rather than a transanal excision; in these instances, preoperative neoadjuvant therapy would probably not be used. Therefore, most surgeons whose practice deals with a high volume of rectal cancer patients rely heavily on the use of rectal ultrasound to determine choice of therapy.

The nomenclature for ultrasound staging of rectal cancers generally parallels histologic staging; however, the prefix "u" is attached to provide clarification. A tumor that is sonographically confined to the mucosa is designated uT1 (Fig. 8). In such instances, a villous adenoma or carcinoma-in-situ is not distinguishable by ultrasound. A cancer that breaches the submucosa but does not cause expansion of the underlying muscularis is also staged uT1. However, if the muscularis propria is thickened relative to the muscularis in other areas of the rectal wall, a stage uT2 designation is given. Penetration into the extrarectal fat is staged as a uT3 (Fig. 9), and invasion of the prostate, seminal vesicles, or vagina merits a uT4 designation (Fig.10).

As stated previously, there has been controversy as to what the five different layers of the rectal wall represent. Initially it was felt that the middle white (hyperechoic) band represents the interface between the submucosa and the muscularis propria (2). However, most rectal sonographers now believe that this represents the submucosa itself. It is probably of academic interest as to what this middle white layer represents because if the muscularis propria is not thickened or expanded by direct tumor invasion then a disruption of the middle white line would be an ultrasound T1 tumor by either definition. Disruption of the hyperechoic layers is easier to sonographically detect than disruption of the hypoechoic layers. The difficulty this poses for accurate staging is compounded by the fact that cancers are usually hypoechoic (3). Failure to recognize expansion of the hypoechoic muscularis propria causes understaging. In a meta-analysis of multiple anorectal ultrasound reports, the sensitivity for determining invasion of the rectal wall was 97% with a specificity of 87%. Positive predictive value was 90%, meaning that 10% of tumors are overstaged by ultrasound. The chief cause for this overstaging is the edema and desmoplastic reaction that some tumors incite; by ultrasound, this may have the appearance of tumor extension. Negative predictive value is 97%, meaning that approximately 3% of patients are understaged by

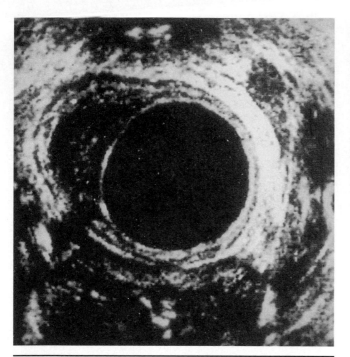

FIGURE 8. Ultrasound T1 lesion. The submucosa (middle white line) has been breached.

ultrasound (4). Table 4 shows accuracy and staging of anorectal ultrasound by several investigators (5–12). When compared with computed tomography (CT) scanning, ultrasound is more sensitive and accurate as one would expect since the probe is placed in direct proximity to the area of interest (5,13). MRI may produce results comparable to those of ultrasound, however, one must

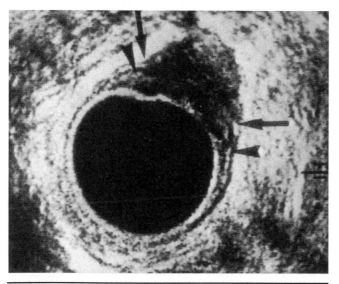

FIGURE 9. Ultrasound T3, penetration into extrarectal fat. Arrowheads indicate muscularis propria, arrows the interface to extrarectal fat.

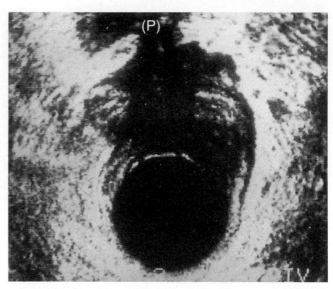

FIGURE 10. Ultrasound T4, invasion into the prostate (P).

keep in mind the relative expense of the examination, as well as the mobility and availability of the test, all of which point in favor of ultrasound.

When scanning for metastatic lymph nodes, it is important to scan above and below the tumor. One must begin above the tumor and progressively withdraw the probe in a caudal direction. If a suspicious structure is visualized, it should be scanned both up and down as this may show that it is a branching blood vessel, which initially may have been seen only on cross-section (Fig. 11). There are debates about ultrasound criteria for benign as opposed to metastatic disease of the lymph nodes. In general, normal lymph nodes are isoechoic with the mesorectal fat and therefore are rarely visible. Inflamed lymph nodes are hyperechoic and oval shaped. Lymph nodes with metastatic disease are usually hypoechoic and spherical (Fig. 12). Positive predictive value, accuracy, and other indices for diagnosing metastatic disease once a node is seen depend on the size of the node, being lowest for nodes smaller than 5 mm and highest for nodes larger than 1 cm. Table 5 shows accuracy of anorectal ultrasound by several investigators (5,6,9,10,12,14).

Preoperative irradiation affects the reliability of anoectal ultrasound because of alterations in tissue density and planes. In one study of 25 patients all of whom had complete pathologic responses, ultrasound correctly predicted no residual cancer in only 17% of patients. Two thirds of patients were over-staged as being T1 cancers and an additional 16% were overstaged as having T2 lesions. In this study, other diagnostic modalities also failed in that digital rectal examination correctly predicted no tumor in only 24% of patients and CT in only 23%. Interestingly, MRI did not correctly predict a complete re-

▶ **TABLE 4** Accuracy and Staging of Anorectal Ultrasound in Diagnosing the Depth of Rectal Cancer Invasion

Reference	Sensitivity	Specificity	Positive Predictive Value	Negative Predictive Value	Overstage	Understage
Herzog, et al (5)	98.3%	75%	89.2%	95.4%	10.2%	0.8%
Sentovitch, et al (6)	79%	—	uT_2: 81% $uT_{3,4}$: 90%	uT_2: 88% $uT_{3,4}$: 100%	17%	4%
Anderson, et al (7)	pT_1: 70% pT_2: 100%	pT_1: 100% pT_2: 44%	uT_1: 100% pT_2: 55%	uT_1: 85% uT_2: 100%	15%	30%
Harnsberger, et al (8)	55%	—	—	—	40%	5%
Orrom, et al (9)	75%	—	—	—	22%	3%
Glaser, et al (10)	96%	—	—	96%	—	—
Hulsmans, et al (11)	97%	24%	—	—	"Extensive"	—
Holdsworth, et al (12)	96%	50%	—	—	—	—

u = ultrasound staging
p = pathology staging

sponse in any of these 25 patients (15). Therefore, many surgeons do not routinely perform preoperative rectal ultrasound following completion of neoadjuvant therapy. Treatment decisions should be made based on the initial ultrasound and clinical examination when cancer was diagnosed and not on the appearance of the tumor following completion of radiation and chemotherapy.

In the postoperative setting, ultrasound can be used to monitor the rectal wall and extrarectal tissue for any sign of recurrent tumor. Since the original surgery will likely have changed the anatomic planes, postoperative treatment decisions should not be based on one abnormal ultrasound alone. Rather, it is essential that the initial ultrasound be obtained shortly after the operation and used as a baseline against which future ultrasound examinations are compared. If changes are seen, such as expansion of a previously noted hypoechoic area within the rectal wall (Fig. 13) or enlargement of extrarectal lymph nodes, then tumor recurrence should be suspected. Needle biopsy of such abnormalities can be performed using ultrasound as a guide. In those instances, it may be necessary to switch from the radial probe to the multiplane probe, which is often used by urologists. This probe has a biopsy guide that greatly facilitates biopsy of either intra-

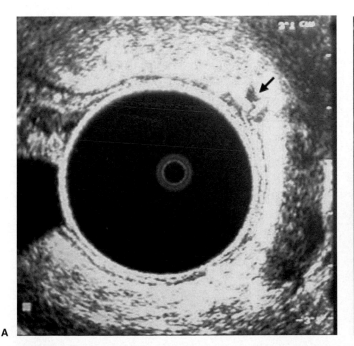
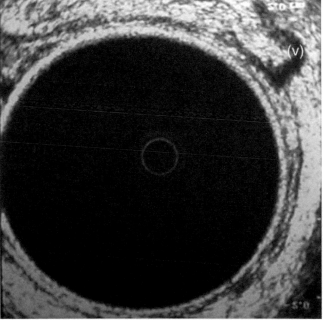

A   B

FIGURE 11. Branching blood vessel (V in **B**), initially appearing as a hypoechoic spherical structure (arrow in **A**).

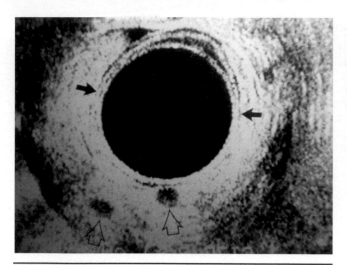

FIGURE 12. Metastatic lymph nodes (*open arrows*). Black arrows indicate rectal wall.

mural or extramural masses. In one study of 338 patients operated on for rectal cancer and followed by ultrasound, 116 recurrences were noted and verified by histologic examination. Of these, 80 had normal proctoscopic examinations and 89 had normal digital examinations. Recurrence was detected by ultrasound alone in 22% of cases (16). In the author's experience, rectal ultrasound is routinely performed at 3-month intervals for the first 2 years in patients who have undergone transanal local excision.

ULTRASOUND IN BENIGN DISEASE

Anorectal ultrasound is an invaluable diagnostic adjunct for various benign diseases, but most notably for fecal incontinence. In this regard, ultrasound has the capability of immediately stratifying patients into either surgical or nonsurgical treatment. Fecal incontinence is a significant social problem, and a significant amount of money is spent annually on hygiene-related incontinence aids. Furthermore, fecal incontinence is a common reason for

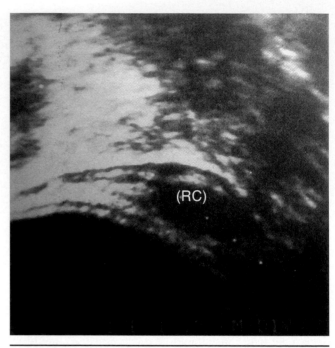

FIGURE 13. Recurrent cancer (RC) noted within the rectal wall.

institutionalizing elderly patients. Unfortunately, many patients are told by their primary care physicians that they must live with this condition and that there is no available treatment. Fortunately, this is not the case; however, before subjecting a patient to reconstructive and possibly radical surgery, an anatomic assessment of the sphincter muscles is important. Hence, the utility of ultrasound is critical.

Minor incontinence, that is, difficulty with flatus or the rare loss of stool that has no impact on lifestyle, can be managed with simple dietary changes as well as with the use of stool-bulking agents and antidiarrheal medications. Patients with major incontinence, which is defined as frequent loss of stool leading to social restrictions and the frequent use of pads and sanitary aids, are referred for physiologic testing. Such testing includes anorectal manometry, electrophysiologic diagnostic testing, and

▶ **TABLE 5** Accuracy of Anorectal Ultrasound in Diagnosing Lymph Node Metastases

Reference	Sensitivity	Specificity	Positive Predictive Value	Negative Predictive Value	Accuracy*
Herzog, et al (5)	89.2%	73.4%	71.2%	90.4%	80.2%*
Sentovitch, et al (6)	0%	100%	—	73%	—
Fleshman, et al (14)	—	—	37.5%	100%	—
Orrom, et al (9)	88%	90%	—	—	88%
Glaser, et al (10)	—	—	—	—	80%
Holdsworth, et al (12)	57%	64%	—	—	61%

*staging accuracy dependent on node size: if nodes were <5 mm, accuracy was lower ($p < .05$)

ultrasound. Of these tests, only ultrasound allows inspection of the anatomy. Anorectal manometry is still a favorite tool of many physicians, and with manometry one is able to assess resting anal canal pressures, squeeze pressures, and sensory thresholds within the rectum. However, manometry has had a dubious impact on clinical decision making with regard to the treatment of patients suffering from fecal incontinence. Diagnostic electrophysiologic tests include measurement of nerve conduction time along the pudendal nerve. This test, known as the pudendal nerve terminal motor latency test, is performed with the use of a special glove inside of which are a stimulating and a sensing electrode. The pudendal nerve is stimulated at the ischial spine and the response is measured at the sphincter muscle. Normal conduction time between these two points is 2 milliseconds; anything longer is considered abnormal. It is possible for a patient to have significant nerve damage but a normal conduction time along the nerve as long as a few of the fast-conducting fibers are still present. It was formally thought that the patients with pudendal neuropathy, as evidenced by prolonged conduction times, were more likely to have an unsatisfactory result following sphincteroplasty. Currently, however, most clinicians do not feel that abnormal conduction times have the prognostic value that was once thought; consequently, sphincteroplasty is not withheld from a patient who has a surgically correctable lesion and abnormal conduction times. Neurologic assessment of the sphincter muscle can also be performed using single-fiber needle electromyography. However, this examination is somewhat painful and is used only in very select instances.

There are many causes of fecal incontinence; obstetric injuries are a common reason patients are referred for surgery. Overall, fecal incontinence is rarely noted after vaginal delivery; however, prolonged labor and instrumented deliveries are associated with sphincter injuries. Approximately 10% of third- and fourth-degree perineal repairs ultimately fail due to factors such as infection, hematoma, or tension on the muscle edges.

Women who have sustained obstetric injuries frequently note impairment in incontinence promptly following delivery. It is interesting to note, however, that of asymptomatic primiparous women, 25% have demonstrable ultrasound evidence of sphincter injury, despite the fact that they have no functional impairment. Many of these women will manifest symptoms later in life. Initial compensatory mechanisms, such as dietary restriction and adjusting the time of defecation around social or athletic events, fail as these women age. For this reason, such women may not experience symptoms until the fifth or sixth decade of life.

At the time of the initial consultation for fecal incontinence, an anal ultrasound scan can be obtained, which immediately stratifies patients into treatment groups. If a defect in the muscle is identified, repair can be offered for the patient who has clinically significant symptoms and disability. If the scan is normal, then further diagnostic testing can be pursued with neurophysiologic testing and manometry to see if the problem is secondary to altered rectal compliance, diminished fecal sensation, or neuropathy. The treatment for these latter patients is primarily nonsurgical and may consist of biofeedback and pelvic floor retraining. Biofeedback consists of muscle-strengthening exercises, with the assistance of auditory or visual input for positive reinforcement. The patient is taught which muscle groups to squeeze and how to sustain a contraction over increasingly longer periods of time. Patients are also taught how to recognize gradually diminishing volumes of air or stool within the rectal vault.

The technique of anal ultrasound is much the same as for the rectal examination. The chief difference is that the end of the probe is covered with a hard, nondeformable plastic cap that permits easy insertion, withdrawal through the anus, and reinsertion. No sedation is required, and preparation is accomplished with a small-volume enema given 2 hours before the test. Interpretation of the sonographic images must be performed taking into account the location of the probe within the anal canal. As stated previously, the upper end of the anal canal is the puborectalis muscle, a horseshoe-shaped configuration of hyperechoic fibers whose open end is located in the anterior quadrant. As such, a lack of muscle fibers anteriorly is a normal finding. The hyperechoic external anal sphincter is located caudad to the puborectalis and therefore is not visualized until one descends in the anal canal. The internal anal sphincter is hypoechoic, easy to identify, and forms a compact circle. Thickness of the internal sphincter does not correlate with gender, body weight or height, or resting pressures as measured manometrically (17,18). The middle anal canal is that point where the internal anal sphincter has reached maximal thickness. The distal anal canal is that point where the internal sphincter begins to disappear and only the external sphincter is detectable. Thickness of the external sphincter does not correlate with manometric anal squeeze pressures; however, defects in the external sphincter correlate with diminished squeeze pressures (19).

The typical obstetrical injury produces a combined defect in the internal and external anal sphincter (Fig. 14). Isolated internal or external sphincter injuries may be seen but are less common. Defects are identifiable as breaks in the continuity of normally circular structures. Regarding the internal sphincter, defects are of mixed echogenicity and are readily apparent in relation to the hypoechoic nature of this muscle. Frequently, the fibers of the internal sphincter are thickened opposite from the defect presumably from retraction of the muscle edges. Defects in the external sphincter may be hypoechoic, hy-

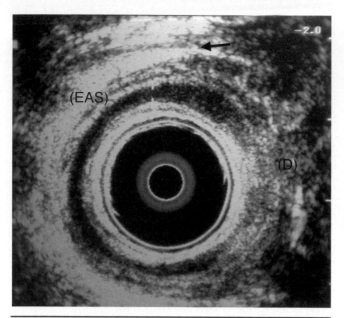

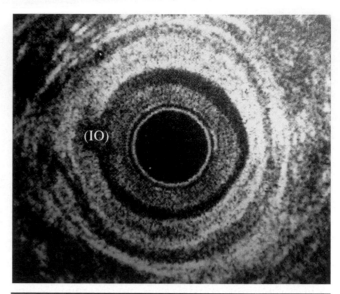

FIGURE 15. Fistula-in-ano. Internal opening (IO) noted in internal anal sphincter.

FIGURE 14. Obstetric injury with defect (D) in the internal and external sphincter (EAS). Arrows indicate severed edges of EAS.

perechoic, or of mixed echogenicity with loss of normal striations. Scar tissue may appear amorphous relative to the external sphincter.

Accuracy of anal ultrasound can best be determined by comparing sonographic with operative findings. In a study of 44 incontinent patients, Deen et al. found a high degree of correlation between ultrasound and subsequent findings at surgery. Twenty-one of 22 internal anal sphincter defects and all external anal sphincter defects were correctly identified (20). In another study, Sultan et al. found that all sonographic abnormalities identified in 12 patients were confirmed at surgery (21).

Ultrasound has also been used to evaluate perianal abscesses and fistulas. It is generally held that these abscesses arise from infections within the anal glands that are located either in the intersphincteric groove or in the internal anal sphincter itself. Infection may stay localized in the groove or may migrate through the external sphincter into the ischiorectal fossa or cephalad to the supralevator space. Most, but not all, abscesses result in a fistula whereby the skin of the anal margin or ischiorectal skin communicates through the fistulous tract with the crypt opening of the responsible anal gland. Most of these can be successfully managed without the need for extravagant imaging tests by unroofing, drainage, and fistulotomy. Despite apparently uneventful surgery, some fistulas persist or recur, and it is for these select instances that ultrasound may prove useful. Persistent sepsis is usually due to failure to identify the internal opening of the fistula (the responsible anal gland and its crypt) and all extensions of the tract itself. Before embarking on re-

operative surgery for these complex or recurrent cases, imaging studies such as fistulography or MRI are frequently ordered.

Sonographic imaging for perianal sepsis is usually initiated with a 10-MHz transducer that is covered with the plastic cap. One may need to switch to the latex balloon for scanning higher up in order to identify all loculations of an abscess. Fistula tracts are hypoechoic and can be followed by passing the ultrasound probe up and down with slow and controlled hand movements in small increments. The internal opening of the fistula may be found by tracing the tract to a hypoechoic defect in the internal sphincter of the anal canal (Fig. 15). Delineation of the fistula may be facilitated by injecting the external opening of the tract with a dilute solution of hydrogen peroxide with a small-caliber plastic cannula. Once inside the tract, the hydrogen peroxide–producing gas imparts a bright hyperechoic image.

CONCLUSIONS

Ultrasound has had a significant impact on the management of malignant and benign conditions of the rectum and anus. With respect to the former, rectal ultrasound can determine depth of tumor penetration in and outside the rectal wall and the presence of metastatic lymph nodes. With this information, the treating physician can individualize treatment, which may consist of transanal excision, prompt transabdominal resection, or preoperative radiation therapy and chemotherapy followed by surgery. Anal ultrasound provides an inexpensive, office-based image of the sphincter muscle and helps to determine whether fecal incontinence is surgically correctable. Ultrasound can also be used to identify fistula tracts and their internal anal opening in cases of complex or recurrent perianal sepsis.

REFERENCES

1. Beynon J, Foy DMA, Temple LN, et al. The endoscopic appearance of normal colon and rectum. *Dis Colon Rectum* 1986;29:810–813.
2. Hildebrandt U, Feifel G. Preoperative staging of rectal cancer by intrarectal ultrasound. *Dis Colon Rectum* 1985;28:42–46.
3. Bartram CI, Burnett SJD. *Atlas of anal endosonography*. Boston: Butterworth Heinemann, 1991:113.
4. Solomon MJ, McLeod RS. Endoluminal transrectal ultrasonography: accuracy, reliability and validity. *Dis Colon Rectum* 1993;36:200–205.
5. Herzog U, von Flüe M. Tondelli P, et al. How accurate is endorectal ultrasound in the preoperative staging of rectal cancer? *Dis Colon Rectum* 1993;36:127–134.
6. Sentovitch SM, Blatchford GJ, Falk PM, et al. Transrectal ultrasound of rectal tumors. *Am J Surg* 1993;166:638–642.
7. Anderson BO, Hann LE, Enker WE, et al. Transrectal ultrasonography and operative selection for early carcinoma of the rectum. *J Am Coll Surg* 1994;179:513–517.
8. Harnsberger JR, Charvat P, Longo WE, et al. The role of intrarectal ultrasound (IRUS) in staging of rectal cancer and detection of extrarectal pathology. *Am Surg* 1994;60:571–577.
9. Orrom WJ, Wong WD, Rothenberger DA, et al. Endorectal ultrasound in the preoperative staging rectal tumors. a learning experience. *Dis Colon Rectum* 1990;33:654–659.
10. Glaser F, Kuntz C, Schlag P, et al. Endorectal ultrasound for control of preoperative radiotherapy of rectal cancer. *Ann Surg* 1993;217:64–71.
11. Hulsmans FJ, Tio TL, Fockens P, et al. Assessment of tumor infiltration depth in rectal cancer with transrectal sonography: caution is necessary. *Radiology* 1994;190:715–720.
12. Holdsworth PJ, Johnston D, Chalmers AG, et al. Endoluminal ultrasound and computed tomography in the staging of rectal cancer. *Br J Surg* 1988;75:1019–1022.
13. Goldman S. Arvidsson H, Norming U, et al. Transrectal ultrasound and computed tomography in preoperative staging of lower rectal adenocarcinoma. *Gastrointest Radiol* 1991; 16:259–263.
14. Fleshman JW, Myerson RJ, Fry RD, et al. Accuracy of transrectal ultrasound in predicting pathologic stage of rectal cancer before and after preoperative radiation therapy. *Dis Colon Rectum* 1992;35:823–829.
15. Kahn H, Alexander A, Rakinic J, et al. Preoperative staging of irradiated rectal cancers using digital rectal examination, computed tomography, endorectal ultrasound, and magnetic resonance imaging does not accurately predict T0, N0 pathology. *Dis Colon Rectum* 1997;40:140–144.
16. Löhnert MSS, Doniec JM, Henne-Bruns D. Effectiveness of endoluminal sonography in the identification of occult local rectal cancer recurrences. *Dis Colon Rectum* 2000;43:483–491.
17. Burnett SJ, Bartram CI. Endosonographic variations in the normal internal anal sphincter. *Int J Colorectal Dis* 1991;6:2–4.
18. Gantke B, Schafer A, Enck P, et al. Sonographic, manometric and myographic evaluation of the anal sphincter's morphology and function. *Dis Colon Rectum* 1993;36:1037–1041.
19. Law PJ, Kamm MA, Bartram CI. Anal endosonography in the investigation of faecal incontinence. *Br J Surg* 1991;78: 312–314.
20. Deen KI, Kumar D, Williams JG, et al. Anal sphincter defects; correlation between endoanal ultrasound and surgery. *Ann Surg* 1993,218:201–205.
21. Sultan AH, Kamm MA, Talbot IC, et al. Anal endosonography for identifying external sphincter defects confirmed histologically. *Br J Surg* 1994;81:463–465.

Endoscopic Ultrasound

Maurice E. Arregui and Mark J. Lybik

Although mostly used for diagnosis, endoscopic ultrasound (EUS) is also a therapeutic tool. Recent curved linear scanheads allow ultrasound-guided needle biopsies, adding the potential for not only diagnostic but also therapeutic applications. EUS is well suited for the gastrointestinal (GI) surgeon as well as the gastroenterologist. As with many endoscopic techniques, this tool was initially used by surgeons but was acquired by gastroenterologists, who have greatly expanded its applications. Because of this, there has been an impetus for manufacturers to refine existing equipment and develop newer and better instruments, thereby increasing the potential for therapeutic uses.

ADVANTAGES AND INDICATIONS

The major advantage of EUS, as with intraoperative ultrasound, is that the transducer is directly on or very close to the organ of interest. This eliminates the interfering abdominal wall, ribs, fat, or bowel gas from acting as an acoustic barrier. Moreover, the proximity allows use of higher frequencies with better resolution providing a very detailed examination (Table 1).

Diagnostic uses of EUS in the foregut include staging esophageal, gastric, pancreatic, biliary, and ampullary cancers (Table 2). The depth of penetration of cancers and identification of nodal metastasis can be determined. Newer indications include staging of lung cancers with mediastinal node evaluation and biopsy. Use for staging rectal neoplasms and diagnosis of benign anorectal lesions is well established (see Chapter 19). The versatility of EUS is especially demonstrated in pancreatic lesions. For pancreatic cancers, a tissue diagnosis can be obtained with the use of EUS-guided needle biopsies. Evaluation of the portal vein, hepatic artery, or superior mesenteric artery encroachment can help determine resectability. EUS can localize islet cell tumors, allow aspiration of cystic neoplasms for diagnosis, and, in the case of pancreatic pseudocyst, help guide endoscopic drainage. EUS-guided celiac ganglion blocks are used to palliate pain from pancreatic cancer or chronic pancreatitis. There are current reports of EUS-guided radiofrequency ablation of nonresectable pancreatic neoplasms (1). As technology evolves, many of the surgical procedures that have been done with open, laparoscopic, or percutaneous approaches will be performed by endoscopic approaches, which in many cases will be guided by EUS.

Although currently few surgeons are performing EUS, it is important that surgeons begin to either get familiar with this tool or, better yet, acquire it; by doing so they may progress in minimally invasive surgery and continue to offer their patients state-of-the-art care.

EQUIPMENT

Scopes and Ultrasound Units

EUS is similar in principle to percutaneous, intraoperative, or laparoscopic ultrasound. The basic difference is that the transducer is on the tip of either a fiberoptic gastroscope or a video endoscope. Because the transducer is on the tip of the scope, the optic is at an angle. The configuration is somewhere between a side-viewing duodenoscope (used for endoscopic retrograde cholangiopancreatography, ERCP) and an end-viewing gastroscope (Fig. 1). The most commonly used diagnostic scope is the radial scope. This is manufactured by Olympus Corporation (Olympus America, Lake Success, NY). The transducer on the Olympus GF-UM20 has an adjustable frequency of 7.5 to 12 MHz. The higher frequency gives better definition of the bowel wall layers. The transducer is made up of a piezoelectric crystal that mechanically spins 360 degrees at a 90-degree angle to the longitudinal axis of the endoscope. Because of this configuration, orientation is improved due to the panoramic view obtained with the 360-degree angle (Fig. 2). The technique of endoscopic ultrasound of the GI tract has been well described using this type of scope. Most endosonographers have learned on this type of scope. Most use this as the primary diagnostic scope and will switch to a curved linear array scope for biopsy or thera-

▶ **TABLE 1 Advantages of Endoscopic Ultrasound**

1. No interferences by abdominal wall, ribs, fat, or gas
2. Higher frequency ultrasound with better image resolution
3. Provision of diagnostic information otherwise not available (particularly preoperatively) by other imaging modalities (e.g., cancer staging, resectability)
4. Therapeutic applications: endoscopic ultrasound guided procedures

▶ **TABLE 2 Indications for Endoscopic Ultrasound**

1. Staging of esophageal, gastric, pancreatic, biliary, and ampullary cancers, (lung cancers): T and N staging, resectability, biopsy
2. Evaluation of pancreatic lesion including cancers, islet cell tumors, cystic neoplasms, and pseudocysts
3. Evaluation of other gastrointestinal diseases such as submucosal tumors, varices, and biliary stones, and assistance in their management
4. Diagnostic or therapeutic guidance of various procedures including biopsy, drainage of pancreatic cyst, celiac ganglion block, and tumor ablation

peutic uses. Recently introduced by Olympus is the GF-UM160 gastrovideoscope, which eliminates the fiberoptic image and increases the frequency range from 5 MHz to 20 MHz.

Increasing in popularity is the linear array or curvilinear array scope manufactured by Pentax (Pentax Precision Instrument Corporation, Orangeburg, NY) and Olympus Corporation. This scope has a transducer that is in line with the endoscope on which it is mounted. Because of this, a needle introduced through the biopsy port can be guided with EUS into the target lesion. The

scanhead frequency of the Pentax scope ranges from 5.0 to 7.5 MHz (Fig. 3). Some scopes have an elevator on the biopsy port that can change the angle of the biopsy needle to improve the accuracy. Solid-state curvilinear array scanheads provide color flow Doppler.

With both types of scanheads, an acoustic coupling is needed because of the air in the GI tract. This is usually provided by a small, water-filled balloon that fits on the

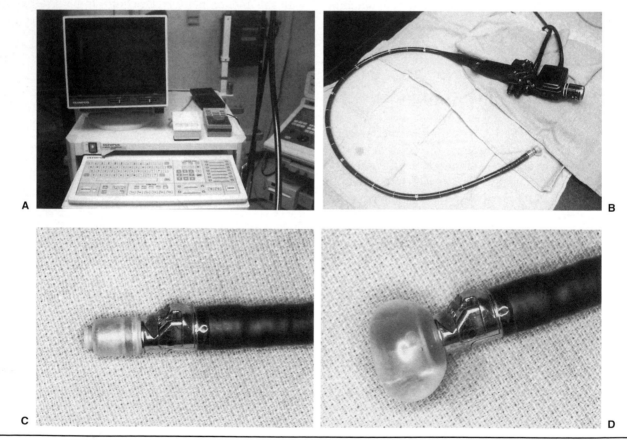

FIGURE 1. **A:** Olympus EUM-20: an ultrasonic processor with a monitor. **B:** Olympus GF-UM20: an upper gastrointestinal endoscopic ultrasound scope with switchable 7.5- and 12-MHz frequencies. **C:** Tip of GF-UM20, consisting of distal end ultrasound transducer and a proximal oblique viewing lens. **D:** Balloon covering the GF-UM20 ultrasound probe and being inflated with water. (From Yiengpruksawan A. Endoscopic ultrasound for surgeons. In: Staren ED, Arregui M, eds. *Ultrasound for the surgeon*. Philadelphia: Lippincott–Raven Publishers, 1997, with permission.)

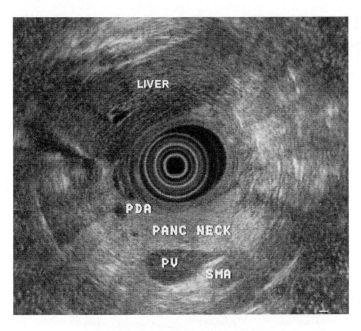

FIGURE 2. A 360-degree image with a radial echoendoscope in the stomach. The liver is anterior and the pancreas posterior. The surrounding vascular structures are as follows: PDA, pancreaticoduodenal artery; PV, portal vein; SMA, superior mesenteric artery.

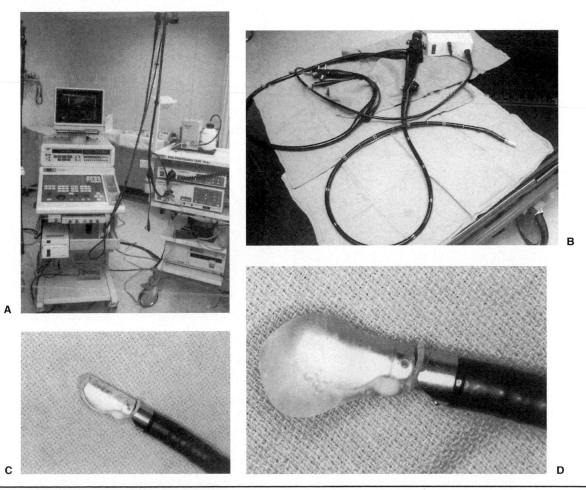

FIGURE 3. **A:** Pentax-Hitachi endoscopic-ultrasound system. **B:** Pentax endoscopic ultrasound scope. **C:** Tip of Pentax endoscopic ultrasound scope consisting of electronic linear array ultrasound transducer and a proximal oblique viewing lens. **D:** Balloon covering the ultrasound probe and being inflated with water. (From Yiengpruksawan A. Endoscopic ultrasound for surgeons. In: Staren ED, Arregui M, eds. *Ultrasound for the surgeon.* Philadelphia: Lippincott–Raven Publishers, 1997, with permission.)

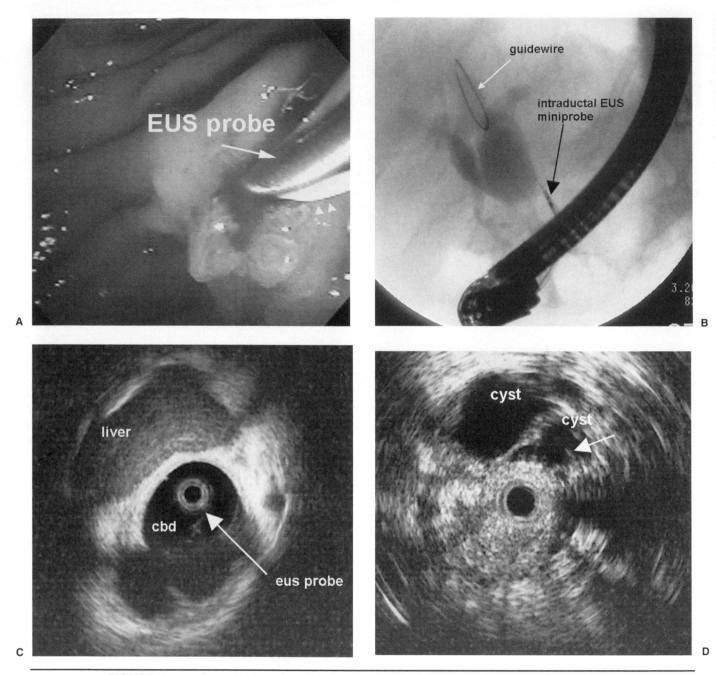

FIGURE 4. A: Endoscopic view of a mini-ultrasound probe being inserted over a guidewire (*arrow*) into the bile duct in a patient with a cystic pancreatic neoplasm. **B:** Fluoroscopic image of the mini-ultrasound probe inserted into the bile duct. **C:** Intraluminal mini-ultrasound probe image in the proximal common bile duct (cbd). The bile duct is dilated. This image is proximal to the obstructing neoplasm. **D:** Intraluminal image in the area of the stricture caused by a malignant cystic pancreatic neoplasm. Note the cysts with septations and irregular walls with projections (*arrow*).

probe. Alternatively or in combination, water with simethicon to reduce bubbles can be infused through the biopsy port.

Newer, thin, catheter-type probes (or mini-ultrasound probes) can be inserted through the biopsy channels of the endoscopes. These are mechanical probes of higher frequency (up to 30 MHz) that can be used to evaluate the bile duct or pancreatic duct or to pass through strictures such as esophageal neoplasms that the regular echoendoscopes cannot traverse (Fig. 4). These higher frequencies allow better resolution of the GI tract wall but have limited sound penetration. Other uses include evaluation of bile duct malignancies and pancreatic lesions.

TABLE 3 Endoscopic Ultrasound–Delineated Gastrointestinal Wall Layers and Corresponding Histologic Layers

Layer	Endoscopic Ultrasound Characteristics	Histology
1	Hyperechoic (bright) band	Superficial mucosa
2	Hypoechoic (dark) band	Deep mucosa
3	Hyperechoic (bright) band	Submucosa
4	Hypoechoic (dark) band	Muscularis propria
5	Hyperechoic (bright) band	Subserosa or serosa (or adventitia)

From Yiengpruksawan A. Endoscopic ultrasound for surgeons. In: Staren ED, Arregui M, eds. *Ultrasound for the surgeon.* Philadelphia: Lippincott–Raven Publishers, 1997, with permission.

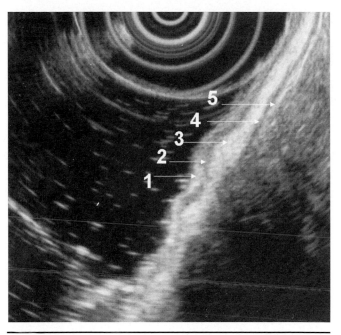

FIGURE 6. Gastric wall layers: 1, Superficial mucosa; 2, deep mucosa; 3, submucosa; 4, muscularis propria; 5, serosal or adventitial layer.

ENDOSCOPIC ULTRASOUND ANATOMY OF THE GASTROINTESTINAL TRACT

Layers of the Gastrointestinal Wall

Perhaps the best tool (other than pathologic evaluation of a resected specimen) to evaluate the normal and pathologic involvement of the various layers of the GI wall is EUS. No other imaging technique can visualize the layers in such detail preoperatively. The greater the frequency, the greater the resolution. With the 12.5-MHz frequency, five layers of the GI tract wall can usually be seen (2) (Table 3 and Fig. 5) These layers include the superficial mucosa (mucosal surface), deep mucosa (muscularis mucosa), submucosa, muscularis propria, and surrounding adventitia or serosal layer (Fig. 6). Higher frequency probes can visualize up to seven layers.

Tumor Staging

The purpose of viewing the layers is to determine the depth of invasion of GI malignancies, which helps to determine resectability and prognosis. Tumor staging is also useful in determining the layer of benign tumor involvement by lesions such as leiomyoma or lipoma. This may help determine excisional technique, which could be an endoscopic, a laparoscopic or an open approach.

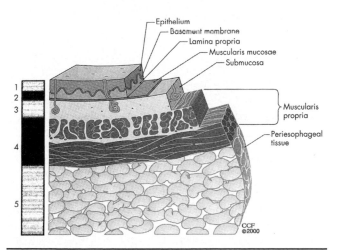

FIGURE 5. The ultrasound layers are correlated to the bowel wall layers. (From Rice TW. Esophageal tumors. In: Cameron JL, ed. *Current surgical therapy*, 7th ed. St. Louis: Mosby; 2001:52, with permission.)

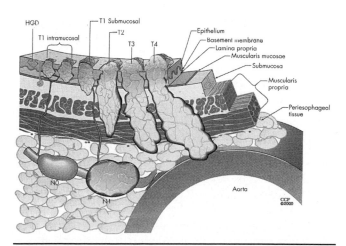

FIGURE 7. T staging of the bowel wall. (From Rice TW. Esophageal tumors. In: Cameron JL, ed. *Current surgical therapy*, 7th ed. St. Louis: Mosby; 2001:52, with permission.)

▶ **TABLE 4** General Characteristics of Normal and Abnormal Lymph Nodes

	Normal Lymph Nodes	Abnormal Lymph Nodes
Shape	Oblong, oval (flat)	Round
Internal echo	Hyperechoic center or hilum with thin hypoechoic rim	Hypoechoic
Border (edge)	Indiscrete	Discrete
Size	Less than 1 cm	More than 1 cm

T Staging

T staging is important for determining the method of resection or the need for neoadjuvant therapy of GI malignancies. The prefix "u" is often attached to the stage to indicate that the staging is performed with EUS. The terminology is uT1, uT2, uT3, uT4 (Fig. 7).

Normal Anatomy of Lymph Nodes

The characteristic features of normal and abnormal lymph nodes are summarized in Table 4. Normally the central part of the lymph node is composed of lymph sinuses, arteries, and veins, making it hyperechoic, and the outer rim or cortex has numerous lymph follicles, making it hypoechoic. A metastatic tumor in the center portion or medulla will make the node hypoechoic in the center and will distort the node, making it rounder. Although some say that any lymph node that can be seen represents a pathologic process, normal lymph nodes are frequently detected by EUS. For example, the suprapancreatic lymph nodes and periportal lymph nodes can be normally found in most patients if carefully looked for. It is important to note that these nodes in particular can be greater than 1 cm (Fig. 8). Inflammatory nodes may be enlarged and hypoechoic. Although EUS can characterize lymph nodes better than computed tomography (CT), distinction of an inflammatory node from a malignant node is still difficult based on ultrasound alone. EUS-guided needle biopsy can be helpful, but it is only useful when the result is positive (Fig. 9). A negative biopsy result does not exclude malignancy.

Surrounding Foregut Anatomy

The surrounding anatomy varies by organ and location. As with other uses of ultrasound, penetration of the ultrasound beam is dependent on the availability of an appropriate acoustic window. Air in the lung and trachea greatly limits viewing structures surrounding the esophagus. A fatty pancreas and the surrounding retroperitoneal fat may also limit ultrasound penetration. Vascular structures are the most easily identifiable landmarks and are

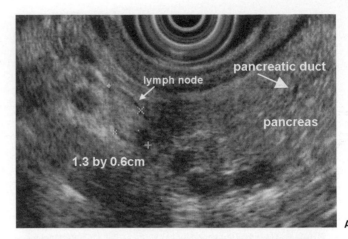

A

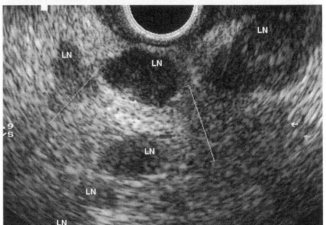

B

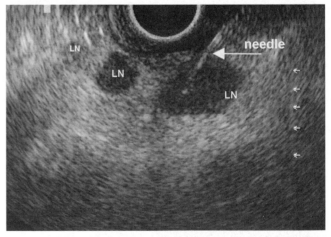

C

FIGURE 8. **A**: Although larger than 1 cm, a suprapancreatic lymph node such as this one (*short arrow, cursors*) is often easily seen with endoscopic and laparoscopic ultrasound. The characteristics of this benign lymph node are the hyperechoic center with hypoechoic rim. This shows a longitudinal view over the body of the pancreas through the posterior gastric wall. **B**: Curvilinear array ultrasound through the third portion of the duodenum in a male patient with recurrent lymphoma. Note the numerous enlarged, hypoechoic, discrete rounded lymph nodes (LN). **C**: Same patient as in (**B**). Ultrasound guided fine needle (*arrow*) lymph node (LN) biopsy revealed malignant lymphoma of follicular origin. *(continued)*

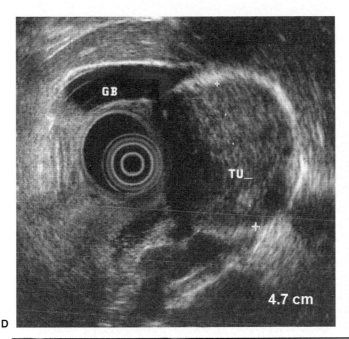

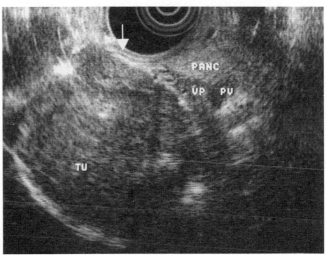

D / E

FIGURE 8. *(Continued)* **D:** A 22-year-old woman with large (4.7 cm) mass adherent to the second portion of the duodenum and pancreatic head. Computed tomography–guided needle and endoscopic ultrasound–guided needle biopsy were inconclusive but showed abundant lymphoid cells. Resection of this retroperitoneal mass revealed Castleman's disease, plasma cell variant. GB, gallbladder; TU, tumor. This view was obtained through the duodenum with a radial echoendoscope. **E:** Same patient as in **(D)**. Note the relationship to duodenum and pancreatic head. This is through the second portion of the duodenum just above the ampulla. Note that the layers of the duodenal wall (*arrow*) are seen and that the tumor is separate. Panc, pancreas; VP, ventral pancreas (hypoechoic relative to the rest of the pancreas); PV, portal vein; TU, tumor.

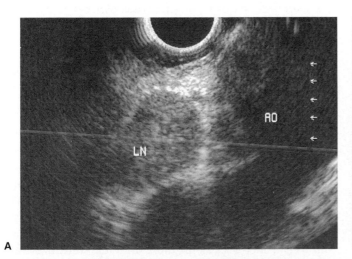

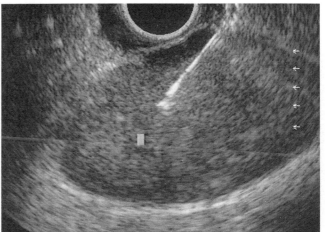

A / B

FIGURE 9. **A:** A patient with lung cancer undergoing preoperative evaluation for suspicious mediastinal nodes. An enlarged node was seen in the aortopulmonary window. AO, aorta; LN, lymph node. **B:** Same patient as in **(A)**. Biopsy of an enlarged subcarinal lymph node was positive for poorly differentiated non–small cell carcinoma.

▶ **TABLE 5 Anatomic Landmarks
in Endoscopic Ultrasound**

In esophagus:
 Gastroesophageal junction, aorta, vena cava, heart, pulmonary
  vein, subclavian vessels, carotids, aortopulmonary window,
  subcarinal node, azygos vein
In stomach:
 Aorta, celiac artery, hepatic artery, splenic artery, left adrenal
  gland, left lobe of liver, caudate lobe, vena cava, portal vein,
  splenic vein, pancreas
In duodenum:
 Gallbladder, common bile duct, pancreatic head, uncinate
  process, ventral pancreas, portal vein, superior mesenteric
  vessels, vena cava

excellent starting points in the search for particular structures. Identifying the aorta at the gastroesophageal junction (GEJ) and following it to the origin of the celiac artery allows identification of the splenic artery, which can be followed to the pancreatic tail and splenic hilum. Similarly, other arterial or venous landmarks can be used. Each area is unique and will be discussed with each organ (Table 5).

Esophagus

The esophagus is best viewed with a slightly distended fluid-filled balloon to obtain a good acoustic window to the esophageal wall and the surrounding structures. The

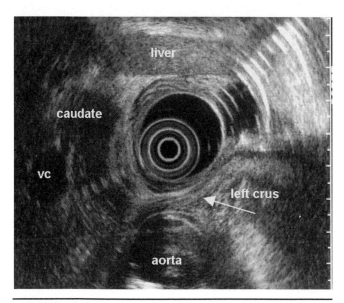

FIGURE 10. Image just below the gastroesophageal junction. The left lobe of the liver is anterior; the caudate lobe of the liver is on the patient's right side. The left crus of the diaphragm is seen between the stomach and aorta. VC, vena cava.

normal esophageal wall is about 2 to 3 mm thick with the balloon gently distended. With a 7.5-MHz transducer, three layers are clearly seen (when optimally scanned, five layers may be seen). The first hyperechoic layer is the interface with the balloon and the mucosa and submucosa. The second layer, which is hypoechoic, represents the muscularis mucosa. The third layer is the hyperechoic interface between the muscularis propria and the surrounding adventitia. With the higher 12-MHz frequency, five layers can be seen. (See the description of the five echo layers of the bowel wall given above.)

It is best to start scanning at the GEJ. With the radial echoendoscope, the orientation should be the same as that on a CT scan with the spine posteriorly on the image and the heart or liver at the top of the image. The patient's right side should be seen on the left side of the image and the patient's left side on the right side of the image. Most patients have undergone CT of the chest, and localization of the lesion in question and orientation are aided by having the CT image available during the procedure. Just below the GEJ, the left crus of the diaphragm can be seen between the esophagus and the aorta (Fig. 10). At the level of the GEJ, the spine is posterior and the aorta is just to the patient's left. The heart is anterior at this level; the left atrium is seen. The vena cava entering the right atrium may also be seen if not obscured by the lung, which is on either side of the esophagus. The azygous vein is posterior or on the patient's right side. As one goes more proximal, the pulmonary veins can be seen, and above this is the subcarinal space where nodes are seen. On either side are the bronchi. As the scope is further pulled proximally, the aortic arch can be seen. Just below this is the aortopulmonary window (Fig. 9A). The subclavian vessels and carotids can be seen above the aortic arch.

Stomach

As with the esophagus, the stomach wall is best seen with a fluid-filled balloon or when filled with water to acquire detail of the gastric wall. The optimal focal distance from the transducer to the gastric wall using the 7.5-MHz probe is 2 to 2.5 cm. This gives the best five-layer image (Fig. 6). The normal gastric wall is about 3 to 4 mm thick but its size increases as the more muscular antrum is approached. The pylorus can be up to 8 mm thick.

The stomach is an excellent acoustic window to the surrounding structures, and through the stomach, the biliary tree, portions of the liver, and most of the pancreas can be visualized. Retroperitoneal structures such as the left adrenal and kidney and vascular structures can be also seen.

Just beyond the level of the GEJ, posteriorly, the aorta is found and the celiac artery is identified. The branching

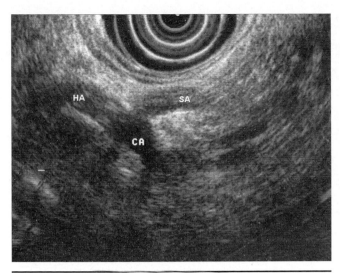

FIGURE 11. Whale's tail. Transverse view. CA, celiac artery; SA, splenic artery; HA, hepatic artery.

of the common hepatic artery and splenic artery forms what has been described as the "whale's tail" (Fig. 11). This is a landmark that is useful when searching for celiac lymph nodes during staging of malignancies. At this level, If the radial scope is turned clockwise, the left adrenal gland is identified (Fig. 12). With the curvilinear scope, an adrenal biopsy can be performed for suspicious lesions. If the radial scope is turned counterclockwise, the common hepatic artery can be identified and followed to the porta hepatis. At this location, the left lobe of the liver (segments 2 and 3) is readily seen (Fig. 13). The caudate lobe of the liver and vena cava is seen medi-

ally (Fig. 10). After the surgeon has found the celiac artery by moving the scope forward, the body of the pancreas is identified, as is the splenic and portal vein. Behind this is the superior mesenteric artery and aorta. This configuration is often described as the golf club sign (Fig. 14). With the scope advanced into the antrum, the biliary tree, porta hepatis, gallbladder, and pancreatic head are identified. The stomach is an excellent window to the lymph nodes during staging of gastric or other GI malignancies. Lymph nodes can be seen in the greater or lesser curvature of the stomach and around the celiac, hepatic, splenic, and left gastric arteries. The splenic hilum and porta hepatis can likewise be assessed for lymphadenopathy. Nodes as small as 3 mm can be identified.

Biliary Tree

The extrahepatic biliary tree, the left hepatic biliary tree, the left lobe of the liver, and the caudate lobe are accessible to EUS. The surrounding portal structures can also be evaluated with EUS. Following placement of the radial EUS scope in the duodenal bulb with a water-filled balloon, the gallbladder is readily identified. The common bile duct can be followed from its extrahepatic location through the head of the pancreas to the ampulla. The surrounding structures, such as the portal vein, hepatic artery, periportal lymph nodes, caudate lobe, and vena cava, are well seen through the duodenal bulb and second portion of the duodenum (Fig. 15). A catheter-type high-frequency probe can be inserted into the bile duct

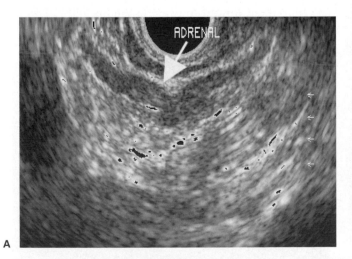

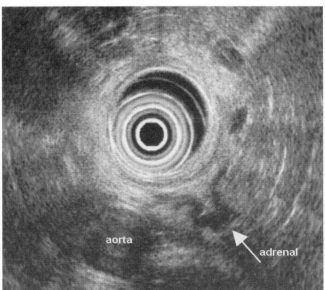

A   B

FIGURE 12. A: Curvilinear ultrasound image of a normal left adrenal gland (*arrow*). **B:** Radial echoendoscopic image of the left adrenal gland (*arrow*) seen just left to the aorta below the level of the crus of the diaphragm. *(continued)*

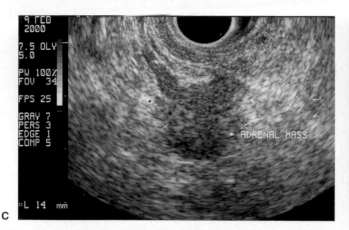

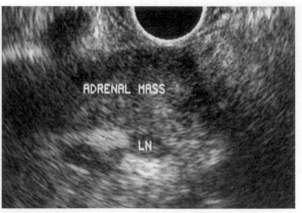

C

D

FIGURE 12. *(Continued)* **C:** Small left adrenal hypoechoic incidentaloma. **D:** A 72-year-old woman who 9 years before had a left pneumonectomy for invasive poorly differentiated adenocarcinoma with a positive regional node. Seven years postoperatively, she was found to have a left adrenal mass and two liver metastases. This endoscopic ultrasound scan of the adrenal gland shows the metastatic lesion with surrounding node (LN). She underwent open left adrenalectomy and radiofrequency ablation of two liver mets, and was asymptomatic until 2 years later when magnetic resonance imaging revealed four liver metastases. There was no evidence of adrenal recurrence. She had laparoscopic ablation of the liver metastases, and currently there is no evidence of extrahepatic disease.

for evaluation in detail. This is called intraductal ultrasound (IDUS) (Table 6).

Pancreas

EUS of the pancreas and retroperitoneal structures is one of the most useful tools available to gastroenterologists, surgeons, and oncologists. This is also one of the most challenging areas in performing EUS.

Identification of pancreatic anatomy starts with locating the aorta at the level of the GEJ. Advancing the radial scope brings the celiac artery into view (Fig. 11). With further movement forward, the splenic vein should come into view. The pancreatic body is anterior to this vein. The body itself should have a homogeneous echo band that is usually more echogenic than the liver. The borders of the pancreas are usually well defined by the gastric wall and splenic vein (Fig. 14). The pancreatic duct can then be located. The duct itself is hypoechoic and is outlined by a slightly brighter border. Once the duct is found, clockwise rotation of the scope, slight deflection, and movement toward the gastric fundus allows visual-

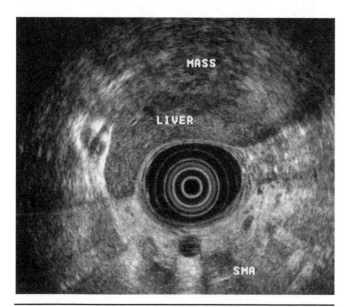

FIGURE 13. Mass in the left lobe of the liver. It was hypoechoic relative to the rest of the liver. This patient had a cancer of the pancreatic tail. SMA, superior mesenteric artery.

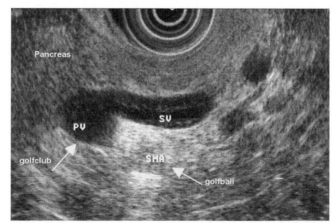

FIGURE 14. Golf club sign. PV, portal vein; SV, splenic vein; SMA, superior mesenteric vein. Transverse view of the pancreas with a radial echoendoscope.

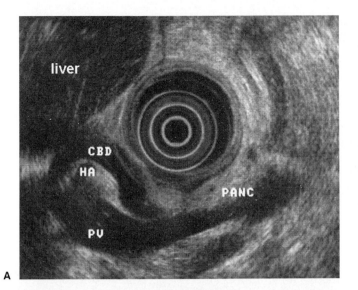

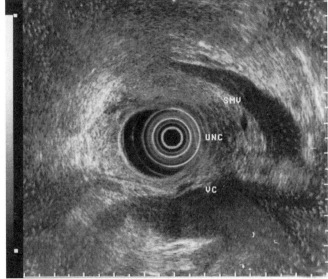

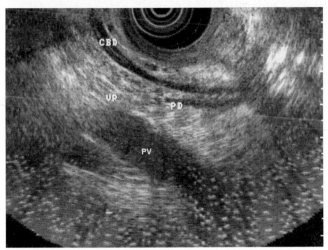

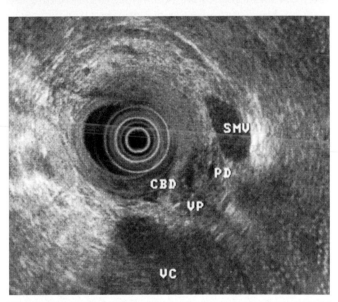

FIGURE 15. A: Common bile duct (CBD) is seen near the hilum of the liver. The hepatic artery (HA) is seen behind it. The portal vein (PV) can be seen going distally behind the pancreatic neck (panc). B: Distal portion of the common bile duct (CBD) coursing through the pancreatic head. The pancreatic duct (PD) is seen behind it and the portal vein (PV) further behind. This is called the "stack sign." VP, ventral pancreas.

FIGURE 16. A: Longitudinal view through the duodenum. The patient's head is on the right. The uncinate process (UNC) is between the superior mesenteric vein (SMV) and vena cava (VC). B: Same patient as in (A). With the radial scope, now in the second portion of the duodenum, a transverse view of the pancreatic head is obtained. The pancreas is between the superior mesenteric vein (SMV) and the vena cava (VC). The ventral pancreas (VP), common bile duct (CBD) and pancreatic duct (PD) are seen.

▶ **TABLE 6 Intraductal ultrasound**

1. Thin catheter-type radial and linear ultrasound: through the biopsy channel of endoscope
2. Higher frequency up to 30 MHz
3. Insert into the bile duct or pancreatic duct (also pass through strictures caused by GI malignancy, such as esophageal cancer)
4. Evaluation of biliary and pancreatic cancers or benign lesions

ization of the tail of the pancreas and the hilum of the spleen. By maneuvering the scope counterclockwise and a gentle push forward, the neck of the pancreas can be seen and the genu of the pancreatic duct can be found.

The head of the pancreas and the uncinate process is best seen through the duodenum. The scope is usually advanced as far into the duodenum as possible and it is slowly pulled out. The thick-walled and sometimes calcified aorta can be identified posteriorly, and often the superior mesenteric artery and superior mesenteric vein can be seen anteriorly. With continued slow pullback, the inferior vena cava can be seen (Fig. 16). The right kidney and uncinate process are then brought into view. With continued withdrawal, the ampulla and the pancreatic duct, which is in the ventral pancreas, can be found. In the majority of patients, the ventral pancreas has a slightly hypoechoic appearance and sometimes is mistaken for a pancreatic carcinoma (Fig. 16). By finding the common bile duct and the pancreatic duct and then tracing them down or filling the duodenum with water, the ampulla, a mildly hypoechoic structure, can be found. The common bile duct is closer to the duodenal wall than the pancreatic duct. Subtle movements of the scope can show the common bile duct and pancreatic duct in a longitudinal view and give an accurate cholangiogram and pancreatogram. The "stack sign" is seen when the common bile duct and pancreatic duct are running parallel to each other. For tumor staging, it is important to find the portal vein as this outlines the posterior border of the pancreatic neck and medial border of the pancreatic head (Fig. 15B).

At times, it is difficult to find all the structures with a pullback approach. An alternative method is to advance the echotip into the duodenal bulb in the long scope position. Inflating the balloon in this location will identify the gallbladder and hilar structures such as the common bile duct, cystic duct, hepatic artery, and portal vein. The common bile duct can then be followed to the head of the pancreas and the pancreatic duct can then be found.

ORGAN-SPECIFIC USES

Esophagus

Esophageal and Gastroesophageal Junction Tumors

EUS is valuable in evaluating patients with esophageal and GEJ tumors who are considered to be candidates for surgical resection. Patients have usually had a CT scan excluding distant metastasis. EUS is more accurate than CT scanning for T and N staging. EUS T staging ranges in accuracy from 59% to 92% and N staging from 55% to 90% (Fig. 17). EUS staging helps to predict survival and

to select patients for nonoperative or neoadjuvant therapy. It is most accurate prior to treatment with chemoradiation. Following neoadjuvant therapy, the accuracy is greatly diminished and EUS is generally unreliable for determining response to treatment. It is also of limited use for identifying recurrent tumor following surgery or neoadjuvant therapy. EUS cannot accurately distinguish inflammation, necrosis, or fibrosis from a malignant node or recurrent disease. It is not useful for guiding clinical decision making after neoadjuvant therapy (3).

Standard echoendoscopes are too large to go through some malignant strictures. The perforation rate for dilation of strictured esophageal malignancies to permit passing of the echoendoscope is about 25%; therefore, such dilation is not recommended. Most of these malignant strictures have stage III or stage IV disease (4). In these cases, thin, catheter-type, high-resolution EUS probes can be used.

Barrett's Esophagus with High-Grade Dysplasia

EUS has been used to detect submucosal invasion and lymph node involvement in patients with Barrett's esophagus with high-grade dysplasia or intramucosal carcinoma who are being considered for nonoperative therapy (5). EUS has also been used to determine the feasibility of endoscopic mucosal resection in patients with high-grade dysplasia or suspected early malignancy (T0 or T1 lesions) (6).

Benign Diseases

EUS is also useful for evaluating benign submucosal lesions of the esophagus. Granular cell tumors, lipomas, hemangiomas, fibroma, leiomyomas, duplication cysts and foregut cysts, or other benign lesions can be evaluated and biopsied. If resection is considered, EUS may be capable of identifying the layer of origin. If a small leiomyoma is submucosal, an endoscopic resection may be performed. If the lesion is found to be in the muscularis propria, a laparoscopic, thoracoscopic, or open approach may be indicated. With the use of EUS, Takada et al. managed five leiomyomas with this endoscopic approach (7). Sun et al. described ultrasound-guided endoscopic enucleation of submucosal tumors from the muscularis mucosa, submucosa, and muscularis propria in 16 patients whose disease is symptomatic without perforation or recurrence (8).

EUS-Guided Biopsy

With linear array EUS scopes, ultrasound-guided biopsy of esophageal and paraesophageal lesions and lymph

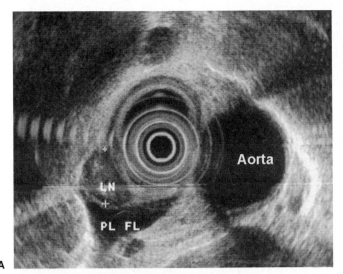

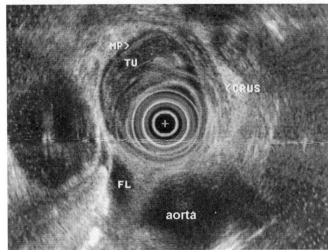

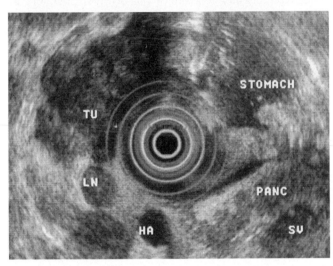

FIGURE 17. A: A 64-year-old man with adenocarcinoma of the gastroesophageal junction. This shows a view above the tumor. The esophagus is normal but there is a suspicious lymph node (LN) and pleural fluid (PL FL) suggesting metastatic disease. B: Same patient as in (A). The tumor (TU) is seen in the esophageal lumen. Note that the muscularis propria (MP) is intact. This is at the level of the diaphragmatic hiatus. The crus can be seen. There is some pleural fluid (FL) at this level as well. C: Same patient as in (A) just below the gastroesophageal junction. Note that the tumor (TU) is invading the surrounding adventitia. There are some suspicious nodes (LN). The hepatic artery (HA), pancreas (panc), and splenic vein (SV) are seen in the oblique view.

nodes can be accomplished to aid in diagnosis and staging (Fig. 9B).

Stomach

As with the esophagus, one of the main indications for EUS of the stomach is for staging of gastric cancers. Other uses of EUS include identifying submucosal lesions, diagnosis of lymphoma, evaluation and management of varices.

Gastric Cancer

As with esophageal cancer, EUS staging of gastric cancer for T and N is more accurate than CT. The accuracy of T staging for EUS ranges from 85% to 92%, which is higher than that of CT (15% to 43%). The accuracy of N staging for EUS is 74% to 87% as compared with 25% to 51% for

CT (9). The five echo layers are very distinctly seen and the depth of tumor penetration determined (Fig. 18). Regional nodes are also more accurately identified. N1 nodes are those within 3 cm of the edge of the tumor and N2 nodes are those beyond 3 cm or along major arteries; celiac, common hepatic, splenic, and left gastric. EUS is not sensitive for distant metastasis, and CT is critical for determining presence of metastasis to the liver or lung. Accurate staging is helpful for determining prognosis and may be useful for deciding on adjuvant therapy. In patients with early gastric cancers limited to the mucosa, endoscopic mucosal resection may be an option. Although more accurate than CT, EUS has a tendency to overstage T1 and T2 lesions because of the inflammation and fibrosis that may accompany ulcerated lesions of the stomach.

EUS can also be quite useful in diagnosing infiltrative cancers, which may have normal mucosal biopsies, such as linitis plastica. EUS-guided deep biopsies may estab-

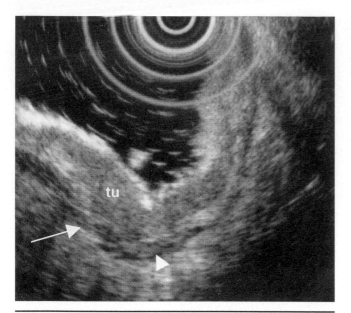

FIGURE 18. A 64-year-old woman with a T2 N0 M0 gastric carcinoma. This endoscopic ultrasound picture shows the tumor (tu) invading the muscularis propria (*arrowhead*). The outer portion of the muscularis propria is intact (*arrow*).

lish the etiologic pathology. Other infiltrative processes such as lymphoma and Ménétrier's disease can be more accurately characterized with EUS.

EUS has not been found useful for distinguishing benign from malignant ulcers. The inflammatory and fi-

brotic changes of an ulcer appear hypoechoic and can mimic an invasive cancer.

Gastric Subepithelial Tumors

Subepithelial or submucosal lesions of the stomach, as in the esophagus, are for the most part benign, and are often incidentally found; however, those that are malignant or symptomatic require an accurate diagnosis and endoscopic or surgical management. EUS provides a more accurate diagnosis than endoscopy, CT, and barium studies. EUS can more accurately distinguish cystic from solid lesions and can identify distinct echo textures. EUS findings can be fairly specific in distinguishing certain lesions, such as a lipoma, which tends to be uniformly hyperechoic and arising in the submucosal layer, from leiomyoma, which tends to be uniformly hypoechoic and is usually found in the muscularis propria (Fig. 19). Both are discrete lesions. The size of the lesion and the layer of the gastric wall are very accurately assessed, which can impact on the surgical approach should the lesion require removal. For more equivocal lesions, EUS-guided biopsy can help to determine the exact pathologic process. Other benign subepithelial lesions include gastric varices, cysts, and aberrant pancreas. Rare lesions include granular cell tumors, fibrovascular polyp, hematoma, carcinoid, hemangioma, granuloma, neurolemmoma, histiocytoma, fibroma, splenic implant, liposarcoma, and Brunner's gland nodule. Malignant lesions

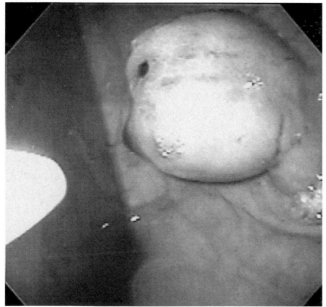

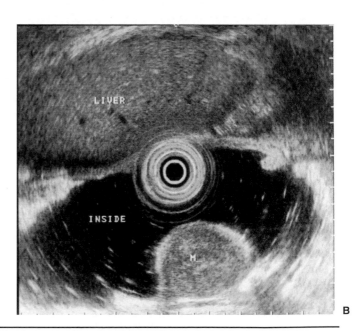

FIGURE 19. A: A 67-year-old man who presented with a gastrointestinal bleed. This endoscopic view shows a submucosal mass with a central ulcer that was the site of bleeding. **B:** Same patient as in **(A).** Endoscopic ultrasound demonstrated the submucosal mass (M). He underwent laparoscopic wedge resection of this lesion, which was a gastrointestinal stromal tumor.

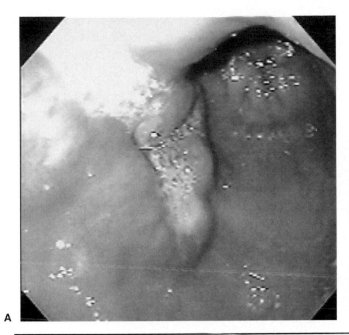

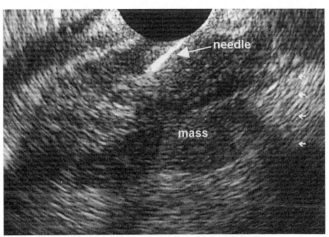

FIGURE 20. A: Endoscopic view of an ulcerated lesion in the stomach, which on multiple biopsies was negative. **B:** Endoscopic ultrasound–guided deep biopsy of lesion in **(A),** which showed abundant lymphoid tissue but was nondiagnostic. Ultimately, this patient underwent gastrectomy and was found to have a mucosa-associated lymphoid tissue (MALT) lymphoma.

presenting as subepithelial lesions can be characterized and EUS-guided biopsy can be performed to aid in diagnosis (Fig. 20).

Gastric Varices

There has been interest in EUS to evaluate esophageal and gastric varices. Although there seems to be minimal advantage of EUS over endoscopy for identifying esophageal varices, EUS evaluation of the size of periesophageal varices and perforators can help predict recurrence following treatment (10). There seems to be additional advantage of EUS in diagnosing gastric varices, which can be difficult to identify by endoscopy alone and may present as submucosal masses or hypertrophic folds. Perforating vessels supplying gastric varices can be identified and mapped (Fig. 21). There are ongoing studies to determine if mapping varices and sclerotherapy with EUS guidance improve the rebleed rate. Konishi et al. recently

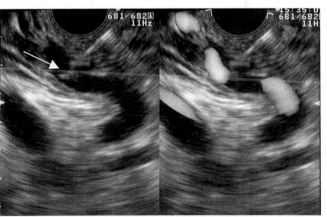

FIGURE 21. A: A 43-year-old man with a history of pancreatitis with splenic vein thrombosis, now with recurring gastrointestinal bleed and gastric varices. This color Doppler imaging (shown in black and white) demonstrates a perforating varix going through the gastric wall. An arrow shows the outer gastric wall. **B:** Same patient as in **(A)** with endoscopic ultrasound–guided needle insertion for sclerotherapy. An arrow shows the needle tip in a perforating vessel. The right image is with color Doppler (shown in black and white).

evaluated 30 patients with bleeding esophageal varices with a 20-MHz catheter-type EUS probe to look for gastric cardia varices. EUS detected varices in the gastric cardia in all patients evaluated, whereas endoscopy detected gastric cardia varices in only 21 of these patients. They also found that patients with severe grade gastric perforators had a significantly higher incidence of rebleeding (90.9%) than those with mild-grade perforators (21.0%) with a *p* value less than 0.01 (11).

Gallbladder and Biliary Tree

Bile Duct Cancer

The diagnosis of cholangiocarcinoma is often difficult to make. Bile duct strictures may represent benign or malignant diseases. ERCP with brush cytology or transpapillary biopsy may not always provide the etiologic information about a bile duct obstruction if the presence of common bile duct stones or an obvious mass is not found. Domagk et al. recently evaluated 60 patients with bile duct strictures of unknown cause with ERCP and transpapillary forceps biopsy as well as with IDUS. Postoperative diagnoses were 30 pancreatic, 17 bile duct, and 3 gallbladder cancers; 10 lesions were benign. ERCP with biopsy gave a correct diagnosis in 60% of cases. IDUS with ERCP had an 83% preoperative accuracy. Combining ERCP with biopsy and IDUS achieved a 98% accuracy rate (12) (Fig. 4).

EUS-guided biopsy using a linear echoendoscope can be helpful in obtaining a tissue diagnosis in patients with suspected cholangiocarcinoma as well as those in whom brush cytology has failed to give a diagnosis. Using a linear echoendoscope and a 20-gauge needle, Fritscher-Ravens et al. obtained adequate tissue in 20 such patients with hilar cholangiocarcinoma and diagnosed seven with cholangiocarcinomas and one with hepatocellular cancer. There was one false negative. Metastatic nodes were confirmed with EUS-guided biopsy in some of these patients (13).

EUS and IDUS is also useful for determining T and N staging to help predict resectability of bile duct tumors. A study by Menzel et al. compared the accuracy of EUS to that of IDUS. For T staging, IDUS was significantly better (IDUS, 77.7%; EUS, 54.1%; *p* < 0.001). For N staging, the accuracy was similar (IDUS 60%, EUS 62.5%). Overall, IDUS was also found to be more accurate and sensitive for diagnosis of bile duct obstruction (14).

Ampullary Cancer

As with bile duct cancers, EUS is helpful to more accurately determine the resectability of ampullary cancers by determining the T and N stage and assessing invasion of the surrounding vascular structures such as the portal vein. It is not so useful in assessing distant metastasis. EUS-guided biopsies can help establish diagnosis of regional and nonregional nodes. Zhang et al. found an 81.8% accuracy of EUS for assessing local extent of ampullary cancer and 59% accuracy in predicting regional lymph node metastasis (15).

Bile Duct Stones

EUS has been used to diagnose common bile duct stones in equivocal cases. ERCP remains the standard procedure for suspected bile duct stones in pre- and postcholecystectomy cases, and it allows therapeutic removal of stones if found. There is an associated morbidity with ERCP; a complication occurs in a duct found to be negative for stones. EUS in this sense is safer, but if a stone is found, either ERCP with endoscopic stone extraction, or laparoscopic or open common bile duct exploration needs to be performed. EUS has also been used to identify small gallstones or microlithiasis in patients with suspected gallbladder disease or pancreatitis of unknown cause who have had a negative transabdominal ultrasound.

Pancreas

Pancreatic Cancer

Pancreatic cancer is one of the most challenging cancers in which an early diagnosis is difficult. EUS is more sensitive than CT in detecting lesions smaller than 3 cm. It is also helpful in staging and determining resectability. In patients who have unresectable tumors, EUS-guided biopsy can obtain a tissue diagnosis and greatly impact manage-

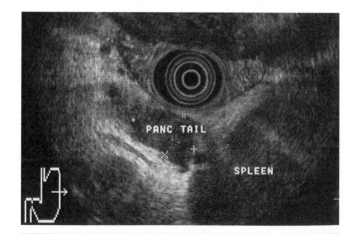

FIGURE 22. Hypoechoic tumor (*cursors*) in the pancreatic tail (panc tail) near the spleen. This patient had liver metastasis found on computed tomography (CT) scan of the abdomen. The pancreatic tumor was not detected on CT scan.

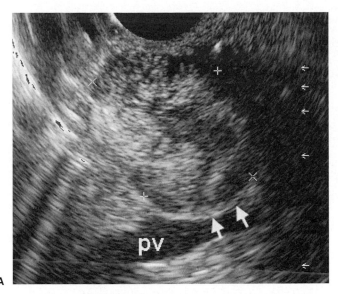
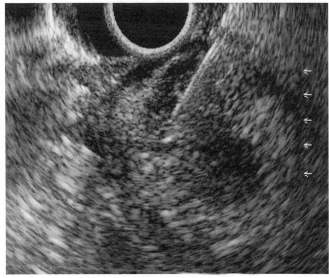

FIGURE 23. A: Image through the duodenum of a tumor (*cursors*) in the head of the pancreas abutting the portal vein (PV). Note that there is a separating white line (*arrows*) indicating impingement but not invasion. This particular cancer is quite discrete and well delineated. **B:** Same patient as **(A)**. Linear endoscopic ultrasound guided biopsy revealing adenocarcinoma of the pancreas.

mont, especially if a lesion is found to be a lymphoma or something other than a pancreatic adenocarcinoma.

The data over the last 10 years have supported the fact that EUS has a higher sensitivity and specificity for diagnosing and determining the resectability of pancreatic cancer than CT, MRI, and ERCP. Most of the studies have compared EUS with older CT imaging equipment and techniques. The newer dual phase helical CT scans are much more accurate and the advantages of EUS are thus diminished (16). Nonetheless, EUS still has a role in obtaining a detailed image and enhancing lymph node detection and biopsy of small or equivocal lesions.

Pancreatic cancer on EUS usually presents as a distinct hypoechoic tumor (Figs. 22 to 24). The diagnosis must be put into a clinical context as inflammation and chronic pancreatitis can often have the same echo texture as a cancer. Pancreatic cancers can also appear inhomogeneous with a mixed hyper- and hypoechoic pattern. This may represent necrosis of parts of the tumor. Cancers can have discrete borders or some tumors can have irregular borders. The size of the tumor usually has some bearing on the pattern of the tumor growth. With obstruction of the pancreatic duct, the uninvolved pancreas may have associated inflammatory changes.

Once the mass is identified, EUS is used to look for metastasis to nonregional and regional nodes. The celiac nodes are readily identified and if suspicious can be biopsied using EUS-guided fine needle aspiration. To a limited extent the liver, especially the left lobe, can be screened for metastasis (Fig. 13). EUS is helpful in determining resectability in terms of involvement of portal venous and major arterial vessels; it can identify portal vein, splenic, or superior mesenteric vein invasion. It can also identify encasement of celiac, hepatic, or superior mesenteric artery. Usually if a vessel is involved, there is

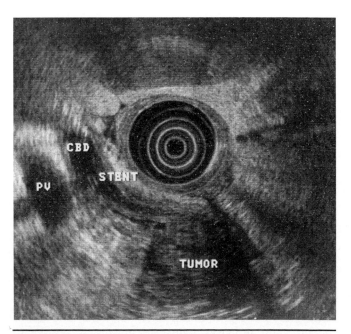

FIGURE 24. Image through the duodenal bulb of a pancreatic head cancer (tumor) with previous stent placement in the common bile duct(CBD). PV, portal vein.

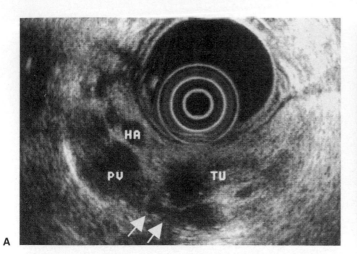

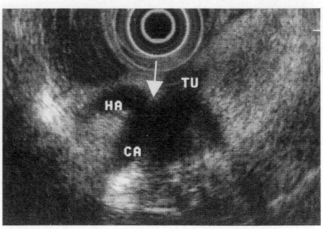

FIGURE 25. **A:** A 76-year-old woman with pancreatic cancer at the neck with portal vein (PV) narrowing (*arrows*) due to impingement from the malignant tumor (TU). HA, hepatic artery. **B:** Same patient as in (**A**). Pancreatic tumor (TU) abutting (*arrow*) the celiac artery (CA) and hepatic artery (HA). The patient was referred for chemoradiation to attempt to downstage the tumor to make it resectable.

loss of the normal border of the vessel. There are times when the ingrowth of tumor into the vessel itself is visualized. It is important to look at the particular vessel in as many planes as possible. It is also important to realize that portal vein invasion itself is not necessarily a contraindication to resection as some surgeons will resect the portal vein if only involved by local tumor invasion (Fig. 25).

Pancreatic Cystic Neoplasms

EUS has led to advances in the diagnosis of cystic lesions of the pancreas. Cystic neoplasms of the pancreas are uncommon. About 1% of all pancreatic malignancies arise from cystic neoplasms. Pancreatic cystic lesions encountered include simple cysts, serous cystadenoma, mucinous cystadenoma, mucinous cystadenocarcinoma, intraductal papillary mucinous tumor (IPMT), and pseudocyst (Fig. 26). The patient history and CT scans usually cannot make the definitive diagnosis. EUS provides a detailed image and the ability to aspirate fluid for analyses to determine the malignant potential of a cystic lesion (Fig. 27). Simple cysts and serous cystadenomas are benign and usually do not require resection unless symptomatic. Mucinous cystadenomas and IPMT can undergo malignant degeneration; therefore, surgery is recommended.

Mucinous cystadenomas make up about 10% of pancreatic cystic lesions and have the highest malignant potential. They are predominantly in the body and tail of the pancreas, and are usually seen in women between 40 and 60 years old. They are hypoechoic with few septations but not as many as serous cystadenomas (Fig. 28).

The aspirated fluid is thick and stains positive for mucin. The carcinoembryonic antigen (CEA) in the fluid analysis tends to be high in these lesions and particularly high in the mucinous cystadenocarcinomas (Figs. 28 and 29). If one of these tumors is found, complete resection can achieve a 70% 10-year survival rate.

Serous cystadenomas are usually multilocated or microcystic and often present in the body, tail, and the uncinate process. On EUS, the cystic lesion has a honeycomb pattern that is quite distinct (Figs. 27A and 30). This le-

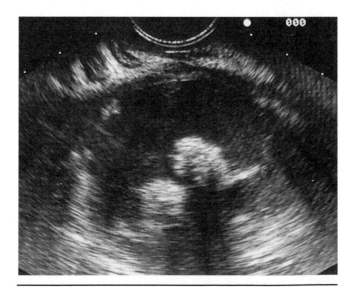

FIGURE 26. A 44-year-old woman with immature pseudocyst from acute pancreatitis due to sphincter of Oddi dysfunction. The projections make this complex cyst mimicking a cystadenocarcinoma. The clinical history is important in the diagnosis.

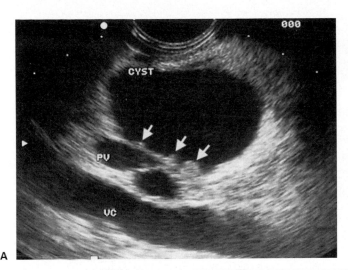 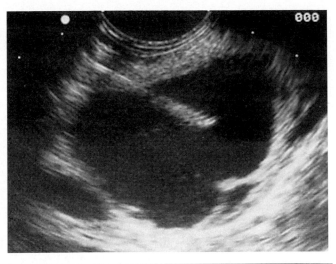

A   B

FIGURE 27. **A:** An 84-year-old woman with a pancreatic cystic neoplasm followed for 4 years. The lesion is somewhat complex with numerous cysts with small projections (*arrows*) on the septations. PV, portal vein; VC, vena cava. **B:** Same patient as in (**A**). Cyst aspiration revealed a low carcinoembryonic antigen level of 17.4 ng/mL, viscosity of 1.2 centipoise U (normal 1.4–1.8), and amylase of 57 U/L, CA 19–9 of 160 U/mL and CA 125 of 7 U/mL. Cytologic examination revealed only inflammatory cells. The patient did not want surgery. The patient has remained asymptomatic for 4 years with no progression of what is presumed to be a serous cystadenoma.

sion can be associated with Von Hippel Lindau disease. Aspirated fluid has a low specific gravity and a low CEA.

IPMT arises from the ducts and produces mucin in the main pancreatic duct or its side branches. EUS usually shows a diffusely dilated pancreatic duct and cystic dilation of the side branch. This is a premalignant lesion or

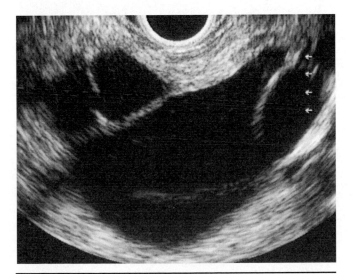

FIGURE 28. A 38-year-old woman with cystic lesion in the pancreatic tail. Endoscopic ultrasound–guided aspiration showed amylase 578 U/L, carcinoembryonic antigen 18421.9 ng/mL. Cytology results were negative. Laparoscopic distal pancreatectomy with splenectomy was performed. Pathologic examination revealed mucinous cystadenoma.

malignant lesion. If found at the time of EUS, it is usually recommended that the patient undergo surgery (Figs. 31 and 32).

Although there are conflicting reports on the value of fluid analysis in distinguishing benign from malignant lesions, it is the most widely used method to help establish the diagnosis (Table 7). EUS images, though helpful, are subject to individual interpretations. The EUS image, CEA, amylase, and mucin analysis combined seem to provide the best information. Cytologic examination in these cystic lesions has a very low yield. Other tumor markers, such as CA 19–9, CA 125, and CA 72–3, are under investigation (17). Its best application is for patients who are poor operative risks. The additional information from EUS may help to clarify if the lesion is a simple cyst or serous cystadenoma, either of which can be safely managed nonoperatively if asymptomatic.

Pancreatic Pseudocysts

Pseudocysts are usually found in the setting of a bout of acute pancreatitis, most commonly from either gallstone or alcoholic pancreatitis. On EUS, the cyst appears anechoic and can have a thick or thin wall. Although the diagnosis is usually made on the basis of clinical and CT findings, sometimes the etiologic factor is equivocal. EUS image and fluid analysis can aid in the diagnosis. Once established, EUS can be used to drain the pseudocyst. These cystic lesions can be drained by two different

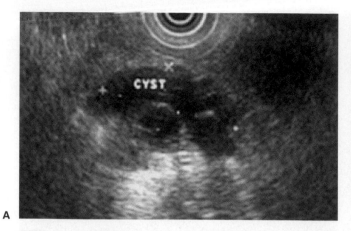

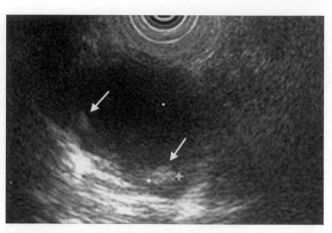

A

B

FIGURE 29. A: A 75-year-old woman with complex pancreatic cyst with multiple septations. This image is similar to that of a patient in Figure 27A. This patient was found to have a mucinous cystadenoma with foci of adenocarcinoma. She underwent resection but had a recurrence with metastasis and died two years following her initial resection. **B:** Different image of same patient as **(A)**. Note the two projections (*arrows*). This has a similar ultrasound picture to that in a patient discussed in Figure 26.

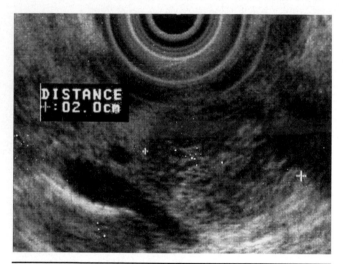

FIGURE 30. A patient referred with an incidentally found asymptomatic mass in the head of the pancreas. This was found on a computed tomography scan of the abdomen. Magnetic resonance imaging suggested a cystic neoplasm consistent with a serous cystadenoma. Transabdominal ultrasound showed a solid mass. This endoscopic ultrasound scan shows what on superficial inspection appears to be a solid mass but on careful inspection shows multiple small cysts (*cursors*). She has been followed for 3 years, and the mass has remained stable.

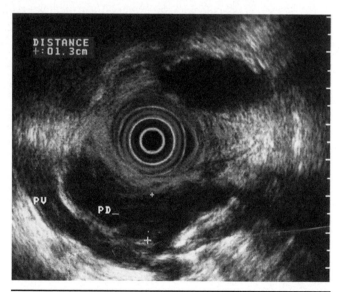

FIGURE 31. A 64-year-old woman with an intraductal papillary mucinous tumor of the pancreas followed for 3 years. Repeat endoscopic ultrasound with biopsy showed suspicious cells and the patient was referred for a Whipple operation. The final pathology result was negative for malignancy. Note that the pancreatic duct (PD) is enlarged at 1.3 cm. PV, portal vein. This image is through the duodenal bulb.

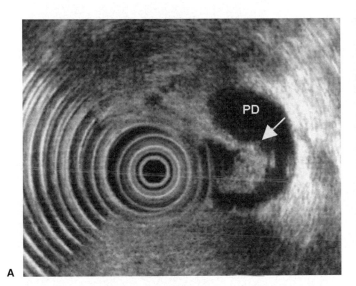
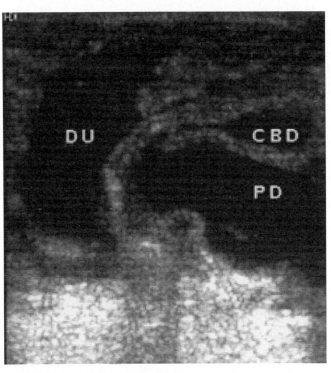

FIGURE 32. **A:** An 85-year old man followed for 2 years with recurring mild episodes of pancreatitis and found to have an intraductal papillary mucinous tumor of the pancreas. Because of his age and health, he did not want to have surgery. Note the papillary projection (*arrow*) in the dilated pancreatic duct (PD). **B:** Same patient as in **(A)**. This image in the second portion of the duodenum (DU) filled with water shows that the mucin distended the pancreatic duct (PD) all the way to the orifice of the ampulla. CBD, common bile duct.

methods. The first method is to perform a needle drainage in cysts that are 6 cm or smaller (Fig. 33). If a lesion is larger than 6 cm, EUS-assisted drainage with endoscopic cystgastrostomy and stent placement is recommended. This is achieved by performing EUS on the suspected lesion and marking a spot that is clear of vessels and with the cyst clearly abutting the gastric wall. Then the scope is changed to a side-viewing duodenoscope, and with a needle knife and cautery a cut is made through the stomach wall into the cyst. A guidewire is then inserted. Over the guidewire, a balloon is used to dilate the tract. Over the same guidewire, stents are then placed extending from the stomach to the pseudocyst

(Fig. 34). With the newer linear video echoendoscopes and their improved images and larger biopsy channels, a stent can be placed without switching to the therapeutic duodenoscope.

Pancreatic Endocrine Tumors

Another valuable use of EUS is to localize islet cell tumors. EUS is a very sensitive tool for finding insulinomas. Ninety percent of insulinomas are under 2 cm and occur within or are attached to the pancreas. The most sensitive tool for finding insulinomas is open surgical exploration and intraoperative ultrasound. More than 90% of islet cell

▶ **TABLE 7 Cystic Fluid Analysis of Pancreatic Cysts**

Diagnosis	Viscosity	Amylase	CA72–4	CEA	CA15–3	Cytology
Pseudocyst	Low	High	Low	Low	Low	Inflammatory
Serous cystadenoma	Low	Variable	Low	Low	Low	50% positive
Mucinous cystadenoma	Often high	Variable	Low	High	High	Usually positive
Mucinous cystadenocarcinoma	High	Variable	High	High	High	Usually positive

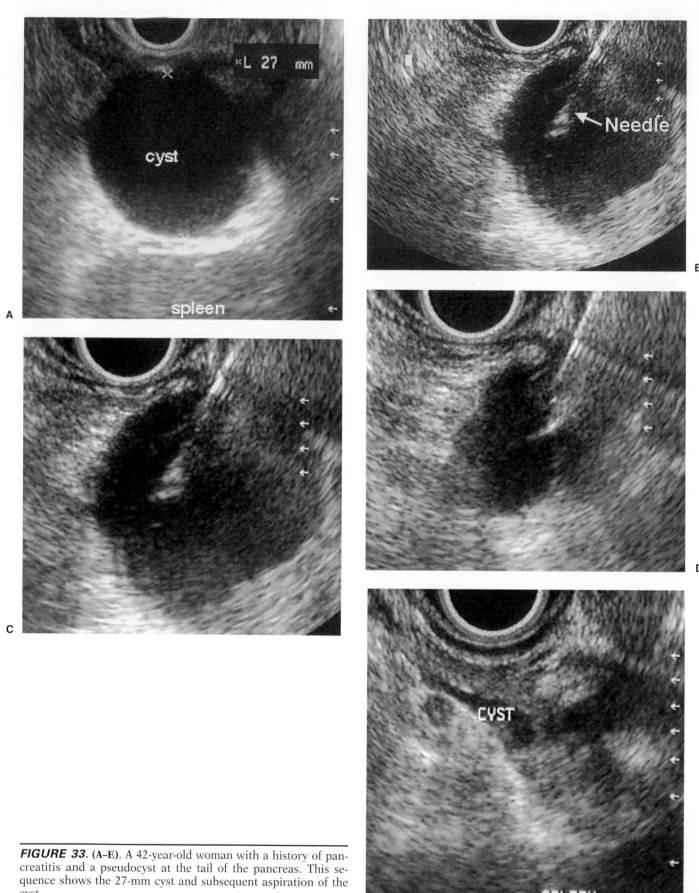

FIGURE 33. (A–E). A 42-year-old woman with a history of pancreatitis and a pseudocyst at the tail of the pancreas. This sequence shows the 27-mm cyst and subsequent aspiration of the cyst.

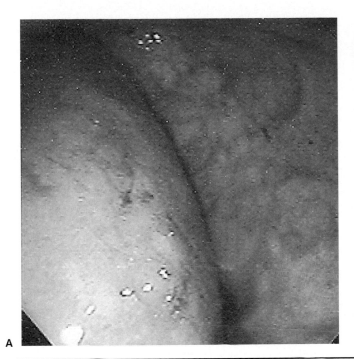
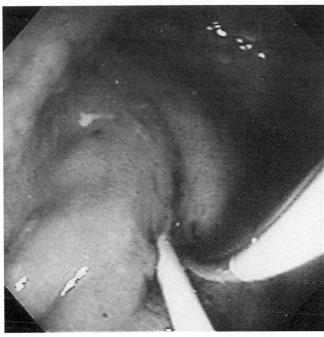

FIGURE 34. A: Endoscopic view of large pancreatic pseudocyst. Note the bulging gastric wall. Endoscopic ultrasound was used to mark a location suitable for puncture. **B:** Same patient as in **(A)**. Note stents placed into pseudocyst for creating endoscopic cystgastrostomy.

tumors are identified in this way. EUS has been found to be nearly as accurate in finding these tumors. Zimmer et al. found that EUS had an overall sensitivity of 93% for localizing insulinomas and 79% for gastrinomas (18). With accurate preoperative evaluation such as location, size of tumor, and proximity to the pancreatic duct, surgical planning can better take place. We have used this approach to plan laparoscopic exploration and enucleation of select tumors (19) (Fig. 35). We have also found it useful in following patients with multiple endocrine neoplasms.

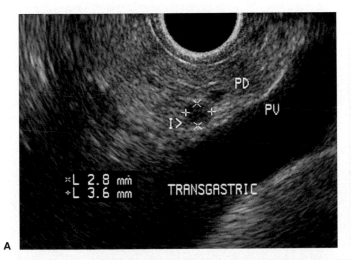
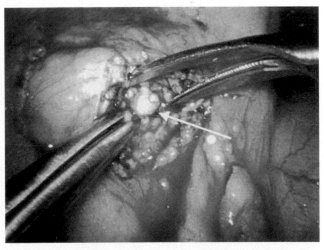

FIGURE 35. A: A 58-year-old nurse found to have hypoglycemia while at work. Workup was consistent with an insulinoma. Endoscopic ultrasound localized a small insulinoma at the pancreatic neck adjacent to the pancreatic duct. The lesion was 3.6 × 2.8 mm. I, insulinoma; PD, pancreatic duct; PV, portal vein. **B:** Same patient as in **(A)**. She underwent laparoscopic ultrasound–guided resection. A needle was placed under ultrasound guidance between the pancreatic duct and the insulinoma. A cutdown was made over the needle to avoid injuring the pancreatic duct. She did not develop a leak. She is now 2 years postresection with no evidence of recurrence and totally asymptomatic. Note the small insulinoma (*arrow*) held in the laparoscopic DeBakey clamp.

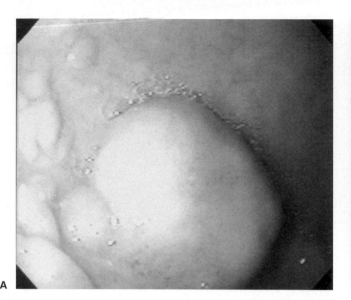

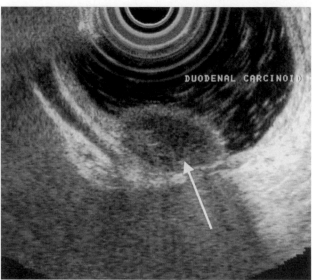

A

B

FIGURE 36. **A:** A man with esophageal cancer found to have a submucosal duodenal nodule that on biopsy revealed a carcinoid. This tumor was not resected due to his advanced esophageal cancer. This shows the endoscopic view of the duodenal carcinoid. **B:** Endoscopic ultrasound image of the same patient as in **(A).** The duodenal hypoechoic carcinoid (*arrow*) is seen in the submucosal layer.

EUS can be used for identifying other pancreatic endocrine tumors such as gastrinomas, as well as other functioning and nonfunctioning tumors of the pancreas. Most islet cell tumors or neuroendocrine tumors are seen as discrete hypoechoic masses (Fig. 36).

Chronic Pancreatitis

EUS can show some very characteristic changes in pancreatitis. Unfortunately, some of these changes, such as ductal dilation and pancreatic fibrosis, can occur in el-

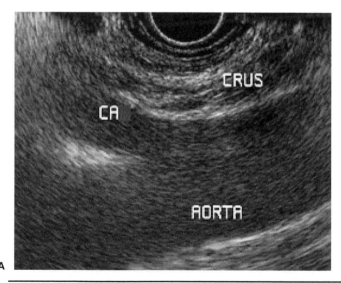

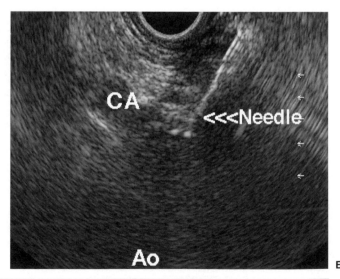

A

B

FIGURE 37. **A:** Celiac artery (CA) coming off the aorta. The crus of the diaphragm can be seen between the stomach and aorta. This is a view with a curvilinear array echoendoscope. **B:** Endoscopic ultrasound–guided insertion of a needle to the side of the celiac artery (CA) for a celiac ganglion block in a patient with pain due to chronic pancreatitis. AO, aorta. **C:** Injection of saline (hypoechoic area) is performed to confirm position of the needle tip. A small amount of air from the needle is seen as a hyperechoic blush.

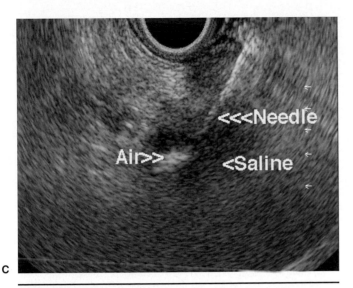

c

FIGURE 37. (Continued)

derly patients and alcoholics without chronic pancreatitis. However, a completely normal EUS can usually exclude chronic pancreatitis.

The features of chronic pancreatitis tend to start in the parenchyma. The echo pattern is irregular and inhomogeneous, and there are intraparenchymal calcifications shown as strong hyperechoic foci. There may also be areas of hypoechogenicity in chronic pancreatitis representing active inflammation and edema. The parenchyma usually has a lobular contour as seen in the elderly patient.

Ductal changes include: dilation of the main pancreatic duct (greater than 3 mm in the head, greater than 2 mm in the body, and greater 1 mm in the tail), irregular contour of the duct, side branch dilation and echo-rich foci in the duct that can represent protein plugs or stones (20).

THERAPEUTIC ASPECTS

Celiac Ganglion Block

Currently, EUS can be used therapeutically for EUS-guided celiac ganglion blocks for treating pain in chronic pancreatitis or pancreatic cancer (21). In benign disease, a combination of local anesthetic and steroid is injected using a linear echoendoscope and a 22-gauge needle directed to either side of the celiac artery. In pancreatic malignancies, absolute alcohol is used for a more permanent block (Fig. 37).

Drainage of Pancreatic Pseudocyst

See the section on pancreatic pseudocysts.

Ablation of Pancreatic Lesions

Preliminary work has been performed on radiofrequency ablation of nonresectable pancreatic cancer in animal studies and in humans using a curvilinear array echoendoscope (1). This therapeutic approach to pancreatic lesions could be extended to islet cell tumors such as insulinomas. Currently percutaneous alcohol ablation of parathyroid tumors with ultrasound guidance is being performed in some centers. Although there are presently no reports of this, it is conceivable that such an approach might be feasible in other endocrine tumors.

Choledochoduodenal Stenting

There is one case report by Giovannini et al. of EUS-guided puncture of a dilated common bile duct and placement of a choledochoduodenal stent in a patient with unresectable pancreatic cancer, in whom repeated ERCP for stent placement was unsuccessful. There were no complications (21). Although this is an extreme case, it does demonstrate the therapeutic potential that EUS may offer in the future.

LIMITATIONS

It is important to know that EUS, as with other ultrasound modalities, is highly user dependent (Table 8). Interpretation depends on experience and understanding of artifacts and pitfalls as well as understanding of ultrasound principles. As mentioned above, one cannot distinguish a malignant from benign gastric ulcer as the inflammation associated with an ulcer is seen as hypoechoic and irregular, and can mimic a cancer penetrating the full wall thickness. Similarly, an inflammatory lymph node can be enlarged, round, hypoechoic, and well demarcated, fulfilling the criteria for a malignant node. If the ultrasound transducer catches the bowel wall in an oblique manner rather than at a 90-degree angle, the wall

▶ **TABLE 8 Limitations or Disadvantages of Endoscopic Ultrasound**

1. Highly user-dependent in EUS scanning and interpretation: requirement of sufficient skills and experiences.
2. Limitation in distinguishing malignant from benign lesions (e.g., benign gastric ulcer versus cancer, inflammatory lymph node versus metastatic node).
3. Limited depth of sound penetration with higher frequency ultrasound [e.g., not good for M-staging (liver metastasis)].
4. Surgeons should understand the limitations and pitfalls in performing EUS or in using information acquired from EUS.

EUS, endoscopic ultrasound.

appears thickened. It is important to obtain images at various angles when evaluating vascular structures around a mass. A pancreatic head mass near the portal vein can appear to invade the portal vein in one view and clearly be seen as noninvasive with a change of angle. The ventral pancreas in some is relatively hypoechoic relative to the dorsal pancreas and can be mistaken for a mass. Blood vessels can be mistaken for the common bile duct or pancreatic duct if viewed longitudinally, as can lymph nodes if viewed transversely. Color Doppler can help make the distinction in such circumstances. As with transabdominal ultrasound, artifacts can mimic sludge or stones in the common bile duct.

CONCLUSION

EUS is a valuable diagnostic tool that is most useful for staging GI and pancreatobiliary malignancies and recently has been extended to the staging of lung malignancies. It is also useful for identifying benign lesions of the GI tract and pancreas. W linear echoendoscopy, EUS-guided needle biopsy, therapeutic celiac ganglion block, drainage of pancreatic cysts, and, more recently, the ablative therapy are important additions to endoscopic surgical options. As with all ultrasound, EUS is highly user dependent. Pitfalls exist in the interpretation of ultrasound images that may lead to overstaging or the mistaken conclusion that a lesion is inoperable when in fact it is operable. It is imperative that the surgeon or gastroenterologist performing the staging be aware of the limitations and pitfalls that could cause them to misread EUS findings. Even in skilled hands, interpretation of images can be difficult, and the EUS report should acknowledge the inability to obtain good images or to interpret equivocal results. It is imperative that surgeons not performing EUS know these limitations and pitfalls when using information acquired from EUS studies (23–27).

REFERENCES

1. Goldberg SN, Mallery S, Gazelle GS, et al. EUS-guided radiofrequency ablation in the pancreas: results in a porcine model. *Gastrointest Endosc* 1999;50:392–401.
2. Rice TW. Esophageal tumors. In: Cameron JL, ed. *Current surgical therapy*, 7th ed. 2001. St. Louis: Mosby, 2001:51–57.
3. Beseth BD, Bedford R, Isacoff WH, et al. Endoscopic ultrasound does not accurately assess pathologic stage of esophageal cancer after neoadjuvant chemoradiotherapy. *Am Surg* 2000;66:827–831.
4. Rice TW, Zuccaro G. Staging esophageal cancer. In: Van Dam J, Sivak MV, eds. *Gastrointestinal endosonography*. Philadelphia: WB Saunders 1999:131–138.
5. Scotiniotis IA, Kochman ML, Lewis JD, et al. Accuracy of EUS in the evaluation of Barrett's esophagus and high-grade dysplasia or intramucosal carcinoma. *Gastrointest Endosc* 2001;54:689–696.
6. Nijhawan PK, Wan KK. Endoscopic mucosal resection for lesions with endoscopic features suggestive of malignancy and high-grade dysplasia within Barrett's esophagus. *Gastrointest Endosc* 2000;52:440–444.
7. Takada N, Higashino M, Osugi H, et al. Utility of endoscopic ultrasonography in assessing the indications for endoscopic surgery of submucosal esophageal tumors. *Surg Endosc* 1999;13:228–230.
8. Sun S, Wan M, Sun S. Use of endoscopic ultrasound-guided injection in endoscopic resection of solid submucosal tumors. *Endoscopy* 2002;34:82–85.
9. Rosch T, Classen M. Staging gastric cancer. In: Van Dam J, Sivak MV, eds. *Gastrointestinal endosonography*. Philadelphia: WB Saunders, 1999:195–200.
10. Irisawa A, Saito A, Obara K, et al. Endoscopic recurrence of esophageal varices is associated with the specific EUS abnormalities: severe periesophageal collateral veins and large perforating veins. *Gastrointest Endosc* 2001;53:77–84.
11. Konishi Y, Nakamura T, Kida H, et al. Catheter US probe EUS evaluation of gastric cardia and perigastric vascular structures to predict esophageal variceal recurrence. *Gastrointest Endosc* 2002;55:197–203.
12. Domagk D, Poremba C, Dietl KH, et al. Endoscopic transpapillary biopsies and intraductal ultrasonography in the diagnostics of bile duct strictures: a prospective study. *Gut* 2002;51:240–244.
13. Fritscher-Ravens A, Broering DC, Sriram PV, et al. EUS-guided fine-needle aspiration cytodiagnosis of hilar cholangiocarcinoma: a case series. *Gastrointest Endosc* 2000;52:534–540.
14. Menzel J, Poremba C, Dietl KH, et al. Preoperative diagnosis of bile duct strictures: comparison of intraductal ultrasonography with conventional endosonography. *Scand J Gastroenterol* 2000;35:77–82.
15. Zhang Q, Nian W, Zhang L, et al. Endoscopic ultrasonography assessment in preoperative staging for carcinoma of ampulla of Vater and extrahepatic bile duct. *Chin Med J (Engl)* 1996;109:622–625.
16. Kochman M. EUS in pancreatic cancer. *Gastrointest Endosc* 2002;56(Suppl):S6–S12.
17. Fernandez-del Castillo C, Warshaw AL. Cystic tumors of the pancreas. *Surg Clin North Am* 1995;75:1001–1016.
18. Zimmer T, Stolzel U, Bader M, et al. Endoscopic ultrasonography and somatostatin receptor scintigraphy in the preoperative localization of insulinomas and gastrinomas. *Gut* 1996;39:562–568.
19. Spitz JD, Lilly MC, Tetik C, et al. Ultrasound-guided laparoscopic resection of pancreatic islet cell tumors. *Surg Laparosc Endosc Percutan Tech* 2000;10:168–173.
20. Sahai AV. EUS and chronic pancreatitis. *Gastrointest Endosc* 2002;56(Suppl):S76–S81.
21. Gunaratnam NT, Wong Gy, Wiersema MJ. EUS-guided celiac plexus block for the management of pancreatic pain. *Gastrointest Endosc* 2000;52(Suppl):S28–S34.
22. Giovannini M, Moutardier V, Pesenti C, et al. Endoscopic ultrasound-guided bilioduodenal anastomosis: a new technique for biliary drainage. *Endoscopy* 2001;33:898–900.
23. Rosch T, Classen M. *Gastroenterologic endosonography*. New York: Thieme, 1992.
24. Staren ED, Arregui M, eds. *Ultrasound for the surgeon*. Philadelphia: Lippincott–Raven Publishers, 1997.
25. Van Dam J, Sivak MV, eds. *Gastrointestinal endosonography*. Philadelphia: WB Saunders, 1999.
26. Van Dam J, ed. *Rec Adv Endosc Ultrasonogr Gastrointest Endosc* 2000;52(6)(Suppl).
27. Lightdale CJ, ed. *Adv Endosc Ultrasound Gastrointest Endosc* 2002;56(4)(Suppl).

Chapter 21

New Ultrasound Technology

R. Stephen Smith and William R. Fry

Diagnostic ultrasound has an important role in essentially every aspect of surgical practice. With further advances in technology, such as miniaturization of ultrasound systems, laparoscopic ultrasound, endoluminal and endocavitary ultrasound, and such innovations as ultrasound contrast materials and ultrasound-mediated delivery of therapeutic agents, it is obvious that the importance of ultrasound to practicing surgeons will continue to increase. As important as new ultrasound technology is the surgeon's ability to acquire and utilize new ultrasound skills. The majority of surgeons in North America received minimal instruction in ultrasound during their residency training. Many surgeons have not yet acquired basic ultrasound skills. Therefore, it is essential that new educational strategies in a variety of ultrasound techniques be given an important role in the education of residents and attending surgeons.

The American College of Surgeons (ACS) has recognized the tremendous importance of ultrasound in the current and future practice of surgery. In February 1998, the Board of Regents of the ACS, through the Committee on Emerging Technologies and Education, published a statement regarding the importance of ultrasound in surgical practice (1). In this statement, it was noted that ultrasound was a technology that was applicable to a variety of surgical procedures and specialties. Thus, the ACS recognized the importance of this emerging technology and its future role in the management of surgical disease processes.

An exhaustive description of all areas of new ultrasound technology is beyond the scope of a single chapter in a textbook. This chapter provides an overview of some recent developments in ultrasound technology and their potential implications for surgical treatments (Table 1).

INNOVATIONS IN ULTRASOUND TRAINING

Perhaps the greatest innovation in the area of surgical ultrasound education is the modular program of ultrasound training developed and presented by the ACS's National Ultrasound Faculty. The surgical community as a whole has embraced this innovative approach to organized ultrasound education. The ACS ultrasound program used the Advanced Trauma Life Support (ATLS) system as a model. The program, which includes both formal lectures and hands-on training, has brought organization and standardization to ultrasound training for surgeons. The ACS program consists of an introductory course referred to as the Basic Ultrasound Module followed by a number of advanced clinical application courses. Advanced courses offered by the ACS include the Acute Module for evaluation of critically ill and injured patients, a Breast Module, a Vascular Module, an Abdominal (transabdominal/intraoperative/laparoscopic) Module, and a Head and Neck Module. The modular design of the ACS ultrasound program allows surgeons to initially gain a basic understanding of ultrasound physics, technology, and clinical applications. These skills are enhanced through advanced courses that emphasize both clinical applications and hands-on training in specific areas applicable to the individual surgeon's practice. Individual course modules have been and will be exported to a number of locations such as specialty societies and residency programs, thereby increasing the availability of ultrasound training. The ACS ultrasound program is detailed in Chapters 1 and 22.

Future advances in ultrasound training will most certainly require simulator and computer-based systems. Ultrasound simulation devices have been available for several years. One of the more widely used simulators is the UltraSim System (MedSim, Ft. Lauderdale, FL), which consists of a torso mannequin and a simulated ultrasound machine. This simulator provides a measure of realism in the assessment of simulated ultrasound findings. The system consists of simulated ultrasound transducers and standard ultrasound machine controls, such as gain, time gain compensation, and depth. The life-sized mannequin provides a realistic anatomic representation of an adult patient so that the student can learn proper transducer locations in reference to external anatomic landmarks. This device has the ability to provide the ultrasound student with consistent findings and can record

> **TABLE 1 New Ultrasound Technology**

1. Ultrasound training
   - Ultrasound simulation device
   - CD-ROM/Web-based multimedia format
2. Clinical applications
   - Miniaturization of ultrasound system
   - Endoluminal and endocavitary transducers: laparoscopic, endoscopic, intravascular, intracardiac ultrasound
3. New imaging and therapeutic innovations
   - Three-dimensional ultrasound
   - Ultrasound contrast and therapeutic agent
   - High-intensity focused ultrasound
   - Harmonic imaging
   - Others: pulse inversion imaging, interval delay imaging, sonic computed tomography, B-color ultrasound, and so forth

student performance for documentation. The ultrasound simulator system coordinates transducer placement on the mannequin via magnetic positioning technology with ultrasound images stored in a data bank. Archived images from actual patients are displayed on the monitor relative to the area scanned. This process emphasizes the anatomic relationships found in both normal and abnormal patient scenarios.

The UltraSim device has been used in a number of ACS ultrasound courses with moderate success. Unfortunately, the UltraSim is relatively expensive, somewhat bulky, and of limited availability. Therefore, its widespread applicability as an ultrasound simulator is limited. However, it is anticipated that this type of simulation device will have a role in ultrasound educational courses in the future.

Paralleling other areas of medicine and science, CD-ROM and web-based ultrasound learning opportunities will play an increasingly important role in providing ultrasound education for surgeons. Recently, the ACS National Ultrasound Faculty endorsed a plan to place the Basic Ultrasound Module in a CD-ROM/web-based multimedia format. Once implemented, this computer-based system will provide surgeons with the experience of the Basic Module at a convenient time utilizing any personal computer. The CD-ROM/web-based format will utilize animation to demonstrate principles of ultrasound physics and instrumentation. Examples of a number of clinical applications of ultrasound will be demonstrated by the use of real-time video clips of ultrasound examinations. In addition to animation and video clips, the CD-ROM/web-based Basic Course will contain all of the lectures and printed material included in the course. Web-based testing will ensure an adequate understanding of basic ultrasound principles, instrumentation, and clinical applications. Upon the student's successful com-

pletion of the computer-based course, a certificate of completion will be immediately available.

It is anticipated that a multimedia presentation of the Basic Ultrasound Module will greatly facilitate understanding of ultrasound principles by practicing general surgeons and will increase accessibility to the variety of advanced modules. The CD-ROM/Web-based course will be made available to residency program directors to provide an introduction to surgical ultrasound for residents (The Basic Ultrasound Module is available in a CD-ROM format as of October 2003).

MINIATURIZATION OF ULTRASOUND TECHNOLOGY

Over the past decade, ultrasound machines have become increasingly small, based on advances in a number of areas of technology. Ultrasound machines have evolved from large devices weighing several hundred pounds and occupying several cubic feet to small hand-held devices weighing as little as 3 pounds. The most common example of successful miniaturization of basic ultrasound systems is a product of the SonoSite Company. In 1998, SonoSite introduced a hand-held device with a number of transducer options. The SonoSite device weighs approximately 6 pounds (Fig. 1). Miniaturization of ultrasound technology has facilitated placement of small ultrasound machines in a variety of new clinical areas including the emergency department and trauma resuscitation area, the intensive care unit, the outpatient clinic, and essentially any other area where clinical assessment is carried out. While image resolution remains superior in larger, more expensive, advanced technology machines, the new miniaturized digital ultrasound technology is adequate for most ultrasound scans performed by surgeons. Recent innovations in technology have assured that ultrasound devices will continue to evolve to smaller and more portable devices. Recently, SonoSite introduced the iLook series of ultrasound machines. These devices have limited applications but are extremely small, weighing approximately 3 pounds (Fig. 2). In addition, a number of other ultrasound manufacturers have introduced miniaturized systems, some of which incorporate lap-top computer technology for storage and image presentation. It is inevitable that in the near future miniaturization will advance to the point where personal ultrasound imaging systems are approximately the same size and weight as traditional stethoscopes. This will allow extensive and widespread bedside application of ultrasound technology for essentially every patient. Ultrasound evaluation may become an essential component of routine physical examination.

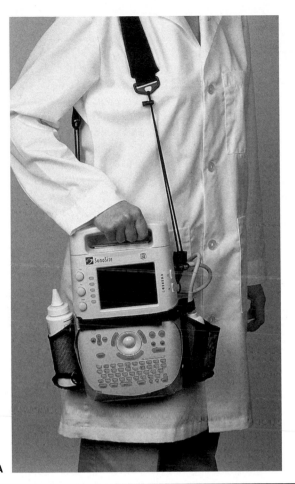
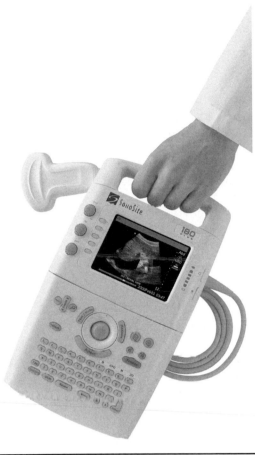

A   B

FIGURE 1. Hand-held small, portable ultrasound machines such as the Sonosite 180 Plus (**A, B**) have greatly enhanced the ability to perform bedside examination.

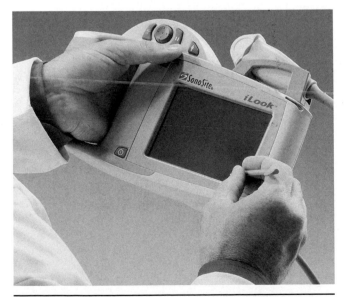

FIGURE 2. Miniaturization of ultrasound systems continues to decrease the size and weight of ultrasound machines. The extremely small Sonosite iLook is commercially available.

LAPAROSCOPIC ULTRASOUND

Laparoscopic ultrasound is a relatively new technology. Intraoperative ultrasound evaluation during open surgical procedures has been a component of the surgeon's diagnostic armamentarium for some time. However, the specialized transducers necessary for laparoscopic ultrasound are a relatively new development. A number of manufacturers have recently advanced laparoscopic ultrasound technology quite significantly. Several laparoscopic ultrasound transducers are now available that allow imaging of intraabdominal structures. In addition, the majority of tertiary centers now have dedicated laparoscopic ultrasound units available in the operating suite for routine use by surgeons.

Current laparoscopic ultrasound transducers are found in a variety of designs and configurations. Most contemporary laparoscopic ultrasound transducers fit easily through a conventional 10-mm laparoscopic operating port. Earlier laparoscopic ultrasound transducers were rigid, which limited the ability of the surgeon to appropriately position the probe to image certain structures. The current generation of laparoscopic ultrasound transducers features a steerable tip in conjunction with a high-frequency (7 to 10 MHz) linear array configuration (see Fig. 2 in Chapter 13).

Laparoscopic ultrasound has been performed extensively and compared with cholangiography in many centers for biliary tract assessment during laparoscopic cholecystectomy. Laparoscopic ultrasound has become an extremely useful modality for assessment of the liver. The greatest utility in this area has involved detection of occult malignant tumors. This technique helps to identify candidates for resection or ablative techniques including cryoablation and radiofrequency ablation (RFA). These ablative procedures are appropriately guided and monitored by laparoscopic ultrasound (2,3). The details of laparoscopic ultrasound are described in Chapter 13 and subsequent chapters.

ENDOSCOPIC ULTRASOUND

A major therapeutic advance in the management of gastrointestinal (GI) malignancy is the relatively new technique of endoscopic mucosal resection. This endoscopic technique provides an exciting new alternative to surgical resection for the management of early GI malignancy. Endoscopic mucosal resection is greatly enhanced by an additional new technology: high-frequency ultrasound probe sonography (HIFUPS) via an endoscope. HIFUPS provides extremely high-resolution imaging of the GI wall (Fig. 3). With HIFUPS, the GI wall appears as a structure with nine distinct layers and interfaces. This technique offers much greater resolution than standard endoscopic ultrasound (EUS) that usually produces images of a five-layered GI wall. HIFUPS has been used to guide and assist endoscopic mucosal resection in the esophagus, the stomach, and the colon.

Conventional EUS transducers are higher frequency (7.5 to 12 MHz) than most transcutaneous transducers. Transducers of these frequencies are most useful for evaluating visible and, in particular, polypoid lesions or advanced tumors. However, 7.5- to 12-MHz transducers are generally not adequate for distinguishing cancers that invade the muscularis mucosa from those that involve the submucosa. However, HIFUPS (20 to 30 MHz) is accurate in assessing these early superficial lesions.

In this new application of EUS, the HIFUPS transducer is introduced through a biopsy port of the endoscope. As would be expected with a very-high-frequency transducer, the depth of ultrasound penetration and thus the depth of the image are limited. Imaging of the GI wall with high-frequency transducers is generally limited to 15 to 20 mm depth (4).

EUS has not only improved diagnostic accuracy of various GI diseases but has also facilitated the development of new therapeutic endoscopic techniques, such as the internal drainage of pancreatic pseudocysts. Studies have shown that a 7.5-MHz curvilinear array echoendoscope (FG-36 UX, Pentex, Orangeburg, NY) produces high-resolution EUS images of pancreatic pseudocysts, allowing one to perform endoscopic cystogastrostomy or cystoenterostomy. Newer echoendoscopes are available that include a therapeutic channel that accelerates insertion of stents into the pseudocyst cavity under real-time ultrasound guidance. The clinical applications of EUS are detailed in Chapter 20 (5).

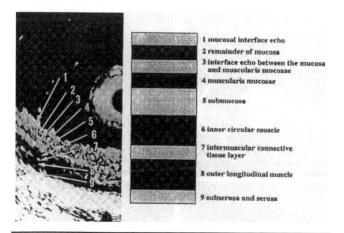

1 mucosal interface echo
2 remainder of mucosa
3 interface echo between the mucosa and muscularis mucosae
4 muscularis mucosae
5 submucosa
6 inner circular muscle
7 intermuscular connective tissue layer
8 outer longitudinal muscle
9 subserosa and serosa

FIGURE 3. High-frequency ultrasound image of the gastrointestinal wall. Note the nine distinct layers. High-resolution images such as this are required for endoscopic mucosal resection.

INTRAVASCULAR AND INTRACARDIAC ULTRASOUND

Ultrasound technology has had an important role in vascular diagnostic imaging for some time. Transcutaneous ultrasound imaging of arterial and venous anatomy is an essential, well-established component in the assessment of the vascular system. Intravascular ultrasound (IVUS) scanning is an exciting new technology that may prove as useful as transcutaneous scanning is at this time. IVUS is a method of ultrasound imaging of vessels from the "inside out." IVUS systems are catheter based and allow for extremely accurate measurement and assessment of diseased and normal arteries. This technology can be used to evaluate the morphology and extent of atherosclerotic plaque as well as delineating the anatomic configuration of branch vessels. In addition, IVUS provides a new and exciting method for imaging vascular anatomy after a therapeutic stent has been placed. This technology allows not only for measurement of the diameter of the vessel undergoing angioplasty and stent placement, but also allows assessment of the accuracy of the stent placement.

IVUS for the assessment of vascular pathophysiology has been performed successfully in a number of vessels, including the coronary arteries. IVUS of coronary vessels is usually performed in the cardiac catheterization laboratory under fluoroscopic guidance. Intracoronary ultrasound assessment is performed with a small catheter-based system utilizing a 30-MHz 360-degree rotating transducer (Ultracross 3.2-Fr, 30-MHz coronary imaging catheter, axial/lateral resolution 0.07 to 0.20 mm, Scimed, Boston Scientific Corp., San Jose, CA). First passing the transducer distal to the area in question and then slowly retracting the transducer through the vessel obtains intracoronary ultrasound images. Once ultrasound data have been obtained, they are digitized and reconstructed into interpretable images. This method of coronary artery assessment has been shown to be one of the most accurate methods for assessment of arterial diameter, but also of atherosclerotic plaque structure and extent. It is anticipated that with the increasing usage of coronary angioplasty and placement of stents with long-term patency, intracoronary ultrasound assessment of the coronary arteries will assume increasing importance.

Intracardiac ultrasound imaging also has the potential to complement the information obtained with other diagnostic modalities. While intracardiac imaging has been used experimentally in a number of animal models in the past, the technique has only recently been introduced into clinical practice to obtain high-resolution images of the heart in both the long and short axis. The ultrasound probe used for this diagnostic study is a 10-Fr 64-element phased-array catheter-based ultrasound system. The catheter is steerable in four directions, allowing imaging of essentially any intracardiac structure or intramural area. The intracardiac transducer permits Doppler assessment of intracardiac hemodynamics and physiology. In addition to delineation of cardiac anatomy, it is anticipated that intracardiac ultrasound will be a viable method for guiding electrophysiologic ablative procedures.

Endovascular treatment for a variety of vascular lesions is assuming an important role in disease management. One of the technical problems that limits the efficacy of intravascular stents is underdeployment. Inadequate expansion and placement of the stent increases the incidence of restenosis or occlusion of a treated vessel. It has recently been demonstrated that IVUS by a catheter-delivered imaging system can prevent underdeployment of stents in many instances. IVUS is an accurate method of defining the diameter of the vessel as well as plaque morphology. In addition, IVUS is an extremely useful method to assess the position of an intravascular stent, once it has been deployed. IVUS is more accurate than arteriography for determining if an expandable vascular stent has been correctly placed in full apposition to the arterial wall.

It has recently been demonstrated that the routine use of IVUS significantly improves long-term patency of iliac artery lesions that have been treated with balloon angioplasty and stenting. The primary benefits obtained by IVUS involve the accurate assessment of angioplasty diameter end point and the adequacy of stent deployment and apposition against the arterial wall. An IVUS system consisting of a catheter-delivered 20- to 30-MHz transducer (Hewlett-Packard Sonos Intravascular, Andover, MD) is utilized for these imaging studies. Using this technology to assess post-stenting anatomic relationships, it was found that IVUS demonstrated underdeployment of stents that were not identified by conventional angiographic assessment in 50% of cases. One of the problems associated with use of a catheter-based IVUS system is increased cost. The disposable, catheter-delivered transducer created an additional cost of approximately $400 per procedure. In addition, an experienced technician and a dedicated ultrasound system were necessary for performance of this procedure routinely.

Intravascular and intracardiac ultrasound represent exciting new fields of surgical ultrasound. It is anticipated that the utilization of extremely small intraluminal transducers will continue to expand and find a number of new surgical applications. Another example is intraductal ultrasound using similar transducers, which can be introduced into the bile ducts or pancreatic duct by means of an endoscope.

THREE-DIMENSIONAL ULTRASOUND

Three-dimensional (3-D) ultrasound is an exciting new technology that permits the creation of images rivaling those created by any other diagnostic imaging modality available. The volume sampling principles of 3-D ultrasound permit the creation of almost life-like images (Fig. 4). The greatest advantage of 3-D ultrasound over 2-D ultrasound is its easy interpretability. Instead of assessing a "slice" of an anatomic structure, this technique presents the entire structure for examination by the clinician. The most dramatic application of this technique thus far has been in fetal and embryonic imaging (e.g., cleft palate and congenital cardiac abnormalities).

From a technical standpoint, 3-D ultrasound involves four components: acquisition, 3-D quantitative multiplanar display, 3-D rendering, and real-time dimensional imaging. As opposed to conventional sonography, 3-D ultrasound depends on volume sampling. This technology

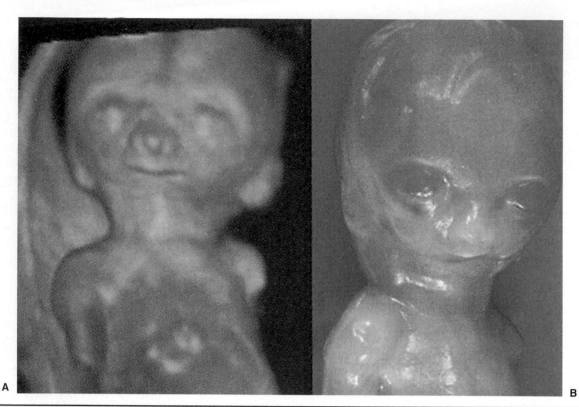

FIGURE 4. Three-dimensional ultrasound image **(A)** of a 15-gestational-week fetus with severe micrognathia and absent upper extremities compared with a postnatal photograph **(B)**.

requires the simultaneous presentation of three scanned planes: horizontal, transverse, and longitudinal. The life-like images created by 3-D ultrasound make interpretation of normal anatomy and pathophysiology much easier for the surgeon. This may be particularly important for localization of lesions of the breast, liver, and other organs and for assessment of the anatomic relationship of a lesion to adjacent ductal or vascular structures. For example, 3-D ultrasound has been used to precisely document the nature and location of bile duct obstructions; 3-D reconstruction of the entire biliary tree with precise localization of areas of obstruction is possible.

CONTRAST AGENTS AND THERAPEUTIC ULTRASOUND

Ultrasound contrast agents have been used to enhance the diagnostic resolution of ultrasound images. Ultrasound contrast agents are primarily substances that contain microbubbles. Microbubbles are elastic and compressible and generally have a much lower density than water. Therefore, intravascular microbubbles create an area of acoustic impedance mismatch with the surrounding tissues through which blood vessels traverse. Microbubbles are extremely efficient reflectors of ultrasound energy and serve as useful ultrasound contrast agents because of this property. Microbubbles also have a much lower threshold to cavitation from ultrasound energy. Cavitation causes the rupture of microbubbles.

Ultrasound contrast agents have been investigated to enhance the reliability of ultrasound in a variety of clinical settings. An example is to determine the effectiveness of ablative procedures, such as percutaneous RFA or alcohol ablation of hepatic lesions (Figs. 5 and 6). Contrast-enhanced color or power Doppler ultrasound examinations following the intravenous injection of a galactose-based microbubble contrast agent (Levovist; Schering, Berlin, Germany) have been done to assess the effectiveness of RFA. Using this technology, power Doppler ultrasound was found to have extremely high accuracy in documenting absence of perfusion in successfully ablated lesions of the liver. The specificity and sensitivity of contrast-enhanced power Doppler examinations equals that of fourth-generation CT scanners for the assessment of RFA. Similarly, real-time contrast-enhanced color Doppler sonography has been successfully used to assess the effect of percutaneous ultrasound-guided ethanol ablation of hepatocellular carcinoma. Transcutaneous power

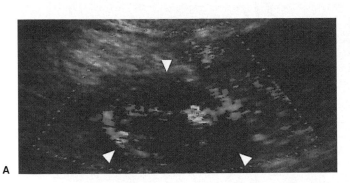
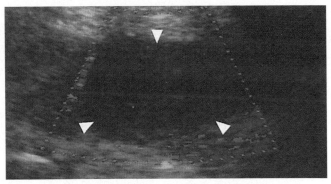

FIGURE 5. A: Contrast-enhanced color Doppler image with Levovist obtained prior to percutaneous ethanol injection of a hepatocellular carcinoma. Note the intratumoral flow signals (*arrowheads*). (See Color Plate 41.) **B:** Contrast-enhanced color Doppler image obtained after percutaneous ethanol injection showing the disappearance of color flow signals in the treated hepatocellular carcinoma (*arrowheads*). (See Color Plate 42.)

Doppler ultrasound with contrast enhancement was found to have equivalent accuracy with CT scan or postablation biopsy for the determination of effectiveness of ethanol ablation. It is anticipated, based on early reports, that contrast-enhanced color or power Doppler examination will be used with increasing frequency for the assessment of therapeutic interventions aimed at ablation of malignant tumors in a variety of organs. Compared with other methods of diagnostic imaging, this modality has the advantage of cost effectiveness and real-time imaging. Contrast-enhanced color or power Doppler assessment can be carried out immediately after the ablative procedure has been performed. With the increasing utilization of ablative procedures for lesions of the liver and other organs, contrast-enhanced color or power Doppler assessment of the effectiveness of this therapy will become increasingly

popular and will serve as a guide to determine the need for additional ablative procedures (6,7).

One of the particular physical properties of microbubbles is their low threshold for cavitation by ultrasound energy. The effects of cavitation easily rupture the microbubbles found in ultrasound contrast material. This unique physical property of microbubbles has led some investigators to use ultrasound contrast agents as a carrier for a variety of therapeutic agents (Figs 7 and 8). The potential advantages of using microbubbles as carriers are obvious. Smaller doses or concentrations of therapeutic materials contained within microbubbles might be injected intravenously with equivalent effects. Ultrasound energy would be focused on the anatomic region of interest during the period when microbubbles are present in the circulatory system. When microbubbles

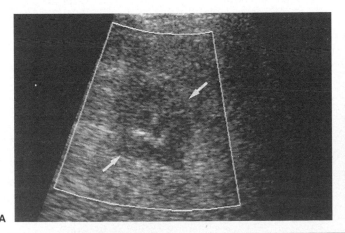
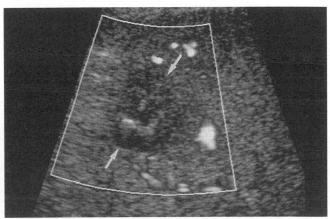

FIGURE 6. Ultrasound images from a patient with hepatocellular carcinoma following radiofrequency ablation. **A:** Unenhanced power Doppler ultrasound image performed after radiofrequency ablation that shows an area of low echogenicity (*arrows*) without intratumoral flow indicative of ablation. (See Color Plate 43.) **B:** Contrast-enhanced power Doppler ultrasound showing no flow signal within the ablated area (*arrows*) but with obvious flow in surrounding tissue. (See Color Plate 44.)

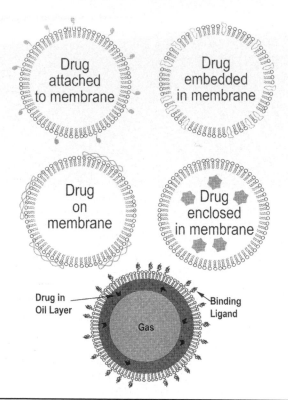

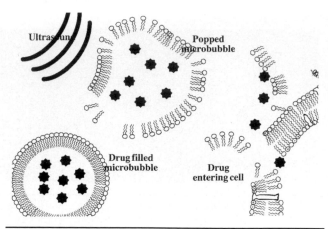

FIGURE 8. Microbubbles are easily ruptured by ultrasound energy. The presence of gas in microbubbles lowers the cavitation threshold that facilitates rupture by insonation. In addition, ultrasound energy promotes passage of drugs, molecules, or genes through the cell membrane.

FIGURE 7. Therapeutic agents may be incorporated into microbubbles in a variety of ways. Agents may be attached to the membrane that stabilizes the microbubble or incorporated into the membrane itself. Using electrostatic interaction, materials may be bound noncovalently to the surface of the microbubbles. Gas-filled microspheres may be formulated to load the interior of the microspheres with both gas and therapeutic agents. Stabilizing membrane materials may be lipids or polymers. A layer of oily material (triacetin) may be used as a film around the microbubble so that hydrophobic drugs can be incorporated.

containing a therapeutic agent pass through the anatomic region undergoing insonation, the microbubbles rupture secondary to cavitation, thereby causing the release of therapeutic agents in a specific capillary bed (Figs. 9 and 10). Also, the effects of cavitation are known

to cause a local shock wave at the cellular level, which improves cellular uptake of a variety of therapeutic agents.

A number of therapeutic agents have been considered for this novel method of delivery, including anticoagulants and gene therapy agents. For example, transcutaneous thoracic ultrasound could be focused on the heart so that an intravenous injection of microbubbles containing genetic material that will cause angiogenesis is selectively delivered to the myocardium. Experimentally, this technique has been shown to produce very high levels of transgenic expression in insonated regions of the myocardium. This type of therapeutic endeavor is particularly attractive for the cardiovascular system. Previous studies have shown encouraging results when the gene for vascular endothelial growth factor is introduced into a local vascular bed. A number of animal studies have shown that when vascular endothelial growth factor is introduced into ischemic tissue, angiogenesis occurs. Angiogenesis under these conditions has significant thera-

FIGURE 9. Cavitation produced by ultrasound increases microvascular permeability. Nanospheres and drugs are delivered to the interstitium as the microbubbles cavitate. This process can be used to enhance local drug delivery.

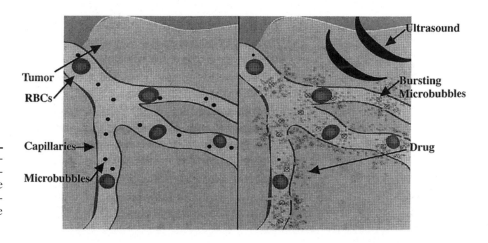

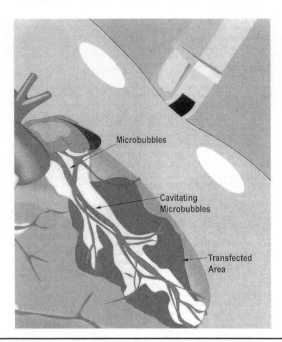

FIGURE 10. Microbubbles may be used to deliver anticoagulants, thrombolytics, or gene therapy to ischemic myocardium. Ultrasound contrast containing a therapeutic agent is given intravenously. As microbubbles enter the region of insonation via the vascular bed, cavitation results in the focused release of the therapeutic agent.

peutic potential to improve perfusion of ischemic cardiac tissue. In addition, the same technique could potentially be used to improve perfusion in patients with severe small vessel peripheral vascular disease. It has been proposed that other antithrombotic agents, such as nitrous oxide synthase, cyclooxygenase, prostacycline synthase, and tissue plasminogen activator, could be delivered by a similar mechanism utilizing microbubbles and focal ultrasound insonation. Delivery of these therapeutic agents via microbubbles has considerable potential advantages in comparison with the alternative, which is the direct injection of these materials into tissue. Delivery of gene therapy or other pharmaceutical agents in a field of ultrasound insonation could obviate the need for an open surgical procedure for direct injection of these materials. In addition, local shock waves created by cavitation have been documented to increase capillary and cellular permeability. Cavitation probably increases the permeability of micropores, thereby increasing the likelihood that molecules and nanoparticles may pass through these structures. Therefore, not only would the effect of ultrasound insonation and cavitation be a release of therapeutic agents contained in microbubbles, there would also be an increase in the likelihood that the therapeutic agents would reach their selected intracellular targets. Microbubble-based contrast agents are available with a low threshold for cavitation that is easily achieved by the ultrasound energy produced from diagnostic transducers

operating at low power levels. In addition, ultrasound contrast agents may be targeted to cell-specific receptors to further localize drug release in a selected anatomic region. It is likely that contrast agents will be used in the future for delivery of a variety of novel therapeutic agents to selected anatomic regions. It is unlikely that specialized ultrasound transducers will be necessary to provide the energy for cavitation and release of therapeutic agents in these selected areas. This novel technique for the delivery of therapeutic agents will reduce the need for more invasive methods of drug or gene delivery (8).

High-intensity focused ultrasound (HIFU) energy has been used as a stand-alone technique for ablation of malignant disease of the brain, liver, and other organs. For example, transrectal HIFU has been used to ablate prostate cancer in clinical trials. A recent series of 82 patients with biopsy-confirmed prostate cancer who underwent transrectal HIFU ablation utilizing the Ablatherm machine (EDAP Technomed, Vaux-en-Velin, France) demonstrated favorable results. This novel approach produces tissue coagulation necrosis in the prostate by causing a sharp temperature increase. Tissue necrosis is produced by a thermal effect linked to the absorption of ultrasound energy and cavitation. Generally, intensities in the range of 500 to 1000 W/cm^2 are used. The Ablatherm machine is a computer-controlled system designed to provide HIFU energy to the prostate gland. The major components of the Ablatherm machine include the patient's bed, a probe-positioning system, an ultrasound generator, and a cooling system that serves to protect the rectal wall from thermal or mechanical ultrasound energy. The ultrasound transducer used in this therapeutic modality incorporates an imaging transducer that allows real-time assessment of the effects of therapeutic HIFU. This procedure is usually performed under general or spinal anesthetic for patient comfort. The technique offers the advantages of a minimally invasive treatment for localized prostate cancer. Other advantages include the avoidance of radiation, a short hospital stay, repeatability, and avoidance of more invasive surgical procedures. Initial studies have shown that this procedure has equivalent results when compared with other therapeutic modalities for stage T1 or T2 prostate cancers (9).

HARMONIC IMAGING

As sound energy interacts with tissue, vibrations of various media occur at frequencies other than the base or fundamental frequency of the sound wave. Resonance or *harmonic* frequencies develop in the tissues. Harmonic frequencies are multiples of the base or fundamental frequency. For example, the first harmonic frequency is double the fundamental frequency, the second harmonic is three times the fundamental frequency, and so forth.

Compared with the fundamental frequency, harmonic frequencies have lower amplitude.

In the past, harmonic frequencies have not been evaluated by conventional clinical ultrasound. However, with currently available computer technology, "tissue harmonic imaging" electronically isolates and evaluates harmonic frequencies. In practice, the selected harmonic frequency is isolated by electronically subtracting the fundamental frequency from the reflected sound energy. Digital encoding of the fundamental frequency facilitates the isolation and analysis of harmonic frequencies by making it possible to "cancel out" the fundamental frequency from returning sound waves. In clinical scanning, the first harmonic frequency is utilized to create an image. For example, if a 3.5-MHz transducer is used, the harmonic frequency that is analyzed has a frequency of 7.0 MHz. The potential advantage of harmonic imaging rests in the greater tissue penetration achieved by a low-frequency transducer, coupled with the greater resolution made possible by interpretation of returning higher frequency harmonic waves.

CONCLUSIONS

Ultrasound technology continues to find utilization in essentially all areas of surgical practice. Despite its wide use, ultrasound technology, and its application to clinical medicine, is at a very early stage of development. It is anticipated that technological advances will bring the further penetration of ultrasound into every aspect of clinical care. Therefore, it is likely that the ultrasound device of the 21st century will continue to be described as a modality as universally applicable as a stethoscope is today. If ultrasound-mediated therapeutic interventions continue to develop, ultrasound may also be thought of as the "scalpel" of the 21st century. Because of the tremendous diagnostic and therapeutic potential of ultrasound technology, it is incumbent on the practicing surgeon to become familiar with ultrasound physics, instrumentation, and new technology.

REFERENCES

1. Committee on Emerging Surgical Technologies and Education. Statement on ultrasound examinations by surgeons (statement 31). *Bull Am Coll Surg* 1998;83:37–40.
2. Nelson TR. Ultrasound into the future. *J Ultrasound Med* 2001;20:1263–1264.
3. Santambrogio R, Bianchi P, Pasta A, et al. Ultrasound-guided interventional procedures of the liver during laparoscopy. *Surg Endosc* 2002;16:349–354.
4. Raju GS, Waxman I. High-frequency US probe sonography assisted endoscopic mucosal resection. *Gastrointest Endosc* 2000;52:(Suppl) S39–S49.
5. Norton ID, Clain JE, Wiersema MJ, et al. Utility of endoscopic ultrasonography in endoscopic drainage of pancreatic pseudocysts in selected patients. *Mayo Clin Proc* 2001;76:794–798.
6. Shirato K, Morimoto M, Tomita N, et al. Hepatocellular carcinoma: therapeutic experience with percutaneous ethanol injection under real-time contrast-enhanced color Doppler sonography with the contrast agent Levovist. *J Ultrasound Med* 2002;21;1015–1022.
7. Choi D, Lim HK, Kim SH, et al. Assessment of therapeutic response in hepatocellular carcinoma treated with percutaneous radio frequency ablation. *J Ultrasound Med* 2002;21: 391–401.
8. Unger EC, Hersh E, Vannan M, et al. Local drug and gene delivery through microbubbles. *Prog Cardiovasc Dis* 2002;44: 45–54.
9. Gelet A, Chapelon JY, Bouvier R, et al. Transrectal high-intensity focused ultrasound: minimally invasive therapy of localized prostate cancer. *J Endourol* 2000;6:519–528.

Chapter 22

Getting Started: Challenges and Strategies

Michael R. Marohn

Surgical ultrasound is a powerful tool that arguably should be in every surgeon's toolbox. Recognizing that challenges are associated with surgeon-performed ultrasound, this chapter is developed to help surgeons get started. The first step is the commitment to engage. Surgeons should identify the types of ultrasound applications desired, equipment necessary, equipment availability, how to keep pace with rapidly evolving technology, how to gain expertise, document training, document patient examinations, how to address credentialing issues, and how to seek reimbursement. Each surgery practice setting is unique, but most surgeons encounter similar problems.

Key topics in getting started in surgical ultrasound are summarized in Table 1. This chapter addresses these specific challenges and offers strategies to help surgeons engage in safe, high-quality, surgeon-performed ultrasound so as to enhance patient care.

SCOPE OF ULTRASOUND AND SURGEON CHALLENGES

Ultrasound traditionally has been the domain of radiology, but it is rapidly evolving as a diagnostic tool with no specialty ownership. Hans Troidl remarked in 1994 that "ultrasound is becoming the modern equivalent of the stethoscope." In surgery, almost every specialty is finding useful ultrasound applications to enhance patient care. For years, obstetricians have tracked pregnancies with serial ultrasound examinations. Vascular surgeons now oversee half of the vascular laboratories in the United States. Trauma surgeons routinely use focused abdominal sonography for trauma (FAST) to guide critical decision making in the trauma bay. Endorectal ultrasound to T-stage rectal cancers is becoming the standard of care and helps guide preoperative chemoradiation therapy for selected rectal cancers. Breast ultrasound is a key adjunct to breast care. Intraoperative ultrasound, whether laparoscopic or "open," is the modality of choice for screening for occult hepatic metastases as well as for guiding hepatic resection. While this book is replete with cutting-edge ultrasound applications appropriate for surgeons and can result in benefits to patients in every surgical specialty, surgeons attempting to utilize ultrasound have faced challenges at multiple levels, making them reluctant to embrace this technology. Until recently, surgical training in ultrasound was limited to interpretation of static images and rarely included real-time image scanning technique and interpretation.

Experience in ultrasound matters. Practicing surgeons and surgeons in training need opportunities to learn ultrasound. What should the short- and long-term strategies be for surgical ultrasound education? Ultrasound machines are expensive; who pays? Are there smart, burden-sharing strategies for buying equipment? Does every specialty need its own ultrasound machine, or can we share? Ultrasound technology evolves rapidly; applications expand; machines and transducers get smarter and smaller, more modular, and more affordable. How do surgeons keep up with changes? Issues regarding the "learning curve" for ultrasound and credentialing continue to evolve. Are there graded strategies for seeking privileges? How should surgeons interface with radiology? How can we gain their support for training and privileges so as to avoid "turf wars"? Finally, what about reimbursement?

INTERNATIONAL PERSPECTIVE

Who performs ultrasound and for what applications changes rapidly. In Germany, radiology board certification does not require demonstration of ultrasound expertise, but surgery board certification does. German surgeons must document 400 ultrasound cases with outcomes. Since 1995, the American Board of Surgery has required "exposure to surgical ultrasound" but has not specified the elements of exposure. In the United States,

▶ **TABLE 1** Key Topics in Getting Started

1. Scope of ultrasound and challenges
2. Surgeon ultrasound education and expertise
3. Equipment and costs
4. Access to ultrasound patients
5. Documentation
6. Credentialing and turf battles
7. Reimbursement

▶ **TABLE 2** ACS Ultrasound Advanced Modules

1. Ultrasound in the Acute Setting [includes the Focused Assessment for the Sonographic examination of the Trauma patient (FAST) and critical care ultrasound applications]
2. Abdominal Ultrasound: Transabdominal/Intraoperative/Laparoscopic
3. Breast Ultrasound
4. Head and Neck Ultrasound
5. Vascular Ultrasound
6. Endorectal Ultrasound, Endoscopic Ultrasound

ultrasound is performed by radiologists, emergency physicians, cardiologists, obstetricians, gynecologists, vascular surgeons, urologists, colorectal surgeons, endocrinologists, general surgeons, family practitioners, and any other specialists who have discovered the diagnostic power of this noninvasive "stethoscope."

EVOLUTION OF SURGEON ULTRASOUND EDUCATION

Until recently, the heritage of ultrasound in U.S. surgical education was limited. Until the late 1990s, few residencies offered more than exposure to static ultrasound image interpretation, and this was not systematic. The resulting population of practicing surgeons lacked ultrasound expertise and had limited access to ultrasound machines, scanning opportunities, and training venues. They faced an ultrasound world largely controlled by radiologists, filled with expensive and intimidating equipment, where expertise was operator dependent and fear of misinterpretation discouraged engagement.

AMERICAN COLLEGE OF SURGEONS LEADERSHIP ROLE

The American College of Surgeons (ACS) has taken a leadership role in identifying the need for a surgical education program. In 1995, the ACS Committee on Emerging Surgical Technology and Education (CESTE) established the ACS National Ultrasound Faculty (NUF), with the mission to develop surgical ultrasound courses, materials, and instructors. The goal of the ACS Surgical Ultrasound Education Program is to promulgate surgeon- performed ultrasound by training surgeons in the effective use of ultrasound for specific surgical problems and/ or diseases.

The ACS Surgical Ultrasound Education Program is modular in concept, building on the basic ultrasound course, which emphasizes ultrasound physics, instrumentation, scanning technique, and interpretation of pitfalls. The basic module is a prerequisite for the advanced modules. Working with several surgical specialty societies, the NUF developed (and continues to develop) advanced modules to address specific surgical applications. In addition, a faculty development program includes an ultrasound instructor course and subsequent instructor candidate monitoring. Several ACS ultrasound advanced modules are currently available or under development (Table 2).

The ACS has also developed a mechanism for exporting these courses to promote surgeon-performed ultrasound education. Several surgical specialty societies have already conducted ACS ultrasound courses. To export an ACS ultrasound course, the College outlines several steps:

1. Identify a course director (either an NUF or an ACS instructor).
2. Identify instructors (ACS certified).
3. Identify the type of ultrasound course.
4. Send completed form to NUF vice-chairperson for education.
5. Use ACS materials: slides, manuals, tests, critiques.
6. Maintain four to six advanced students per instructor ratio or less.
7. Complete postcourse report.

Following the Advanced Trauma Life Support (ATLS) model, the ACS Surgical Ultrasound Education Program courses have been carefully developed by the NUF in cooperation with surgical specialty societies, and a standardized, "each course is the same" approach is encouraged.

To further encourage exposure to surgical ultrasound, the College has provided ultrasound questions to the American Board of Surgery. Some of these have already been included in the written qualifying examination for general surgery.

LONG-TERM KEY TO SURGEON-PERFORMED ULTRASOUND: RESIDENT EDUCATION

Beyond training practicing surgeons, promulgation of surgeon-performed ultrasound requires integration of ultrasound education into surgery residencies, using the strategy:

- Train the trainers
- Train attending surgeons
- Train surgery residents

Following a "boot strap" strategy, these steps can be concurrent. The ACS Basic Module can be introduced early in surgery residency, including hands-on ultrasound scanning technique and interpretation orientation. Several residencies have already established resident ultrasound training, including the University of Vermont, Emory University, Medical College of Ohio, University of California at San Francisco, and Walter Reed Hospital, among others. ACS ultrasound instructors are standing by.

VERIFICATION OF TRAINING

As with ATLS, the ACS does not verify experience or competence in surgeon-performed ultrasound. It does document attendance and successful testing at its ultrasound courses. The College verification model addresses ultrasound education, not expertise:

Level 1: Verification of attendance
Level 2: Verification of satisfactory completion of course objectives
Level 3: Instructor level

Level 1 documents only a surgeon's attendance at an ultrasound course; level 2 documents a surgeon's success at meeting ultrasound course objectives (being "proctor ready"); and level 3 documents a surgeon's monitored clinical experience including outcomes, completion of the ultrasound instructor course, and teaching experi-

▶ **TABLE 3 Documentation: Key for Surgeons Performing Ultrasound**

1. Certification verifying taking a course
2. Training and proctoring
3. Ultrasound findings and outcomes
4. Continuing medical education and continuous quality improvement
5. Adequate facility and equipment (calibration and maintenance)
6. Certification of specialty society performance guidelines

ence. The importance of documentation of each step of ultrasound training and experience is critical for local credentialing, maintaining continuing medical education (CME), continuing quality improvement (CQI), and fulfilling specialty society performance guidelines (which continue to evolve). Key advice for surgeons performing ultrasound is to document all activities, as listed in Table 3.

GUIDELINES FOR DOCUMENTING EXPERIENCE AND CERTIFYING COMPETENCE

Surgical specialty societies have worked with the ACS NUF in developing educational courses, materials, and faculty. The College has encouraged surgical specialty societies to develop ultrasound performance guidelines for documenting experience and certifying competence, which are keys to credentialing.

EXAMPLE OF SPECIALTY SOCIETY CERTIFICATION GUIDELINES

The American Society of Breast Surgeons (ASBS) has been a model group in two ways: First, its members worked closely with (or were members of) the NUF in developing the ACS Breast Ultrasound module course, materials, and faculty. Second, the ASBS has developed an exemplary set of requirements for breast ultrasound certification.

The ASBS provides a 5-year certification for breast surgeons who meet established standards. The standards are based on a framework of the general principles for proper performance and interpretation of diagnostic ultrasound and appropriate application of interventional breast ultrasound. The completed certification includes recognition and assessment of the surgeon's training, clinical experience, and quality assurance in diagnostic and interventional breast ultrasound. The process involves both a clinical and written examination, given twice annually. While membership in the ASBS is not required for certification, the candidate must agree to comply with ASBS standards, policies, and procedures. Eligibility criteria include:

- Medical education certificate
- Ultrasound training certificate
- Medical licensure
- American Board of Surgery certificate
- At least 1 year of breast ultrasound performance
- A statement of the scope of practice of the candidate

More specifics are available from the ASBS (see resources section at end of this chapter). Such rigid certification requirements for breast ultrasound help meet increasing societal demands for performance-based credentialing.

Other surgical specialty societies are developing ultrasound application specific certification guidelines to help surgeons navigate "turf war" and credentialing challenges.

EQUIPMENT QUALITY ASSURANCE

Ultrasound facilities must meet safety and quality assurance standards. The ACS outlined in Statement 31, June 1998 (1) the importance of quality assurance policies and procedures not only for an individual surgeon's ultrasound experience but for ultrasound facilities. Ultrasound facilities should define:

- Medical direction and policies for scope of ultrasound privileges
- Electrical safety policies and testing
- Appropriate equipment
- Quality control of instruments, equipment, and images (including, for example, annual calibration guidelines with phantoms)

National organizations, including the American Institute of Ultrasound in Medicine (AIUM) (see resources section at the end of this chapter), have developed ultrasound facilities and certification processes that are beyond the scope of this chapter. However, familiarization with this requirement is important for any sonographer.

PRACTICAL STEPS TO GETTING STARTED

The remainder of this discussion focuses on practical tips for getting started. The general steps are the same, regardless of ultrasound application, as summarized in Table 4.

> **TABLE 4** **Steps to Getting Started**

1. Find an ultrasound machine
2. Scan, scan, scan
3. Identify a mentor
4. Start simply, then add complexity
5. Gain experience and expertise, *then* worry about billing
6. Document everything
7. Plan credentialing strategies based on your ultrasound application
8. Learn coding and billing documentation guidelines (do this *last*)

Ultrasound scanning and interpretation are operator dependent, and experience matters. To gain experience, surgeons need access to ultrasound machines, ultrasound patients, mentoring, and, most of all, experience in obtaining and interpreting ultrasound scans.

ACCESS TO ULTRASOUND MACHINES

Who has ultrasound equipment? In most hospitals, access to ultrasound equipment requires either purchase of a machine or partnering with a group that already has one. Ultrasound machines are more available that most providers think. Throughout a typical community hospital, there may be 15 or more different ultrasound machines in various locations: radiology, cardiology, obstetrics, emergency room (ER), breast center, endocrinology, vascular surgery, urology, colorectal surgery, general surgery, and operating room (OR).

COSTS: BURDEN SHARING

In the OR, burden sharing is a smart, cost-effective strategy for ultrasound machine purchasing that also improves efficiency and machine utilization. Instead of each service vying for limited funds to purchase their own ultrasound unit, multiple services can share through "team buying" to distribute equipment cost and use. As an example, when one community hospital's radiology department upgraded its ultrasound machines, a replaced unit was given to the ER, which shares the machine with the OR. The OR purchases were limited to intraoperative open and laparoscopic probes, which matched the shared ultrasound machines in the ER and radiology department.

GAINING EXPERIENCE: SCAN, SCAN, SCAN (Table 5)

Three steps are required for surgeons to gain ultrasound experience (Table 6).

Experience matters. Scan yourself, friends, phantoms, homemade models, then patients. Use ultrasound screen-

> **TABLE 5** **How to Gain Ultrasound Experience**

1. Scan, scan, scan: Experience matters
2. Five phases of learning ultrasound
3. Identification of a mentor
4. Support from radiologists
5. Ultrasound "creep"

▶ **TABLE 6** Three Steps to Gain Experience

1. Need access to ultrasound machines
2. Need access to ultrasound patients
3. Need access to experienced guidance
4. Most of all, *need experience*

ing as a diagnostic and learning aid. In the ER, use the department's ultrasound machine when consulting for a patient with probable acute cholecystitis to scan the right upper quadrant in an effort to find gallstones. While learning, obtain a follow-up ultrasound study in radiology to confirm findings and provide feedback on your examination. A similar strategy can be adopted for breast evaluation. Scan what appears to be a simple breast cyst in the office, then request a radiology breast ultrasound to assess the accuracy of your examination. In the OR, any open abdomen is an ultrasound examination opportunity. With increased availability of laparoscopic probes, almost any operation is a potential opportunity for ultrasound examination.

Learning ultrasound can be divided into five phases, paralleling the ACS Ultrasound Education Program:

1. Learning basic ultrasound concepts (cognitive)
   ■ Basic ultrasound physics (pulse-echo principle, propagation speeds, impedance, attenuation, reflection, resolution, etc.)
   ■ Basic ultrasound instrumentation (machine components, "knobology")
   ■ Basic ultrasound scanning techniques (probe orientation, ultrasound planes, probe handling [sliding, tilting, rotating, rocking, etc.])
   ■ Basic ultrasound interpretation principles [machine assumptions, hypoechoic, hyperechoic, isoechoic, artifacts (shadowing, enhancement, reverberation, mirror image, etc.)]
2. Learning advanced ultrasound applications (cognitive)
   ■ Advanced concepts for specific ultrasound applications
3. Learning real-time ultrasound scanning (practical, hands-on experience)
   ■ Supervised experience to guide learning of specific scanning techniques, interpretive skills, and interventions
4. Mentored/monitored practice of specific ultrasound applications
5. Independent, credentialed practice of specific ultrasound applications

The first three phases can be achieved through ultrasound courses, whereas the fourth phase requires a local proctor or mentor. The College's Ultrasound Education Program verifies completion of the first three phases and

makes a surgeon "proctor ready" for the fourth phase, which is preparation for independent ultrasound practice.

IDENTIFY A MENTOR: FIND ONE LOCALLY, IMPORT ONE, OR EXPORT YOURSELF

Mentoring matters. Identify an ultrasound mentor, ideally an experienced surgeon in your own department. If ultrasound expertise is not available in your department, import a mentor or, if necessary, export yourself. Critical to gaining experience is guidance from an expert surgical colleague or radiologist to act as a mentor, teach scanning techniques, monitor your interpretations, and shape your skills to accelerate the learning curve. Even after you are credentialed to perform ultrasound, you should continue to enlist a mentor to help compare results to outcomes [e.g., to compare FAST findings with computed tomography (CT) scans and operative findings in trauma patients], to periodically review real-time scanning tapes, and to discuss missed findings so as to continually hone your imaging and interpretive skills.

GAINING SUPPORT FROM RADIOLOGISTS

How do you cajole radiologists to support surgeon-performed ultrasound? Ideally, partner with them; they are often essential in helping a surgeon get started in the performance of ultrasound. As above, enlist them as mentors. Develop an environment of mutual support in which the radiologist recognizes that surgeon-performed ultrasound can solve problems of radiologist availability (e.g., in the trauma bay, in the OR, and so forth) and can extend effective applications of ultrasound beyond the radiology department. Then, when your skills are established, help the radiologists understand that they do not want to do ultrasound when and where you do. If you tell a radiologist that you need him or her to monitor your adequacy in performing FAST examinations in the trauma bay at 3 o'clock in the morning, that individual will quickly recognize that FAST is a basic ultrasound skill that you can rapidly master. There are places that radiologists may not want to be:

■ Trauma room at 3 o'clock in the morning
■ OR at anytime
■ Anorectal canal at anytime

The above examples are intended as playful. Nonetheless, it is important to recognize that radiologists can be valuable allies in starting your ultrasound experience but that certain ultrasound applications fall uniquely in the surgeon's domain.

START SIMPLY, THEN ADD COMPLEXITY: ULTRASOUND "CREEP"

The concept of ultrasound creep is one of accretion. Begin with simple tasks and add complexity, knowing that embedded in the simple tasks are opportunities to acquire complex skills. As you gain experience with one ultrasound task, you gain expertise in others, "creeping" your experience from simple to more complex skills with each scan. Several examples follow.

The purpose of a FAST examination is to determine the presence or absence of intraabdominal fluid (likely blood). This is a relatively simple ultrasound question, with a "yes" or "no" answer. While answering the FAST question is simple, each examination requires identification of the kidneys, liver, spleen, pericardium, diaphragm, and urinary bladder. The more you image these structures, the sharper your interpretive skills become.

When evaluating an ER consult for cholecystitis, the surgeon may ask a "yes" or "no" question with a right upper quadrant ultrasound for gallstones (assuming that a confirmatory follow-up radiology ultrasound study is planned), but the gallbladder scan requires identification of the liver, the gallbladder, and acoustic shadowing from the gallstones, and is an opportunity to recognize gallbladder wall thickening, pericholecystic fluid, biliary anatomy, even the presence of choledocholithiasis.

Laparoscopic ultrasound of the gallbladder and biliary tree is not only useful in diagnosing or ruling out choledocholithiasis (another "yes" or "no" question), but also helps the surgeon acquire skills essential for liver scanning for metastatic tumor screening, hepatic surgery resection planning, and other advanced ultrasound applications.

The strategy of ultrasound creep reflects the fact that every simple ultrasound skill is a gateway to more complex ultrasound skills.

GAIN EXPERIENCE AND EXPERTISE: HOW MUCH EXPERIENCE IS ENOUGH?

How much ultrasound experience does someone need to gain ultrasound expertise? This is not a simple question. Specialty societies and institutions have already established reference numbers (Table 7). One problem with setting numbers is that the required experience should vary depending on the complexity of the task (this is further addressed in the discussion about tiered credentialing). Simple scanning to address simple questions is easy

▶ **TABLE 7** Reference Numbers for Needed Experience in Ultrasound

Institution	Ref. No.
American Institute of Ultrasound Medicine	400 cases
German Board of Surgery	400 cases
Emory/Grady Memorial	32 hours
University of California at San Francisco	25 cases
University of Vermont	15 normal, then 25 cases
Radiologists	4-year residency

to learn quickly. Requisite experience learning FAST examinations will be different from the learning curve for breast imaging or hepatic scanning.

KNOWLEDGE IS POWER: SURGEONS ARE TRAINABLE

Surgeons are quick learners. Published data have demonstrated that surgeons can learn to perform the FAST examination rapidly and accurately. Furthermore, comparative studies suggest that surgeons can learn to perform the FAST examination as accurately as radiologists (Table 8) (2–6). In a collected series of 4,941 patients, surgeons have performed FAST with a sensitivity of 93.4%, a specificity of 98.7%, and an accuracy of 97.5% in detecting both hemoperitoneum and visceral injury (7).

DOCUMENTATION

Document everything. The documentation of ultrasound didactic and hands-on training, monitored ultrasound experience, and correlation of ultrasound findings with clinical outcomes is critical in securing privileges for surgeon-performed ultrasound.

Documentation of the basic elements of ultrasound examinations is essential to good patient care, continuing quality improvement, and reimbursement (see reimbursement discussion below). Key elements of an ultrasound ex-

▶ **TABLE 8** Comparative Study of Surgeons and Radiologists in Acquiring FAST Expertise

Surgeons performing FAST	93.4% sensitivity	98.7% specificity
Radiologists performing FAST	90.7% sensitivity	99.2% specificity

FAST, focused abdominal sonography for trauma.

ULTRASOUND EXAMINATION Date: Patient ID: Age: Sex:	Institution: Location:
Type of ultrasound examination:	Machine:
Transducer:	Frequency:
Findings: (include appropriate areas, both normal & abnormal, & measurements)	Outcome:
Comments: Images recorded:	Examiner: Signature

FIGURE 1. Sample ultrasound examination record.

amination include patient demographics (e.g., patient identification, date, location of examination, ultrasound machine, probe, frequency), key findings (e.g., FAST site-specific positive or negative result), relevant documented freeze-frame/static images of real-time scan (e.g., images of positive FAST fluid, gallstones, common bile duct, etc.), and outcomes (e.g., correlation with CT Scan or operating room findings). Figure 1 shows a sample ultrasound examination form that includes these minimal elements. Your form should be tailored to your specific ultrasound application. An original should be placed in the patient's medical record and a copy maintained by the sonographer.

CREDENTIALING: PRINCIPLES (Table 9)

Credentialing for any procedure is a local control issue, but guiding principles help. Granting and renewal of privileges is a local control, department-based, hospital-

▶ **TABLE 9 Credentialing Strategies**

1. Local control issue: hospital-approved process
2. Surgeons credential surgeons
3. Avoid "turf battles"; instead co-opt
4. "Tiered" credentialing
Level I ultrasound: simple
Level II ultrasound: complex

approved process. Surgeons should set the guidelines for surgeons. Uniform standards should apply. Standards should be criterion based and should address formal training, experience, documented competence, monitored performance, CME, and maintenance of skills verification.

The ACS Ultrasound Education Program helps surgeons verify ultrasound education. Certification of experience and competence is a more demanding and involved process. The complexity of the ultrasound skills required for specific tasks may help stratify this process.

As surgical specialty societies proffer specific ultrasound application certification guidelines, surgeons will have guidelines to help with local credentialing decisions. In the interim, the following tactics may help. A key tactical principle is that surgeons should credential surgeons.

STRATEGIES FOR DEALING WITH CREDENTIALING "TURF BATTLES"

The initial focus for getting started with ultrasound should be gaining expertise, not credentialing, and certainly not billing. Particularly in the civilian sector, turf battles exist regarding who should perform ultrasound. In vascular ultrasound in the United States, radiologists run 50% of vascular laboratories and vascular surgeons run the remaining 50%. Breast ultrasound, traditionally the province of radiology, is increasingly a surgical modality. Surgeons and emergency physicians now routinely perform FAST examinations. Radiologists rarely perform endorectal ultrasound, deferring to general and colorectal surgeons. Intraoperative ultrasound, particularly laparoscopic ultrasound, is uniquely the surgeon's domain.

So how do you get started to work toward ultrasound privileges? Initially, partner with radiology. You need them, particularly if they have the machines, patients, and expertise. They hold the keys to your ultrasound access and can help you learn "knobology," scanning techniques, and image interpretation. Use the creep strategy. Start with simple imaging questions and focus on gaining experience. Remember the FAST examination question: is there fluid present? Learn quickly to master the scanning and interpretive skills to assess the four FAST "listening" sites. Remember, while learning these skills, you are learning about scanning the liver, kidneys, spleen, diaphragm, pericardium, and urinary bladder.

To gain radiology support, help them discover that your ultrasound applications often represent simple tasks for which they may not want or need to be available (e.g., as discussed before, a FAST examination in the trauma bay at 3 o'clock in the morning). Surgical ultrasound expands the effective use of ultrasound in the hospital and supplements radiology ultrasound applications.

"TIERED" CREDENTIALING FRAMEWORK

Paralleling the "start simple, then add complexity" ultrasound learning strategy, we favor a tiered credentialing format to help avoid credentialing confrontation.

TIERED CREDENTIAL REQUIREMENTS FOR ULTRASOUND

Level I ultrasound skills require basic knowledge, scanning techniques, and interpretive skills. Ultrasound applications for level I privileges ask simple questions requiring simple interpretive answers. FAST privileges would fit this level, where the abdominal ultrasound scanning technique asks the sonographer to answer a simple yes-or-no question (e.g., is there fluid present)? Documentation of level I training, experience, and competence should be a simple process.

Level II ultrasound skills require advanced scanning techniques, interpretive, even interventional skills, as for breast, thyroid, vascular, hepatic, or laparoscopic ultrasound. Documentation of level II training, experience and competence will be more demanding.

Proposing a tiered credentialing system can avoid confrontation about simple ultrasound application privileges and can accelerate surgeon-performed ultrasound practice.

STAYING CURRENT: CONTINUING MEDICAL EDUCATION

No guidelines exist yet, but maintenance of ultrasound knowledge and skills requires ongoing use of the skills and requires continuing medical education. The ACS encourages surgical specialty societies to develop CME guidelines. Recommended ultrasound skill maintenance and CME requirements might include:

- 25 ultrasound cases and outcomes per year
- 3 hours of CME (Category I) per year

REIMBURSEMENT: CODING AND BILLING

All ultrasound examinations include professional and technical components. Reimbursement codes for professional and technical components are available for all surgeon-performed ultrasound examinations. See Chapter 23 describing coding and billing information in detail.

Medicare has been paying physicians, regardless of specialty, for diagnostic and therapeutic ultrasound services. To receive reimbursement, adequate documentation is required, as outlined previously, including images of appropriate scans (both normal and abnormal), measurements, and patient demographics (date, patient identification, and image orientation), with a copy provided for the patient's medical record.

CONCLUSIONS (Table 10)

Surgeon-performed ultrasound is one of the most promising and powerful emerging tools in the surgeon's toolbox. More powerful than the stethoscope, and becoming as portable, ultrasound is an affordable, repeatable, bedside extension of the surgeon's eyes, hands, and ears that can improve how surgeons care for their patients.

Because surgeons use ultrasound in clinical practice, they are primed to find new ultrasound applications. As an example, while conducting a recent ultrasound course, one of the ACS National Ultrasound Faculty was scanning a patient model's neck while the patient spoke, and noted that the vocal cords could easily be visualized, with the recognition that this represents an easy, noninvasive way to assess recurrent laryngeal nerve function before and after head and neck surgery.

▶ **TABLE 10 ABCs of Getting Started with Ultrasound**

A. Attend ultrasound education courses. The American College of Surgeons Ultrasound Education Program is an excellent resource.
B. Buy an ultrasound machine or at least find a way to share access to one.
C. "Creep" your ultrasound experience from simple to complex, with a mentor.
D. Document every step of your ultrasound experience and every examination.
E. Engage.

Key to gaining mastery in using ultrasound is to start using ultrasound. Below are listed a few helpful resources.

RESOURCES

American College of Surgeons
National Ultrasound Faculty
633 North Saint Clair Street
Chicago, IL 60611–3211
(312) 202–5415
website: *http://www.facs.org*

American Institute of Ultrasound in Medicine
14750 Sweitzer Lane
Suite 100
Laurel, MD 20707–5906
(301) 498–4100
(800) 638–5352
website: *http://www.aium.org*

American Society of Breast Surgeons
585 Main Street
Suite 243
Laurel, MD 20707
(301) 362–1722
(877) 362–1722
website: *http://www.breastsurgeons.org*

REFERENCES

1. American College of Surgeons: Statement 31—Ultrasound examinations by surgeons. *Bull Am Coll Surg* 1998;83:35.
2. Rozycki GS, Ochsner MG, Jaffin JH, et al. Preoperative evaluation of surgeons' use of ultrasound in the evaluation of trauma patients. *J Trauma* 1993;34:516–521.
3. Rozycki GS, Ochsner MG, Schmidt JA, et al. A prospective study of surgeon-performed ultrasound as the primary adjutant modality for injured patient assessment. *J Trauma* 1995;39:492–498.
4. Rozycki GS, Ballard RB, Feliciano DV, et al. Surgeon-performed ultrasound for the assessment of truncal injuries. *Ann Surg* 1998;228:557–567.
5. Shackford SR, Ricci MA, Herbert JC. Education and credentialing. *Probl Gen Surg* 1997;14:226–232.
6. Shackford SR, Rogers FB, Osler TM, et al. Focused abdominal sonogram for trauma: the learning curve of non-radiologist clinicians in detecting hemopneumoperitoneum. *J Trauma* 1999;46:553–564.
7. Rozycki GS, Shackford SR. Ultrasound: what every trauma surgeon should know. *J Trauma* 1996;40:1–4.

Coding and Billing for Ultrasound Examinations for Surgeons

Junji Machi and Edgar D. Staren

Once the surgeon becomes proficient in performing independent ultrasound examination and the credentialing for performing ultrasound is achieved locally, he or she can consider billing for ultrasound examinations. It is not necessary to hesitate in billing for the procedure as long as ultrasound examinations are adequately performed and for appropriate indications. Table 1 summarizes some important points for coding and billing for ultrasound examinations.

DOCUMENTATION OF ULTRASOUND FINDINGS

Adequate documentation is an essential component to high-quality patient care, but it is also required for billing. There should be a permanent record of the ultrasound examination and its interpretation. Comparison with previous relevant imaging studies may prove helpful. Images of all appropriate areas, both normal and abnormal, should be recorded in imaging or storage format. Variations from normal size should be accompanied by measurements. Images should be labeled with the examination date, patient identification, and image orientation. A report of the ultrasound findings should be included in the patient's medical record, regardless of where the study is performed.

CODING AND BILLING

First of all, documentation is essential. In addition to ultrasound findings, appropriate indications for examinations should be documented. For the process of billing, the correct coding with appropriate modifiers must be used. The coding may change, and therefore the surgeon should update the coding using the current "CPT" and "ICD-9." Like all procedures in today's environment, surgeons or their billers must follow up on reimbursement for ultrasound. If appropriate reimbursement is not received, the surgeon should discuss the issue with the insurer and, when necessary, with local or national professional societies.

For all ultrasound examinations, there are professional and technical components. Surgeons performing office ultrasound (e.g., breast ultrasound, transabdominal ultrasound, etc.) by themselves using their own equipment can code for both the professional and the technical components. In such a case, no modifier is required. For surgeons performing ultrasound in a facility or hospital (e.g., ultrasound in the emergency room, intensive care unit, or operating room) the situation is more complex. If a surgeon performs ultrasound examinations (with or without a technician) using the hospital's machine, he or she should use *modifier –26* to charge only for the professional component. In a facility or hospital, a surgeon performing ultrasound by himself or herself (without the help of a hospital technician) using his or her own machine can charge only for the professional component for Medicare patients. In this case, the surgeon must add *modifier –26* (they must include this; otherwise the claim will be rejected) because Medicare pays only for the professional component on the HCFA 1500. For other insurers (such as Blue Cross/Blue Shield), both components may be paid; however, the surgeon should first discuss this issue with a medical director of the insurance company. Otherwise the *modifier –26* should be used for the professional charge only.

Table 2 is a list of coding for ultrasound examinations commonly performed in a surgical practice, including office-based ultrasound and hospital-based ultrasound.

Surgeons who evaluate a patient, determine that an ultrasound examination is indicated, and perform the ultrasound by themselves can charge for both the evaluation and management (E/M) service and the ultrasound examination. E/M services are separately payable if the

▶ **TABLE 1** Coding and Billing for Ultrasound Examinations

1. Proficiency and credentialing
2. Adequate ultrasound examination for appropriate indications
3. Adequate documentation: indications and ultrasound findings
4. Use of correct coding and modifier
5. Updating of coding using current "CPT" and "ICD-9"
6. Follow-up of reimbursement

documentation indicates that the visit led to the decision to perform a procedure (the ultrasound examination). Generally, when a procedure is performed (e.g., incision and drainage) after an E/M service, it is reported by adding the *modifier –25* to the appropriate level of E/M service. However, it is not necessary to add –25 for an ultrasound examination. For example, if the surgeon is asked (consulted) to evaluate a patient with right upper

▶ **TABLE 2** Coding for Ultrasound Examinations Frequently Performed by Surgeons and Medicare Reimbursement[a]

| Code | Procedure (Ultrasound Examination) | Medicare Reimbursement of 2004 (Average of All States) | |
		Total Service	Professional Component
76536	US of head and neck, including thyroid, parathyroid, and parotid	$85.13	$28.75
76604	US of chest (including pleural cavity, mediastinum)	$79.53	$28.00
76645	US of breasts (unilateral or bilateral)	$70.19	$28.38
76700	US of abdomen, including liver, biliary, pancreas, and spleen, <u>complete</u>	$120.23	$42.19
76705	US of abdomen, <u>limited</u> (e.g., <u>single organ, quadrant, follow-up</u>)	$87.37	$30.99
	76700 and 76705 are frequently used by surgeons performing abdominal US, including FAST. Use 76705 for US of abdominal wall (e.g., hernia evaluation).		
76770	US of retroperitoneum (e.g., renal, aorta, nodes), <u>complete</u>	$116.49	$38.46
76775	US of retroperitoneum, <u>limited</u>	$86.62	$30.24
	76770 and 76775 are not commonly used by surgeons. Instead, 76700 and 76705 are used, because the retroperitoneum US is usually performed as part of the abdominal US.		
76856	US of pelvis (nonobstetric)	$96.33	$35.84
	76856 is not frequently used. A possible utility for surgeons is the pelvic US during evaluation of appendicitis or lower abdominal pain. In such circumstances, 76700 or 76705 may be a better code.		
76870	US of scrotum and contents	$93.72	$33.23
76872	Transrectal US	$109.40	$36.22
76880	US of extremity, nonvascular	$87.37	$30.99
76942	US guidance for needle placement (biopsy, aspiration, injection, localization device, etc.)	$133.67	$35.10
	US guidance (76942) is just for the US portion of the procedure and is added to the procedure itself.		
	Examples: 60001 and 76942: US-guided thyroid cyst aspiration		
	19000 and 76942: US-guided breast cyst aspiration		
	10022 and 76942: US-guided FNA of breast lump or thyroid nodule		
	19102 and 76942: US-guided core needle biopsy of breast lump		
	49080 and 76942: US-guided paracentesis		
	47000 and 76942: US-guided percutaneous liver biopsy		
	47001 and 76942: US-guided open liver biopsy		
76970	US study follow-up	$62.35	$26.54
	This code is used for repeat US for follow-up of specific organs.		
76975	Gastrointestinal endoscopic US	$102.68	$42.19
76986	US guidance, intraoperative	$165.78	$62.73
	This code is used when US is performed to guide procedures (e.g., hepatic resection) during surgery. However, for open liver biopsy, it is better to use 76942.		
76999	Unlisted US procedure		
	Like other unlisted procedures, a procedure report must be submitted when using 76999.		
93875 to 93990	Noninvasive vascular diagnostic studies including US or Doppler US		

(continued)

▶ **TABLE 2** Coding for Ultrasound Examinations Frequently Performed by Surgeons and Medicare Reimbursement*a* *(Continued)*

| Code | Procedure (Ultrasound Examination) | Medicare Reimbursement of 2004 (Average of All States) | |
		Total Service	Professional Component
76700	Intraoperative abdominal US and laparoscopic US	$120.23	$42.19
	76986 used to be the code for "echography, intraoperative." However, it was changed for "ultrasonic guidance, intraoperative." Therefore, currently there is no code specific for "intraoperative abdominal US" and "laparoscopic US." For this reason, 76700 is used for intraoperative abdominal US and laparoscopic US, as well as transabdominal US. This code is for diagnostic US, and if you perform US guidance (e.g., US-guided open liver biopsy) during an operation, you can add these codes. Example: 76700, 47001, 76942, 47130: Intraoperative US for evaluation or diagnosis, then US-guided liver biopsy, then hepatic lobectomy. Laparoscopic US during laparoscopic cholecystectomy is coded as 47562 and 76700.		
76940	US guidance for tissue ablation	$171.38	$103.80
	This is a new code (as of October 2001). When US is used for guidance of tissue ablation, such as radiofrequency thermal ablation and cryoablation, 76940 is used. Do not report 76986 in addition to 76940. For ablation procedures (radiofrequency and cryo) themselves, see codes 47370–47382.		

*a*Coding and reimbursement shown here are based on information (Medicare Reimbursement of 2004) as of April 2004.
US, ultrasound; FAST, focused abdominal sonography for trauma; FNA, fine needle aspiration.

quadrant abdominal pain and performs ultrasound after E/M service, the codes are as follows:

9924X Office consultation
76700 Ultrasound of abdomen

The surgeon should make sure that the information in the documentation is substantive enough to demonstrate medical necessity for the ultrasound examination.

For multiple surgical procedures, generally the *modifier –51* is added. However, it is not necessary to add –51 for additional ultrasound coding. For example, when billing for the professional component of intraoperative ultrasound, ultrasound guidance for liver biopsy, followed by right hepatic lobectomy, the codes are:

47130 Hepatic lobectomy
47001–51 Open liver biopsy
76700–26 Intraoperative ultrasound
76942–26 Ultrasound guidance for biopsy

Medicare has been paying physicians for diagnostic and therapeutic ultrasound services regardless of specialty. To receive reimbursement for ultrasound services, it may be necessary to submit documentation of credentialing for performing ultrasound in accordance with the local insurer's policies.

The above guidelines regarding coding and billing are applicable to Medicare. Other insurers may use a slightly different coding system, and therefore one may have to confirm each insurer's policy regarding ultrasound practice.